Essentials of Hematology

Essentials of Hematology

Edited by Martha Roper

hayle medical
New York

Hayle Medical,
750 Third Avenue, 9th Floor,
New York, NY 10017, USA

Visit us on the World Wide Web at:
www.haylemedical.com

ISBN: 978-1-63241-496-0

The publisher's policy is to use permanent paper from mills that operate a sustainable forestry policy. Furthermore, the publisher ensures that the text paper and cover boards used have met acceptable environmental accreditation standards.

Printed in China.

Cataloging-in-Publication Data

Essentials of hematology / edited by Martha Roper.
p. cm.
Includes bibliographical references and index.
ISBN 978-1-63241-496-0
1. Hematology. 2. Blood--Diseases. I. Roper, Martha.
RC633 .E43 2018
616.15--dc23

Table of Contents

Preface

One of the most important parts of our body is the fluid that flows in it to provide necessary nutrients and oxygen to all parts of the body i.e. blood. It is made up of blood cells that contain blood plasma. Other important components of blood are glucose, hormones, mineral oils, dissipated proteins, carbon dioxide, etc. The branch of medicine that studies the diseases and disorders related to blood is called hematology. It aims to provide readers with a thorough understanding of this vast subject. The topics included herein are of utmost significance and bound to provide incredible insights to readers. It will serve as a valuable source of reference for graduate and post-graduate students.

All of the data presented henceforth, was collaborated in the wake of recent advancements in the field. The aim of this book is to present the diversified developments from across the globe in a comprehensible manner. The opinions expressed in each chapter belong solely to the contributing authors. Their interpretations of the topics are the integral part of this book, which I have carefully compiled for a better understanding of the readers.

At the end, I would like to thank all those who dedicated their time and efforts for the successful completion of this book. I also wish to convey my gratitude towards my friends and family who supported me at every step.

Editor

1

Detection of Tumor Cell-Specific mRNA and Protein in Exosome-Like Microvesicles from Blood and Saliva

Jieping Yang, Fang Wei, Christopher Schafer, David T. W. Wong*

School of Dentistry, University of California Los Angeles, Los Angeles, California, United States of America

Abstract

The discovery of disease-specific biomarkers in oral fluids has revealed a new dimension in molecular diagnostics. Recent studies have reported the mechanistic involvement of tumor cells derived mediators, such as exosomes, in the development of saliva-based mRNA biomarkers. To further our understanding of the origins of disease-induced salivary biomarkers, we here evaluated the hypothesis that tumor-shed secretory lipidic vesicles called exosome-like microvesicles (ELMs) that serve as protective carriers of tissue-specific information, mRNAs, and proteins, throughout the vasculature and bodily fluids. RNA content was analyzed in cell free-saliva and ELM-enriched fractions of saliva. Our data confirmed that the majority of extracellular RNAs (exRNAs) in saliva were encapsulated within ELMs. Nude mice implanted with human lung cancer H460 cells expressing hCD63-GFP were used to follow the circulation of tumor cell specific protein and mRNA in the form of ELMs *in vivo*. We were able to identify human GAPDH mRNA in ELMs of blood and saliva of tumor bearing mice using nested RT-qPCR. ELMs positive for hCD63-GFP were detected in the saliva and blood of tumor bearing mice as well as using electric field-induced release and measurement (EFIRM). Altogether, our results demonstrate that ELMs carry tumor cell–specific mRNA and protein from blood to saliva in a xenografted mouse model of human lung cancer. These results therefore strengthen the link between distal tumor progression and the biomarker discovery of saliva through the ELMs.

Editor: Muy-Teck Teh, Queen Mary University of London, United Kingdom

Funding: This study was supported by a Ruth L. Kirschstein National Research Service Award (grant T32-DE07296) and the National Institute of Dental and Craniofacial Research/National Institutes of Health (grants UO1-DE017790 and RO1-DE15970). The project described was also supported by the National Center for Research Resources and the National Center for Advancing Translational Sciences, National Institutes of Health (grant UL1TR000124). It was also supported by the California Tobacco-Related Diseases Research Program (TRDRP) 20PT-0032, 21RT-0112 and also DoD grant LS110207. Support was also received from a Faculty Seed Grant from the Univerity of California, Los Angeles School of Dentistry (grant 441901-69749-FWEI-FY11DR). The funders had no role in study design, data collection and analysis, decision to publish, or preparation of the manuscript.

Competing Interests: David Wong is co-founder of RNAmeTRIX Inc., a molecular diagnostic company. He holds equity in RNAmeTRIX, and serves as a company Director and Scientific Advisor. The University of California also holds equity in RNAmeTRIX. Intellectual property that David Wong invented and which was patented by the University of California has been licensed to RNAmeTRIX.

* Email: dtww@ucla.edu

Introduction

Human saliva is a clear, slightly acidic (pH 6.0–7.0) biofluid known to contain a diverse range of proteins [1], over 3000 unique mRNAs [1,2,3], and 700 bacterial species [4]. In recent years, a number of investigations evaluating the constituency of oral fluid have discovered that it may actually reflect an individual's physiological condition. In fact, multiple groups have identified saliva-based proteomic, transcriptomic, and microbiological markers for Sjögren's syndrome, inflammatory bowel disease, and even cancers [5,6,7,8,9,10,11,12,13]. Although promising, the novelty of using saliva as an effective evaluator of local and systemic health has not found widespread acceptance. Significant skepticism remains regarding how these unique molecular indicators are developed in saliva.

Exosomes are small, lipid-bound, spherical structures measuring approximately 30 to 100 nm in diameter [14,15]. Randomly formed from the invagination of intracellular vesicles, exosomes often contain biologically active host cell lipids, proteins, miRNAs, mRNAs, ncRNAs, and other cellular constituents [14,16,17, 18,19,20,21]. Microvesicles containing similar host cell biomolecules and heterogeneous in size may also be formed by the budding-off the cellular membrane [22,23]. Majority of vesicles isolated from body fluids are referred as exosomes based on their exosomal protein markers [24,25]. However, the microvesicles do be co-isolated using current available purification method [24,25]. We, therefore, collectively refer these vesicles as exosome-like microvesicles (ELMs) here. ELMs are known to shed continuously from multiple cell types including: hematopoietic, intestinal epithelial, Schwann, fat, neuronal, fibroblasts, and several tumor cell lines [26]. Many types of cancer cells release ELMs and tumor-derived ELMs carry a wide range of nucleic acids, including miRNA, mRNA, ncRNA and DNA [21]. ELMs containing these nucleic acids have been shown to reflect the genetic status of tumor, and be able to travel to distant site and transfer their cargo to the recipient cells and to induce phenotypic changes [27,28,29]. Previous investigations have revealed that tumors are often the primary source of circulating membrane vesicles and increased amount of tumor derived protein, RNA and DNA were found in the blood of cancer patients [30,31,32,33].

In addition to their presence in blood, ELMs are also present in urine, saliva, breast milk, malignant and pleural effusions, synovial fluid, epididymal fluid, and amniotic fluid [21,26]. Therefore, tissue-specific exosomes with their constituent tissue-specific biomarkers can serve as a biomarker source for the diagnosis, prognosis, and monitoring of disease [34,35,36].

Recent evidence has emerged describing a role for ELMs in the processes that govern the induction of discriminatory salivary biomarkers [17,37,38]. However, the mechanisms underpinning the etiology and biogenesis of saliva-based biomarkers have not been clearly explained. Understanding how these markers come to exist in oral fluids will both shed light on the body's capacity for extracellular communication and help credential salivary biomarkers as an acceptable mode for personalized medical assessment.

In this study, we demonstrated that exRNA in cell-free saliva were largely encapsulated and protected from degradation by ELMs. A novel human lung cancer mouse xenograft model in which implanted human lung cancer H460 cells consistently express exosomal marker hCD63-GFP was developed to study whether ELMs contribute to the emergency of discriminatory salivary biomarkers during systemic disease progression. We were able to identify hCD63-GFP positive ELMs and human GAPDH mRNA in hCD63 positive ELMs in the blood and saliva of tumor bearing mice. Our evidence indicates that ELMs play a critical role in this process by acting to protect and transport tumor-specific molecular information throughout the vasculature, as well as in bodily fluids. This study represents a substantial discovery, describing the induction of discriminatory saliva-based biomarkers, Understanding these phenomena may facilitate the development of novel strategies for diagnostics, monitoring, and therapeutics.

Materials and Methods

Ethics Statement

Human saliva samples were obtained from healthy volunteers under the institutional review board protocol (IRB#10-000431) approved by the University of California Los Angeles IRB. Written informed consent forms were obtained from all participants.

All mouse procedures were approved by the UCLA Animal Research Committee in compliance with the Association for Assessment and Accreditation of Laboratory Care (AAA-LAC) International.

Saliva Collection and Salivary ELMs Isolation

Unstimulated saliva samples were obtained and processed according to previously established protocols [2]. ELMs were isolated using Exoquick precipitation solution (System Biosciences, Inc.). Three hundred microliters of cell-free saliva was thoroughly mixed with an equal volume Exoquick solution, incubated at 4°C overnight, and centrifuged at 1500×*g* for 15 min at 4°C. The pellets were then resuspended in water [39] and used for RNA isolation and immunoblotting via electron microscopy (EM).

Isolation of RNA from Saliva and ELMs

Cell-free saliva, salivary ELMs, and ELM-depleted saliva supernatant were treated with RNase cocktail (final concentration 100 U/ml) with or without 1% Triton X-100 (Tx) at room temperature for 20 min. RNA was extracted from these processed samples using the RNeasy Mini Kit (Qiagen) according to the manufacturer's instructions. The isolated RNA was quantified using the RiboGreen RNA quantification Kit (Invitrogen) and analyzed by reverse transcription PCR (RT-PCR) followed by quantitative PCR (qPCR).

Cell Culture

The human non-small cell lung cancer cell line H460 and mouse Lewis lung cancer cell line LLC1 were obtained from ATCC. Cells were grown in DMEM medium with glutamax-I supplemented with 10% (v/v) FBS and Pen/Strep in an atmosphere of 95% air and 5% CO_2 at 37°C. H460 cells were transfected with the plasmid encoding hCD63-GFP, pCT-CD63-GFP (SBI, USA). Stable H460-hCD63-GFP cells were selected and maintained in puromycin-containing medium at 1 μg/ml. Dimethyl amiloride (DMA) (Sigma, MO) was used to inhibit ELM secretion in H460-hCD63-GFP cells [40]. Cells were treated with 1 μmol or 10 μmol DMA for 48 h, and the amount of ELMs secreted into medium in the presence of DMA was determined and compared to untreated controls using an acetylcholinesterase activity assay. The trypan blue exclusion assay was used to determine the cytotoxity of DMA using a Beckman Coulter Vi-Cell (Beckman Coulter Inc., CA).

Western blotting

H460 hCD63-GFP and H460 cells were grown in serum-free DMEM supplemented with 1% non-essential amino acids for 48 h. ELMs were collected from the conditioned media and lysed along with both H460 hCD63-GFP and H460 cells. The H460 hCD63-GFP and H460 cell and ELM lysates (5 μg protein) were denatured at 95°C for 10 min and loaded onto 12% sodium dodecyl sulfate–polyacrylamide gel electrophoresis (SDS-PAGE). Proteins were transferred to a nitrocellulose membrane and probed with rabbit anti-GFP HRP-conjugated antibody (Invitrogen). ELMs were isolated from human saliva using exoquick precipitation (System Biosciences, Inc.). Exoquick precipitated pellets were lysed and then separated by SDS-PAGE. Proteins were transferred to a nitrocellulose membrane and probed with rabbit anti-CD63 (Santa Cruz Biotechnology, Santa Cruz, CA) followed by an incubation with a secondary antibody (Invitrogen).

Isolation and Quantification of ELMs from Condition Medium

ELMs were prepared using differential ultracentrifugation methods, as described previously [41]. Briefly, cell-free conditioned media was centrifuged at 10,000×*g* for 30 min at 4°C, then at 100,000×*g* for 2 h at 4°C. The ELM pellet was washed and resuspended in PBS. The Amplex Red acetylcholinesterase assay kit was used to measure the total amount of ELMs according to the manufacturer's protocol (Invitrogen, USA).

Characterization of ELMs Using Electron Microscopy

Isolated ELMs were loaded onto carbon-coated grids; fixed in 2% paraformaldehyde; washed in PBS; and immunolabeled with anti-hCD63 (BD Biosciences, US) or anti-CopGFP primary antibodies (Evrogen, Moscow, Russia) and goat anti-mouse or rabbit IgG coupled to 10-nm or 15-nm gold particles (Sigma, US). The grids were post-fixed in 2.5% glutaraldehyde, washed, and contrasted with 2% uranyl acetate, as previously described [42]. The ELMs were then examined with a JEOL 100GX transmission electron microscope (JEOL USA, Inc. Peabody, MA) (Electron Microscopy Service Center, Brain Research Institute, UCLA).

Mouse Lung Cancer Xenograft Model

Male athymic BALB/c nude mice were obtained from Charles River (MA, USA) and weighed 20–22 g at the start of the experiments. The mice were housed in sterilized filter-topped cages and maintained in sterile conditions. A total of 1×10^6 H460 hCD63-GFP cells, or 100 µl saline were injected into the left chest cavity of nude mice. Briefly, mice were anesthetized using 1–3% isoflurane in oxygen from a precision vaporizer. Mice were placed in the right lateral decubitus position. One hundred microliters of cells or saline were injected slowly into the left intercostal space at the dorsal mid-axillary line just below the inferior border of the scapular using a 30-gauge needle attached to a 1-ml syringe. The needle was advanced approximately 5 mm through the chest wall into the pleural space. After injection, the needle was retracted and mice were turned to the left lateral decubitus position for recovery. Some tumor-bearing mice were treated with daily intrapleural injection of 1 µmol/kg DMA (Sigma) or PBS control for 1 week before sacrifice [43].

Collection of Mouse Saliva, Blood, and Tumor Tissue

Twenty days after tumor implantation, saliva was collected and mice were sacrificed. Mild anesthesia was induced by intramuscular (IM) injection of 1 µl/kg body weight of a solution containing 60 mg/ml ketamine (Phoenix Scientific, St. Joseph, MO) and 8 mg/ml xylazine (Phoenix Scientific, CA). To stimulate saliva secretion, mice were subcutaneously injected between the ears with pilocarpine (0.05 mg pilocarpine/100 g body weight). Collection was completed in 20 min using a micropipette, and samples were immediately placed in pre-chilled 1.5-ml microcentrifuge tubes. Samples were centrifuged at 3500 rpm for 30 min at 4°C and supernatant was collected and stored at −80°C until analysis. Blood was collected in BD vacutainer tubes containing clot activator (BD Biosciences, CA) and centrifuged at 1000×*g* for 10 min after mice were sacrificed. Salivary glands and tumor tissues were removed from mice, snap-frozen in liquid nitrogen, and stored at −80°C.

Detection of hCD63/GFP-Positive ELMs Using EFIRM Technology

The human hCD63/GFP-positive ELMs were quantified using immuno-adsorption and an electrochemical sensor detection technology, called electric field-induced release and measurement (EFIRM) [44,45]. Briefly, saliva, serum or conditioned media were centrifuged at 1000 rpm at 4°C for 10 min. The cell-free supernatant was further centrifuged at 3500 rpm at 4°C for 30 min, to eliminate cellular debris. Five microliters of streptavidin-coated magnetic beads (Invitrogen, USA) were mixed with 1 µl of biotinylated anti-human CD63 (hCD63) antibody (Ancell, USA) on a HulaMixer Sample Mixer (Invitrogen) for 30 min at room temperature. Then, 1 ml of conditioned medium, or 10 µl of saliva or serum diluted in 990 µl of casein-PBS (Invitrogen, USA), was incubated with the anti-hCD63-conjugated magnetic beads for 2 h at room temperature to form ELMs–magnetic bead complexes. Beads were then washed twice with casein-PBS and incubated with rabbit anti-GFP HRP-conjugated polyclonal antibody for 1 h at room temperature. After incubation, the beads were washed twice with casein-PBS and accumulated onto an electrochemical sensor by applying a magnetic field [44,45].

Confocal Microscopy

The tumor sections were examined using a Leica TCS-SP2 confocal microscope with Plan APO 63×1.4 NA oil objective lens and LCS confocal software.

RT-qPCR Assay

RT-PCR followed by separate qPCR (hereafter termed RT-qPCR) was performed to detect salivary mRNAs. Multiplex RT-PCR preamplification of three mRNAs was performed using a SuperScript III platinum qRT-PCR System (Invitrogen) with a pool of outer primer sets, and conducted using a GeneAmp PCR-System 9700 (Applied Biosystems) with a fixed thermal-cycling program. SYBR Green qPCR was performed to quantitatively detect the expression levels of salivary mRNAs. The qPCR sample was prepared by combining 2× qPCR Mastermix (Applied Biological Materials), inner primers (900 nmol/l; Table S1 in Supporting information S1), and 2 µl cDNA template. The total volume of each reaction was 10 µl, adjusted with nuclease-free water. The qPCR associated with melting-curve analysis was conducted using an AB-7500HT System (Applied Biosystems) with a fixed thermal-cycling program. Each gene was tested in triplicate for all samples, including the negative control, in which the cDNA template was the product of the RT-PCR preamplification negative control.

Human GAPDH Nested RT-PCR Detection

hCD63-positive ELMs from mouse saliva or blood were adsorbed onto anti-human anti-CD63 antibody-coated magnetic beads, as previously described [44,45]. Beads were washed twice with PBS and resuspended in 10 µl TE buffer (Ambion, USA). Human GAPDH RNA was reverse transcribed using 4 µl of ELM-bead complex and the SuperScript III One-Step RT-PCR System (Invitrogen, USA). Nested PCR reactions for human GAPDH were performed using the following primer sets:

5′-TCAAGTGGGGCGATGCTGGC-3′ and 5′-TGGGGG-CATCAGCAGAGGGG-3′, 5′-GCTGGCGCTGAGTACGTC-GT-3′ and 5′-CCTGCAAATGAGCCCCAGCC-3′. PCR clean-up was performed using ExoSAP-IT after the initial RT-PCR reaction (Affymetrix, CA, USA). Native -PAGE (15%) was used to reveal the 72-bp human GAPDH PCR product.

Statistical Analysis

All statistical analyses were conducted using the IBM SPSS Statistics version 21; mean values, and standard deviations were calculated using descriptive statistics. One-way analysis of variance, two-sample *t* tests were used for testing the difference between expression values. *P* values <0.05 were considered significant. Post-hoc comparisons were conducted by using Tukey's analysis. Data are expressed as mean ± SD.

Results

Salivary ExRNAs are Predominantly Contained Within ELMs

Previous studies have demonstrated that cell-free saliva supernatant contains more than 3000 different mRNA species [1,2,3], and the exRNAs remain stable unless they are exposed to detergents [46]. Lipidic vesicles, exosomes, protected the breakdown of exRNAs in saliva [42]. To evaluate whether all exRNAs in saliva are subject to this type of vesicular protection, we compared exRNAs in cell-free saliva and salivary ELMs. We first isolated salivary ELMs from the cell-free saliva of seven healthy subjects, which were characterized by the expression of exosomal surface marker CD63 (Fig. 1a, b). exRNAs in salivary ELMs and cell-free salivary were quantified and found to range from from 74 to 300 ng/ml and 87 to 350 ng/ml, respectively, with no statistically significant difference (Fig. 1c). Consistent with previous observation [42], the exRNAs in salivary ELMs is protected from RNase degradation. Quantitative PCR analysis of extracted RNAs revealed no notable differences in C_t values of the reference genes GAPDH, ß-actin, or RPS9 between cell-free saliva, salivary ELMs, and salivary ELMs with RNase treatment (Fig. 1e). 1% Triton X-100 (Tx) solution compromised structural integrity of salivary ELMs (Fig. 1d). ELMs with Triton X-100 plus RNase treatment or ELMs-depleted saliva exhibited substantially higher C_t values of reference genes GAPDH, ß-actin, or RPS9 (Fig. 1e) These results indicate that exRNAs in cell-free saliva are largely encased within salivary ELMs.

Next, we sought to compare the transcriptome content of salivary ELMs vs. cell-free saliva using microarray expression analysis (Affymetrix HU133 plus 2.0). Approximately 2938 and 2040 mRNA transcripts were detected in cell-free saliva and isolated salivary ELMs respectively. Categorizing each group ontologically revealed similar mRNA profiles (Fig. S1a in Supporting information S1). Eight mRNAs were abundant across each data set (Fig. S1b in Supporting information S1). These overlapping molecular characteristics suggest that the transcriptomic constituency of saliva may exclusively reside within ELMs, a structure whose integrity is critical for the stability of salivary RNA.

Establishment of an ELM-Labeling Xenograft Lung Cancer Mouse Model

To help determine whether ELMs function as a conduit for long-range transportation of tissue-specific biomolecules, we

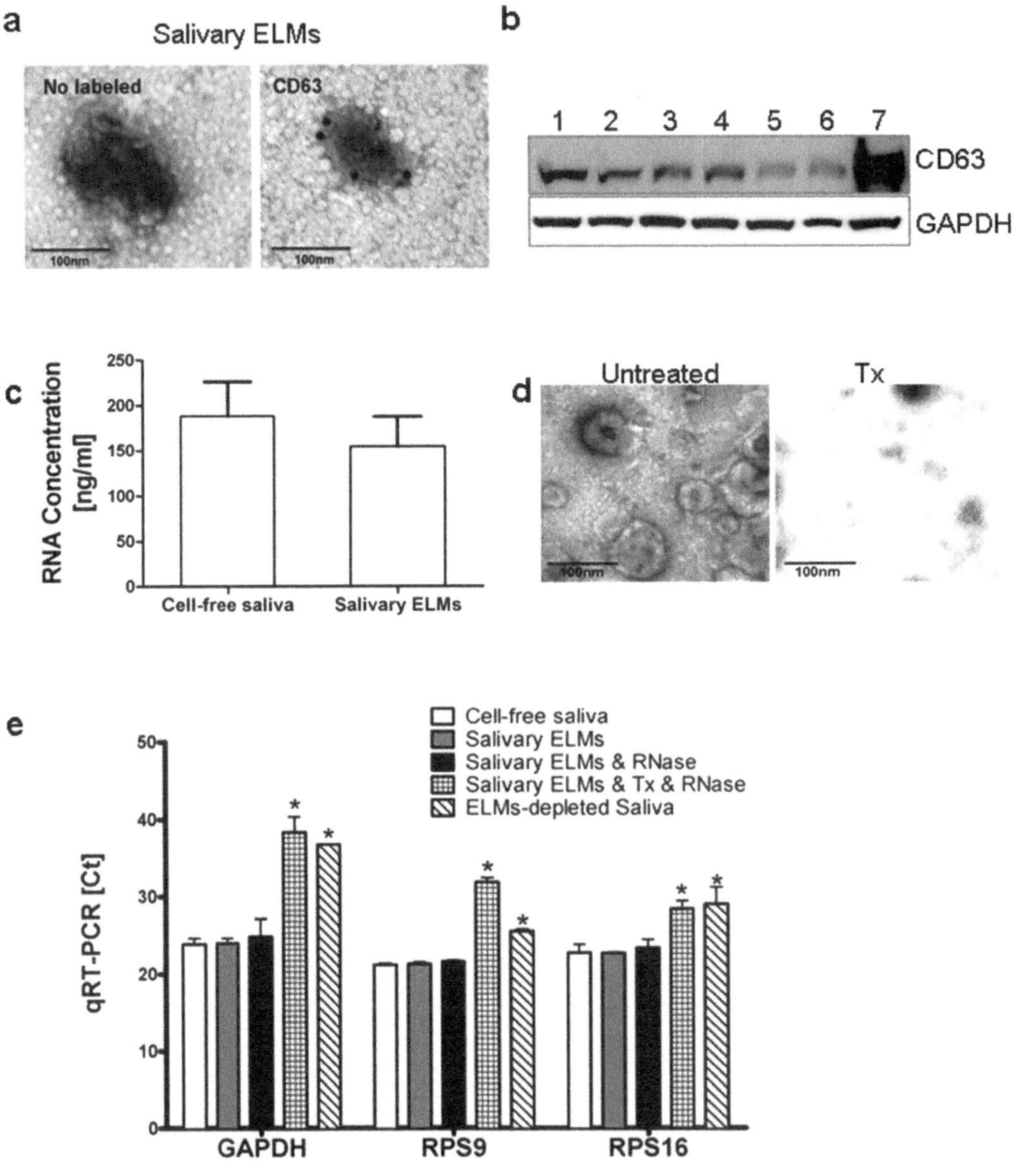

Figure 1. Salivary RNAs reside within salivary ELMs. (a) Representative electron microscopy images of salivary ELMs, and anti-CD63 immunogold-labeled ELMs in human saliva. (b) Western blot analysis of salivary ELMs using antibodies against human CD63 and GAPDH. Lane 1 to 7 are protein extracts of the salivary ELM pellets obtained from seven donors using Exoquick precipitation. (c) Ribogreen RNA quantitation from seven donors. Error bars represent means ± SD. (d) Representiave electron microscopy images of salivary ELMs and salivary ELMs treated with Tx. (e) RT-qPCR results of three reference genes from the following samples: cell-free saliva; salivary ELMs; salivary ELMs treated with RNase; salivary ELMs treated with Tx and RNase and ELM-depleted saliva. Data are expressed as means ± SD. *$P<0.05$, statistically significant difference from the saliva group.

labeled and tracked tumor-derived ELMs *in vivo*. We implanted nude mice with H460 human non-small cell lung cancer (hNSCLC) cells that stably expressed a well-known exosomal surface protein, hCD63 [20] fused to GFP (Fig. 2a–d). Prior to implantation, GFP-labeled H460-derived ELMs were confirmed by Western blotting and immuno-electron microscopy (Fig. 2d, e). The presence of tumors 20 days after implantation were confirmed by H&E section showing tumor nodule attached to the pleural surface and tumor nodule in the lung parenchyma (Fig. 2f, g). Together, these results confirm the establishment of human lung cancer xenograft mouse model with trackable tumor cell derived ELMs.

Tumor-Specific mRNA in Blood and Salivary ELMs from Tumor-Bearing Mice

With our *in vivo* model in place, we chose to explore its ability to determine the capacity of ELMs to shuttle tumor-specific mRNAs throughout the body. To effectively employ this model, we found it imperative to identify ELM-derived transcriptomic indicators of our implanted tumor cells. Given that GAPDH mRNA is abundant in ELMs [47], we elected to pursue it as a potential marker of ELMs exRNA transport. Using anti-hCD63 magnetic beads, we captured hCD63-positive ELMs from both the blood and the saliva of mice implanted with human H460-hCD63-GFP cells (Fig. 3a). To assess the specificity of our primers, we compared human GAPDH RT-PCR results on RNA extracted from H460-hCD63-GFP cells, murine Lewis lung carcinoma LL2/LLC1 cells, and their respective ELMs. Nested RT-PCR revealed that only H460 hCD63-GFP cells and their ELM derivatives were positive for human GAPDH mRNA (Fig. 3b). These results suggest that human GAPDH mRNA is an acceptable marker to detect H460 hCD63-GFP tumor cell-specific mRNA carried by hCD63-positive ELMs.

Next, we evaluated the efficacy of human GAPDH mRNA as an acceptable indicator of ELM-mediated exRNA transportation

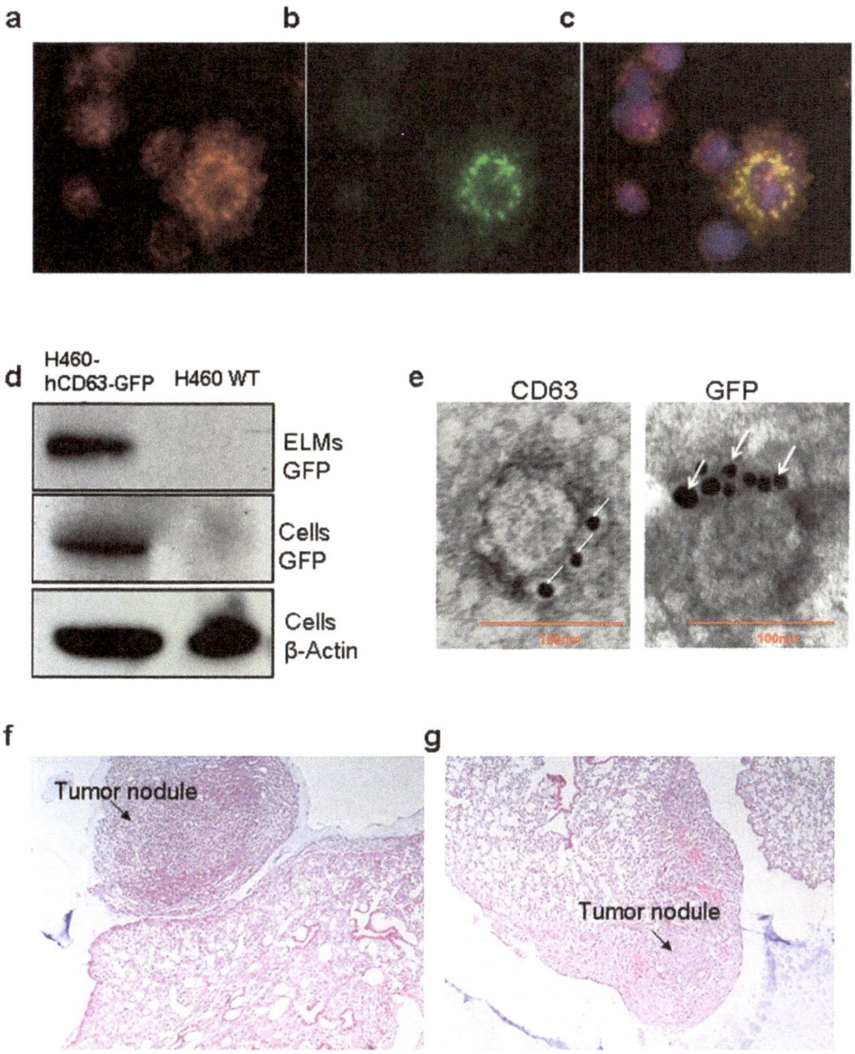

Figure 2. Establishment of a human lung cancer xenograft mouse model. To generate our xenograft lung cancer mouse model, H460 human lung cancer cells that stably express hCD63-GFP were orthotopically injected into male athymic BALB/c nude mice. CD63 immunolabeled (a, red) and GFP-postive (b, green) H460 CD63-GFP cells are shown. (c) Merge image of CD63, GFP, and DAPI staining. (d) Anti-CD63 and anti-GFP Western blot of ELMs and cell lysates from H460 CD63-GFP and H460 cells. (e) Electron microscopy images of anti-CD63-labeled and anti-GFP-labeled ELMs isolated from the conditioned medium of H460 CD63-GFP cells. Scale bar = 100 nm. (f, g) Nude mice were intrapleurally injected with 1×10^6 H460 hCD63-GFP cells. H&E staining of pulmonary tumor tissue shows (f) tumor nodule attached to the pleural surface and (g) tumor nodule in the lung parenchyma.

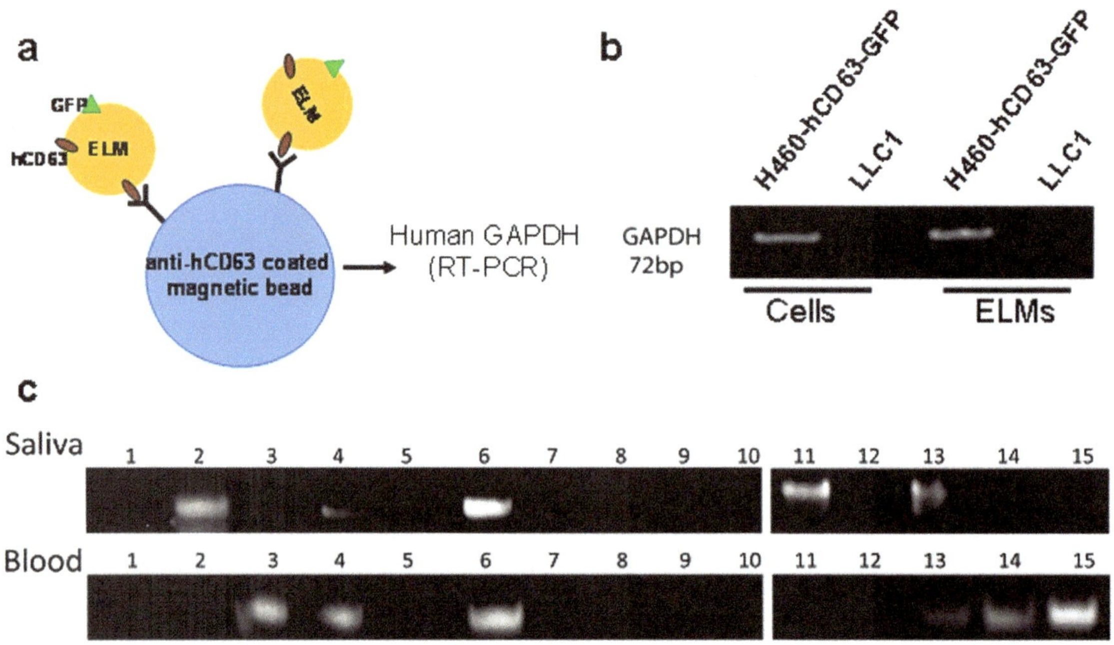

Figure 3. Detection of human GAPDH mRNA in tumor-bearing mice. (a) Illustration of anti-hCD63-coated magnetic beads used to isolate hCD63-positive ELMs from saliva, and blood. (b) This native PAGE analysis depicts the 72-bp nested RT-PCR products for human GAPDH from H460-hCD63-GFP cells, LLC1 cells, and (c) the blood and saliva of 15 H460-hCD63-GFP tumor-bearing or control mice.

in our mouse model. Previous works report that mice that have been intrapleurally implanted with 1×10^6 H460 cells subsequently developed lung tumor nodules within 20 days post-injection [48]. Accordingly, human GAPDH was detected in the blood and salivary ELMs of experimental mice within 20 days of implantation (Fig. 3c and g). 40% and 33% of all tumor-bearing mice carried the human GAPDH mRNA in their blood and salivary ELMs respectively (Fig. 3c; Table 1). These findings suggest that ELMs present in blood and saliva hold tissue-specific, viable, transcriptomic information, and support the hypothesis that ELMs might serve as potential targets of biomarker discovery and development.

Detection of Tumor-Specific Pprotein in the Blood and Salivary ELMs of Tumor-Bearing Mice

After demonstrating that ELMs contain tissue-specific exRNA molecules, we further probed these microvesicles to determine the likelihood that they contain additional molecular constituents. We focused on the proteomic content of hCD63-GFP-positive ELMs from saliva and blood. In doing so, we employed EFIRM technology (Fig. 4c) [45] to evaluate the blood and salivary hCD63-GFP-positive ELMs from H460 hCD63-GFP tumor-bearing mice exposed to either the ELMs secretion inhibitor dimethyl amiloride (DMA) [43] or PBS. Compared with PBS, DMA-treated H460 hCD63-GFP cells exhibited a non-cytotoxic, dose-dependent decrease in the ELM concentration of conditioned media (Fig. 4a, b). These results were echoed *in vivo* when, after 7 days of DMA or PBS treatment, the concentration of blood hCD63-GFP-positive ELMs was significantly decreased in DMA-treated mice compared with control animals (Fig. 4d). Salivary hCD63-GFP-positive ELMs was lower in DMA treated mice but not significant (Fig. 4e).

Collectively, these outcomes suggest a role for ELMs as conduits of tissue-specific molecular information. Furthermore, this finding highlights the concerted utility of EFIRM as a diagnostic tool and saliva as a diagnostic medium.

Discussion

Discovering saliva-based biomarkers of oral and systemic disease [1,2] has suggested the possibility of a paradigm shift in the field of molecular diagnostics. Identifying and validating disease-specific molecules in oral fluids could be of great interest to scientists and clinicians alike, and may facilitate the development of early disease diagnostic procedures and screening programs worldwide. Despite the inherent significance here, the mechanism by which markers of distal pathologies come to exist in salivary secretions currently eludes us. Here we show that small secretory lipidic vesicles called ELMs may have a substantial role in contributing to this phenomenon. We demonstrate that ELMs, secreted from distal tissues, encase and protect cell-specific RNAs and proteins within extracellular environments, including blood and saliva. Overall, our results suggest that ELMs play a significant part in transmitting biochemical information from remote cell populations to the oral cavity.

In agreement with our evidence, a recent publication showed that seven validated pancreatic cancer-specific mRNA markers and GAPDH have been detected in mouse salivary and blood-derived exosomes in a pancreatic cancer mouse model, and some of these mRNA markers were abolished when tumor cell exosome biogenesis was blocked [38]. Another interesting study found that mice bearing melanoma tumors have overlapping transcriptomic signatures in two tissues: the tumor itself, and the salivary gland [49]. Yet, it was concluded that salivary transcriptomic regulation was achieved through tumor cell-released mediators, such as growth factors and other inducers [49].

However, whether the induction of salivary molecular signatures were disease specific biomolecules directly shuttled into saliva through ELMs, or the result of a synergistic interplay between

Table 1. Detection of human GAPDH mRNA in saliva and blood from mice bearing hCD63-GFP tumors.

Mouse ID	Blood	Saliva
1	ND	ND
2	ND	D
3	D	ND
4	D	D
5	ND	ND
6	D	D
7	ND	ND
8	ND	ND
9	ND	ND
10	ND	ND
11	ND	D
12	ND	ND
13	D	D
14	D	ND
15	D	ND

salivary glands and tumor-derived mediators, including growth factor and ELMs, remain largely unknown. Our mouse model was injected with human H460-hCD63-GFP lung cancer cells, which subsequently produced species-specific CD63 proteins and GAPDH mRNA, the very markers we detected and reported in blood and saliva. Accordingly, identification of these unique markers in distant tissues and fluids most likely happens after their excretion from xenograft hosts. Moreover, the appearance of saliva-based protein marker in our model showed a small decrease upon inhibition of ELM secretion, detracting from theories suggesting other means of regulation (Fig. 4e).

We however could not completely exclude the possibility that some of them were from metastatic tumor cells. To the best of our knowledge, no evidence of oral metastasis was seen in this widely used NCI-H460 human tumor xenograft model by previous publication [31,48]. In addition, we did not observe lung metastasis at oral cavity by gross examination in this study. Therefore, we are inclined to conclude that H460-hCD63-GFP tumor-derived ELMs played a formative role in the generation of salivary biomarkers in our model.

Our present results in combination with previous reports demonstrate that ELMs thwart the enzymatic degradation of RNAs by providing a protective milieu [42,50,51,52]. However, previous publication noted an ancillary mechanism of extracellular RNA transport by insinuating that circulating RNAs are associated with and sheltered from destruction by large protein complexes called ribonucleoproteins [53]. We have previously shown that approximately 30% of most common salivary exRNAs contain AU-rich elements (ARE) in their 3′ untranslated regions, which complex with ARE binding protein and protect salivary exRNAs from degradation [54]. In this study, 69% exRNAs identified from saliva of healthy individuals were present in salivary ELMs (Fig.S1a in Supporting information S1). We therefore speculate that most salivary exRNAs reside within ELMs. However, we cannot rule out the possibility of ribonucleoprotein contamination in our ELM samples. Our method of isolation employed the commercially available Exoquick kit to precipitate ELMs from bodily fluids [39], a technology that is relatively new and has not been thoroughly characterized [39]. Therefore, we cannot conclude that our ELM preparations were ribonucleoprotein-free, which may have affected our results. To overcome this issue, future experiments should employ ultracentrifugation-based ELM isolation protocols. Although this procedure requires larger volumes of fluid [42], it is the gold standard for purifying microvesicles and should quell any contamination concerns.

As mentioned previously, a number of tumor cells commonly shed ELMs into the peripheral circulation [55,56]. It has also been demonstrated that ELMs exist within salivary secretions and carry transcriptomic information [42]. Although the origin of salivary ELMs remains unknown, here we provide evidence for their etiology by illustrating that peripherally secreted ELMs traverse the vasculature and land on oral cavity. We reveal this phenomenon by verifying that existence of seven salivary mRNA markers [57] in the malignant pleural effusion derived ELMs under same clinical setting (Table S2 in Supporting information S1). Four of these markers (BRAF [58], EGFR [59], LZTS1 [60], and FGF19 [61,62]) have been directly correlated with lung cancer development and progression. These findings implicate ELMs as carriers of tissue-specific biomolecules throughout the vasculature and within bodily fluids.

To effectively investigate our hypothesis, we found it most convincing to pursue an animal model whose ELM constituents would be undeniably discriminatory. Using xenograft mice for this purpose is an ideal way to establish the fundamentals of our proposed mechanism, as implanted H460A cells should release species-specific ELMs that contain human molecular information. Identifying these markers in murine blood and saliva provides sufficient credence for the concept of ELM-based biomarker discovery using saliva.

Despite the strength of our design, a number of issues must be considered when determining the collective significance of the experimental outcomes. First, although we revealed species-specific ELM protein and transcript in the blood and saliva of our xenograft mouse model, we cannot justifiably conclude that they are identical. In other words, the structure and molecular constituency of ELMs respectively derived from blood or saliva may be fundamentally unique. Blood-based ELMs and their contents may be altered prior to their subsequent introduction into the oral cavity. Although our observations are in agreement with previous reports [47], we concede that the data presented here does not eliminate or definitively describe the interplay of ELMs within salivary gland tissues. Comprehensive proteomic and transcriptomic characterizations of hCD63-GFP–positive ELMs found in bodily fluids are needed to shed light on these issues. Future studies using patient-derived lung cancer xenograft mouse model containing a variety of genetic aberrations, and comprehensively proteomic and transcriptomic characterizations of blood and saliva ELMs could further our understanding of the role of ELMs in the circulation of tumor-specific bimolecules as well as the biogenesis of salivary biomarkers.

Second, detecting ELMs in oral fluids presented a substantial obstacle. Current assays, including Western blotting and acetylcholinesterase assay, proved unreliable owing to the small volumes of blood and saliva samples that are obtainable from murine subjects. Our solution, EFIRM, involves two antibodies that bind to non-overlapping hCD63-GFP fusion protein [45]. Because ELMs are commonly characterized by their CD63 membrane-bound proteins, there is an inherent concern of non-specific binding by murine ELMs to anti-human CD63 magnetic beads. To address this issue, we tested the specificity of EFIRM and found that mouse salivary ELMs produced a signal similar to

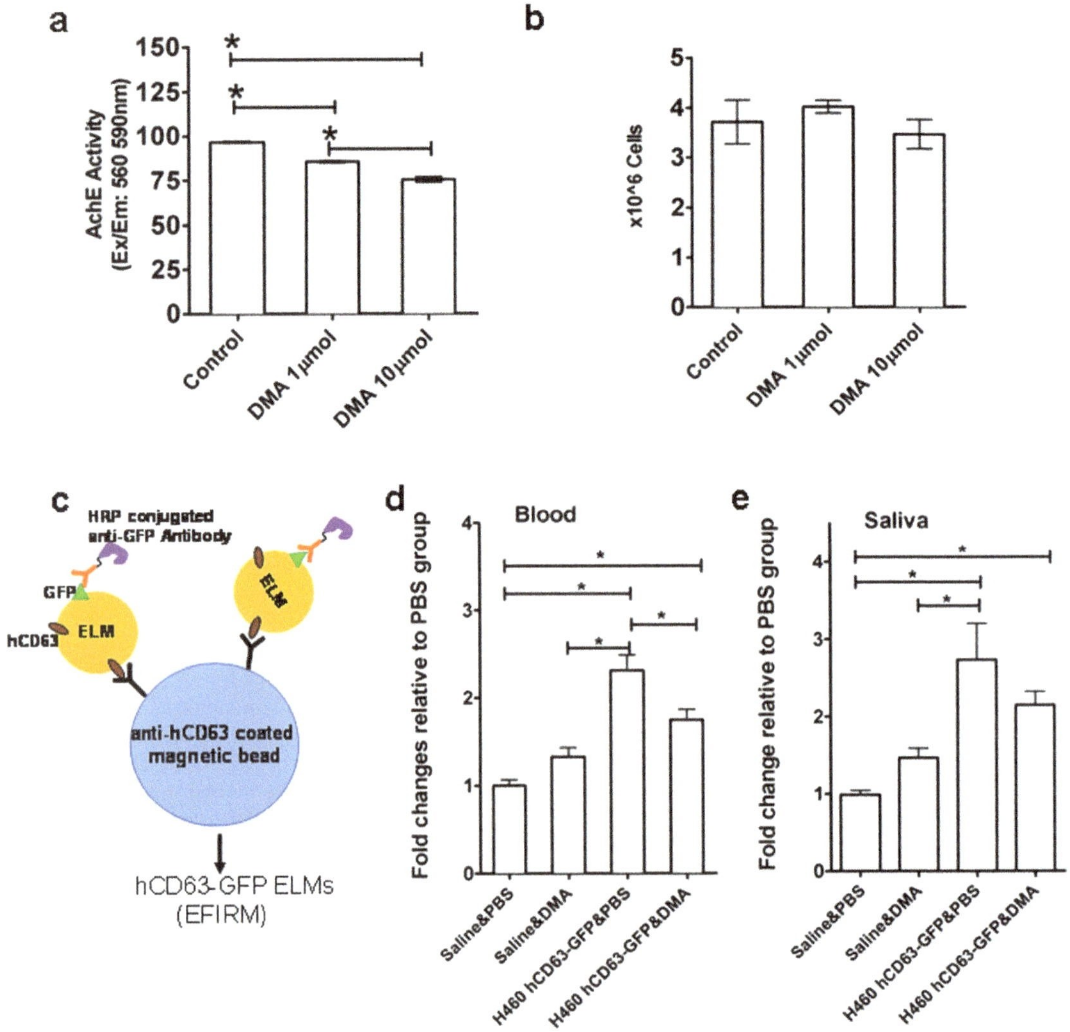

Figure 4. hCD63-GFP-positive ELMs in saliva and blood from tumor-bearing mice. (a) Acetylcholinesterase quantification of ELMs from the conditioned media of H460-hCD63-GFP cells treated with 1 μmol or 10 μmol DMA for 48 h. (b) Trypan blue exclusion assay of H460-hCD63-GFP cells after 48 h DMA treatment. (c) Illustration of the measurement of hCD63-positive ELMs in saliva and blood using EFIRM technology, allowing the detection of hCD63-GFP positive ELMs by electrochemical sensors. Samples of (d) blood and (e) saliva from control or tumor-bearing mice treated with PBS or DMA for 1 week and assayed for hCD63-GFP-positive ELMs using EFIRM technology. $N = 9–11$ per group; *$P < 0.05$, statistically significant differences.

background [45]. This outcome substantiates the specificity of this technique, and more importantly supports our aforementioned EFIRM data indicating the existence of human-specific molecules in the saliva and blood of our xenograft mouse model.

When the data is considered in its totality, one interesting value presents itself as somewhat of an aberration. Two tumor-bearing mice had human GAPDH mRNA in their saliva, but not their blood. While we speculate that distant pathologies secrete ELMs into the vasculature, these data insinuate that might not be the case. One possible explanation for this inconsistency may be the location of the tumorigenic cells. As it turns out, sputum (a respiratory expectorate used in lung cancer biomarker analysis [63,64]) might be a means of bypassing the circulatory system. In this scenario, cancer cells or microvesicles could travel to the oral cavity via the pharynx, leaving the blood absent of disease-specific markers. This eventuality may be enhanced by the anatomical position of the neoplasm within the lungs. Hence, a lack of blood-derived lung cancer markers would not disqualify our model; on the contrary, it would strengthen the suggested efficacy of oral fluids as a diagnostic medium. In any case, additional investigations will be required to delineate the communicative interaction between the oral cavity and distant diseases.

Although our report does not definitively explain the etiology of salivary biomarkers, here we describe the detection of tumor cell-specific molecules in ELMs derived from saliva. Overall, our data suggest that ELMs released from distant tissues are involved in this process by serving as protective conduits of biochemical information. Considering this information, we put forth the idea that saliva is an effective source of discriminatory biomarkers and suggest that salivary ELMs are instrumental in their presentation.

Supporting Information

Supporting information S1 Supporting information, figure and tables.

Author Contributions

Conceived and designed the experiments: JY DTWW. Performed the experiments: JY FW. Analyzed the data: JY FW. Wrote the paper: JY CS.

References

1. Hu S, Wang J, Meijer J, Ieong S, Xie Y, et al. (2007) Salivary proteomic and genomic biomarkers for primary Sjogren's syndrome. Arthritis Rheum 56: 3588–3600.
2. Li Y, St John MA, Zhou X, Kim Y, Sinha U, et al. (2004) Salivary transcriptome diagnostics for oral cancer detection. Clin Cancer Res 10: 8442–8450.
3. Lee YH, Wong DT (2009) Saliva: an emerging biofluid for early detection of diseases. Am J Dent 22: 241–248.
4. Dewhirst FE, Chen T, Izard J, Paster BJ, Tanner ACR, et al. (2010) The Human Oral Microbiome. Journal of Bacteriology 192: 5002–5017.
5. Zhang L, Budiman V, Day AS, Mitchell H, Lemberg DA, et al. (2010) Isolation and detection of Campylobacter concisus from saliva of healthy individuals and patients with inflammatory bowel disease. J Clin Microbiol 48: 2965–2967.
6. Zhang L, Farrell JJ, Zhou H, Elashoff D, Akin D, et al. (2010) Salivary transcriptomic biomarkers for detection of resectable pancreatic cancer. Gastroenterology 138: 949–957 e941–947.
7. Zhang L, Xiao H, Karlan S, Zhou H, Gross J, et al. (2010) Discovery and preclinical validation of salivary transcriptomic and proteomic biomarkers for the non-invasive detection of breast cancer. PLoS One 5: e15573.
8. Streckfus C, Bigler L, Dellinger T, Dai X, Kingman A, et al. (2000) The Presence of Soluble c-erbB-2 in Saliva and Serum among Women with Breast Carcinoma: A Preliminary Study. Clinical Cancer Research 6: 2363–2370.
9. Brinkmann O, Wong DT (2011) Salivary transcriptome biomarkers in oral squamous cell cancer detection. Advances in clinical chemistry 55: 21–34.
10. Ciravolo V, Huber V, Ghedini GC, Venturelli E, Bianchi F, et al. (2012) Potential role of HER2-overexpressing exosomes in countering trastuzumab-based therapy. J Cell Physiol 227: 658–667.
11. Farrell JJ ZL, Zhou H, Chia D, Elashoff D, Akin D, Paster BJ, Joshipura K, Wong DT. (2012) Variations of oral microbiota are associated with pancreatic diseases including pancreatic cancer. Gut 61: 582–588.
12. Hu S, Vissink A, Arellano M, Roozendaal C, Zhou H, et al. (2011) Identification of autoantibody biomarkers for primary Sjögren's syndrome using protein microarrays. PROTEOMICS 11: 1499–1507.
13. Lee Y-H, Kim J, Zhou H, Kim B, Wong D (2012) Salivary transcriptomic biomarkers for detection of ovarian cancer: for serous papillary adenocarcinoma. Journal of Molecular Medicine 90: 427–434.
14. Thery C, Ostrowski M, Segura E (2009) Membrane vesicles as conveyors of immune responses. Nat Rev Immunol 9: 581–593.
15. Yang C, Robbins PD (2011) The Roles of Tumor-Derived Exosomes in Cancer Pathogenesis. Clinical and Developmental Immunology 2011: 11.
16. Dimov I, Jankovic Velickovic L, Stefanovic V (2009) Urinary Exosomes. TheScientificWorldJOURNAL 9: 1107–1118.
17. Lotvall J, Valadi H (2007) Cell to Cell Signalling via Exosomes Through esRNA. Cell Adhesion & Migration 1: 156–158.
18. Putz U, Howitt J, Doan A, Goh C-P, Low L-H, et al. (2012) The Tumor Suppressor PTEN Is Exported in Exosomes and Has Phosphatase Activity in Recipient Cells. Sci Signal 5: ra70-.
19. Thery C, Zitvogel L, Amigorena S (2002) Exosomes: composition, biogenesis and function. Nat Rev Immunol 2: 569–579.
20. Valadi H, Ekstrom K, Bossios A, Sjostrand M, Lee JJ, et al. (2007) Exosome-mediated transfer of mRNAs and microRNAs is a novel mechanism of genetic exchange between cells. Nat Cell Biol 9: 654–659.
21. Vlassov AV, Magdaleno S, Setterquist R, Conrad R (2012) Exosomes: Current knowledge of their composition, biological functions, and diagnostic and therapeutic potentials. Biochimica et Biophysica Acta (BBA) - General Subjects 1820: 940–948.
22. Cocucci E, Racchetti G, Meldolesi J (2009) Shedding microvesicles: artefacts no more. Trends Cell Biol 19: 43–51.
23. Marzesco AM, Janich P, Wilsch-Brauninger M, Dubreuil V, Langenfeld K, et al. (2005) Release of extracellular membrane particles carrying the stem cell marker prominin-1 (CD133) from neural progenitors and other epithelial cells. J Cell Sci 118: 2849–2858.
24. Webber J, Clayton A (2013) How pure are your vesicles? J Extracell Vesicles 2.
25. Raposo G, Stoorvogel W (2013) Extracellular vesicles: exosomes, microvesicles, and friends. J Cell Biol 200: 373–383.
26. Record M, Subra C, Silvente-Poirot S, Poirot M (2011) Exosomes as intercellular signalosomes and pharmacological effectors. Biochemical Pharmacology 81: 1171–1182.
27. Hess C, Sadallah S, Hefti A, Landmann R, Schifferli JA (1999) Ectosomes released by human neutrophils are specialized functional units. J Immunol 163: 4564–4573.
28. MacKenzie A, Wilson HL, Kiss-Toth E, Dower SK, North RA, et al. (2001) Rapid secretion of interleukin-1beta by microvesicle shedding. Immunity 15: 825–835.
29. Wolfers J, Lozier A, Raposo G, Regnault A, Thery C, et al. (2001) Tumor-derived exosomes are a source of shared tumor rejection antigens for CTL cross-priming. Nat Med 7: 297–303.
30. Rabinowits G, Gercel-Taylor C, Day JM, Taylor DD, Kloecker GH (2009) Exosomal microRNA: a diagnostic marker for lung cancer. Clin Lung Cancer 10: 42–46.
31. Taylor DD, Lyons KS, Gercel-Taylor C (2002) Shed membrane fragment-associated markers for endometrial and ovarian cancers. Gynecol Oncol 84: 443–448.
32. Logozzi M, De Milito A, Lugini L, Borghi M, Calabro L, et al. (2009) High levels of exosomes expressing CD63 and caveolin-1 in plasma of melanoma patients. PLoS One 4: e5219.
33. Ogata-Kawata H, Izumiya M, Kurioka D, Honma Y, Yamada Y, et al. (2014) Circulating exosomal microRNAs as biomarkers of colon cancer. PLoS One 9: e92921.
34. Bland J (2008) The Importance of Functional Biomarkers in the Management of Chronic Illness. Altern Ther Health Med 14: 18–21.
35. Bossuyt PM (2011) THe thin line between hope and hype in biomarker research. JAMA: The Journal of the American Medical Association 305: 2229–2230.
36. Frangogiannis NG (2012) Biomarkers: hopes and challenges in the path from discovery to clinical practice. Translational Research 159: 197–204.
37. Lasser C, Seyed Alikhani V, Ekstrom K, Eldh M, Torregrosa Paredes P, et al. (2011) Human saliva, plasma and breast milk exosomes contain RNA: uptake by macrophages. Journal of Translational Medicine 9: 9.
38. Lau C, Kim Y, Chia D, Spielmann N, Eibl G, et al. (2013) Role of pancreatic cancer-derived exosomes in salivary biomarker development. J Biol Chem.
39. Taylor DD, Zacharias W, Gercel-Taylor C (2011) Exosome isolation for proteomic analyses and RNA profiling. Methods Mol Biol 728: 235–246.
40. Sreekumar PG, Kannan R, Kitamura M, Spee C, Barron E, et al. (2010) alphaB crystallin is apically secreted within exosomes by polarized human retinal pigment epithelium and provides neuroprotection to adjacent cells. PLoS One 5: e12578.
41. Raposo G, Nijman HW, Stoorvogel W, Liejendekker R, Harding CV, et al. (1996) B lymphocytes secrete antigen-presenting vesicles. J Exp Med 183: 1161–1172.
42. Palanisamy V, Sharma S, Deshpande A, Zhou H, Gimzewski J, et al. (2010) Nanostructural and transcriptomic analyses of human saliva derived exosomes. PLoS One 5: e8577.
43. Chalmin F, Ladoire S, Mignot G, Vincent J, Bruchard M, et al. (2010) Membrane-associated Hsp72 from tumor-derived exosomes mediates STAT3-dependent immunosuppressive function of mouse and human myeloid-derived suppressor cells. J Clin Invest 120: 457–471.
44. Wei F, Patel P, Liao W, Chaudhry K, Zhang L, et al. (2009) Electrochemical sensor for multiplex biomarkers detection. Clin Cancer Res 15: 4446–4452.
45. Wei F, Yang J, Wong DT (2013) Detection of exosomal biomarker by electric field-induced release and measurement (EFIRM). Biosens Bioelectron 44C: 115–121.
46. Lee YH, Zhou H, Reiss JK, Yan X, Zhang L, et al. (2011) Direct saliva transcriptome analysis. Clin Chem 57: 1295–1302.
47. Skog J, Wurdinger T, van Rijn S, Meijer DH, Gainche L, et al. (2008) Glioblastoma microvesicles transport RNA and proteins that promote tumour growth and provide diagnostic biomarkers. Nat Cell Biol 10: 1470–1476.
48. Kraus-Berthier L, Jan M, Guilbaud N, Naze M, Pierre A, et al. (2000) Histology and sensitivity to anticancer drugs of two human non-small cell lung carcinomas implanted in the pleural cavity of nude mice. Clin Cancer Res 6: 297–304.
49. Gao K, Zhou H, Zhang L, Lee JW, Zhou Q, et al. (2009) Systemic disease-induced salivary biomarker profiles in mouse models of melanoma and non-small cell lung cancer. PLoS One 4: e5875.
50. Sharma S, Rasool HI, Palanisamy V, Mathisen C, Schmidt M, et al. (2010) Structural-mechanical characterization of nanoparticle exosomes in human saliva, using correlative AFM, FESEM, and force spectroscopy. ACS Nano 4: 1921–1926.
51. Keller S, Ridinger J, Rupp AK, Janssen JW, Altevogt P (2011) Body fluid derived exosomes as a novel template for clinical diagnostics. J Transl Med 9: 86.
52. Park NJ, Li Y, Yu T, Brinkman BM, Wong DT (2006) Characterization of RNA in saliva. Clin Chem 52: 988–994.
53. Arroyo JD, Chevillet JR, Kroh EM, Ruf IK, Pritchard CC, et al. (2011) Argonaute2 complexes carry a population of circulating microRNAs independent of vesicles in human plasma. Proc Natl Acad Sci U S A 108: 5003–5008.
54. Palanisamy V, Park NJ, Wang J, Wong DT (2008) AUF1 and HuR proteins stabilize interleukin-8 mRNA in human saliva. J Dent Res 87: 772–776.
55. De la Pena H, Madrigal JA, Rusakiewicz S, Bencsik M, Cave GWV, et al. (2009) Artificial exosomes as tools for basic and clinical immunology. Journal of Immunological Methods 344: 121–132.
56. Andre F, Schartz NE, Movassagh M, Flament C, Pautier P, et al. (2002) Malignant effusions and immunogenic tumour-derived exosomes. Lancet 360: 295–305.

57. Zhang L, Xiao H, Zhou H, Santiago S, Lee JM, et al. (2012) Development of transcriptomic biomarker signature in human saliva to detect lung cancer. Cell Mol Life Sci 69: 3341–3350.
58. Pao W, Girard N (2011) New driver mutations in non-small-cell lung cancer. Lancet Oncol 12: 175–180.
59. Paez JG, Janne PA, Lee JC, Tracy S, Greulich H, et al. (2004) EGFR mutations in lung cancer: correlation with clinical response to gefitinib therapy. Science 304: 1497–1500.
60. Nonaka D, Fabbri A, Roz L, Mariani L, Vecchione A, et al. (2005) Reduced FEZ1/LZTS1 expression and outcome prediction in lung cancer. Cancer Res 65: 1207–1212.
61. Desnoyers LR, Pai R, Ferrando RE, Hotzel K, Le T, et al. (2008) Targeting FGF19 inhibits tumor growth in colon cancer xenograft and FGF19 transgenic hepatocellular carcinoma models. Oncogene 27: 85–97.
62. Sawey ET, Chanrion M, Cai C, Wu G, Zhang J, et al. (2011) Identification of a therapeutic strategy targeting amplified FGF19 in liver cancer by Oncogenomic screening. Cancer Cell 19: 347–358.
63. Petty TL (2000) The early identification of lung carcinoma by sputum cytology. Cancer 89: 2461–2464.
64. Gray RD, Duncan A, Noble D, Imrie M, O'Reilly DS, et al. (2010) Sputum trace metals are biomarkers of inflammatory and suppurative lung disease. Chest 137: 635–641.

2

Behavioral Responses to Mammalian Blood Odor and a Blood Odor Component in Four Species of Large Carnivores

Sara Nilsson[1], Johanna Sjöberg[1], Mats Amundin[2], Constanze Hartmann[3], Andrea Buettner[3], Matthias Laska[1]*

1 Department of Physics, Chemistry and Biology, Linköping University, Linköping, Sweden, **2** Kolmården Wildlife Park, Kolmården, Sweden, **3** Department of Chemistry and Pharmacy, Friedrich-Alexander-Universität Erlangen-Nürnberg, Erlangen, Germany

Abstract

Only little is known about whether single volatile compounds are as efficient in eliciting behavioral responses in animals as the whole complex mixture of a behaviorally relevant odor. Recent studies analysing the composition of volatiles in mammalian blood, an important prey-associated odor stimulus for predators, found the odorant trans-4,5-epoxy-(E)-2-decenal to evoke a typical "metallic, blood-like" odor quality in humans. We therefore assessed the behavior of captive Asian wild dogs *(Cuon alpinus)*, African wild dogs *(Lycaon pictus)*, South American bush dogs *(Speothos venaticus)*, and Siberian tigers *(Panthera tigris altaica)* when presented with wooden logs that were impregnated either with mammalian blood or with the blood odor component trans-4,5-epoxy-(E)-2-decenal, and compared it to their behavior towards a fruity odor (iso-pentyl acetate) and a near-odorless solvent (diethyl phthalate) as control. We found that all four species displayed significantly more interactions with the odorized wooden logs such as sniffing, licking, biting, pawing, and toying, when they were impregnated with the two prey-associated odors compared to the two non-prey-associated odors. Most importantly, no significant differences were found in the number of interactions with the wooden logs impregnated with mammalian blood and the blood odor component in any of the four species. Only one of the four species, the South American bush dogs, displayed a significant decrease in the number of interactions with the odorized logs across the five sessions performed per odor stimulus. Taken together, the results demonstrate that a single blood odor component can be as efficient in eliciting behavioral responses in large carnivores as the odor of real blood, suggesting that trans-4,5-epoxy-(E)-2-decenal may be perceived by predators as a "character impact compound" of mammalian blood odor. Further, the results suggest that odorized wooden logs are a suitable manner of environmental enrichment for captive carnivores.

Editor: Nadine Ravel, Université Lyon, France

Funding: The authors have no support or funding to report.

Competing Interests: The authors have declared that no competing interests exist.

* Email: malas@ifm.liu.se

Introduction

The hunting behavior of a variety of mammalian predators suggests that they may use the odor of blood to home in on wounded prey [1–3]. The behavior of mammalian prey species, in turn, suggests that the odor of conspecific blood may serve as a warning signal and elicits adaptive behavioral responses such as increased vigilance or flight [4–8]. The odor of blood may also be an important indicator of the reproductive status in female mammals [9]. Furthermore, mammalian prey species have been observed to display behavioral responses to heterospecific blood odors [10,11] suggesting that there may be a common olfactory motive in mammalian blood odor that is recognized across species.

Despite the presumed importance of blood odors for both predator/prey relationships and intraspecific chemical communication, surprisingly little is known about the volatiles that comprise the odor of blood in mammals, and even less is known about the constituents of blood odor that elicit behavioral responses in predators and/or prey species. Such knowledge, however, would be useful for both theoretical and practical purposes: it would, for example, allow ethologists to better understand the chemosensory dimension of predator/prey relationships and of intraspecific chemical communication [3]. It would also allow olfactory researchers to further explore the concept of "key compounds" in naturally occurring odor mixtures [12]. Finally, it may allow for the development of more effective chemical repellents, for example along highways or around plantations [13], or more effective environmental enrichment for captive carnivores [14].

Using sophisticated chemo-analytical methods such as gas chromatography-mass spectrometry (GC-MS) and gas chromatography-olfactometry (GC-O), a recent study analyzed the composition of volatiles in mammalian blood and found one substance, trans-4,5-epoxy-(E)-2-decenal, to evoke a typical "metallic, blood-like" odor quality in humans [15]. Humans are extremely sensitive to this odorant and have an extraordinarily low detection threshold of 0.078 ppt –0.33 ppt (parts per trillion) for this aldehyde [16].

It was therefore the aim of the present study (1) to assess behavioral responses of four large carnivore species to mammalian blood odor and to the mammalian blood odor component trans-4,5-epoxy-(E)-2-decenal, (2) to compare their behavioral responses to those towards a fruity odor and a near-odorless control, (3) to compare the behavioral responses between the four species, and (4) to assess the suitability of these odor stimuli as environmental enrichment for captive carnivores.

Materials and Methods

Ethics Statement

The experiments reported here comply with the *Guide for the Care and Use of Laboratory Animals* (National Institutes of Health Publication no. 86-23, revised 1985) and also with current Swedish laws. They were performed according to a protocol approved by the ethical board of the Swedish Board of Agriculture (Jordbruksverket, protocol # 31-2647/10).

Animals

The study was conducted at Kolmården Wildlife Park, near Norrköping, Sweden. The four species studied were:

Asian wild dogs *(Cuon alpinus)*. A group of 12 animals, comprising seven females and five males ranging from 1–8 years of age, was observed. The group was composed of one breeding pair plus their offspring. The Asian wild dogs, also known as dholes, were housed in an outdoor enclosure of 2900 m^2 which contained dens, trees, bushes, and rocks, but mainly consisted of open grassland with a 0.5 m deep water moat along one of its sides.

African wild dogs *(Lycaon pictus)*. A group of 12 animals, comprising one female and eleven males ranging from 2–9 years of age, was observed. Nine of the eleven males were offspring of the female. The African wild dogs, also known as painted dogs, were housed in an outdoor enclosure of 5200 m^2 which consisted of a rocky area in the center with surrounding open grassland areas.

South American bush dogs *(Speothos venaticus)*. A group of 10 animals, comprising five females and five males ranging from 1–6 years of age, was observed. The group was composed of one breeding pair plus their offspring. The South American bush dogs were housed in an outdoor enclosure of 1000 m^2 which contained dens, trees, bushes, and rocks, but mainly consisted of open grassland.

Siberian tigers *(Panthera tigris altaica)*. A group of 6 animals, comprising three females and three males ranging from 2–11 years of age, was observed. One of the males was the father of the three females and of one of the males, and he was the brother of the remaining male. The Siberian tigers were housed in an outdoor enclosure of 4800 m^2 which contained dens, trees, rocks, an area with steep rocky cliffs, and an area with open grassland with both an artificial stream and a water moat along one of its sides.

The outdoor enclosures of all four species were connected to indoor enclosures into which the animals were locked in for cleaning the outdoor enclosures and for removing the odor stimuli after the end of an experimental day.

Odor stimuli

The four odor stimuli used were:

Blood from a domestic horse *(Equus caballus)*. The rationale for using horse blood was that horse meat is a regular part of the food that all four carnivore species studied here are provided with at Kolmården Wildlife Park. The blood was collected in April 2012 directly after the horse was euthanized and immediately deep-frozen in aliquots of 0.5 ml at –20°C. On the morning of each testing day, five aliquots of horse blood were thawed and warmed up to approximately 25°C.

Trans-4,5-epoxy-(E)-2-decenal (CAS# 134454-31-2). This odorant has been identified as a volatile component in mammalian blood and evokes a typical "metallic, blood-like" odor quality in humans [15]. It was presented at a dilution of 1:100 (in diethyl phthalate) from a stock solution of 5 mg/ml.

iso-pentyl acetate (CAS# 123-92-2). This odorant has been identified as a volatile component in a variety of fruits and evokes a typical "banana-like" odor quality in humans [17]. It was presented at a dilution of 1:1,000 (in diethyl phthalate).

Diethyl phthalate (CAS# 84-66-2). This organic solvent is near-odorless and was used both for diluting the two monomolecular odorants mentioned above and as a blank stimulus.

The concentrations mentioned above for the blood odor component and for the fruity odor were chosen in order to provide stimuli that were clearly detectable for humans, but not overwhelmingly strong so that a relatively close contact to the odor source was necessary to detect them.

Experimental procedure

The four different odor stimuli were presented to the animals using wooden (spruce) logs of 48×7×4.5 cm. Each log was impregnated with 0.5 ml of a given odor stimulus immediately prior to each presentation. The odor stimulus was applied on the two largest surfaces of a log using a micropipette and then spread over the surface using a paint brush. Plastic gloves were used whenever the logs were handled to avoid that they were contaminated with human odor. Five logs, impregnated with the same odor stimulus, were used during a given experimental day.

At the start of each experimental day, five freshly odorized wooden logs were thrown into the outdoor enclosure of a species. Care was taken to present the wooden logs to the animals at positions that differed between experimental days and, at the same time, allowed the experimenter to see all five logs at least at the start of the observation. Immediately after the logs were put in place, the animals were allowed access into the outdoor enclosure and were observed for three hours in the morning and three hours in the afternoon (between 08:00 a.m. and 16:00 p.m.). Experiments were only performed on non-rainy days to prevent the odor stimuli from being washed away by the rain. Similarly, experiments were only performed on non-feeding days to prevent the animals from losing interest for the wooden logs due to the presence of food and postprandial inactivity. At least two days were interspersed between consecutive presentations of odorized wooden logs with a given species and care was taken to remove used logs from an enclosure prior to the start of the next presentation. Each of the four odor stimuli was presented to each of the four species for a total of five times in a pseudo-randomized order which resulted in a total of 20 experimental days per species. The experiments were carried out between May and October 2012 (with the South American bush dogs and the Siberian tigers), and between May and October 2013 (with the Asian wild dogs and the African wild dogs).

Continuous sampling was used to record the occurrence of each interaction with a wooden log which was visible to the experimenter. A total of ten behaviors involving different kinds of interaction with or immediate behavioral responses to the inspection of an odorized wooden log were considered (Table 1). During one experimental day per odor stimulus and species, the duration of the behaviors was also recorded using a stopwatch.

Figure 1 illustrates some of the behaviors considered in the present study.

Table 1. Ethogram of all behaviors considered in the present study.

functional term	description
sniffing	using the nose to investigate a wooden log
licking	using the tongue to investigate a wooden log
biting	using the teeth to investigate a wooden log
pawing	using the paw or claws to scratch a wooden log
toying	moving or otherwise manipulating a wooden log
flehmen	curling of the upper lip and "grimacing" when investigating a wooden log
self-impregnating	rubbing the face or other body part at a wooden log
scent-marking	urinating or defecating or spraying onto a wooden log
orientating	turning head (or ears or eyes) following an interaction with a wooden log
vocalizing	producing sounds during or following an interaction with a wooden log

Data analysis

Differences in the frequency of occurrence of behavioral responses between odor stimuli and between species were assessed using the Chi-square test. Between-species comparisons in the duration of behavioral responses were performed using the Mann-Whitney U-test for independent samples. Within-species comparisons of the duration of behavioral responses were performed using the Wilcoxon signed-rank test for related samples. Correlational

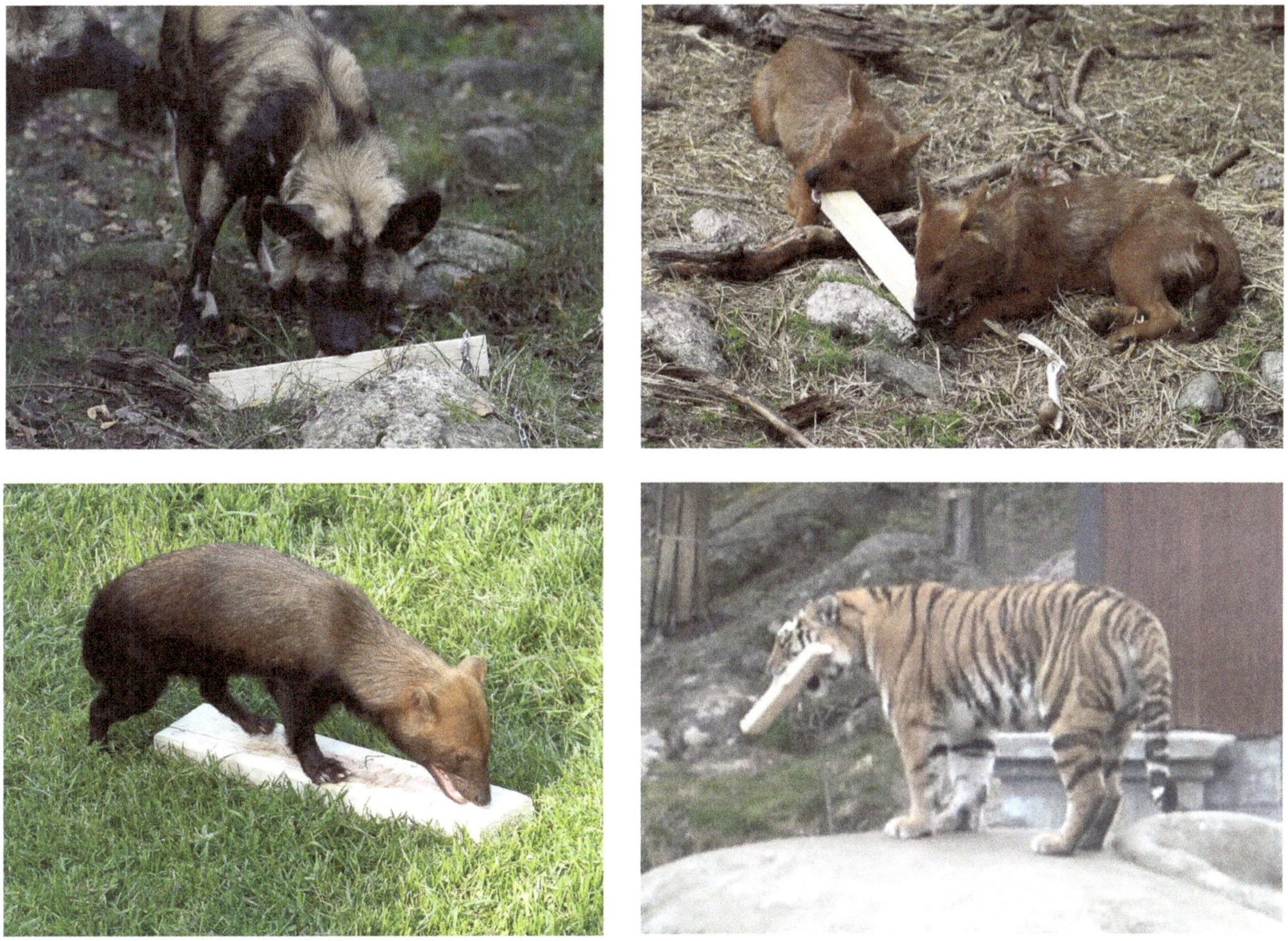

Figure 1. Some of the behaviors considered in the present study. *upper left*: an African wild dog *(Lycaon pictus)* sniffing at an odorized wooden log; *upper right*: two Asian wild dogs *(Cuon alpinus)* biting an odorized wooden log; *lower left*: a South American bush dog *(Speothos venaticus)* performing flehmen on an odorized wooden log; *lower right*: a Siberian tiger *(Panthera tigris altaica)* "toying" with (in this case: carrying) an odorized wooden log.

analyses were performed by calculating Spearman rank-order coefficients r_s which were teseted for significance by computing z-scores. As the number of animals differed between species, we calculated the number of interactions per animal by dividing the total number of interactions observed in a given species by the number of animals.

Results

Asian wild dogs

Across the 20 experimental days, a total of 458 interactions with the odorized logs was observed. Sniffing was, by far, the most frequently displayed behavior and accounted for 54.6% of all observations, followed by biting (26.0%) and toying (12.4% of all observations). Three of the behaviors, flehmen, scent-marking, and vocalizing were not observed at all (Table 2).

A comparison between the four odor stimuli showed that the Asian wild dogs displayed a significantly higher number of interactions with the odorized logs when presented with the real blood odor compared to the fruity odor ($\chi^2 = 15.02$, $P<0.0001$) and the blank control ($\chi^2 = 29.49$, $P<0.0001$). Similarly, the animals displayed a significantly higher number of interactions when presented with the blood odor component compared to the fruity odor ($\chi^2 = 17.86$, $P<0.0001$) and the blank control ($\chi^2 = 33.39$, $P<0.0001$). There was no significant difference in the number of interactions between the real blood odor and the blood odor component ($\chi^2 = 0.07$, $P = 0.786$), and between the fruity odor and the blank control ($\chi^2 = 2.10$, $P = 0.147$), respectively.

African wild dogs

A total of 647 interactions with the odorized logs was observed across the 20 experimental days. Sniffing was, by far, the most frequently displayed behavior and accounted for 64.3% of all observations, followed by licking (16.5%) and biting (12.4% of all observations). Four of the behaviors, flehmen, scent-marking, orientating, and vocalizing were not observed at all (Table 3).

A comparison between the four odor stimuli showed that the African wild dogs displayed a significantly higher number of interactions with the odorized logs when presented with the real blood odor compared to the blank control ($\chi^2 = 4.31$, $P = 0.038$), but not to the fruity odor ($\chi^2 = 0.31$, $P = 0.575$). In contrast, the animals displayed a significantly higher number of interactions when presented with the blood odor component compared to the fruity odor ($\chi^2 = 30.01$, $P<0.0001$), the blank control ($\chi^2 = 48.78$, $P<0.0001$), and the real blood odor ($\chi^2 = 23.37$, $P<0.0001$). There was no significant difference in the number of interactions between the fruity odor and the blank control ($\chi^2 = 2.04$, $P = 0.154$).

South American bush dogs

Across the 20 experimental days, a total of 1582 interactions with the odorized logs was observed. Sniffing was, by far, the most frequently displayed behavior and accounted for 82.5% of all observations, followed by biting (6.6%) and orientating (4.6% of all observations). Two of the behaviors, self-impregnating and vocalizing were not observed at all (Table 4).

A comparison between the four odor stimuli showed that the South American bush dogs displayed a significantly higher number of interactions with the odorized logs when presented with the real blood odor compared to the fruity odor ($\chi^2 = 35.44$, $P<0.0001$) and the blank control ($\chi^2 = 67.41$, $P<0.0001$). Similarly, the animals displayed a significantly higher number of interactions when presented with the blood odor component compared to the fruity odor ($\chi^2 = 30.70$, $P<0.0001$) and the blank control ($\chi^2 = 60.82$, $P<0.0001$). There was no significant difference in the number of interactions between the real blood odor and the blood odor component ($\chi^2 = 0.14$, $P = 0.712$). Finally, the number of interactions with the odorized logs was significantly higher when the animals were presented with the fruity odor compared to the blank control ($\chi^2 = 4.86$, $P = 0.028$).

Siberian tigers

A total of 392 interactions with the odorized logs was observed across the 20 experimental days. Sniffing was, by far, the most frequently displayed behavior and accounted for 49.7% of all observations, followed by biting (14.5%) and toying (11.2% of all observations). Only one of the behaviors, vocalizing, was not observed at all (Table 5).

A comparison between the four odor stimuli showed that the Siberian tigers displayed a significantly higher number of interactions with the odorized logs when presented with the real blood odor compared to the fruity odor ($\chi^2 = 47.41$, $P<0.0001$) and the blank control ($\chi^2 = 53.31$, $P<0.0001$). Similarly, the animals displayed a significantly higher number of interactions when presented with the blood odor component compared to the fruity odor ($\chi^2 = 45.85$, $P<0.0001$) and the blank control

Table 2. Number of interactions with the odorized logs in Asian wild dogs (n = 12).

behavior	real blood	blood component	fruity odor	blank control	Total
sniffing	75	110	41	24	250
licking	17	3	0	0	20
biting	51	28	24	16	119
pawing	2	3	1	0	6
toying	13	23	10	11	57
flehmen	0	0	0	0	0
self-impregnating	2	2	0	0	4
scent-marking	0	0	0	0	0
orientating	1	1	0	0	2
vocalizing	0	0	0	0	0
Total	161	170	76	51	458

Table 3. Number of interactions with the odorized logs in African wild dogs (n = 12).

behavior	real blood	blood component	fruity odor	blank control	Total
sniffing	104	173	85	54	416
licking	10	47	32	18	107
biting	14	44	7	15	80
pawing	1	1	0	0	2
toying	13	8	3	4	28
flehmen	0	0	0	0	0
self-impregnating	0	10	0	4	14
scent-marking	0	0	0	0	0
orientating	0	0	0	0	0
vocalizing	0	0	0	0	0
Total	142	283	127	95	647

($\chi^2 = 51.67$, $P<0.0001$). There was no significant difference in the number of interactions between the real blood odor and the blood odor component ($\chi^2 = 0.01$, $P = 0.969$), and between the fruity odor and the blank control ($\chi^2 = 0.07$, $P = 0.789$), respectively.

Comparison between species

The four predator species differed in their total number of interactions with the odorized wooden logs (see Tables 2–5). However, as the number of animals that we studied differed between the four species, we have to consider the number of recorded interactions with an odorized log *per animal* for between-species comparisons.

The South American bush dogs displayed the highest number of interactions with the odorized logs with 158 interactions per animal, and the Asian wild dogs displayed the lowest number of interactions with the odorized wooden logs with only 38 interactions per animal. The Siberian tigers and the African wild dogs fell in between with 65 and 54 interactions with the odorized logs per animal, respectively. Accordingly, the South American bush dogs displayed a significantly higher number of interactions with the odorized logs per animal compared to the three other species ($\chi^2 \geq 19.41$, $P<0.0001$ with all three comparisons). In contrast, the African wild dogs, the Asian wild dogs, and the Siberian tigers did not differ significantly in their number of interactions with the odorized logs per animal ($\chi^2 \leq 3.09$, $P>0.05$ with all three comparisons).

In all four species sniffing was the most frequently displayed behavior and accounted for at least 49% (Siberian tigers) and up to 82% (South American bush dogs) of all observations. Similarly, in all four species licking, biting, pawing, and toying were among the next most frequently displayed behaviors and together with sniffing these five behaviors accounted for more than 90% of all observations. Finally, vocalizing during or following an interaction with an odorized log was not observed in any of the four species. Accordingly, the rankings from most frequent to least frequent behaviors correlated positively between all four species (Spearman, $+0.41 \leq r_s \leq +0.93$ with all six comparisons), and in four of the six cases this correlation was even statistically significant (Asian wild dogs vs. African wild dogs: $r_s = +0.93$, $P = 0.0052$; Asian wild dogs vs. Siberian Tigers: $r_s = +0.91$, $P = 0.0063$; African wild dogs vs. Siberian tigers: $r_s = +0.76$, $P = 0.0222$; South American bush dogs vs. Siberian tigers: $r_s = +0.77$, $P = 0.0201$).

Duration of interactions

Table 6 summarizes the average duration of interactions with the odorized logs in the four species. The Siberian tigers displayed

Table 4. Number of interactions with the odorized logs in South American bush dogs (n = 10).

behavior	real blood	blood component	fruity odor	blank control	Total
sniffing	467	371	261	206	1305
licking	6	2	2	0	10
biting	17	70	9	9	105
pawing	2	8	0	0	10
toying	5	40	6	1	52
flehmen	9	0	1	0	10
self-impregnating	0	0	0	0	0
scent-marking	7	1	8	2	18
orientating	27	29	10	6	72
vocalizing	0	0	0	0	0
Total	540	521	297	224	1582

Table 5. Number of interactions with the odorized logs in Siberian tigers (n = 6).

behavior	real blood	blood component	fruity odor	blank control	Total
sniffing	64	93	16	22	195
licking	22	12	1	1	36
biting	31	17	7	2	57
pawing	22	15	4	2	43
toying	21	15	6	2	44
flehmen	1	2	0	0	3
self-impregnating	1	0	0	0	1
scent-marking	1	0	0	0	1
orientating	3	9	0	0	12
vocalizing	0	0	0	0	0
Total	166	163	34	29	392

significantly longer interactions with the odorized logs compared to the three other species (Mann-Whitney U-test, $P<0.05$ with all three comparisons). This was true both when considering the four odor stimuli together and when considering the real blood odor, the blood odor component, and the fruity odor separately. In contrast, the Asian wild dogs, African wild dogs, and South American bush dogs did not differ significantly in the duration of their interactions with the odorized logs (Mann-Whitney U-test, $P>0.05$ with all three comparisons).

The South American bush dogs and the Siberian tigers spent a significantly longer time per interaction with the odorized logs when presented with the real blood odor compared to the other three stimuli (Wilcoxon, $P<0.05$ with all three comparisons per species). The African wild dogs displayed significantly longer interactions with the odorized logs when they were impregnated with the real blood odor or the blood odor component compared to the fruity odor (Wilcoxon, $P<0.05$ with both comparisons), but not with the blank control (Wilcoxon, $P>0.05$). The Asian wild dogs did not differ in the duration of interactions with the odorized logs with any of the four stimuli (Wilcoxon, $P>0.05$ with all six comparisons).

Variability between sessions

Figure 2 illustrates the number of interactions with the odorized logs per animal across the five sessions performed per odor stimulus and species. In all four species, and with all four odor stimuli, a considerable session-to-session variability in the number of interactions per animal was observed. Correlational analyses showed a significant decrease in the number of interactions per animal across sessions in the South American bush dogs (Spearman $r_s = -0.54$, $P = 0.0193$), but not in the Asian wild dogs, African wild dogs, and Siberian tigers (Spearman, $-0.44 \leq r_s \leq -0.24$, $P>0.05$ with all three correlations).

Discussion

The results of the present study demonstrate that a single blood odor component can be as efficient in eliciting behavioral responses in large carnivores as the odor of real blood. Further, the results show that all four predator species tested here responded differently to prey-associated odors and non-prey-associated odors, respectively. Finally, the results suggest that odorized wooden logs are a suitable manner of environmental enrichment for captive carnivores.

Our finding that trans-4,5-epoxy-(E)-2-decenal was at least as efficient in eliciting behavioral responses in large carnivores as the odor of real blood is not trivial considering that there are hardly any examples so far showing that animals may respond in the same manner to a single food odor component as they do to the real complex odor of a food item. Combined analytical and sensory studies in humans have shown that the complex odor of some, but not all, foods is characterized by so-called "key compounds" (sometimes also referred to as "character impact compounds") [12]. However, when presented alone, these "key compounds" often resemble, but hardly ever are perceived as being identical with the natural complex odor of the food, thus emphasizing the importance of other components of the mixture as contributors to the odor "gestalt" and identifiability of a food item [18,19].

In animal studies, nonhuman primates showed no indication at all of associating "key compounds" of natural food items such as acetic esters or monoterpene alcohols found in the odor of tropical fruits with the food items themselves [20–22]. Rather, the animals

Table 6. Duration of interactions with the odorized logs (in seconds).

species	real blood	blood component	fruity odor	blank control	Total
Asian wild dogs	4.7±3.0	3.6±2.6	3.9±3.1	4.3±3.6	4.2±2.9
African wild dogs	3.6±1.8	4. 2±3.0	2.7±2.2	4.6±4.3	3.8±3.0
Bush dogs	7.8±7.7	3.2±4.0	3.7±3.3	3.0±2.1	5.6±3.5
Siberian tigers	17.4±7.1	6.2±4.0	7.6±6.6	1.8±0.5	12.6±7.1

given are mean values ± standard deviations.

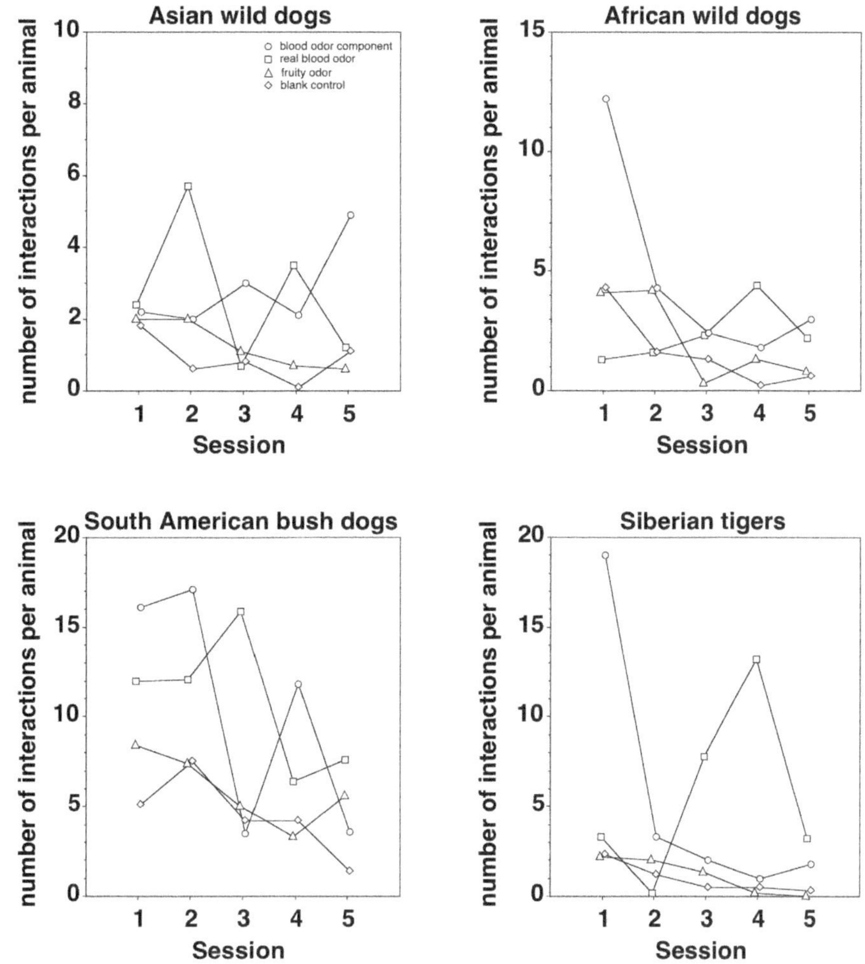

Figure 2. The number of interactions with the odorized logs per animal across the five sessions performed per odor stimulus and species. circles: blood odor component (trans-4,5-epoxy-(E)-2-decenal); squares: real blood odor (horse blood); triangle: fruity odor (iso-pentyl acetate); diamond: blank control (diethyl phthalate).

behaved in the same manner as towards other monomolecular odorants that are found in the same fruits, but belong to different chemical classes and are considered not to be "character impact compounds" [23,24], or to non-food-associated odorants [25].

The same phenomenon that single components of behaviorally relevant odors are usually less effective in animals than the complex odor mixture they are normally part of has been reported repeatedly with predator odors and pheromones: the natural body, faecal or urine odors of predators are usually more effective in eliciting avoidance responses in prey species compared to single components of these odors [26,27]. Testosterone-dependent volatiles from the urine of male mice that increase aggression among males have been found to be perceptible, but behaviorally ineffective when presented to mice in an aqueous solution and thus outside of a complex urine background odor [28].

Although we cannot be sure that the four predator species tested here indeed associated the odor of trans-4,5-epoxy-(E)-2-decenal with prey or perceived it – similar to humans – as "blood-like", at the moment this is the most straightforward interpretation of our results. This notion is supported by our finding that three of our four species responded in the same manner to both real horse blood and to the blood odor component – with the fourth species even displaying more interactions with the former compared to the latter stimulus – and differently to the two non-prey-associated odors (the fruity iso-pentyl acetate and the solvent diethyl phthalate). This, too, is not a trivial finding if we consider that mammalian carnivores are known to strongly rely on their sense of smell and therefore generally display a high interest in odor stimuli in their environment [3,29]. Further, a number of carnivores, particularly members of the canid family, have been reported to regularly self-impregnate with smelly material that is not food-associated [30–32]. Additional support for the notion that the four predator species of the present study may indeed have associated the odor of trans-4,5-epoxy-(E)-2-decenal with prey comes from the following observation: all four species tended to guard or to rest close to (or even on top of) odorized wooden logs when they were impregnated with the real blood odor or the blood odor component, but not when they were impregnated with the fruity odor or the blank control (Figure 3). Interestingly, the animals showed a similar behavior on feeding days and tended to guard or rest close to left-overs of their food such as bones.

Future studies are needed to elucidate whether other blood odor components may be equally effective as trans-4,5-epoxy-(E)-2-decenal in eliciting behavioral responses in carnivores or whether this odorant is perhaps indeed the character impact compound of

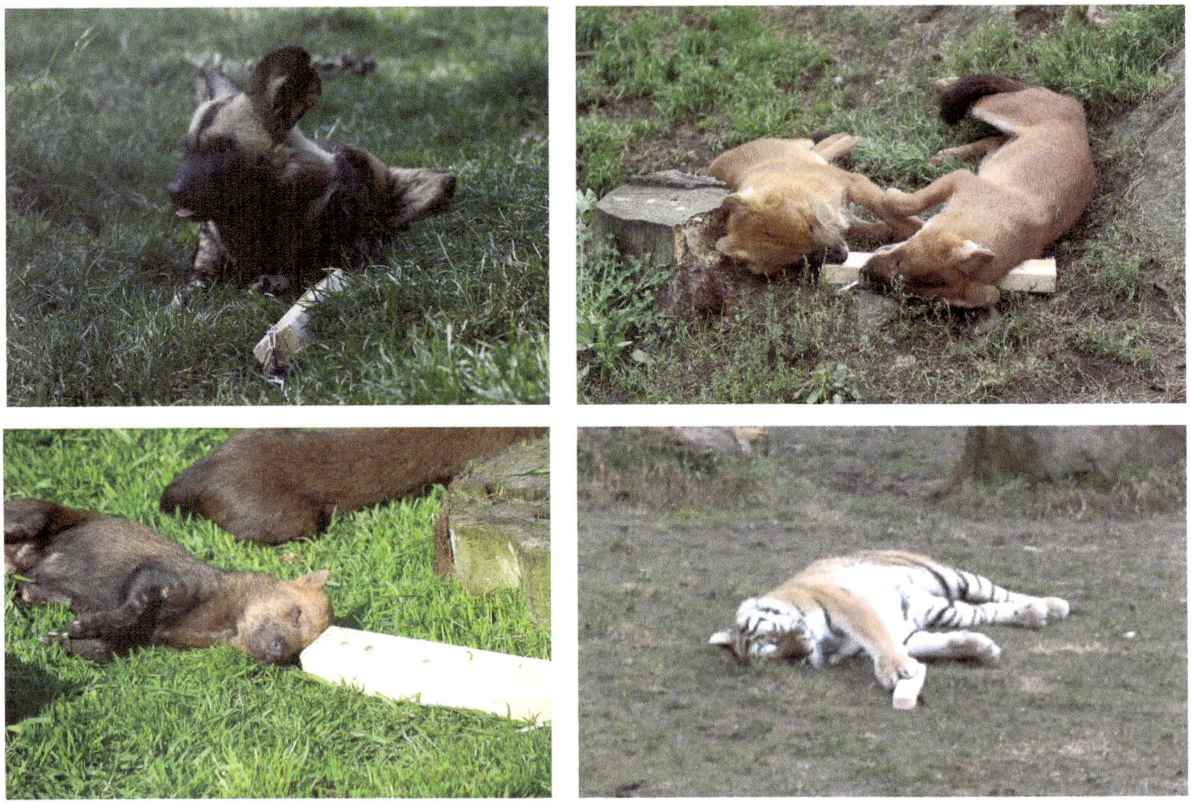

Figure 3. Guarding of or resting close to odorized wooden logs impregnated with either real blood odor or with the blood odor component trans-4,5-epoxy-(E)-2-decenal. *upper left*: an African wild dog *(Lycaon pictus)*; *upper right*: two Asian wild dogs *(Cuon alpinus)*; *lower left*: a South American bush dog *(Speothos venaticus)*; *lower right*: a Siberian tiger *(Panthera tigris altaica)*.

mammalian blood odor, not only in humans [15,16], but also in nonhuman mammals.

Our finding that the South American bush dogs displayed a significantly higher number of interactions with the odorized logs per animal compared to the other three species raises the question as to possible reasons underlying this difference. Although we cannot rule out the possibility that between-species differences in overall interest in odor stimuli or in behavioral relevance of olfactory information for a given species may account for our data, this seems unlikely because all four species studied here are known to rely on their sense of smell in a variety of behavioral contexts such as hunting and food selection, social communication, mate choice, reproduction, kin recognition, and territoriality [33–36]. Rather, it could well be that differences in relative enclosure size might explain the observed between-species difference in the number of interactions with the odorized logs. This notion is supported by the fact that the South American bush dogs had the smallest relative enclosure size with 100 m^2 per animal and thus they had clearly the highest statistical chance of finding or being close to the odorized logs and thus to interact with them. The Siberian tigers, in contrast, had the largest relative enclosure size with 800 m^2 per animal. Another possible explanation for our finding that the South American bush dogs displayed significantly more interactions with the odorized logs per animal than the Asian wild dogs, the African wild dogs, and the Siberian tigers is that these species may differ in their overall activity levels in captivity.

We also found that the four predator species differed in the average duration of the interactions with the odorized logs. The Siberian tigers displayed significantly longer interactions with the odorized logs than the other three predator species (see Table 6). Here, too, it seems unlikely that this finding reflects between-species differences in overall interest in odor stimuli or in behavioral relevance of olfactory information for a given species. Rather, these differences may simply reflect the fact that the Siberian tigers displayed the highest proportion of behaviors such as toying and biting (see Tables 1–4) which in all four species lasted longer on average than sniffing, for example.

Finally, the results of the present study suggest that odorized wooden logs are a suitable manner of environmental enrichment for captive predators. This, too, is not a trivial finding if we consider that inactivity or stereotypies are a big problem for zoos keeping large mammalian predators [37].

Environmental enrichment is commonly defined as "an animal husbandry practice that aims to increase species-specific behaviors, increase explorative and interactive behaviors with the environment and reduce abnormal behaviors of captive animals" [38]. A review of olfactory-based enrichment attempts in zoos reported that the presentation of olfactory stimuli can indeed stimulate explorative behaviors and reduce inactivity in a variety of species including large carnivores [14]. However, it was also found that the success of olfactory enrichment may strongly depend on the type of odor used and on the mode of odor presentation and its spatial and temporal distribution. Inappropriate odor stimuli or a continuous odor presentation may be counterproductive and even lead to increased levels of stereotypy and neophobia [39].

The wooden logs used in the present study turned out to be a particularly suitable way of presenting odor stimuli as environmental enrichment for captive predators as they allowed the animals to move the odorized objects and to interact with them in multiple ways (see Figure 1) which would not have been possible if stationary objects such as rocks would have been impregnated with an odor stimulus. Further, the use of wooden logs which can easily be removed from an enclosure (again, as opposed to stationary objects) allowed us to control the temporal distribution of odor presentations and thus to avoid habituation to a given stimulus. In this context it is important to mention that only one of the four species tested here displayed a significant decrease in the number of interactions with the odorized logs across sessions (see Figure 2) and that, in all four species, the number of interactions with the odorized logs did not go down to zero even on the 20th and last test day of testing. None of the four odor stimuli employed here led to an apparent increase in undesirable behaviors such as stereotypies or neophobia, but rather had the desired effect of increasing explorative behaviors and interaction with the environment. We therefore conclude that the presentation of odorized wooden logs is a suitable, cheap and easily applicable manner of environmental enrichment for captive carnivores that may contribute to a sustainable increase in animal welfare, particularly when a larger number of odor stimuli and a pseudorandomized scheme of presentation is employed.

Acknowledgments

The animal caretakers at Kolmården Wildlife Park involved in this study are gratefully acknowledged for their help and support.

Author Contributions

Conceived and designed the experiments: ML SN JS MA. Performed the experiments: SN JS. Analyzed the data: ML SN JS MA CH AB. Contributed reagents/materials/analysis tools: ML MA CH AB. Contributed to the writing of the manuscript: ML SN JS MA CH AB.

References

1. Stoddart DM (1980) Detection of food. In: Stoddart DM, editor. The ecology of vertebrate olfaction. London: Chapman & Hall. 63–83.
2. Rogers LL, Wilker GA, Scott SS (1991) Reactions of black bears to human menstrual blood. J Wildl Mgmt 55: 632–634.
3. Conover RM (2007) Predator-prey dynamics: the role of olfaction. Boca Raton: CRC Press.
4. Stevens DA, Saplikoski NJ (1973) Rats' reactions to conspecific muscle and blood: evidence for an alarm substance. Behav Biol 8: 75–82.
5. Hornbuckle PA, Beal T (1974) Escape reactions to the blood of selected mammals by rats. Behav Biol 12: 573–576.
6. Mackay-Sim A, Laing D (1981) Rats' responses to blood and body odors of stressed and nonstressed conspecifics. Physiol Behav 27: 503–510.
7. Sandnabba NK (1997) The effect of blood signals on aggressive behaviour in mice. Behav Proc 41: 51–56.
8. Terlouw EMC, Boissy A, Blinet P (1998) Behavioural responses of cattle to the odours of blood and urine from conspecifics and to the odour of faeces from carnivores. Appl Anim Behav Sci 57: 9–21.
9. Wyatt TD (2003) Pheromones and animal behaviour. Cambridge: Cambridge University Press.
10. March KS (1980) Deer, bears and blood: a note on non-human animal responses to menstrual odor. Am Anthropol 82: 125–126.
11. Nunley MC (1981) Responses of deer to human blood odor. Am Anthropol 82: 630–634.
12. Dunkel A, Steinhaus M, Kotthoff M, Nowak B, Krautwurst D, et al. (2014) Nature's chemical signatures in human olfaction: a foodborne perspective for future biotechnology. Angew Chem Int Ed 53: 7124–7143.
13. Hone J (2007) Analysis of vertebrate pest control. Cambridge: Cambridge University Press.
14. Clark F, King AJ (2008) A critical review of zoo-based olfactory enrichment. In: Hurst JL, Beynon RJ, Roberts SC, Wyatt TD, editors. Chemical Signals in Vertebrates 11. New York: Springer. 391–398.
15. Rachamadugu SK (2012) Characterization of specific volatiles of blood with the potential as predator chemoattractants and as prey warning signals. M.Sc. thesis, Linköping University, Linköping, Sweden.
16. Buettner A, Schieberle P (2001) Aroma properties of a homologous series of 2,3-epoxyalkanals and trans-4,5-epoxy-2-enals. J Agric Food Chem 49: 3881–3884.
17. Burdock GA (2009) Fenaroli's Handbook of Flavor Ingredients, 6th edition. Boca Raton: CRC Press.
18. Grosch W (2001) Evaluation of the key odorants of foods by dilution experiments, aroma models and omission. Chem Senses 26: 533–545.
19. McGorrin RJ (2012) Character-impact flavor and off-flavor compounds in foods. In: Marsili R, editor. Flavor, fragrance, and odor analysis. Boca Raton: CRC Press. 207–262.
20. Laska M, Seibt A (2002) Olfactory sensitivity for aliphatic esters in squirrel monkeys and pigtail macaques. Behav Brain Res 134: 165–174.
21. Hernandez Salazar LT, Laska M, Rodriguez Luna E (2003) Olfactory sensitivity for aliphatic esters in spider monkeys, *Ateles geoffroyi*. Behav Neurosci 117: 1142–1149.
22. Laska M, Höfelmann D, Huber D, Schumacher M (2006) The frequency of occurrence of acyclic monoterpene alcohols in the chemical environment does not determine olfactory sensitivity in nonhuman primates. J Chem Ecol 32: 1317–1331.
23. Løtvedt PK, Murali SK, Hernandez Salazar LT, Laska M (2012) Olfactory sensitivity for "green odors" (aliphatic C6 alcohols and C6 aldehydes) – A comparative study in male CD-1 mice *(Mus musculus)* and female spider monkeys *(Ateles geoffroyi)*. Pharmacol Biochem Behav 101: 450–457.
24. Laska M, Rivas Bautista RM, Hernandez Salazar LT (2006) Olfactory sensitivity for aliphatic alcohols and aldehydes in spider monkeys *(Ateles geoffroyi)*. Am J Phys Anthropol 129: 112–120.
25. Wallén H, Engström I, Hernandez Salazar LT, Laska M (2012) Olfactory sensitivity for six amino acids: a comparative study in CD-1 mice and spider monkeys. Amino Acids 42: 1475–1485.
26. Apfelbach R, Blanchard CD, Blanchard RJ, Hayes RA, McGregor IS (2005) The effects of predator odors in mammalian prey species: a review of field and laboratory studies. Neurosci Biobehav Rev 29: 1123–1144.
27. Sarrafchi A, Odhammer AME, Hernandez Salazar LT, Laska M (2013) Olfactory sensitivity for six predator odorants in CD-1 mice, human subjects, and spider monkeys. PLoS ONE 8: e80621.
28. Novotny M, Harvey S, Jemiolo B, Alberts J (1985) Synthetic pheromones that promote intermale aggression in mice. PNAS 82: 2059–2061.
29. Gorman ML, Trowbridge BJ (1989) The role of odor in the social lives of carnivores. In: Gittleman JL, editor. Carnivore behavior, ecology and evolution. New York: Chapman and Hall. 57–88.
30. Ryon J, Fentress JC, Harrington FH, Bragdon S (1986) Scent rubbing in wolves *(Canis lupus)*: the effect of novelty. Can J Zool 64: 573–577.
31. Gosling LM, McKay HV (1990) Scent-rubbing and status signaling by male mammals. Chemoecology 1: 92–95.
32. Drea CM, Vignieri SN, Cunningham SB, Glickman SE (2002) Responses to olfactory stimuli in spotted hyenas *(Crocuta crocuta)*: I. Investigation of environmental odors and the function of rolling. J Comp Psychol 116: 331–341.
33. Apps P, Mmualefe L, McNutt JW (2013) A reverse-engineering approach to identifing which compounds to bioassay for signalling activity in the scent marks of African wild dogs *(Lycaon pictus)*. In: East ML, Dehnhard M, editors. Chemical Signals in Vertebrates 12. NewYork: Springer. 417–432.
34. Fox MW (1984) The whistling hunters: field studies of the Asiatic wild dog (Cuon alpinus). Albany: SUNY Press.
35. Porton I (1983) Bush dog urine-marking: its role in pair formation and maintenance. Anim Behav 31: 1061–1069.
36. Barja I, Miguel FJ (2010) Chemical communication in large carnivores: urine-marking frequencies in captive tigers and lions. Polish J Ecol 58: 397–400.
37. Clubb R, Mason GJ (2007) Natural behavioural biology as a risk factor in carnivore welfare: how analysing species differences could help zoos improve enclosures. Appl Anim Behav Sci 102: 303–328.
38. Shepherdson DJ, Mellen JD, Hutchins M (1999) Second nature: Environmental enrichment for captive animals. Washington: Smithsonian Institution Press.
39. Young RJ (2003) Environmental enrichment for captive animals. Oxford: Blackwell.

Elevated Soluble CD163 Plasma Levels Are Associated with Disease Severity in Patients with Hemorrhagic Fever with Renal Syndrome

Junning Wang[1], Weijuan Guo[2], Hong Du[1], Haitao Yu[1], Wei Jiang[1], Ting Zhu[1], Xuefan Bai[1]*, Pingzhong Wang[1]*

1 Department of Infectious Diseases, Tangdu Hospital, Fourth Military Medical University, Xi'an, Shaanxi Province, China, **2** Department of Obstetrics and Gynecology, Chang An Hospital, Xi'an, Shaanxi Province, China

Abstract

Background: Hantaan virus is a major zoonotic pathogen that causesing hemorrhagic fever with renal syndrome (HFRS). Although HFRS pathogenesis has not been entirely elucidated, the importance of host-related immune responses in HFRS pathogenesis has been widely recognized. CD163, a monocyte and macrophage-specific scavenger receptor that plays a vital function in the hosts can reduce inflammation, is shed during activation as soluble CD163 (sCD163). The aim of this study was to investigate the pathological significance of sCD163 in patients with HFRS.

Methods: Blood samples were collected from 81 hospitalized patients in Tangdu Hospital from October 2011 to January 2014 and from 15 healthy controls. The sCD163 plasma levels were measured using a sandwich ELISA, and the relationship between sCD163 and disease severity was analyzed. Furthermore, CD163 expression in 3 monocytes subset was analyzed by flow cytometry.

Results: The results demonstrated that sCD163 plasma levels during the HFRS acute phase were significantly higher in patients than during the convalescent stage and the levels in the healthy controls ($P<0.0001$). The sCD163 plasma levels in the severe/critical group were higher than those in the mild/moderate group during the acute ($P<0.0001$). A Spearman correlation analysis indicated that the sCD163 levels were positively correlated with white blood cell, serum creatine, blood urea nitrogen levels, while they were negatively correlated with blood platelet levels in the HFRS patients. The monocyte subsets were significantly altered during the acute stage. Though the CD163 expression levels within the monocyte subsets were increased during the acute stage, the highest CD163 expression level was observed in the CD14++CD16+ monocytes when compared with the other monocyte subsets.

Conclusion: sCD163 may be correlated with disease severity and the disease progression in HFRS patients; however, the underlying mechanisms should be explored further.

Editor: Jianming Qiu, University of Kansas Medical Center, United States of America

Funding: This work was supported by the National Basic Research Program of China (973 Program) (No. 2012CB518905) and National Natural Science Foundation of China (No. 81373118). The funders had no role in study design, data collection and analysis, decision to publish, or preparation of the manuscript.

Competing Interests: The authors have declared that no competing interests exist.

* Email: wangpz63@126.com (PZW); xfbai2011@163.com (XFB)

Introduction

Hantaviruses are negative-sense, single-stranded, ribonucleic acid (RNA) viruses that belong to the Bunyaviridae family [1]. These viruses cause two obvious syndromes in humans: hemorrhagic fever with renal syndrome (HFRS) in Europe and Asian and hantavirus pulmonary syndrome (HPS) in the Americas. Currently, there are as many as 150,000 cases of HFRS reported annually worldwide [2]. HFRS is endemic in all 33 provinces of the People's Republic of China, where it is a significant public health problem, in which 20,000–50,000 human cases are diagnosed annually [3]. Notably, Xi'an city, which is the central district of the Shaanxi province, had an increasing HFRS incidence and mortality rate due to HFRS over the last three years [4]. There are five successive clinical phases in typical HFRS patients. These include the fever, hypotensive shock, oliguric, polyuric and convalescent phases. Additionally, some of these phases frequently overlap in severe cases, and several phases are frequently ignored in some mild cases of the disease [5]. The most remarkably pathological characteristics of HFRS are endothelial inflammation, loss of endothelial barrier function, immune cell migration and increased vascular permeability; however, HFRS pathogenesis is not entirely clear. Previous studies revealed that a "cytokine storm", increased immune responses, complement activation and platelet dysfunction might be involved in pathogenesis of HFRS [2,6]. Monocytes and macrophages bridging innate and adaptive immunity, high expression of cytokines activating monocytes and macrophages in the early phase of HFRS supports the immune-mediated pathogenesis [1].

Monocytes and macrophages constitute a significant component of the immune responses against viruses. These cells trigger inflammation as well as bridging innate and adaptive immunity following viral infections [7,8]. Monocytes in circulation represent a heterogeneous population. Three major subsets of monocytes have been identified based upon the relative expression of the lipopolysaccharide co-receptor, CD14 and the FcγRIII receptor, CD16. "Classical" monocytes (CD14++CD16−, Mon1) account for 80–90% of the monocytes in circulation, whereas the "intermediate" (CD14++CD16+, Mon2) and "non-classical" (CD14+CD16++, Mon3) monocyte subsets, of which the latter two subsets are summarized as CD16+ monocytes, account for 10 to 20% of the circulating monocytes [9,10]. The relative monocyte distribution that is observed in circulation is dynamic and changes as a function of the inflammatory and metabolic drivers that impact the differentiation between the subsets and their functions. CD16+ monocytes increase significantly in some inflammatory and immune disorders as well as in infectious conditions. These range from arthritis [11], inflammatory bowel disease [12], acute ischaemic heart failure [13], sepsis [14] to virus infections, such as HIV infection [15] and dengue fever [16].

CD163 is a specific scavenger receptor for hemoglobin/heme in vivo. It includes nine scavenger-receptor cysteine-rich domains that are located on the extracellular side of the monocytes and macrophages membrane [17]. One of its primary and well-described functions is the clearance of extracellular hemoglobin by a means of hemoglobin–haptoglobin complex endocytosis, which thus avoids the oxidative stress associated with free hemoglobin by liberating free iron, bilirubin, and carbon monoxide [18]. CD163 expression levels on monocytes down-regulation by inflammatory cytokines, such as tumor necrosis factor α (TNF-α) and granulocyte–macro-phage colony-stimulating factor (GM-CSF) [19,20]. A soluble form of CD163 is constituted by proteolytic cleavage of the extracellular part of the protein and is shed into circulation. Increased sCD163 levels are associated with both monocyte activation and proliferation during the course of infection or inflammation [21]. The shedding of CD163 is a constitutive process, but it can be increased by various stimuli, such as lipopolysaccharide (LPS), IL-6, and IL-10 [19]. Increased sCD163 serum concentrations have been reported in patients who suffer from various infectious and inflammatory diseases, such as sepsis, tuberculosis, diabetes, acquired immune deficiency syndrome, liver disease, dengue fever, rheumatoid arthritis and hemophagocytosis [22,23]; however, the physiological role of sCD163 was unknown, until now.

This aims of this study were to observe the CD163 expression levels on peripheral blood monocyte subsets and the plasma sCD163 levels in HFRS patients and to further analyze the correlation among CD163, sCD163 and disease severity.

Methods

Ethics Statement

The study protocol conformed with the Declaration of Helsinki (2008 version) and was approved by the Ethics Committee of Tangdu Hospital, the Fourth Military Medical University. Written informed consent was obtained from all study participants.

Patients

Eighty-one hospitalized HFRS patients were enrolled in the study from October 2011 to January 2014 at Tangdu Hospital, the Fourth Military Medical University (Xi'an, China) (see Table 1). The clinical HFRS diagnosis was confirmed serologically by detection of IgM and IgG antibodies that were specific to the HTNV nucleocapsid protein [24]. Fifteen healthy volunteers were also included in the study as normal controls. Blood samples were collected from the patients during their hospitalization. All of the blood samples were separated into plasma and peripheral blood mononuclear cells (PBMC), then they were frozen at −80°C or liquid nitrogen until further use. The clinical parameters were collected during the patient hospitalizations, using routine hospital laboratory techniques.

According to the laboratory parameters and symptoms, such as body temperature, hemorrhage, edema, blood pressure and urine volume, the degree of HFRS disease severity was classified into the four clinical types, as formerly described [25]. These types were classified as: (1) mild, which included mild renal failure without an obvious oliguric stage and hypotension; (2) moderate, which included evident uremia, effusion (bulbar conjunctiva), hemorrhage (skin and mucous membrane) and acute renal failure with an obvious oliguric stage; (3) severe, which included severe uremia, effusion (bulbar conjunctiva and either pleura or peritoneum), hemorrhage (skin and mucous membrane), and acute renal failure with oliguria (a urine output of 100–500 ml/day) for ≤5 days or anuria (a urine output of <100 ml/day) for ≤2 days; and (4) critical, which were cases with one or more of the following symptoms compared with the severe patients: refractory shock (≥2 days), visceral hemorrhage, heart failure, pulmonary edema, brain edema, severe secondary infection and severe acute renal failure with oliguria (a urine output of 50–500 ml/day) for >5 days or anuria (a urine output of <100 ml/day) for >2 days, or a blood urea nitrogen level of >42.84 mmol/L. The exclusion criteria were: (1) any other kidney disease, (2) diabetes mellitus, (3) autoimmune disease, (4) hematological disease, (5) cardiovascular disease, (6) viral hepatitis (types A, B, C, D or E), and (7) any other liver disease. In addition, none received corticosteroids or other immunomodulatory drugs during the study period.

PBMC Isolation

PBMC from the healthy controls and HFRS patients were obtained from 20 ml of heparinized venous blood using density gradient centrifugation with lymphoprep 1.077 g/ml (d = 1.077 g/ml; Sigma-Aldrich, America). The PBMCs were harvested from the interface and washed twice in RPMI-1640. The PBMC viability was >95% after Trypan Blue exclusion. The PBMCs were then aliquoted and resuspended in 1 ml fetal calf serum and freeze media (10% DMSO in RPMI-1640) and stored initially at −70°C for 24 hours before introduction into liquid nitrogen cryopreservation for later analysis. All PBMC samples were obtained at the same time as the plasma samples that were used to measure sCD163.

Flow cytometry

Frozen PBMCs were quickly thawed in a 37°C water bath, until only a small crystal remained, and washed twice in 10 ml of heated RPMI with 10% fetal bovine serum. The thawed cells that were used for staining were incubated with 10% FCS at 37°C for 30 minutes prior to staining. The cells were then resuspended at a final concentration of 1×10^6 PBMCs/ml. A separate aliquot of cells were stained with a cocktail composed of 20 μl CD14 (anti-CD14-FITC, clone M5E2, BD Biosciences, San Jose, CA, USA), 5 μl CD16 (anti-CD16-APC, clone B73.1 BD Biosciences, San Jose, CA, USA), and 20 μl CD163 (anti-CD163-PE, clone GHI/61, BD Biosciences, San Jose, CA, USA). The cells were incubated in the dark for 30 min at 4°C. Following incubation, the cells were

Table 1. The HFRS Patient Clinical Characteristics.

	Mild	Moderate	Severe	Critical
Demographic characteristics				
Patient number	12	21	25	23
Sample number	19	39	49	38
Age (years)	40 (34–45)	41 (31–51)	44 (36–52)	39 (38–58)
Males (%)	63.6	70.8	70.0	82.6
The clinical parameters at acute stage				
sCD163 (mg/l)	2.07 (1.76–2.73)	3.31 (2.67–3.70)	3.93 (2.96–5.82)	5.03 (4.43–9.34)
WBC ($\times10^3/\mu L$)	8.2 (5.5–13.3)	10.3 (8.8–18.7)	16.8 (10.9–22.4)	16.5 (12.8–35.2)
IFN-γ (pg/ml)	40.4 (24.7–54.8)	31.7 (22.2–77.3)	63.1 (41.8–118.1)	115.4 (32.6–180.1)
IL-6 (pg/ml)	24.5 (13.6–36.4)	30.5 (19.1–59.3)	48.8 (25.4–110.0)	114.5 (38.7–216.2)
PLT ($\times10^3/\mu L$)	88.5 (62.7–103.5)	48.5 (34.3–98.3)	35.0 (23.5–44.5)	26.2 (16.3–60.2)
BUN (μmol/L)	5.5 (3.6–10.6)	15.1 (9.3–20.2)	22.7 (17.1–27.1)	16.6 (11.5–27.1)
Cr (μmol/L)	78 (69–219)	216 (135.5–299)	330 (243–544)	271 (189–398)
Monocyte ($\times10^9$/L)	0.68 (0.48–2.12)	1.21 (0.88–1.88)	2.31 (1.51–2.96)	2.32 (1.34–3.91)

Values represent medians with their corresponding interquartile ranges. Acute stage include the febrile, hypotensive and oliguria phases.
Abbreviations: sCD163, soluble CD163; IL-6, Interleukin-6; IFN-γ, interferon-γ; WBC, white blood cells; PLT, platelet count; BUN, blood urea nitrogen; Scr, serum creatinine.

washed in 2 ml of cold PBS, pH 7.4. The flow cytometric analysis was performed within 1 hour using a FACS Aria II analyzer (BD Biosciences, San Jose, CA, USA). Monocytes were identified based on their forward and side scatter appearance. We recorded 100,000 events for each sample, CD14 and CD16 were used as monocyte markers, isotype-matched controls were used according to the manufacturer's recommendations, and the percentage of positive cells for each individual marker were obtained after monocyte gating. The percentage of CD163 positive monocytes out of the total monocyte population was recorded and analyzed. The data were analyzed with FlowJo software, version 7.6.1 (Oregon, USA).

ELISA assays

One hundred and forty-five plasma samples were obtained from 81 HFRS patients and 15 healthy control subjects and were stored at −80°C until later use. The sCD163, IL-6 and IFN-γ concentration measurements were obtained by a double antibody sandwich ELISA (Human sCD163 ELISA Ready-SET Go! eBioscience Products, Catalog Number: 88-50360; IL-6 and IFN-γ, Mabtech Products, Catalog Number: 3424-1H-2, 3460-1H-2). In this study, duplicate wells were used to detect the plasma sCD163, IL-6 and IFN-γ concentrations. Each examination step was carried out strictly following the product manual.

Statistical analyses

The analyses were performed with the SPSS 17.0 (SPSS Inc, Chicago, IL, USA) and GraphPad Prism 5 software packages (GraphPad Software, San Diego CA). Medians and interquartile ranges were calculated for the continuous variables and numbers and percentages were calculated for the categorical variables. A Kruskal-Wallis test performed for analysis of variation among multiple groups. Mann–Whitney U tests were used to compare the sCD163 levels between the two independent groups. Correlations were compared with a Spearman's correlation analysis. All of the tests were two-sided and P values that were less than 0.05 were considered to be statistically significant.

Results

Clinical parameters and demographic conditions of HFRS patients

A total of 81 patients were confirmed to be HFRS following HTNV IgM and IgG specific antibody detection evaluations from the patients' serum specimens. From these patients, 145 plasma samples were collected during the febrile/hypotensive (Febr/Hypo), oliguric (Olig), diuretic (Diur), and convalescent (Conv) disease stages. On the basis of the clinical records and diagnostic criteria, 12, 21, 25, and 23 patients were classified as having mild, moderate, severe, and critical HFRS types, respectively. The clinical parameter specifics that were detected during the HFRS patient hospitalizations are summed in Table 1.

Changes in the soluble CD163 plasma level in the HFRS patients

The median sCD163 levels during the febrile/hypotensive, oliguric, diuretic, and convalescent stages, as well as in the normal controls, were 3.75 mg/l, 3.58 mg/l, 2.43 mg/l, 1.80 mg/l, and 0.81 mg/l, respectively. On the basis of the clinical disease course classification criteria, the acute phase comprised the febrile, hypotensive and oliguric stages, and the convalescent phase comprised the diuretic and convalescent stages [26]. During the acute phase, the sCD163 in the HFRS patient plasma samples was obviously higher than the levels observed in the normal controls (febrile/hypotensive or oliguric vs. NC, $P<0.0001$). The plasma sCD163 level in the HFRS patients decreased during the convalescent phase (febrile/hypotensive vs. diuretic or convalescent, $P<0.0001$; oliguric vs. convalescent, $P=0.001$); however, it was still higher than the levels observed in the normal controls (diuretic vs. NC, $P=0.004$) (Figure 1A). The plasma sCD163 levels in the patients with different disease severities displayed a similar change trend; however, a more distinct decline was observed in the severe/critical patient group (Figure 1B and 1D, $P<0.0001$). The sCD163 concentration in the acute phase was higher than the level that was observed during the convalescent phase in the HFRS patients (Figure 1C, $P<0.001$). The sCD163 concentration was also obviously higher during the acute and convalescent phases in the HFRS patients compared with those in the normal controls ($P<0.0001$), (Figure 1C and 1D). The sCD163 plasma levels in the severe/critical group were higher than those in the mild/moderate group during the acute ($P<0.0001$) (Figure 1E). The plasma sCD163 levels in the mild/moderate group were compared with those in the severe/critical group, and only 4 (13.7%) of the 29 mild/moderate group cases had plasma sCD163 levels that were over 4 mg/l, while 28 (60.8%) of the 46 severe/critical group cases had sCD163 levels that were over 4 mg/l (a 4.3-fold change between the high vs. mild/moderate groups). These results demonstrate that there was some kind of an association between the plasma sCD163 concentrations and the disease severity during the HFRS course.

The correlation between the sCD163 levels and clinical parameters

The relationships between the plasma sCD163 concentrations in the HFRS subjects and the key clinical parameters that can represent the disease severity were analyzed. A Spearman correlation analysis showed that the increased sCD163 concentration was positively correlated with the increased WBC (Figure 2A, $r=0.5322$, $P<0.0001$), Crea (Figure 2C, $r=0.3718$, $P<0.0001$), BUN (Figure 2D, $r=0.38$, $P<0.0001$) levels, and negatively correlated with the decreased PLT counts (Figure 2B, $r=-0.6109$, $P<0.0001$) in the HFRS patients.

Monocyte subsets were altered in patients with HFRS

Monocytes and their subsets were identified by flow cytometry based on their forward and side scatter characteristics and by their CD14 and CD16 expression levels [27]. The gating strategy used to identify the classical (CD14++CD16−), intermediate (CD14++CD16+), and non-classical monocytes (CD14+CD16++) is shown in Figure 3C. Additionally, summary figures are displayed in Figures 3D, 3E, and 3F. The intermediate monocyte proportions (CD14++CD16+) were significantly increased during the patients of acute phase (median = 18.5%, interquartile range IQR = 15.3%–24.9%, $P<0.0001$) compared with the patients of convalescent phase (median = 6.5%, IQR = 5.1%–8.5%) and the healthy control (median = 5.0%, IQR = 3.3%–7.1%). However, no significant differences ($P>0.05$) were observed between the convalescent phase and healthy control proportions, (Figures 3E). The classical (CD14++CD16−) and non-classical (CD14+CD16++) monocyte proportions were both significantly decreased during the acute phase (median = 68.4%, IQR = 61.8%–75.1%, and median = 1.6%, IQR = 1.1%–2.58%, $P<0.0001$) compared with those during the convalescent phase (median = 80.0%, IQR = 76.5%–81.6% and median = 3.6%, IQR = 2.5%–5.5%) and in the healthy controls (median = 83.0%, IQR = 80.1%–84.7% and median = 4.5%, IQR = 3.2%–6.1%); however no significant differences between both monocyte subsets ($P>0.05$) were observed between the patients of convalescent phase and the healthy controls, (Figures 3D and 3F).

The CD163 expression on the monocyte subsets

As is known, the CD163 expression on the monocyte subsets surface is different [15]. In this study, we confirmed that the CD163 expression on the CD14++CD16+ monocyte subset was most highly expressed compared with less expression on the CD14++CD16− monocyte subset and lower levels on the CD14+CD16++ monocyte subset (Figure 4B). CD163 expression on the CD14++CD16+ monocyte was more remarkable during the acute phase (median = 64.2%, IQR = 38.8%–88.5%, $P<0.0001$) than during the convalescent phase (median = 17.3%, IQR = 11.3%–24.5%) in the HFRS patients and healthy controls (median = 16.3%, IQR = 9.4%–21.3%); however no significant ($P>0.05$) differences were observed during the convalescent phase and in the healthy controls. CD163 expression on the classical and non-classical monocytes were increased during the acute phase (median = 43.6%, IQR = 25.9%–68.8% and median = 30.0%, IQR = 22.4%–48.6%, $P<0.0001$) when compared with the convalescent phase (median = 14.0%, IQR = 8.1%–16.5% and median = 12.3%, IQR = 9.1%–21.1%) and healthy control findings (median = 11.6%, IQR = 8.3%–16.2% and median = 9.6%, IQR = 6.7%–15.4%); however, no significant differences ($P>0.05$) were observed in the convalescent phase and healthy control samples, (Figure 4B).

The sCD163 levels correlated with frequency of monocytes

There was a correlation between the sCD163 levels and the absolute monocyte counts, increased CD14++CD16+ monocyte percentage, and the CD163 expression on CD14++CD16+ monocyte. A Spearman correlation analysis demonstrated that the increasing sCD163 level was positively correlated with the increasing monocyte absolute counts (Figure 5A, $r=0.6673$, $P<0.0001$), CD14++CD16+ monocytes (Figure 5B, $r=0.5779$, $P<0.0001$) and the CD163 expression on CD14++CD16+ monocyte (Figure 5C, $r=0.6245$, $P<0.0001$) in the HFRS patients.

The correlation between the sCD163 levels and cytokine

There was a correlation between the sCD163 plasma levels and IL-6 and IFN-γ plasma levels in the HFRS patients. A Spearman correlation analysis showed that the increased sCD163 concentration was positively correlated with the increased IL-6 (Figure 6A, $r=0.4837$, $P<0.0001$), IFN-γ (Figure 6B, $r=0.4929$, $P<0.0001$) concentration in the HFRS patients.

Discussion

Our study reports that the plasma levels of sCD163, a surface marker that is shed by monocytes, were significantly higher in HFRS patients during the acute phase than in the healthy controls and during patients of the convalescent stage. Importantly, the sCD163 plasma levels in the severe/critical group were higher than those in the mild/moderate group during the acute. The plasma sCD163 level elevation was also closely related to the clinical parameters in the present study. Additionally, we demonstrated that CD14++CD16+ monocyte ratio increased significantly during the acute phase. However, the CD14++CD16− and CD14+CD16++ monocyte ratios were reduced. Though the CD163 expression on the three monocyte subsets was increased during the acute stage, the CD163 expression on the CD14++CD16+ monocytes was the highest levels compared with the CD163 expression on the other monocyte subsets. This is consistent with research that evaluated HIV infection [15]. Additionally, the plasma sCD163 levels correlated with expansion of the CD14++CD16+ monocytes and increased CD163 expression on CD14++CD16+ monocyte. Overall, these results suggest that sCD163 is a novel marker for HFRS, and likely, the monocyte-mediated disease progression that is associated with Hantaviruses infection.

In our study, sCD163 levels were elevated during the acute stage; however, they fell gradually during the recovery stage. This is in agreement with a previous observation in malaria patients [28]. The sCD163 plasma levels in the severe/critical group were

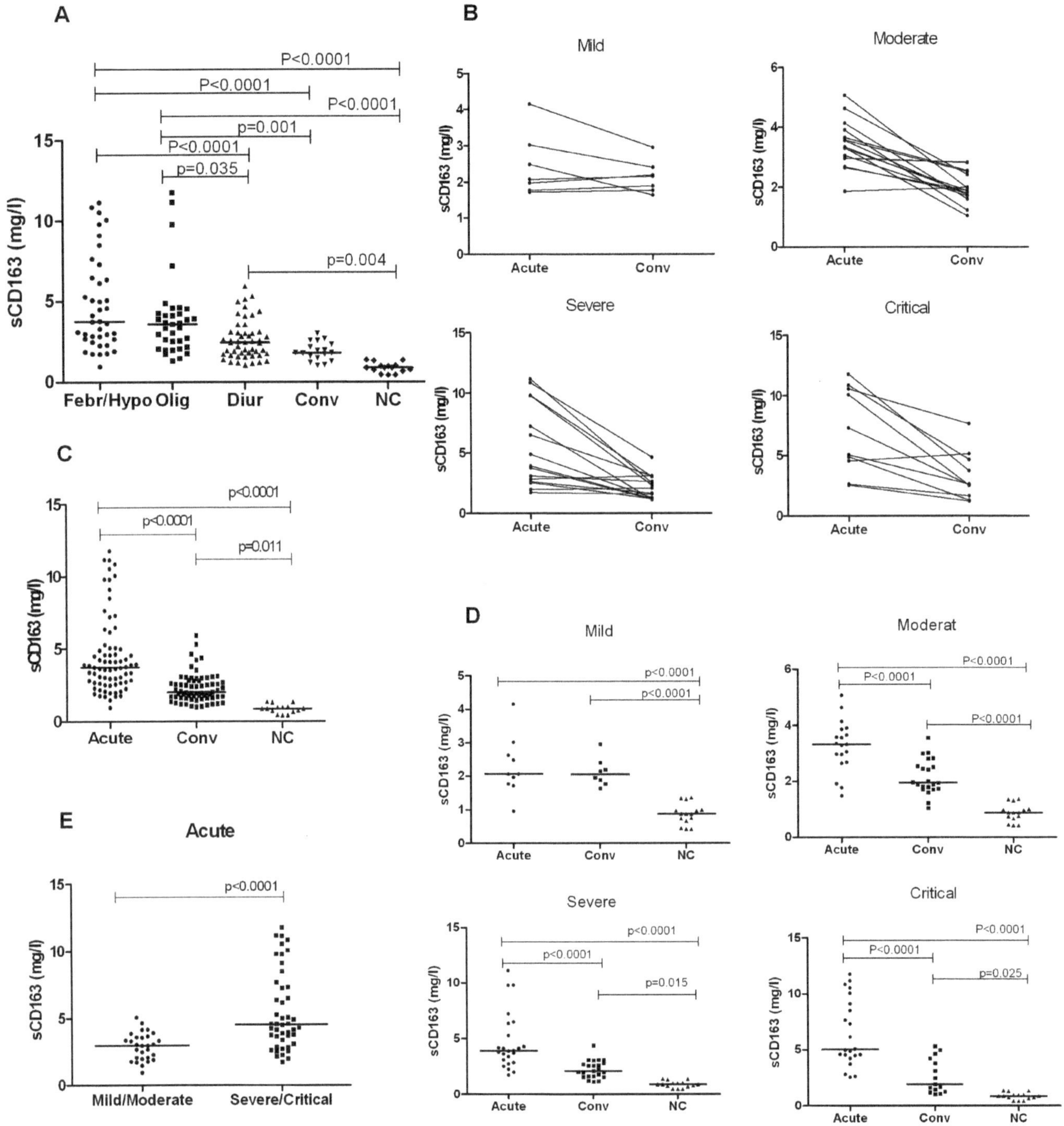

Figure 1. The obvious changes in the soluble CD163 (sCD163) plasma levels in the different HFRS severity patient groups. (A) Comparison of plasma sCD163 levels at the different HFRS stages in the patients. Data were obtained from 145 plasma samples that were collected during the febrile/hypotensive (Febr/Hypo), oliguric (Olig), diuretic (Diur), and convalescent (Conv) HFRS phases in the patients and from 15 healthy subject plasma samples that were used as normal controls (NC). Significant differences were observed between the following stage comparisons: febrile/hypotensive or oliguric vs. NC ($P<0.0001$); febrile/hypotensive vs. diuretic or convalescent ($P<0.0001$); oliguric vs. diuretic ($P=0.035$), oliguric vs. convalescent ($P=0.001$); and diuretic vs. NC ($P=0.004$). (B) The plasma sCD163 level changes in the acute (which included the febrile, hypotensive, and oliguric stages) and convalescent phase samples (which included the diuretic and convalescent stages) of the same patient in the different disease severity groups are represented. (C) The changes in the patient sCD163 plasma levels of the acute and convalescent phases when compared with the normal controls. (D) The changes in the sCD163 plasma levels during the acute phase and convalescent phases when compare with the normal controls in the different disease severity groups. (E) Comparison of the acute phase sCD163 levels between the mild/moderate and the severe/critical groups. The significance of the differences among the multiple groups was determined with the Kruskal-Wallis test. The significance of the differences between the two groups was determined with the Mann–Whitney U test. Black lines represent medians and the *P* values are plotted in each graph.

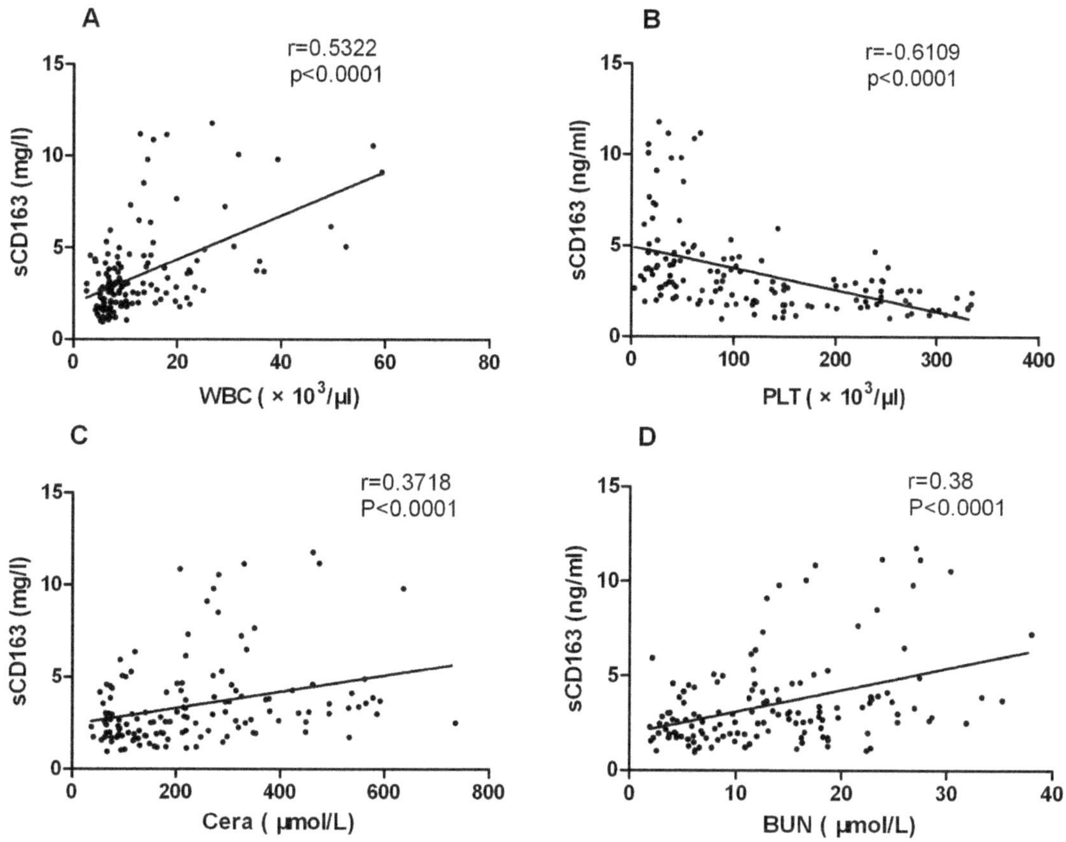

Figure 2. The relationship between elevated sCD163 plasma levels and the clinical parameters. The values are derived from the same blood sample from the HFRS subjects during hospitalization. The Spearman correlation test was used to test the correlation between the sCD163 levels and clinical parameters. The serum sCD163 concentrations were positively correlated with the white blood cells (WBC) (A), creatinine (Crea) (C), and the blood urea nitrogen (BUN) (D) levels for the entire group of subjects while they were negatively correlated with the platelet count (PLT) (B) levels. The r and *P* values are indicated in the graphs.

higher than those in the mild/moderate group during the acute, and interestingly, the mild/moderate group still had elevated sCD163, which suggested that monocyte activation occurs even with moderate disease during the acute stage, albeit to a lower extent. The sCD163, but not the membrane-bound form, might have anti-inflammatory functions because it inhibits T lymphocyte activation and proliferation in vitro [29]. The binding of Hb-Hp complexes to sCD163 has been shown to inhibit the supply of heme iron that is available for hemolysis that is caused by a bacterial infection [30]. Furthermore, during the innate immune response, CD163 plays a vital function in the hosts ability to reduce inflammation [31]. Interestingly, several inflammatory processes are associated with elevated sCD163 levels [31,32,33,34,35]. Because HFRS is associated with a higher inflammatory response and many inflammatory cytokines and chemokines are involved in the process, our research team [36] evaluated the serum TNF-α, IL-6, IL-4, IL-8,interferon (IFN)-γ, IP-10, and chemokine (C–C motif) ligand 5 levels in HFRS patients. The data showed that significant changes in serum TNF-α, IL-8, IFN-γ, IL-6, IP-10 and RANTES concentrations occurred in patients as they progressed through the different HFRS phases. In this experimental study, our found that increased sCD163 concentration was positively correlated with the increased IL-6 and IFN-γ. It seems that Hantaan virus infections induced over production of many inflammatory cytokines, known as a "cytokine storm" during the early stage. The increased sCD163 concentration during the acute stage most likely serves as a counter regulatory mechanism against inflammation. These results could be interpreted together with previous reports to suggest that CD163 might have a key position in the infectious diseases [23]. The membrane-bound CD163 receptor itself has anti-inflammatory capabilities by scavenging plasma hemoglobin and the products formed from toxic heme decomposition [37].

There was also a positive correlation observed between elevated plasma sCD163 levels and BUN and Cr levels, which was previously shown to predict kidney dysfunction in HFRS patients [25]. This suggests that sCD163 might be involved in renal dysfunction. In fact, studies have shown that in PUUV infected patients, acute hantavirus infection was associated with immune reaction-induced renal tissue damage [38]. Sustained inflammation can lead to renal dysfunction, and vice-versa, renal dysfunction can fuel the inflammatory response; therefore, it is not surprising that sCD163 in our study kept rising in patients who developed kidney dysfunction. Elevated sCD163 levels have been reported in chronic kidney disease patients [39]. Hemolysis, disseminated intravascular coagulation (DIC), and bleeding are characteristic clinical manifestations for HFRS [1,24] and result in hemoglobin/heme release, which yields ferrous ions. At the same time, oxidation reduction reactions that catalyze hydrogen peroxide give rise to oxygen free radical release, which causes injury to the kidney and other organs [40]. Therefore, timely hemoglobin/heme clearance is required to avoid its excessive

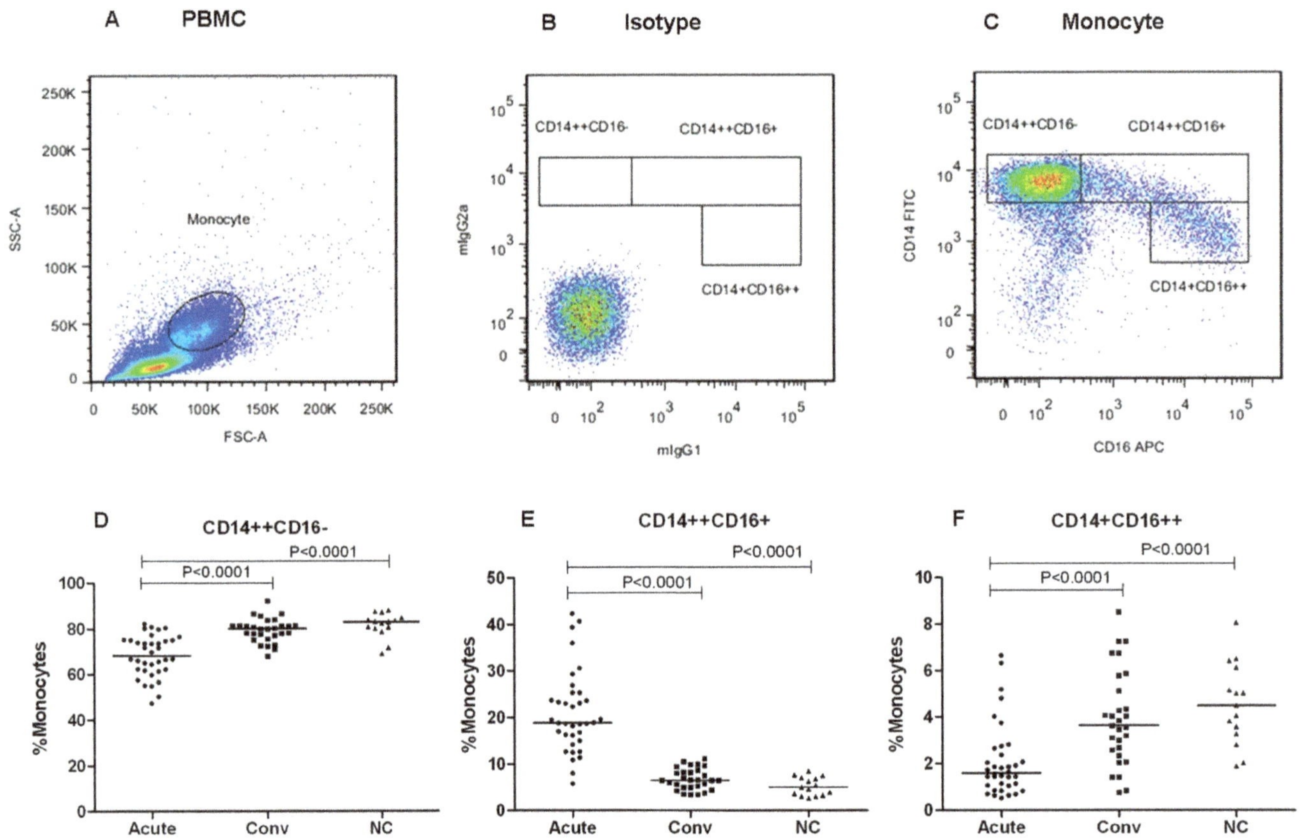

Figure 3. The monocyte subset proportions were altered in the HFRS subjects. A representative example of the monocyte subset analysis procedure is displayed (A, B, and C). (A) Monocytes from the total PBMC population were identified by forward (FSC) and side scatter (SSC) property analysis. (B) The isotypic negative control staining of CD14 and CD16 is displayed. (C) Using surface CD14 and CD16 expression, monocyte gated populations were further divided into three monocyte subsets, which were classic (CD14++CD16−), intermediate (CD14++CD16+) and non-classical monocytes (CD14+CD16++). A summary of the monocyte subset distribution analyses during the acute and convalescent HFRS phases and in the healthy subjects is displayed (D, E, and F). The significance of the differences among the multiple groups was determined by the Kruskal-Wallis test, Black lines represent medians and *P* values are plotted in each graph.

discharge into the blood and the outbreak of critical pathological responses. Hemoglobin/heme can only be cleared by monocyte/macrophage phagocytes when combined with haptoglobin and CD163 recognition [18]. sCD163 is shed from monocyte surfaces and, for this reason, we speculate that plasma sCD163 is likely to be highly expressed during HFRS and reflects kidney injury during this disease. However, there are no reports regarding this issue.

In the acute stage, CD163 expression on monocyte subset was increased. We showed that CD163 is more highly expressed on CD14++CD16+ monocytes compared with CD14++CD16− and CD14+CD16++ monocytes. Additionally, we showed a significant correlation between plasma sCD163 levels and the percentage of CD14++CD16+ monocytes and CD163 expression on CD14++CD16+ monocyte. This suggests that the sCD163 that is shed during Hantavirus infection is likely from CD14++CD16+ monocytes. These results may be support the hypothesis that CD14++CD16+ monocytes contribute to reduce inflammation reaction through anti-inflammatory mediator production that, in turn, inhibits T-cell differentiation and maturation. Other study found that CD14++CD16+ monocyte expansion also corresponded with disease progression in other diseases, including HIV infection [15], and in acute coronary syndrome [27]. Additionally, in the patients of convalescent phase, plasma sCD163 levels were still higher than the normal control levels; however, the membrane-bound CD163 levels were not significantly different between the HFRS and normal control groups. Thus, it is possible that plasma sCD163 also comes from activated tissue macrophages [33]. Monocytes stay in circulation for only 1 to 3 days and then migrate to peripheral tissues either spontaneously or upon stimulation [41]. Monocytes are known to migrate to the vascular endothelium, secrete cytokines, and be involved in endothelial dysfunction, which leads to increased endothelial permeability [42]. There are several conflicting reports regarding CD163 protein expression on monocytes. Some studies have shown that during chronic inflammation, surface CD163 expression is decreased [32,43]. However, during acute inflammation, surface CD163 expression is increased [44,45]. Additionally, through CD163 shedding, decreased surface CD163 expression was followed by the recovery and induction of surface CD163 to higher levels [46]. We speculate that surface CD163 expression might vary according to different inflammatory states in patients and during different inflammation stages.

Although we obtained some significant results, the present study has limitations. It has to be emphasized that this study only shows associations without providing evidence for possible causal mechanisms. Additionally, there were a relatively small number of patients in this study. More research is needed, with a large

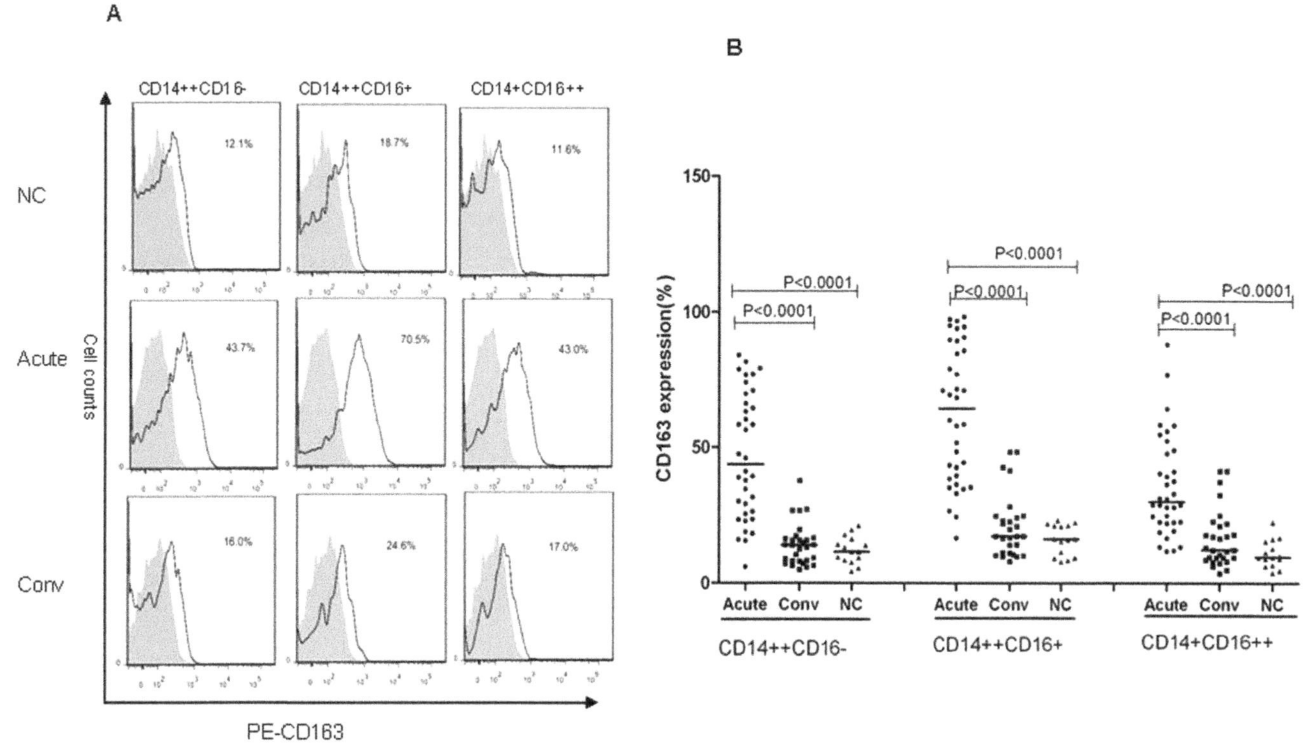

Figure 4. CD163 was differentially expressed on the monocyte subsets. (A) CD163 protein expression (black lines) in each monocyte subset is shown compared with the matched isotype control (shaded histograms) in the histograms. The data illustrate results from a representative experiment. (B) The CD163 expression summary data for the three monocyte subsets during the acute and convalescent phases and in the normal controls. The significance of the differences among the multiple groups was determined with the Kruskal-Wallis test. The black lines represent medians and *P* values are plotted for each graph.

sample and multi-center study, to improve our insight into the physiology and time course of sCD163 release and its relation with HFRS. This may be helpful for us to further understand the pathogenesis of the disease and to offer some useful information for HFRS prevention and treatment.

In conclusion, we have identified the presence of the protein marker, sCD163, in HFRS patients, which is shed from monocytes and macrophages and is related to monocyte expansion. Additionally, sCD163 levels may be useful in predicting Hantavirus disease progression. This is the first observation that evaluated Hantaviruses infected patients with a plasma marker that is both exclusive to monocytes and an innate immune system activation marker that parallels severity and reflects the clinical parameters. Our findings indicate that sCD163 may serve as a useful biomarker for HFRS, but the underlying mechanisms should be explored further.

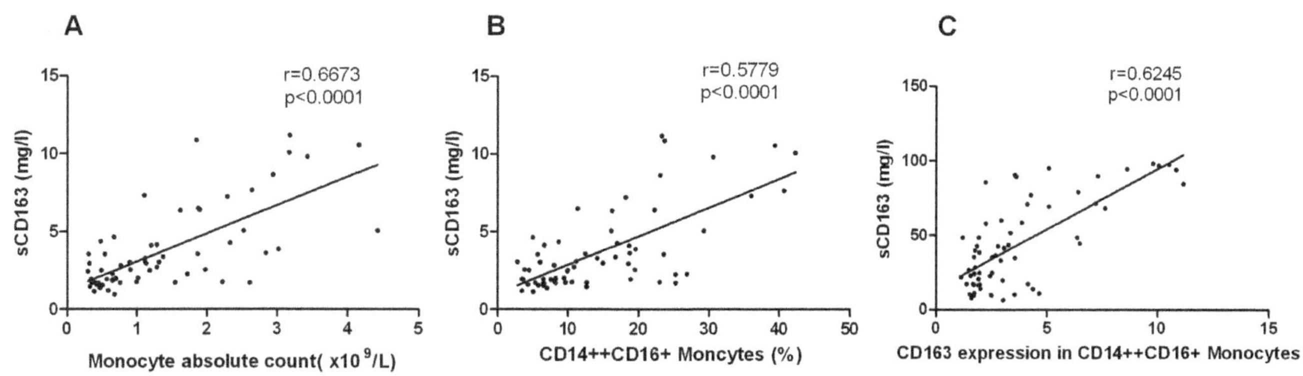

Figure 5. The sCD163 levels correlated with frequency of monocytes. Relationship between elevated plasma sCD163 levels and the absolute monocyte counts (A), intermediate (CD14++CD16+) monocyte percentage (B), and CD163 expression on the intermediate (CD14++CD16+) monocytes (C) evaluated by the Spearman correlation test, The values were derived from the same HFRS patient blood samples during their hospitalizations. The r and *P* values are indicated in the graphs.

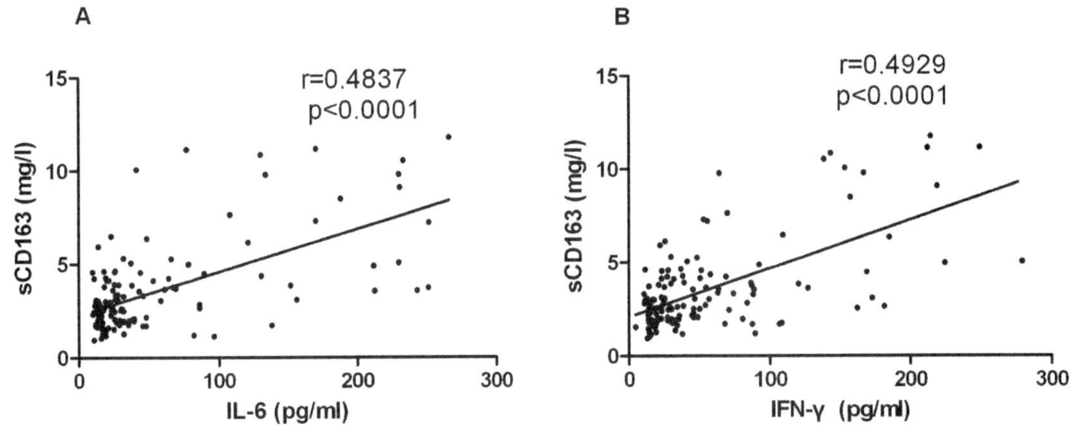

Figure 6. The sCD163 levels correlated with IL-6 and IFN-γ. Relationship between elevated plasma sCD163 levels and IL-6 (A) and IFN-γ (B) plasma levels evaluated by the Spearman correlation test. The values were derived from the same HFRS patient blood samples during their hospitalizations. The r and *P* values are indicated in the graphs.

Acknowledgments

The authors would like to express thanks to their colleagues from the Center of Infectious Diseases for their valuable support during this study.

Author Contributions

Conceived and designed the experiments: JNW HTY XFB. Performed the experiments: JNW TZ. Analyzed the data: JNW HD. Contributed reagents/materials/analysis tools: WJ. Wrote the paper: JNW WJG XFB PZW.

References

1. Mustonen J, Makela S, Outinen T, Laine O, Jylhava J, et al. (2013) The pathogenesis of nephropathia epidemica: new knowledge and unanswered questions. Antiviral Res 100: 589–604.
2. Jonsson CB, Figueiredo LT, Vapalahti O (2010) A global perspective on hantavirus ecology, epidemiology, and disease. Clin Microbiol Rev 23: 412–441.
3. Zhang YH, Ge L, Liu L, Huo XX, Xiong HR, et al. (2014) The epidemic characteristics and changing trend of hemorrhagic Fever with renal syndrome in hubei province, china. PLoS One 9: e92700.
4. Du H, Li J, Jiang W, Yu H, Zhang Y, et al. (2014) Clinical study of critical patients with hemorrhagic fever with renal syndrome complicated by acute respiratory distress syndrome. PLoS One 9: e89740.
5. Schmaljohn C, Hjelle B (1997) Hantaviruses: a global disease problem. Emerg Infect Dis 3: 95–104.
6. Penttinen K, Lahdevirta J, Kekomaki R, Ziola B, Salmi A, et al. (1981) Circulating immune complexes, immunoconglutinins, and rheumatoid factors in nephropathia epidemica. J Infect Dis 143: 15–21.
7. Cassetta L, Cassol E, Poli G (2011) Macrophage polarization in health and disease. ScientificWorldJournal 11: 2391–2402.
8. Barbosa RR, Silva SP, Silva SL, Tendeiro R, Melo AC, et al. (2012) Monocyte activation is a feature of common variable immunodeficiency irrespective of plasma lipopolysaccharide levels. Clin Exp Immunol 169: 263–272.
9. Pedraza-Sanchez S, Hise AG, Ramachandra L, Arechavaleta-Velasco F, King CL (2013) Reduced frequency of a CD14+ CD16+ monocyte subset with high Toll-like receptor 4 expression in cord blood compared to adult blood contributes to lipopolysaccharide hyporesponsiveness in newborns. Clin Vaccine Immunol 20: 962–971.
10. Ghigliotti G, Barisione C, Garibaldi S, Brunelli C, Palmieri D, et al. (2013) CD16(+) monocyte subsets are increased in large abdominal aortic aneurysms and are differentially related with circulating and cell-associated biochemical and inflammatory biomarkers. Dis Markers 34: 131–142.
11. Coulthard LR, Geiler J, Mathews RJ, Church LD, Dickie LJ, et al. (2012) Differential effects of infliximab on absolute circulating blood leucocyte counts of innate immune cells in early and late rheumatoid arthritis patients. Clin Exp Immunol 170: 36–46.
12. Koch S, Kucharzik T, Heidemann J, Nusrat A, Luegering A (2010) Investigating the role of proinflammatory CD16+ monocytes in the pathogenesis of inflammatory bowel disease. Clin Exp Immunol 161: 332–341.
13. Wrigley BJ, Shantsila E, Tapp LD, Lip GY (2013) CD14++CD16+ monocytes in patients with acute ischaemic heart failure. Eur J Clin Invest 43: 121–130.
14. Zhang D, He J, Shen M, Wang R (2014) CD16 inhibition increases host survival in a murine model of severe sepsis. J Surg Res 187: 605–609.
15. Tippett E, Cheng WJ, Westhorpe C, Cameron PU, Brew BJ, et al. (2011) Differential expression of CD163 on monocyte subsets in healthy and HIV-1 infected individuals. PLoS One 6: e19968.
16. Azeredo EL, Neves-Souza PC, Alvarenga AR, Reis SR, Torrentes-Carvalho A, et al. (2010) Differential regulation of toll-like receptor-2, toll-like receptor-4, CD16 and human leucocyte antigen-DR on peripheral blood monocytes during mild and severe dengue fever. Immunology 130: 202–216.
17. Moestrup SK, Moller HJ (2004) CD163: a regulated hemoglobin scavenger receptor with a role in the anti-inflammatory response. Ann Med 36: 347–354.
18. Van Gorp H, Delputte PL, Nauwynck HJ (2010) Scavenger receptor CD163, a Jack-of-all-trades and potential target for cell-directed therapy. Mol Immunol 47: 1650–1660.
19. Etzerodt A, Moestrup SK (2013) CD163 and inflammation: biological, diagnostic, and therapeutic aspects. Antioxid Redox Signal 18: 2352–2363.
20. Thomsen HH, Moller HJ, Trolle C, Groth KA, Skakkebaek A, et al. (2013) The macrophage low-grade inflammation marker sCD163 is modulated by exogenous sex steroids. Endocr Connect 2: 216–224.
21. Andersen MN, Abildgaard N, Maniecki MB, Moller HJ, Andersen NF (2014) Monocyte/macrophage-derived soluble CD163: a novel biomarker in multiple myeloma. Eur J Haematol.
22. Kjaergaard AG, Rodgaard-Hansen S, Dige A, Krog J, Moller HJ, et al. (2014) Monocyte Expression and Soluble Levels of the Haemoglobin Receptor (CD163/sCD163) and the Mannose Receptor (MR/sMR) in Septic and Critically Ill Non-Septic ICU Patients. PLoS One 9: e92331.
23. Buechler C, Eisinger K, Krautbauer S (2013) Diagnostic and prognostic potential of the macrophage specific receptor CD163 in inflammatory diseases. Inflamm Allergy Drug Targets 12: 391–402.
24. Manigold T, Vial P (2014) Human hantavirus infections: epidemiology, clinical features, pathogenesis and immunology. Swiss Med Wkly 144: w13937.
25. Du H, Wang PZ, Li J, Bai L, Li H, et al. (2014) Clinical characteristics and outcomes in critical patients with hemorrhagic fever with renal syndrome. BMC Infect Dis 14: 191.
26. Zhang Y, Liu B, Ma Y, Yi J, Zhang C, et al. (2014) Hantaan virus infection induces CXCL10 expression through TLR3, RIG-I, and MDA-5 pathways correlated with the disease severity. Mediators Inflamm 2014: 697837.
27. Funderburg NT, Zidar DA, Shive C, Lioi A, Mudd J, et al. (2012) Shared monocyte subset phenotypes in HIV-1 infection and in uninfected subjects with acute coronary syndrome. Blood 120: 4599–4608.
28. Mendonca VR, Luz NF, Santos NJ, Borges VM, Goncalves MS, et al. (2012) Association between the haptoglobin and heme oxygenase 1 genetic profiles and soluble CD163 in susceptibility to and severity of human malaria. Infect Immun 80: 1445–1454.
29. Frings W, Dreier J, Sorg C (2002) Only the soluble form of the scavenger receptor CD163 acts inhibitory on phorbol ester-activated T-lymphocytes, whereas membrane-bound protein has no effect. FEBS Lett 526: 93–96.
30. Weaver LK, Hintz-Goldstein KA, Pioli PA, Wardwell K, Qureshi N, et al. (2006) Pivotal advance: activation of cell surface Toll-like receptors causes shedding of the hemoglobin scavenger receptor CD163. J Leukoc Biol 80: 26–35.

31. Etzerodt A, Rasmussen MR, Svendsen P, Chalaris A, Schwarz J, et al. (2014) Structural basis for inflammation-driven shedding of CD163 ectodomain and tumor necrosis factor-alpha in macrophages. J Biol Chem 289: 778–788.
32. Burdo TH, Lentz MR, Autissier P, Krishnan A, Halpern E, et al. (2011) Soluble CD163 made by monocyte/macrophages is a novel marker of HIV activity in early and chronic infection prior to and after anti-retroviral therapy. J Infect Dis 204: 154–163.
33. Burdo TH, Soulas C, Orzechowski K, Button J, Krishnan A, et al. (2010) Increased monocyte turnover from bone marrow correlates with severity of SIV encephalitis and CD163 levels in plasma. PLoS Pathog 6: e1000842.
34. Kazankov K, Barrera F, Moller HJ, Bibby BM, Vilstrup H, et al. (2014) Soluble CD163, a macrophage activation marker, is independently associated with fibrosis in patients with chronic viral hepatitis B and C. Hepatology.
35. Su L, Feng L, Song Q, Kang H, Zhang X, et al. (2013) Diagnostic value of dynamics serum sCD163, sTREM-1, PCT, and CRP in differentiating sepsis, severity assessment, and prognostic prediction. Mediators Inflamm 2013: 969875.
36. Wang PZ, Li ZD, Yu HT, Zhang Y, Wang W, et al. (2012) Elevated serum concentrations of inflammatory cytokines and chemokines in patients with haemorrhagic fever with renal syndrome. J Int Med Res 40: 648–656.
37. Possamai LA, Antoniades CG, Anstee QM, Quaglia A, Vergani D, et al. (2010) Role of monocytes and macrophages in experimental and human acute liver failure. World J Gastroenterol 16: 1811–1819.
38. Klingstrom J, Hardestam J, Stoltz M, Zuber B, Lundkvist A, et al. (2006) Loss of cell membrane integrity in puumala hantavirus-infected patients correlates with levels of epithelial cell apoptosis and perforin. J Virol 80: 8279–8282.
39. Simoni J, Simoni G, Griswold JA, Moeller JF, Tsikouris JP, et al. (2006) Role of free hemoglobin in 8-iso prostaglandin F2-alpha synthesis in chronic renal failure and its impact on CD163-Hb scavenger receptor and on coronary artery endothelium. ASAIO J 52: 652–661.
40. Nielsen MJ, Moestrup SK (2009) Receptor targeting of hemoglobin mediated by the haptoglobins: roles beyond heme scavenging. Blood 114: 764–771.
41. Geissmann F, Manz MG, Jung S, Sieweke MH, Merad M, et al. (2010) Development of monocytes, macrophages, and dendritic cells. Science 327: 656–661.
42. Kundumani-Sridharan V, Dyukova E, Hansen DR, Rao GN (2013) 12/15-Lipoxygenase mediates high-fat diet-induced endothelial tight junction disruption and monocyte transmigration: a new role for 15(S)-hydroxyeicosatetraenoic acid in endothelial cell dysfunction. J Biol Chem 288: 15830–15842.
43. Ye H, Wang LY, Zhao J, Wang K (2013) Increased CD163 expression is associated with acute-on-chronic hepatitis B liver failure. World J Gastroenterol 19: 2818–2825.
44. Kjaergaard AG, Rodgaard-Hansen S, Dige A, Krog J, Moller HJ, et al. (2014) Monocyte expression and soluble levels of the haemoglobin receptor (CD163/sCD163) and the mannose receptor (MR/sMR) in septic and critically ill non-septic ICU patients. PLoS One 9: e92331.
45. West SD, Goldberg D, Ziegler A, Krencicki M, Du Clos TW, et al. (2012) Transforming growth factor-beta, macrophage colony-stimulating factor and C-reactive protein levels correlate with CD14(high)CD16+ monocyte induction and activation in trauma patients. PLoS One 7: e52406.
46. Davis BH, Zarev PV (2005) Human monocyte CD163 expression inversely correlates with soluble CD163 plasma levels. Cytometry B Clin Cytom 63: 16–22.

Effects of Increased Von Willebrand Factor Levels on Primary Hemostasis in Thrombocytopenic Patients with Liver Cirrhosis

Andreas Wannhoff[1], Oliver J. Müller[2], Kilian Friedrich[1], Christian Rupp[1], Petra Klöters-Plachky[1], Yvonne Leopold[1], Maik Brune[3], Mirja Senner[1], Karl-Heinz Weiss[1], Wolfgang Stremmel[1], Peter Schemmer[4], Hugo A. Katus[2], Daniel N. Gotthardt[1]*

1 Department of Internal Medicine IV, University Hospital Heidelberg, Heidelberg, Germany, **2** Department of Internal Medicine III, University Hospital Heidelberg, Heidelberg, Germany, **3** Department of Internal Medicine I and Clinical Chemistry, University Hospital Heidelberg, Heidelberg, Germany, **4** Department of General and Transplant Surgery, University Hospital Heidelberg, Heidelberg, Germany

Abstract

In patients with liver cirrhosis procoagulant and anticoagulant changes occur simultaneously. During primary hemostasis, platelets adhere to subendothelial structures, via von Willebrand factor (vWF). We aimed to investigate the influence of vWF on primary hemostasis in patients with liver cirrhosis. Therefore we assessed in-vitro bleeding time as marker of primary hemostasis in cirrhotic patients, measuring the Platelet Function Analyzer (PFA-100) closure times with collagen and epinephrine (Col-Epi, upper limit of normal ≤165 s) or collagen and ADP (Col-ADP, upper limit of normal ≤118 s). If Col-Epi and Col-ADP were prolonged, the PFA-100 was considered to be pathological. Effects of vWF on primary hemostasis in thrombocytopenic patients were analyzed and plasma vWF levels were modified by adding recombinant vWF or anti-vWF antibody. Of the 72 included cirrhotic patients, 32 (44.4%) showed a pathological result for the PFA-100. They had mean closure times (± SD) of 180±62 s with Col-Epi and 160±70 s with Col-ADP. Multivariate analysis revealed that hematocrit ($P = 0.027$) and vWF-antigen levels ($P = 0.010$) are the predictors of a pathological PFA-100 test in cirrhotic patients. In 21.4% of cirrhotic patients with platelet count ≥150/nL and hematocrit ≥27.0%, pathological PFA-100 results were found. In thrombocytopenic (<150/nL) patients with cirrhosis, normal PFA-100 results were associated with higher vWF-antigen levels (462.3±235.9% vs. 338.7±151.6%, $P = 0.021$). These results were confirmed by multivariate analysis in these patients as well as by adding recombinant vWF or polyclonal anti-vWF antibody that significantly shortened or prolonged closure times, respectively. In conclusion, primary hemostasis is impaired in cirrhotic patients. The effect of reduced platelet count in cirrhotic patients can at least be partly compensated by increased vWF levels. Recombinant vWF could be an alternative to platelet transfusions in the future.

Editor: Ferruccio Bonino, University of Pisa, Italy

Funding: AW received a grant from the Dekanat der Medizinischen Fakultät Heidelberg (Medical faculty Heidelberg). DNG was supported by a grant from Deutsche Forschungsgemeinschaft (German Research Foundation). The funders had no role in study design, data collection and analysis, decision to publish, or preparation of the manuscript.

Competing Interests: The authors have declared that no competing interests exist.

* Email: Daniel_Gotthardt@med.uni-heidelberg.de

Introduction

Patients with liver cirrhosis suffer from complex abnormalities of the hemostatic system that affect primary and secondary hemostasis and fibrinolysis. Changes in procoagulant and anticoagulant proteins occur simultaneously [1,2], and yet it has not been understood if an individual patient currently is in favor of bleeding or thrombosis. Thus, these patients can clinically present with an increased bleeding risk or an increased rate of venous thrombosis as well as develop portal vein thrombosis [3,4].

During primary hemostasis, platelets adhere to the subendothelium via the von Willebrand factor (vWF) [5]. Thrombocytopenia, thrombocytopathy, or impaired function of vWF can disrupt primary hemostasis. Thrombocytopenia is common in liver cirrhosis, occurring in up to 70% of patients even though the underlying pathomechanisms are most likely multifactorial and not yet fully understood [6]; it is assumed that an imbalance between the production and survival of platelets is its most likely cause. Thrombocytopenia can be due to bone marrow suppression or decreased thrombopoietin levels. Hypersplenism, platelet consumption, and platelet autoantibody action might decrease survival of platelets in cirrhotic patients [7]. Data on concomitant thrombocytopathy is not clear and in part controversial. As an example of thrombocytopathy, impaired platelet activation has been reported, while other results indicate hyperactivation of platelets in end-stage liver disease [7]. Levels of vWF are elevated in cirrhosis, which may be due to different causes. Endotoxemia in patients with liver cirrhosis has shown to increase vWF-levels [8].

Further, vWF mRNA levels in hepatic tissue are increased as well, indicating increased hepatic synthesis of vWF [9].

In hemostasis, von Willebrand factor binds to glycoprotein Ib on the platelet surface and to the subendothelial matrix. Besides this, vWF was recently recognized as playing important roles during angiogenesis, inflammation, cell proliferation and tumor cell growth [10]. Further, vWF levels were shown to correlate with the degree of portal hypertension as measured by hepatic venous pressure gradient and vWF levels were predictive of survival free of portal hypertension-related events and liver transplantation [11]. They were as well associated with development of hepatopulmonary syndrome [12] and in a further study prediction of mortality in patients with end-stage liver disease was equal to MELD score [13]. vWF is cleaved by the protease ADAMTS13 (a disintegrin-like and metalloprotease with thrombospondin type 1 motif 13), which is mainly synthesized in the liver and found to be reduced in cirrhosis [14,15].

Measurement of the in-vitro bleeding time using the Platelet Function Analyzer (PFA-100) is an established method for assessing primary hemostasis. It shows almost no intra-assay variability and has a high accuracy for detection of platelet function defects with an area under the ROC curve of 0.977 [16]. It successfully aids detection of patients with platelet function defects or von Willebrand's disease [17].

We assessed the PFA-100, a test that closely represents the in-vivo setting, in cirrhotic patients to investigate primary hemostasis. Therefore, we aimed to study the effect of increased levels of vWF on the in-vitro bleeding time in thrombocytopenic patients.

Materials and Methods

Patients

Patients with end-stage liver disease on the waiting list for liver transplantation at the Heidelberg University Hospital (Germany) were eligible for inclusion, regardless of etiology, platelet count, or hematocrit levels. Patients who had taken either antiplatelet drugs, non-steroidal anti-inflammatory drugs (NSAID), or other anticoagulant agents within the last ten days were excluded; patients were also excluded if no information on these drugs was available.

We measured a complete blood count as well as PFA-100 closure-times after stimulation with epinephrine or ADP, vWF-antigen, and vWF-activity as well as the ratio vWF-activity:vWF-antigen and ADAMTS13 activitiy. Analyses were separately conducted for the whole study cohort, for patients without thrombocytopenia and without anemia (defined as platelet count ≥150/nL and hematocrit ≥27%) and for patients with thrombocytopenia (<150/nL). Analysis was as well performed for patients with a platelet count <60/nL, which is an accepted cut-off for performing invasive procedures, such as transcutaneous liver biopsy. A platelet concentration of 50–0/nL in cirrhotic patients is sufficient to preserve thrombin generation at a level equivalent to the lower 10% of the normal range [18]. To investigate the effect of vWF-levels on platelet aggregation further, we measured vWF levels within a subset of cirrhotic patients as described below. Data on patient demographic and health characteristics, including age, sex, etiology of liver disease, Child-Turcotte-Pugh (CTP) score, and MELD score were obtained.

Ethics Statement

All patients provided written informed consent, and the study was previously approved by the local ethics committee of the medical faculty of the University Hospital Heidelberg and the study was performed in accordance with the Declaration of Helsinki.

Blood samples

Blood was drawn from the cubital or antecubital vein with a 21-gauge butterfly needle. The first milliliters of blood was collected into an EDTA-tube (ethylenediaminetetraacetic acid) and used for complete blood count. Then, citrated blood was collected for analysis of vWF. Finally, 3.8 ml of blood was collected into a tube containing 0.129 mol/l citrate (S-Monovette for PFA 100, Sarstedt AG & Co., Germany) for analysis of PFA-100 closure times.

Modification of vWF

In patients with thrombocytopenia (platelet count <150/nL), vWF levels were modified as follows to proof the hypothesis that increased vWF can compensate for reduced platelet count in patients with liver cirrhosis: Four tubes containing 0.129 mol/l citrate (S-Monovette for PFA 100) were collected per patient. Immediately after collection, 66 µg or 165 µg of a polyclonal anti-human vWF antibody (Haematologic Technologies, Inc., U.S.A.) was added to two tubes, respectively. A third tube was prepared with 25 µg of recombinant vWF (r-vWF) (Haematologic Technologies, Inc.). We aimed to add the amount of vWF that usually is found in healthy individuals and which thus would increase vWF in healthy individuals by 100%. Based on a concentration of 10µg vWF in 1 mL plasma of healthy controls [19] and an estimated hematocrit of 35% in cirrhotic patients, 25µg r-vWF are needed to meet these assumptions. A fourth tube was used as a control. All tubes were then incubated for 60 min at 37°C in a water bath. Next, PFA-100 was performed in all samples to measure closure times using collagen-epinephrine (Col-Epi) and collagen-ADP (Col-ADP). Additionally, plasma from these same samples was used to measure vWF-antigen levels.

Use of PFA-100 and determination of closure time

Without shaking, the samples were immediately brought to the central laboratory of the Heidelberg University Hospital, and were analyzed within 3 h after being drawn. Samples that underwent modification of vWF were analyzed immediately after incubation in a water bath.

For PFA-100 closure time analysis, a whole blood sample, collected in a tube with 3.8% sodium citrate, was used for input. It is aspirated through a capillary tube and exposed to a collagen membrane, coated with either epinephrine or ADP, at a shear rate of 5000–6000/s. Activation of platelets is caused by shear stress and exposure to the coated membrane, thus initiating the formation of a platelet plug. The time until full occlusion (and blood flow discontinuation) is measured; this is called the closure time and is a parameter for primary hemostasis [20].

PFA-100 (Siemens Healthcare, Germany) was performed using standard cartridges containing Col-Epi and Col-ADP (both Siemens Healthcare) and results for closure times were measured in seconds. Closure time >165 s with Col-Epi and that >118 s with Col-ADP were considered pathological. The test was stopped, if no clotting was achieved after 300 s; in this case, 300 s was recorded as closure time. According to recommendations and clinical practice, the PFA-100 was analyzed as following[16]: If the test with Col-Epi was prolonged, than Col-ADP was as well included for analysis. Only if this was prolonged as well, the PFA-100 was considered to be pathological.

Analysis of vWF and ADAMTS13

vWF-antigen levels and vWF-activity were determined turbidimetric assays on a Siemens BCS XP system applying appropriate reagents (vWF Ag and INNOVANCE vWF Ac kits, respectively,

Table 1. Characteristics of patients with liver cirrhosis.

	Child A	Child B	Child C	Total
Patients, n (%)	19 (26.4%)	31 (43.1%)	22 (30.6%)	72
Female, n (%)	6 (31.6%)	11 (35.5)	11 (50.0%)	28 (38.9%)
Age, yrs. (±SD)	48.5 (±8.9)	51.3 (±11.1)	52.8 (±9.4)	51.0 (±10.1)
Etiology of cirrhosis				
Cryptogenic, n (%)	1 (5.3%)	4 (12.9%)	3 (13.6%)	8 (11.1%)
Alcoholic, n (%)	8 (42.1%)	14 (45.2%)	13 (59.1%)	35 (48.6%)
Viral hepatitis, n (%)	5 (26.3%)	6 (19.4%)	5 (22.7%)	16 (22.2%)
Autoimmune hepatitis, n (%)	0	3 (9.7%)	0	3 (4.2%)
Cholestatic[a], n (%)	3 (15.8%)	4 (12.9%)	0	7 (9.7%)
Other[b], n (%)	2 (10.5%)	0	1 (4.5%)	3 (4.2%)
LabMELD, median (range)	8 (7–12)	12 (7–21)	19 (13–37)	12 (7–37)

Description of baseline parameters such as age, sex, and etiology of patients with liver cirrhosis and labMELD-score; grouped by Child-Turcotte-Pugh score.
[a]Including primary sclerosing cholangitis and biliary atresia.
[b]Including Wilson disease and polycystic liver disease.

all by Siemens Healthcare). Normal ranges of vWF-antigen and vWF-activity were 70–120% and 61–179%, respectively, in patients with all blood types; normal vWF-activity was 46–146% in patients with blood type O.

For measurement of ADAMTS13 activity, citrate plasma samples of 50 patients were kept in aliquots at −20°C before analysis in the central laboratory. ADAMTS13 activity was determined applying the Technozym ADAMTS-13 Activity ELISA kit (Technoclone, Heidelberg, Germany) on a Biochrom EZ Read 400 ELISA Microplate Reader at 450 nm according to the manufacturer's instructions.

Statistical analysis

Results for closure times, vWF-antigen, vWF-activity, ADAMTS13, hematocrit, and platelet counts are reported as means with standard deviations (SD). Student's *t*-test and one way ANOVA were used to compare results of parametric data. For comparison of categorical variables, Fisher's exact test was used. Closure times, hematocrit, platelet count, vWF, and ADAMTS13 were evaluated on the basis of CTP and MELD scores. Multivariate analysis was done using a logistic regression model. Only variables showing a $P<0.1$ in univariate analysis were included for multivariate analysis. Results of the vWF-modification experiments were analyzed using the *t*-test for paired samples. Statistical analyses were performed using IBM SPSS version 21 (IBM Corp, Armonk, NY). Significance was defined as $P<0.05$. Original data can be found in Tables S1 and S2.

Results

Study cohort

A total of 95 patients with liver cirrhosis were screened between January 2012 and October 2013; of these, 23 were excluded because of anti-platelet drugs or NSAIDs intake. PFA-100 closure time using Col-Epi was determined in the remaining 72 patients; of these, Col-ADP was available in 62 patients.

Among the included 72 cirrhotic patients, 19 (26.4%) had Child A cirrhosis, 31 (43.1%), Child B cirrhosis, and 22 (30.6%), Child C cirrhosis; labMELD score ranged from 7 to 37 (median: 12). Further details on patient characteristics are given in Table 1. Enrolment details of the study population are shown in Figure 1.

PFA-100 closure times and basic laboratory values in cirrhotic patients

The mean PFA-100 closure time with Col-Epi in cirrhotic patients was 180±62 s and that with Col-ADP was 160±70 s. Of the 72 samples tested with Col-Epi, 35 (48.6%) had results within the normal range, while 37 (51.4%) had pathological results. Of the 62 samples tested with Col-ADP, 22 (35.5%) had results within the normal range and 40 (64.5%) had pathological results. Of the patients with prolonged Col-Epi, measurement of Col-ADP was pathological in 32 (86.5%), thus a total of 32 of the 72 patients (44.4%) were classified as having a pathological test results for the PFA-100.

All patients had a mean platelet count of 109/nL (±63) and mean hematocrit of 34.2% (±6.9). Mean vWF-antigen was

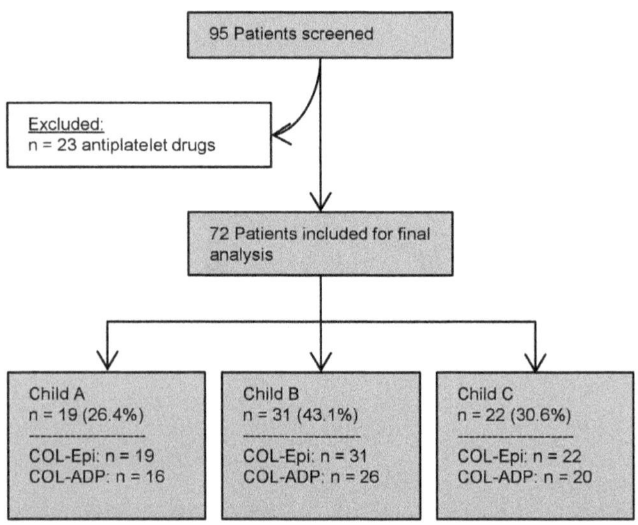

Figure 1. Selection of the study population. The enrolment details of the study population are shown, including the number of patients excluded because of the use of antiplatelet drugs or because there was no information on use of these drugs. For all subgroups, the number of available test results for PFA-100 with Col-Epi and Col-ADP is given.

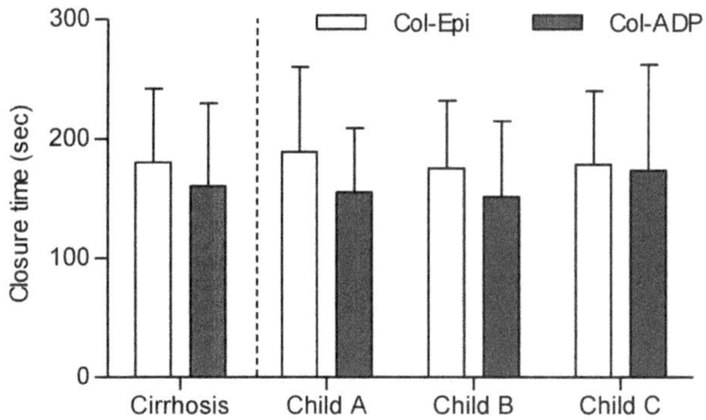

Figure 2. Results for PFA-100 in cirrhotic patients. Overall, mean closure times were above the upper limit of normal for Col-Epi (>165 s) and Col-ADP (>118 s) in cirrhotic patients. There were no significant differences between patients with different Child-Turcotte-Pugh scores.

383.9% (±200.6) mean vWF-activity was 313.5% (±168.7) and mean vWF-activity:vWF-antigen ratio was 0.83 (±0.14). Mean ADAMTS13 activity was 67.9% (±24.0).

Analysis by Child-Turcotte-Pugh score revealed no significant differences for mean closure times after induction with either Col-Epi or Col-ADP (Figure 2) nor in the rate of pathological PFA-100 test results. Yet there were significant differences in hematocrit, vWF-antigen and vWF-activity and a strong trend towards reduced ADAMTS13 activity in CTP B ($P = 0.050$) and CTP C ($P = 0.070$) compared to CTP A patients was observed (Table 2). Additionally, there were no significant differences in PFA-100 closure times between patients with Child-Turcotte-Pugh A, B, and C, if only patients with a platelet count ≥150/nL and hematocrit ≥27.0% were included (data not shown).

Analysis of PFA-100 closure times in thrombocytopenic patients with liver cirrhosis

A total of 58 patients with thrombocytopenia (<150/nL) were included, among which were 29 (50.0%) with a pathological result for the PFA-100 test. This resembles a strong trend towards an increased rate of pathological results in these patients compared to the non-thrombocytopenic group (3 out of 11, $P = 0.053$). Compared to the 14 non-thrombocytopenic patients, patients with a platelet count <150/nL had prolonged closure times for Col-Epi (187±62 s vs. 149±53 s; $P = 0.037$) and Col-ADP (164±70 s vs. 140±70 s; $P = 0.281$). There were significantly more pathological results for Col-ADP (58.1% vs. 6.5%; $P = 0.019$) in the thrombocytopenic group compared to the non-thrombocytopenic patients, but this was not significant for Col-Epi (44.4% vs. 6.9%; $P = 0.240$).

Thrombocytopenic patients had significantly more advanced liver cirrhosis (median MELD 13 [range 7–37] vs. 11 [range 7–20]; $P = 0.040$ according to Mann-Whitney-*U* test), but did not show a significant difference in hematocrit (33.7±6.9% vs. 36.4±6.5%; $P = 0.184$). Levels of vWF-antigen were higher in the thrombocytopenic group (400.5±206.2% vs. 310.0±160.0%; $P = 0.143$) as were levels of vWF-activity (333.6±176.5% vs. 223.7±86.0%, $P = 0.033$).

In patients with a platelet count of less 60/nL (n = 12) closure time was 201±66 s for Col-Epi. After performing Col-ADP in the 8 (66.7%) patients with prolonged results for Col-Epi, all these patients were diagnosed with a pathological PFA-100. There was no statically significant difference in PFA closure times compared to patients with a platelet count ≥60/nL (Col-Epi: $P = 0.203$, Col-ADP: $P = 0.341$), but there was a trend towards a higher rate of pathological PFA-100 test in these patients compared to those with a platelet count ≥60/nL ($P = 0.090$).

Analysis of vWF in thrombocytopenic patients

Analysis of vWF in thrombocytopenic patients (defined as platelet count <150/nL) revealed an association with closure times: vWF-antigen was significantly higher in those thrombocy-

Table 2. Results for PFA-100, full blood count, and vWF.

	Child A	Child B	Child C	P<0.05
Col-Epi, n (%)	19	31	22	
Closure time, s (±SD)	189 (±71)	175 (±57)	178 (±62)	n.s.
Pathological, n (%)	10 (52.6%)	15 (48.4%)	12 (54.5%)	n.s.
Col-ADP n (%)	16	26	20	
Closure time, s (±SD)	155 (±54)	151 (±64)	173 (±89)	n.s.
Pathological, n (%)	12 (75.0%)	15 (57.7%)	13 (65.0%)	n.s.
PFA-100 test result				
Pathological, n (%)	8 (42.1%)	13 (41.9%)	11 (50.0%)	n.s.
Laboratory values				
Platelet count,/nL (±SD)	122 (±50)	115 (±80)	91 (±40)	n.s.
Hematocrit, % (±SD)	38.9 (±5.9)	34.0 (±5.9)	30.4 (±6.8)	A/B, A/C
vWF-antigen, % (±SD)	274.1 (±111.1)	358.5 (±148.6)	513.5 (±252.3)	A/C, B/C
vWF-activity, % (±SD)	223.1 (±101.7)	301.9 (±132.2)	407.3 (±212.3)	A/C
vWF-activity:vWF-antigen ratio (±SD)	0.81 (±0.11)	0.85 (±0.14)	0.83 (±0.14)	n.s.
ADAMTS13, % (SD)	81.0 (±18.9)	64.5 (±23.2)	63.7 (±26.2)	n.s.

Results for PFA-100 and basic laboratory values are grouped by Child-Turcotte-Pugh classification. The 'P<0.05'-column indicates significant differences between groups according to one-way ANOVA or Fisher's exact test. For example, A/C indicates a significant difference between CTP groups A and C.

topenic patients with a normal PFA-100 (462.3±235.9%) compared to those with pathological results (338.7±151.6%, $P=0.021$). A similar trends was as well found for vWF-activity (376.2±209.7% vs. 291.0±125.1%, $P=0.065$). Regarding vWF-activity:vWF-antigen ratio and ADAMTS13 activity no differences were found ($P=0.161$ and $P=0.628$, respectively). These results on the differences in vWF-antigen and vWF-activity were as well present when separately analyzed for Col-Epi and Col-ADP (Table 3, Figure 3A).

Results after modification of vWF

In 21 patients with a platelet count <150/nL, plasma vWF levels were modified with a polyclonal antibody or with recombinant vWF. Mean closure times were 197±60 s (Col-Epi) and 159±61 s (Col-ADP) in the unmodified samples. Compared to these, closure times were 178±57 s (Col-Epi; $P=0.019$) and 149±60 s (Col-ADP; $P=0.189$) after addition of recombinant vWF and we found a significant increase in vWF antigen levels in all 21 samples ($P<0.001$). Addition of 66 µg of anti-vWF-antibody resulted in closure times of 247±49 s for Col-Epi ($P=0.016$) and 213±45 s for Col-ADP ($P=0.091$); addition of 165 µg resulted in closure times of 274±33 s for Col-Epi ($P=0.005$) and 277±32 s for Col-ADP ($P=0.006$). Results are shown in Figure 3B-D and summarized in Table 4.

Detection of thrombocytopathy in patients with normal platelet count and hematocrit

Overall, 14 patients with liver cirrhosis had a platelet count ≥ 150/nL and hematocrit ≥27%. Mean closures time were 149±53 s for Col-Epi. Pathological results for Col-Epi were found in 5 (35.7%) patients and after measurement of Col-ADP in these patients, a total of 3 (21.4%) patients were diagnosed with a pathological PFA-100 test. There were no differences regarding platelet count, hematocrit, or vWF between patients with normal and pathological results.

Analysis of independent predictors of pathologic results for the PFA-100 test

The influence of the following variables on the outcome of the PFA-100 was investigated: age, sex, labMELD score, serum albumin, platelet count, hematocrit, vWF-antigen, vWF-activity:vWF-antigen ratio, and ADAMTS13. In univariate analysis only platelet count ($P=0.086$), hematocrit ($P=0.054$) and vWF-antigen ($P=0.064$) levels were associated ($P<0.1$) with the outcome of the PFA-100. In a multivariate analysis including these three variables, only hematocrit ($P=0.027$) and vWF-antigen ($P=0.010$) turned out to significantly influence the PFA-100 test results, yet there was a strong trend for platelet count as well ($P=0.069$). The same analysis was performed in thrombocytopenic patients (<150/nL), which revealed again hematocrit ($P=0.026$) and vWF-antigen ($P=0.013$) as independent predictors of the test outcome (Table 5 and 6).

Discussion

Over the past years, knowledge about hemostasis in patients with cirrhosis has greatly expanded and revealed that conventional coagulation parameters as International Normalized Ratio (INR), prothrombin time, or platelet count are not as reliable to indicate an increased risk of bleeding as assumed previously. Especially with regard to platelet transfusions or supplementation with coagulation factors, clinicians are in need of tests that determine the actual hemostatic balance in these patients more accurately [21]. Therefore, we conducted a study to evaluate primary

Table 3. Analysis of the effect of vWF on results of PFA-100 in thrombocytopenic patients.

	PFA-100			Col-Epi			Col-ADP		
	norm.	path.	*P*	norm.	path.	*P*	norm.	path.	*P*
vWF-antigen, % (±SD)	462.3 (±235.9)	338.7 (±151.6)	0.021	467.8 (±248.7)	345.8 (±146.3)	0.033	470.6 (±252.3)	358.3 (±171.8)	0.077
vWF-activity, % (±SD)	376.2 (±209.7)	291.0 (±125.1)	0.065	383.7 (±220.7)	292.9 (±119.1)	0.067	401.2 (±241.3)	300.9 (±135.8)	0.068
vWF-activity:vWF- antigen ratio	0.82 (±0.13)	0.87 (±0.14)	0.161	0.83 (±0.14)	0.86 (±0.14)	0.372	0.84 (±0.11)	0.86 (±0.14)	0.712

Comparison of vWF-antigen and vWF-activity in thrombocytopenic (<150/nL) patients with liver cirrhosis and the effect of vWF on results of PFA-100 measured with Col-Epi and Col-ADP (norm. = normal test result, path. = pathological test result).

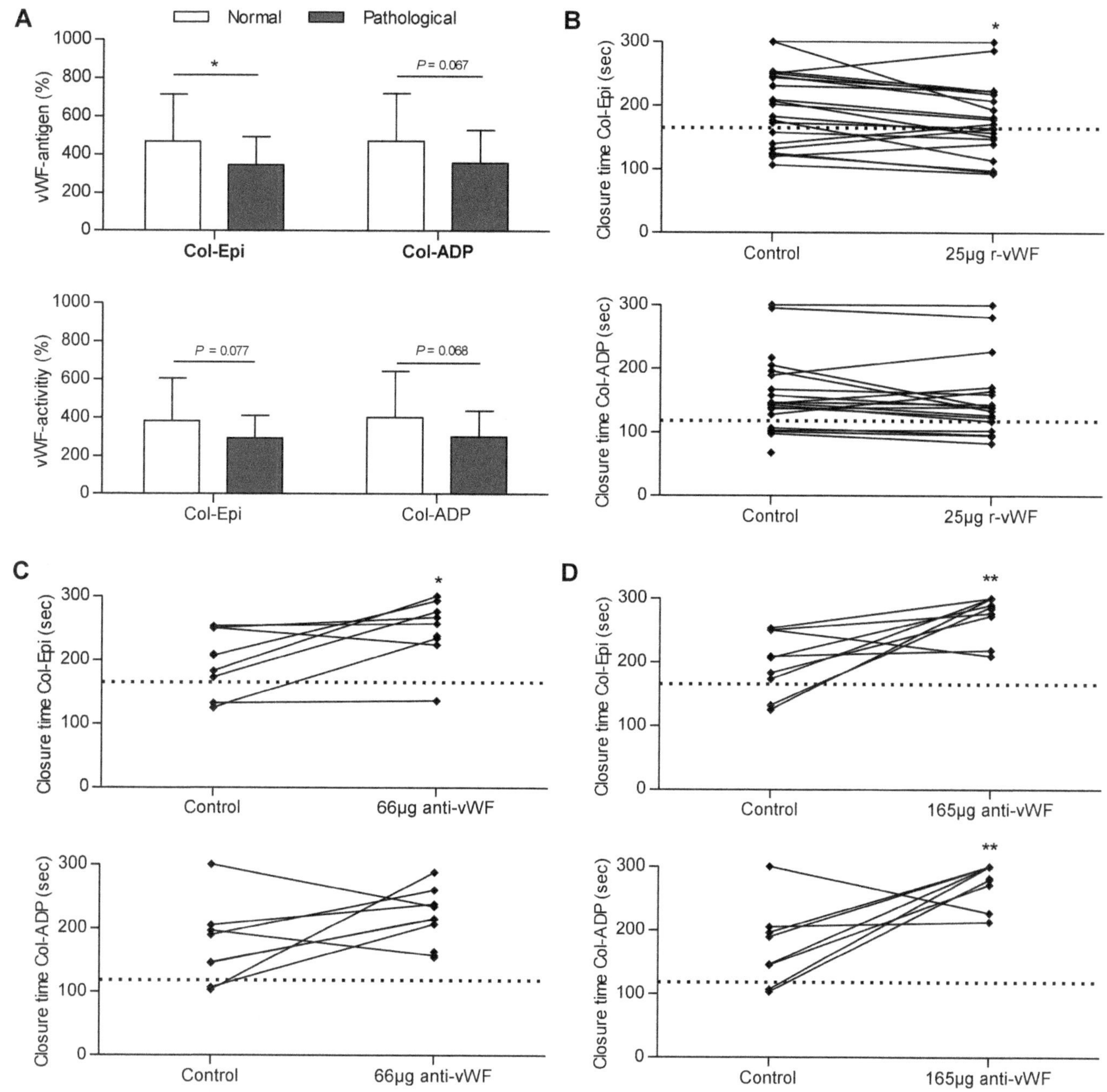

Figure 3. Effect of von Willebrand factor on primary hemostasis in thrombocytopenic patients with liver cirrhosis. Increased levels of vWF were associated with maintained normal primary hemostasis in patients with liver cirrhosis and reduced platelet count (<150/nL). vWF-antigen and vWF-activity were higher in patients with normal results for PFA-100 after measuring with Col-Epi and Col-ADP (A+B). Substitution of recombinant vWF (r-vWF) resulted in improved primary hemostasis as compared to unmodified samples (C). Addition of a 66-µg or 165-µg polyclonal anti-vWF-antibody levels led to prolonged closure times compared to unmodified control samples (D+E). Horizontal lines represent the upper limit of normal for closure times with Col-Epi or Col-ADP [**: $P<0.01$, *: $P<0.05$].

hemostasis in patients with liver cirrhosis by means of PFA-100 closure times. On the one hand side our results indicate that primary hemostasis is impaired in a large number of patients and we found a high rate of results indicating thrombocytopathy. On the other hand side we also demonstrated that increased vWF levels can compensate for reduced platelet count.

PFA-100 is a validated test for screening of platelet function disorders and von Willebrand's disease [17,22] and has been used to detect platelet-related defects of primary hemostasis in dialysis patients as well [23]. Until now, data on its use in patients with liver cirrhosis is only available from two smaller studies. The first study reported increased closure times in 20 patients with Child A or B cirrhosis. An improvement of closure times was shown after experimentally increasing hematocrit [24]. Since we found pathological results in patients with a hematocrit ≥27% in the present study, we esteem that transfusion of packed red blood cells may only improve primary hemostasis in some patients. The second study focused on differences between cholestatic and non-

Table 4. Effect of vWF levels on primary hemostasis in thrombocytopenic patients with cirrhosis.

	25 μg r-vWF	66 μg anti-vWF	156 μg anti-vWF
Col-Epi	↓	↑	↑
Col-ADP	↔	↑	↑

Overview of the main results: changes in closure times after addition of either recombinant vWF or anti-vWF-antibody (↔: no change, ↓: improved, ↑: worsened).

cholestatic causes of liver diseases. Closure times for patients with primary biliary cirrhosis and primary sclerosing cholangitis were less compared to patients with non-cholestatic causes of cirrhosis [25]. Despite including more patients, especially with end-stage liver disease, to our knowledge, this is the first study to acknowledge platelet count, hematocrit, and vWF in the analysis. The latter two were as well identified as independent predictors of maintained primary hemostasis in multivariate analysis, yet a strong trend was found for platelet count as well. Our study results support the hypothesis that cirrhosis disrupts primary hemostasis, which does seem independent on the stage of cirrhosis.

Within our samples of non-thrombocytopenic, non-anemic patients, we obtained pathological results for the PFA-100 in 21.4% of cases. Platelet dysfunction is the most likely reason for these pathological results, since patients with low hematocrit and low platelet count were not included in this analysis and vWF-antigen and vWF-activity were increased. Until now, data on the presence of thrombocytopathy in cirrhotic patients is still controversial [7]. Possible causes of thrombocytopathy in liver cirrhosis are signal transduction defects, storage pool disorders, or impaired thromboxane A2 synthesis [26,27,28]. According to our findings, in a system closely mimicking in-vivo primary hemostasis, platelet function defects are present in cirrhotic patients and might contribute to prolonged primary hemostasis.

Analysis of the PFA-100 test results and results for Col-Epi and Col-ADP in thrombocytopenic patients only revealed a higher rate of pathological results in some of the analysis in these patients with reduced platelet count, but results did show no differences for the other analyses. This was true for either of two cut-offs used in our analysis, namely 150/nL and 60/nL. This strengthens the hypothesis that platelet count alone as a static parameter does not resemble of the current state of coagulation in cirrhotic patients. This is further supported by a ROC (receiver operating characteristic) analysis performed to analyze whether platelet count predicts PFA-100 results. This revealed an area under the curve of 0.716 and thus showing only moderate capability of discriminating between normal and pathological PFA-100 results. The assessment of bleeding risk before medical interventions probably is not well predicted based upon a static parameter, such as platelet count [29]. Therefore tests globally and dynamically assessing primary hemostasis should be further investigated, especially since other factors, as vWF or hematocrit, might

Table 5. Results for univariate analysis of predictors of a pathological PFA-100 test result.

Variable	Exp(B)	95% KI für Exp(B)	*P*
All patients			
Age	0.981	0.936–1.028	0.418
Sex	0.900	0.346–2.339	0.829
MELD	1.019	0.943–1.101	0.627
Albumin	0.984	0.916–1.057	0.661
Platelet count	0.992	0.983–1.001	0.086
Hematocrit	0.930	0.864–1.001	0.054
vWF-antigen	0.997	0.994–1.000	0.064
vWF-activity:vWF-antigen ratio	13.528	0.409–447.335	0.145
ADAMTS13	0.991	0.967–1.014	0.437
Platelets <150/nL			
Age	0.969	0.920–1.022	0.246
Sex	1.161	0.398–3.392	0.785
MELD	0.998	0.920–1.083	0.967
Albumin	0.994	0.916–1.079	0.888
Platelet count	0.990	0.974–1.006	0.223
Hematocrit	0.932	0.860–1.010	0.086
vWF-antigen	0.996	0.993–1.000	0.032
vWF-activity:vWF-antigen ratio	17.371	0.309–967.333	0.165
ADAMTS13	0.994	0.969–1.019	0.619

Univariate analysis of the following variables was performed to identify predictors of a pathological PFA-100 test results in the whole study cohort and in thrombocytopenic cirrhotic patients. Multivariate analysis was then performed with variables showing a *P*-value ≤0.1 in univariate analysis.

Table 6. Results for multivariate analysis of predictors of a pathological PFA-100 test result.

Variable	Exp(B)	95% KI für Exp(B)	*P*
All patients			
Platelet count	0.990	0.980–1.001	0.069
Hematocrit	0.909	0.834–0.989	0.027
vWF-antigen	0.995	0.992–0.999	0.010
Platelets <150/nL			
Hematocrit	0.901	0.822–0.987	0.026
vWF-antigen	0.995	0.992–0.999	0.013

Variables with a P≤0.1 in univariate analysis were included in multivariate analysis, which was separately performed for the whole study cohort and for patients with a platelet count y 150/nL.

compensate for a reduced platelet count. These studies should as well evaluate if bleeding complications are related to pathological test result. Our study indicates that the PFA-100 might be useful to characterize the interplay of increased vWF and reduced platelet count in cirrhotic patients. Thus, PFA-100 should be examined in cirrhotic patients undergoing medical interventions.

In patients with cirrhosis and thrombocytopenia, maintenance of normal primary hemostasis seems to depend greatly on concomitantly increased vWF levels and reduced levels of the vWF cleaving protease ADAMTS13 [15,30]. Evidence for this was first reported by Lisman et al. [31] and is supported by our analysis of thrombocytopenic patients and the vWF-modification experiment. In addition to the important work by Lisman et al., who used pooled plasma from healthy controls and patients with liver cirrhosis we further decided to directly modify plasma vWF levels. We were thus able to directly identify vWF as the important coagulation factor responsible for maintained primary hemostasis. We found that higher vWF-antigen and higher vWF-activity in thrombocytopenic patients were associated with normal closure times. Since there were no differences in vWF-activity:vWF-antigen ratio, we conclude that the difference is due to an increase in vWF-antigen and not due to differences in functionality of vWF. Further no influence of ADAMTS13 was noted in this setting and in the multivariate analysis performed. A decrease of ADAMTS13 in decompensated cirrhosis is in line with previous results [15]. Further, in Line with Lisman et al., we found a negative correlation between ADAMTS13 and the vWF-activity:vWF-antigen ratio (Pearson's $r = -0.350$, $P = 0.013$), indicating increased vWF proteolysis in some patients with consequently reduced vWF activity [31]. Yet neither ADAMTS13 nor the vWF-activity:vWF-antigen ratio were predictive of the PFA-100 test results, which was only true for vWF-antigen, which did not correlate to ADAMTS13. We thus suspect that a decrease in ADAMTS13 is not the solitary reason for increased vWF levels and thereby maintained normal primary hemostasis in cirrhotic patients. In thrombocytopenic patients, the addition of r-vWF significantly improvement closure times while addition of an anti-vWF-antibody yielded significantly prolonged closure times. Yet, it remains unclear whether there is physiological connection between increased vWF and decrease platelet count or not, but most interestingly both changes are commonly found in portal hypertension [11]. PFA-100 has previously been shown to correlate well with vWF [32]; therefore, we assume that it is an appropriate test to measure the effect of different vWF levels. Whether measurement of the PFA-100 or supplementation of vWF could be an option in clinical practice needs to be further evaluated. The test could be used to identify patients with impaired primary hemostasis who might benefit from increased platelet counts or vWF levels and to differentiate them from patients with risk of thrombosis due to use of pro-coagulant drugs. This is of importance, since the substitution of thrombopoietin is associated with increased rate of thrombosis [33] and platelet transfusion during liver transplantation is associated with increased mortality [21]. With regard to the supplementation of vWF, previous studies on the administration of desmopressin, able to induce vWF release from the endothelium, resulted in an improved in-vivo bleeding time, thereby supporting this approach [34,35]. Yet, before this can be implemented in clinical practice further studies are needed to determine the optimal dose of r-vWF and to actually show an improvement compared to platelet transfusion in a clinical trial.

In conclusion, we found that primary hemostasis is impaired in cirrhotic patients probably because of reduced platelet count or hematocrit, but also because of thrombocytopathy. Increased vWF levels can partially compensate for reduced platelet count and the supplementation with r-vWF should further be investigated and compared with platelet transfusion.

Supporting Information

Table S1 Results for PFA-100 in patients with liver cirrhosis.

Table S2 Results of the vWF modification experiment.

Acknowledgments

We would like to thank Bärbel Calvo for her assistance with PFA-100 analyses.

Author Contributions

Conceived and designed the experiments: AW OJM KHW WS PS HAK DNG. Performed the experiments: AW KF CR PK YL MB MS DNG. Analyzed the data: AW OJM KF CR PK YL MB MS KHW DNG. Contributed reagents/materials/analysis tools: AW OJM MB WS DNG. Wrote the paper: AW OJM KF CR MS DNG. Critically revised the manuscript for important intellectual content: MB KHW WS PS HAK. Approved the final version of the article: AW OJM KF CR PK YL MB MS KHW WS PS HAK DNG.

References

1. Tripodi A, Mannucci PM (2011) The coagulopathy of chronic liver disease. N Engl J Med 365: 147–156.
2. Lisman T, Porte RJ (2010) The role of platelets in liver inflammation and regeneration. Semin Thromb Hemost 36: 170–174.
3. Sogaard KK, Horvath-Puho E, Gronbaek H, Jepsen P, Vilstrup H, et al. (2009) Risk of venous thromboembolism in patients with liver disease: a nationwide population-based case-control study. Am J Gastroenterol 104: 96–101.
4. Amitrano L, Guardascione MA, Brancaccio V, Margaglione M, Manguso F, et al. (2004) Risk factors and clinical presentation of portal vein thrombosis in patients with liver cirrhosis. J Hepatol 40: 736–741.
5. Sakariassen KS, Bolhuis PA, Sixma JJ (1979) Human blood platelet adhesion to artery subendothelium is mediated by factor VIII-Von Willebrand factor bound to the subendothelium. Nature 279: 636–638.
6. Giannini EG, Savarino V (2008) Thrombocytopenia in liver disease. Curr Opin Hematol 15: 473–480.
7. Violi F, Basili S, Raparelli V, Chowdary P, Gatt A, et al. (2011) Patients with liver cirrhosis suffer from primary haemostatic defects? Fact or fiction? J Hepatol 55: 1415–1427.
8. Ferro D, Quintarelli C, Lattuada A, Leo R, Alessandroni M, et al. (1996) High plasma levels of von Willebrand factor as a marker of endothelial perturbation in cirrhosis: relationship to endotoxemia. Hepatology 23: 1377–1383.
9. Hollestelle MJ, Geertzen HG, Straatsburg IH, van Gulik TM, van Mourik JA (2004) Factor VIII expression in liver disease. Thromb Haemost 91: 267–275.
10. Lenting PJ, Casari C, Christophe OD, Denis CV (2012) von Willebrand factor: the old, the new and the unknown. J Thromb Haemost 10: 2428–2437.
11. La Mura V, Reverter JC, Flores-Arroyo A, Raffa S, Reverter E, et al. (2011) Von Willebrand factor levels predict clinical outcome in patients with cirrhosis and portal hypertension. Gut 60: 1133–1138.
12. Horvatits T, Drolz A, Roedl K, Herkner H, Ferlitsch A, et al. (2014) vWF, a screening tool for detection of hepatopulmonary syndrome in patients with liver cirrhosis. J Hepatol.
13. Ferlitsch M, Reiberger T, Hoke M, Salzl P, Schwengerer B, et al. (2012) von Willebrand factor as new noninvasive predictor of portal hypertension, decompensation and mortality in patients with liver cirrhosis. Hepatology 56: 1439–1447.
14. Levy GG, Motto DG, Ginsburg D (2005) ADAMTS13 turns 3. Blood 106: 11–17.
15. Mannucci PM, Canciani MT, Forza I, Lussana F, Lattuada A, et al. (2001) Changes in health and disease of the metalloprotease that cleaves von Willebrand factor. Blood 98: 2730–2735.
16. Mammen EF, Comp PC, Gosselin R, Greenberg C, Hoots WK, et al. (1998) PFA-100 system: a new method for assessment of platelet dysfunction. Semin Thromb Hemost 24: 195–202.
17. Harrison P, Robinson MS, Mackie IJ, Joseph J, McDonald SJ, et al. (1999) Performance of the platelet function analyser PFA-100 in testing abnormalities of primary haemostasis. Blood Coagul Fibrinolysis 10: 25–31.
18. Tripodi A, Primignani M, Chantarangkul V, Clerici M, Dell'Era A, et al. (2006) Thrombin generation in patients with cirrhosis: the role of platelets. Hepatology 44: 440–445.
19. Mannucci PM (1998) von Willebrand factor: a marker of endothelial damage? Arterioscler Thromb Vasc Biol 18: 1359–1362.
20. Kundu SK, Heilmann EJ, Sio R, Garcia C, Davidson RM, et al. (1995) Description of an in vitro platelet function analyzer—PFA-100. Semin Thromb Hemost 21 Suppl 2: 106–112.
21. Saner FH, Gieseler RK, Akiz H, Canbay A, Görlinger K (2013) Delicate Balance of Bleeding and Thrombosis in End-Stage Liver Disease and Liver Transplantation. Digestion 88: 135–144.
22. Buyukasik Y, Karakus S, Goker H, Haznedaroglu IC, Ozatli D, et al. (2002) Rational use of the PFA-100 device for screening of platelet function disorders and von Willebrand disease. Blood Coagul Fibrinolysis 13: 349–353.
23. Zupan IP, Sabovic M, Salobir B, Ponikvar JB, Cernelc P (2003) Utility of in vitro closure time test for evaluating platelet-related primary hemostasis in dialysis patients. Am J Kidney Dis 42: 746–751.
24. Escolar G, Cases A, Vinas M, Pino M, Calls J, et al. (1999) Evaluation of acquired platelet dysfunctions in uremic and cirrhotic patients using the platelet function analyzer (PFA-100): influence of hematocrit elevation. Haematologica 84: 614–619.
25. Pihusch R, Rank A, Gohring P, Pihusch M, Hiller E, et al. (2002) Platelet function rather than plasmatic coagulation explains hypercoagulable state in cholestatic liver disease. J Hepatol 37: 548–555.
26. Laffi G, La Villa G, Pinzani M, Ciabattoni G, Patrignani P, et al. (1986) Altered renal and platelet arachidonic acid metabolism in cirrhosis. Gastroenterology 90: 274–282.
27. Laffi G, Marra F, Failli P, Ruggiero M, Cecchi E, et al. (1993) Defective signal transduction in platelets from cirrhotics is associated with increased cyclic nucleotides. Gastroenterology 105: 148–156.
28. Laffi G, Marra F, Gresele P, Romagnoli P, Palermo A, et al. (1992) Evidence for a storage pool defect in platelets from cirrhotic patients with defective aggregation. Gastroenterology 103: 641–646.
29. Vieira da Rocha EC, D'Amico EA, Caldwell SH, Flores da Rocha TR, Soares ESCS, et al. (2009) A prospective study of conventional and expanded coagulation indices in predicting ulcer bleeding after variceal band ligation. Clin Gastroenterol Hepatol 7: 988–993.
30. Lisman T, Porte RJ (2010) Rebalanced hemostasis in patients with liver disease: evidence and clinical consequences. Blood 116: 878–885.
31. Lisman T, Bongers TN, Adelmeijer J, Janssen HL, de Maat MP, et al. (2006) Elevated levels of von Willebrand Factor in cirrhosis support platelet adhesion despite reduced functional capacity. Hepatology 44: 53–61.
32. Haubelt H, Anders C, Vogt A, Hoerdt P, Seyfert UT, et al. (2005) Variables influencing Platelet Function Analyzer-100 closure times in healthy individuals. Br J Haematol 130: 759–767.
33. Tripodi A, Primignani M (2013) Nontransfusional approach to increased platelet count in patients with cirrhosis and thrombocytopenia. Hepatology 58: 1177–1180.
34. Burroughs AK, Matthews K, Qadiri M, Thomas N, Kernoff P, et al. (1985) Desmopressin and bleeding time in patients with cirrhosis. Br Med J (Clin Res Ed) 291: 1377–1381.
35. Mannucci PM, Vicente V, Vianello L, Cattaneo M, Alberca I, et al. (1986) Controlled trial of desmopressin in liver cirrhosis and other conditions associated with a prolonged bleeding time. Blood 67: 1148–1153.

5

Cell Fate Decisions in Malignant Hematopoiesis: Leukemia Phenotype Is Determined by Distinct Functional Domains of the MN1 Oncogene

Courteney K. Lai[1,2], Yeonsook Moon[3], Florian Kuchenbauer[4,5], Daniel T. Starzcynowski[6], Bob Argiropoulos[7], Eric Yung[1], Philip Beer[1], Adrian Schwarzer[8], Amit Sharma[8], Gyeongsin Park[9], Malina Leung[1], Grace Lin[1], Sarah Vollett[1], Stephen Fung[1], Connie J. Eaves[1,2], Aly Karsan[10,11], Andrew P. Weng[1,11], R. Keith Humphries[1,2*¶], Michael Heuser[12¶]

1 Terry Fox Laboratory, BC Cancer Agency Research Centre, Vancouver, BC, Canada, **2** Department of Medicine, Faculty of Medicine, University of British Columbia, Vancouver, BC, Canada, **3** Department of Laboratory Medicine, Medical School of Inha University, Incheon, Korea, **4** Department of Internal Medicine III, University Hospital of Ulm, Ulm, Germany, **5** Institute of Experimental Cancer Research, Comprehensive Cancer Centre, University Hospital of Ulm, Ulm, Germany, **6** Department of Pediatrics, Cincinnati Children's Hospital Medical Center, Cincinnati, Ohio, United States of America, **7** Department of Medical Genetics, University of Calgary, Calgary, AB, Canada, **8** Institute of Experimental Hematology, Hannover Medical School, Hannover, Germany, **9** Department of Hospital Pathology, Catholic University of Korea, Seoul, Korea, **10** Genome Sciences Centre, BC Cancer Agency, Vancouver, BC, Canada, **11** Department of Pathology and Laboratory Medicine, University of British Columbia, Vancouver, BC, Canada, **12** Department of Hematology, Hemostasis, Oncology, and Stem Cell Transplantation, Hannover Medical School, Hannover, Germany

Abstract

Extensive molecular profiling of leukemias and preleukemic diseases has revealed that distinct clinical entities, like acute myeloid (AML) and T-lymphoblastic leukemia (T-ALL), share similar pathogenetic mutations. It is not well understood how the cell of origin, accompanying mutations, extracellular signals or structural differences in a mutated gene determine the phenotypic identity of leukemias. We dissected the functional aspects of different protein regions of the MN1 oncogene and their effect on the leukemic phenotype, building on the ability of MN1 to induce leukemia without accompanying mutations. We found that the most C-terminal region of MN1 was required to block myeloid differentiation at an early stage, and deletion of an extended C-terminal region resulted in loss of myeloid identity and cell differentiation along the T-cell lineage in vivo. Megakaryocytic/erythroid lineage differentiation was blocked by the N-terminal region. In addition, the N-terminus was required for proliferation and leukemogenesis in vitro and in vivo through upregulation of *HoxA9*, *HoxA10* and *Meis2*. Our results provide evidence that a single oncogene can modulate cellular identity of leukemic cells based on its active gene regions. It is therefore likely that different mutations in the same oncogene may impact cell fate decisions and phenotypic appearance of malignant diseases.

Editor: Ken Mills, Queen's University Belfast, United Kingdom

Funding: This study was supported by grants from the Terry Fox Foundation, Canada (http://www.terryfox.org/TerryFox/The_Terry_Fox_Foundation.html) (grant Nos. 18006 and 122869), the Cancer Research Society, Canada (http://www.crs-src.ca/), the Stem Cell Network of Canada (http://www.stemcellnetwork.ca/index.php?page=funding-opportunities), Deutsche Krebshilfe e.V (grant No. 109003, 110284, 110292, and 111267) (http://www.krebshilfe.de/metanavigation/english.html), grant No. DJCLS H09/1f, R 10/22, and R13/14 from the Deutsche-José-Carreras Leukämie-Stiftung e.V (http://www.carreras-stiftung.de/); grant No. M 47.1 from the H. W. & J. Hector Stiftung (http://www.hector-stiftung.de/), the German Federal Ministry of Education and Research grant 01EO0802 (IFB-Tx) (http://www.bmbf.de/en/14580.php), and DFG grants HE 5240/4-1, HE 5240/5-1 (http://www.dfg.de/en/research_funding/programmes/individual/research_grants/). CKL was supported by studentships from the Canadian Institute of Health Research (http://www.cihr-irsc.gc.ca/e/193.html#), the University of British Columbia (https://www.grad.ubc.ca/awards/four-year-doctoral-fellowship-4yf), and the BC Cancer Agency (http://www.bccancer.bc.ca/default.htm). FK was supported by grants from Deutsche Krebshilfe grant 109420 (Max-Eder program) (http://www.krebshilfe.de/metanavigation/english.html); fellowship 2010/04 by the European Hematology Association (http://www.ehaweb.org/career/career-development-grants/eha-research-fellowships-and-the-jose-carreras-foundation-eha-young-investigator-fellowship/); and by the Deutsche Forschungsgemeinschaft (grant D.3955 (SFB 1074)) (http://www.dfg.de/en/research_funding/programmes/individual/). PB was supported by an intermediate fellowship from the Kay Kendall Leukaemia Fund (http://www.kklf.org.uk/intermediate.html). GL was supported by a BC Cancer Studentship from the BC Cancer Agency (http://www.bccancer.bc.ca/default.htm). SV was supported by a studentship from the Stem Cell Network of Canada (http://www.stemcellnetwork.ca/index.php?page=co-op-award). The funders had no role in study design, data collection and analysis, decision to publish, or preparation of the manuscript.

* Email: khumphri@bccrc.ca

¶ RKH and MH are senior authors on this work.

Introduction

The postulated requirement for induction of leukemogenesis has long been the combination of class I and II mutations [1], although recent insights into the genetic composition of acute myeloid leukemia (AML) cells has revealed additional pathogenetic mechanisms including changes in epigenetic regulation. On average, 13 coding genes are mutated per AML genome [2], suggesting that several events are required for leukemogenesis. Despite the heterogeneity of cells that can give rise to AML, only a small proportion of AML cells show clonogenic activity in culture and only a small fraction of AML blast cells are able to confer disease to immune-deficient mice [3]. While such disease-propagating or leukemia-initiating cells (LICs) may be rare, they are not necessarily restricted to the most primitive cells within the hematopoietic hierarchy but rather, can include committed progenitor cells such as common myeloid progenitors (CMPs) or common lymphoid progenitors (CLPs) [4–7]. The high level of heterogeneity seen in AML and within an individual patient underscores the importance of understanding the molecular mechanisms underlying this disease and the functional consequences on leukemic cells.

While there is a high degree of cellular heterogeneity within the cells of an individual leukaemia [8], there is striking redundancy of mutated genes in distinct diseases like AML [9], T-lymphoblastic leukemia (T-ALL) [10], and primary myelofibrosis [11], including mutations in *DNMT3A* and several other genes. Explanations for how mutations in the same gene can cause different diseases may include: differing cells of origin [12] or cell-extrinsic signals [13], as illustrated by the ability of the MLL-AF9 fusion gene to cause myeloid and lymphoid leukemias; the influence of the microenvironment, such as the ability of abnormal stroma cells to induce myelodysplasia in hematopoietic stem cells (HSCs) [14]; and the ability of mutations to change the lineage potential of the oncogene and possibly the phenotype of the disease, as in EZH2 mutations in B-non-Hodgkin lymphoma and myeloid disorders [15,16]. The meningioma (disrupted in balanced translocation) 1 (*MN1*) model of leukemogenesis constitutes a simple and ideal model to test this latter hypothesis due to its ability to induce leukemia as a single hit through constitutive overexpression [17].

The ability of MN1 to induce rapid onset leukemia on its own highlights its central regulatory role in hematopoietic transformation. MN1 has been shown to be most highly expressed in murine CMPs, but is downregulated upon differentiation [17] and is capable of enhancing proliferation of human CD34+ cord blood cells [18]. High MN1 expression has been associated with both acute myeloid and lymphoid leukemias [19] as well as other AML characteristics such as inv(16) [20] or overexpression of EVI-1 [21]. Significantly, it also has been identified as an independent prognostic factor in patients with AML with normal cytogenetics, associated with shorter relapse-free survival, overall survival, and resistance to ATRA-induced differentiation [19,22–25]. As loss of MN1 expression has been shown to impair proliferation and significantly decrease clonogenic activity of human leukemic cells, it is a potential therapeutic target in AML patients [26].

MN1 has been shown to rapidly induce leukemia in mice [20,22]. We have recently shown that MN1 is capable of transforming single CMP cells as the cell of origin [17]. Significantly, GMPs required co-overexpression of *Meis1* for in vitro transformation, and the additional co-overexpression of HOXA9 or HOXA10 to induce leukemia in vivo [17]. Loss of MEIS1 expression abrogated leukemic activity in MN1 cells, suggesting that, combined with co-localization of MN1 and MEIS1 at a large proportion of MEIS1 target sites, MEIS1 and its cofactor HOXA9 are essential to MN1 leukemogenesis [17]. In addition, MN1 cells are arrested at an immature stage of myelopoiesis and are highly resistant against all-trans retinoic acid (ATRA) [22], a potent inducer of myeloid differentiation, although ectopic CEBPα expression, which MN1 is thought to repress, can abrogate the leukemogenic activity of MN1 [18].

We hypothesize that multiple functions are encoded in this protein and can be localized to different regions. Thus, delineation and localisation of these functions at a structural level will provide insight into the key mechanisms required for leukemic transformation by a single central regulator such as MN1. Despite the established role of MN1 overexpression in leukemia, little is known about the protein itself. The MN1 protein is highly conserved between different species, but largely lacks recognised protein domains excepting two proline-glutamine stretches and a single 28 residue-long glutamine stretch. Here, we systematically localise known properties of MN1 leukemia using both *in vitro* and extensive *in vivo* studies to specific physical regions of wildtype MN1 through a detailed structure-function analysis of MN1. We demonstrate that the proliferative ability and self-renewal activity, and the inhibition of megakaryocyte/erythroid, myeloid, and lymphoid differentiation are localised to distinct regions within MN1 and provide evidence that different mutations of a single oncogene can induce distinct diseases such as myeloid and lymphoid leukemia and myeloproliferative disease.

Materials and Methods

Retroviral vectors and vector production

Retroviral vectors for expression of MN1 [22] and NUP98HOXD13 (ND13) [27] have been previously described. Primers were designed for each MN1 mutant truncation construct to ensure the N- and C-termini of the final construct were flanked by *Not*I sites, then subcloned into the expression vector pSF91 [28] upstream of the internal ribosomal entry site (IRES) and the enhanced green fluorescent protein (GFP) gene. MN1 Strategy 1 constructs were generated by PCR amplification of the N- (proximal) and C-terminal (distal) regions of the construct with *Hind*III sites at the internal sites. The proximal and distal fragments were then subcloned into the pSF91-IRESeGFP vector. As a control, the pSF91 vector carrying only the IRES-enhanced GFP cassette was used. Constructs were validated by sequencing and correct expression and transmission were confirmed by qRT-PCR and PCR. Primer sequences can be found in Table S1. For HA-tagged constructs, full-length and MN1 mutant deletion constructs were cut to ensure the N- and C-termini of the final construct were flanked by *BglII* or *BamHI* (for constructs lacking the N-terminal region) and *NotI* sites, respectively, then subcloned into the MSCV-IRES-GFP expression vector [29], and an HA-tag was cloned to the N-terminus of MN1 or the deletion constructs. Helper-free recombinant retrovirus was generated by using supernatants from the transfected ecotropic Phoenix packaging cell line to transduce the ecotropic GP + E86 packaging cell line [30].

Clonogenic progenitor assays

Colony-forming cells (CFCs) were assayed in methylcellulose (MethoCult M3434 or MegaCult-C, Catalog No. 04964; STEMCELL Technologies, Vancouver, BC, Canada). For each assay freshly isolated and transduced unsorted bone marrow cells were plated in duplicate in Methocult medium (1000 cells/well). Colonies were evaluated microscopically 10 days after plating using standard criteria. To assay megakaryocyte progenitor frequency, freshly isolated and transduced bone marrow cells were sorted for GFP expression, and 1×10^5 cells were suspended in MegaCult-C medium containing recombinant human thrombopoietin (50 ng/mL), recombinant human IL6 (20 ng/mL), recombinant human IL11 (50 ng/mL), and recombinant mouse IL3 (10 ng/mL), mixed with collagen and dispensed in chamber slides (all from STEMCELL Technologies, Vancouver, BC, Canada). Cultures were incubated at 37°C for 7 days. Slides were stained with acetylthiocholiniodide according to manufacturer's instructions, and colonies were counted manually under a microscope, as previously described [31].

Quantitative real-time RT-PCR

Total RNA from stored, frozen cell pellets was isolated using TRIZOL reagent (Life Technologies, Burlington, ON, Canada). Total RNA was converted into cDNA using the SuperScript VILO cDNA synthesis kit (Life Technologies, Burlington, ON, Canada) using 500 ng of total RNA. Quantitative real-time PCR was performed as previously described using the 7900 HT Fast Real-Time PCR system (Applied Biosystems, Foster City, CA, USA) [32] and Fast SYBR Green Master Mix (Life Technologies, Burlington, ON, Canada) [32]. Relative expression was determined with the $2^{-\Delta\Delta CT}$ method, and the housekeeping gene transcript *Abl1* was used to normalize the results. Primers were manufactured by Life Technologies. Primer sequences can be found in Table S2.

Western blot analysis

For Western blot analysis, 1×10^6 cells were lysed with 150 µL lysis buffer (50 mM Tris-HCl [pH 8], 0,1% Tween-20, 0.1% SDS, 150 mM NaCl, 0.5 mM EDTA, 10 mM DTT, and 1 mM PMSF, plus protease inhibitor cocktail; Sigma, Oakville, ON, Canada) and incubated for 20 minutes on ice. NuPage LPS loading buffer (4x) and NuPage Sample Reducing Agent (10x) (Life Technologies, Burlington, ON, Canada) were added and samples were heated for 15 minutes at 95°C. Lysates were loaded onto 4%-12% NuPage Novex BIS-Tris SDS-polyacrylamide gels (Life Technologies, Burlington, ON, Canada) and electroblotted in MOPS transfer buffer to nitrocellulose membrane (Life Technologies, Burlington, ON, Canada). Rabbit polyclonal anti-HA (Abcam, Cambridge, England) or mouse monoclonal anti-beta-actin (abm, Richmond, BC, Canada) and Mouse TrueBlot ULTRA HRP-conjugated anti-mouse (Rockland Inc., Gilbertsville, PA, USA) or goat anti-rabbit IgG antibodies (Jackson ImmunoResearch Laboratories Inc., PA, USA) in 1:5000 dilutions of 0.1% Tween-20, 5% bovine serum albumin (BSA), Tris-buffered saline (TBS) were used for protein detection. Proteins were visualised using Clarity Western enhanced chemiluminescence (ECL) Substrate (Bio-Rad, Hercules, CA, USA).

ATRA cytotoxicity assay

To ensure that cells proliferated in vitro even if a MN1 mutation was non-functional, MN1 deletion constructs were transduced in bone marrow cells immortalized by retroviral expression of the fusion gene ND13. In vitro cytotoxicity assays were performed in Dulbecco's modified Eagle medium (DMEM) supplemented with 15% fetal bovine serum (FBS), 6 ng/mL murine interleukin 3 (mIL3), 10 ng/mL human interleukin 6 (hIL6), and 20 ng/mL murine stem-cell factor (mSCF; all from STEMCELL Technologies, Vancouver, BC, Canada). Cells were seeded at a cell density of 1×10^4/mL in a 96 well plate, and incubated under light-protective conditions. ATRA (Sigma, Oakville, ON, Canada) was dissolved in DMSO (Sigma) and added to the culture medium at the specified concentrations as 1/1000th of the final volume. After 64 hours, cells were stained with Alamar Blue (Sigma) for 8 hours and fluorescence was measured with a Tecan Safire^2 microplate reader (Life Technologies, Burlington, ON, Canada). Viability was determined as percentage of DMSO-treated cells after background subtraction of fluorescence in wells with medium only. The 50% inhibitory concentration was determined as the concentration of ATRA that reduced cell viability to 50% of DMSO-treated cells.

Mice and retroviral infection of primary bone marrow cells and bone marrow transplantation

Primary mouse bone marrow cells from 5-fluorouracil treated C57BL/6J donor mice (Faulding, Underdaler, Australia) were prestimulated for 48 hours, transduced by co-cultivation with viral producers for 48 hours, then harvested and plated into CFC media or directly transplanted into lethally irradiated syngeneic recipient mice, as previously described [32]. Recipient mice were exposed to a single dose of 750 to 810 cGy total-body irradiation accompanied by a life-sparing dose of 1×10^5 freshly isolated bone marrow cells from syngeneic mice, and were monitored daily. Engraftment of transduced cells in peripheral blood was monitored every 4 weeks by fluorescence-activated cell-sorter (FACS) analysis and quantification of GFP-positive cells. Sick or moribund mice were sacrificed, spleens weighed, and red blood cells and white blood cells were counted using the scil Vet abc blood analyser (Vet Novations, Barrie, ON, Canada).

Ethics Statement

C57BL/6J mice were bred and maintained in the Animal Research Centre of the British Columbia Cancer Agency as approved by the University of British Columbia Animal Care Committee (the Institutional Animal Care and Use Committee, IACUC). Experimental studies were approved by the University of British Columbia Animal Care Committe under experimental protocol numbers A04-0380 and A09-0009, and all efforts were made to minimise suffering.

FACS analysis

Lineage distribution was determined by FACS analysis (FACSCalibur; Becton Dickinson, Mississauga, ON, Canada) as previously described [27]. Monoclonal antibodies used were phycoerythrin (PE)-labeled Gr1 (clone Ly6G-6C), B220 (CD45R), CD4, Ter119, and Sca-1 (Ly6A/E) and allophycocyanin (APC)-labeled CD11b, CD8, and c-kit (CD117) (BD Biosciences, Mississauga, ON, Canada).

Bone marrow morphology

Cytospin preparations were stained with Wright-Giemsa stain. Images were visualised using a Nikon Eclipse 80i microscope (Nikon, Mississauga, ON, Canada) and a 20x/0.40 numerical aperture objective, or a 100x/1.25 numerical aperture objective and Nikon Immersion Oil (Nikon). A Nikon Coolpix 995 camera (Nikon) was used to capture images.

Confocal microscopy

Twenty-four hours prior to fixation, micro growth glass cover slips (VWR International, Mississauga, ON, Canada) were coated in Cultrex Poly-L-Lysine (Trevigen, Gaithersburg, MD, USA). GP + E86 expressing cell lines expressing MN1, MN1Δ1, and MN1Δ5-7 were then plated. Cells were fixed in 4% paraformaldehyde in phosphate-buffered saline (PBS) for 10 minutes at room temperature, incubated with a 1:500 dilution of rabbit anti-HA primary antibody followed by a 1:300 dilution of anti-rabbit Alexa eFluor 594 secondary antibody (Life Technologies, Burlington, ON, Canada) and then stained with DAPI at 1 µg/mL (Sigma-

Aldrich, St Louis, MO, USA). Slides were then mounted with DABCO mounting medium (Sigma-Aldrich, St Louis, MO, USA) and Z-stack photographs were taken 0.13 µm apart using a Leica TCS SP5 Confocal microscope (100x objective). Images were captured using LAS AF software (Leica Microsystems, Inc., Exton, PA, USA) and deconvoluted using Real-time GPU-based 3D Deconvolution [33] and DeconvolutionLab [34] in ImageJ.

Gene expression profiling and gene set enrichment analysis

RNA was extracted using TRIZOL reagent (Life Technologies, Burlington, ON, Canada) from GFP+ cells that were sorted from mouse bone marrow cells four weeks after transplantation. Quality and integrity of the total RNA isolated was controlled by running all samples on an Agilent Technologies 2100 Bioanalyzer (Agilent Technologies, Mississauga, ON). Extracted RNA from MN1, MN1Δ1, and MN1Δ7 leukemia cells and Gr1+/CD11b+ bone marrow cells were hybridized to the Affymetrix GeneChip Mouse 430 2.0 (43.000 probes) microarray ($n = 2$) according to the manufacturer's instructions. Experiments were performed at the British Columbia Genome Sciences Centre, Vancouver, Canada. Gene expression can be found at the Gene Expression Omnibus database (GEO accession number GSE46990; http://www.ncbi.nlm.nih.gov/geo/query/acc.cgi?token=zhedbmoeuqcksli&acc=GSE46990). Data were analyzed using R and Bioconductor [35]. Quality was assessed with the ArrayQualityMetrics package [36]. Arrays were preprocessed using RMA [37]. Differentially expressed probesets were calculated with the LIMMA package [38] applying Benjamini-Hochberg multiple testing correction at an FDR of 0.05. For gene set enrichment the Broad Institute GSEA software package was used [39]. The datasets were collapsed into single genes and rank-ordered by signal to noise ratio. Gene set permutations were used to estimate statistical significance. Analyzed gene ontology sets were obtained from MSigDB v3.1 [39]. The gene set enrichment analysis software [39] (http://www.broad.mit.edu/gsea/index.jsp) was used to compare gene enrichment of Gene Ontology gene sets (dataset C5, available from the Molecular Signature database v3.1 [39]) between MN1Δ1 vs MN1 and MN1Δ7 vs. MN1.

Statistical analysis

Comparisons were performed by unpaired T-tests. The two-sided level of significance was set at P less than 0.05. Comparison of survival curves were performed using the Kaplan-Meier method and log-rank test. Statistical analyses were performed with Excel (Microsoft Canada, Mississauga, ON, Canada) and GraphPad Prism 6 (GraphPad Software, La Jolla, CA, USA).

Results

The N-terminal region of MN1 is required for immortalization of bone marrow cells in vitro

To elucidate the relationship between the structure of MN1 and the characteristics of MN1 leukemia, MN1 deletion mutants were generated in three strategies. Wildtype MN1 was divided into seven regions, each approximately 200 amino acids in length and numbered sequentially from the N-terminus. In an internal deletion series (strategy 1), distinct 200 amino acid regions were deleted (Figure 1A). Due to technical difficulties the construct lacking the third region from the N-terminus (MN1Δ3) did not express and was excluded from further analysis. Progressive N-terminal deletions (strategy 2) included six mutant constructs in which approximately 200 amino acid-regions were cumulatively deleted starting from the MN1 N-terminus. For progressive C-terminal deletions (strategy 3), stretches of approximately 200 amino acids were cumulatively deleted starting from the MN1 C-terminus (Figure 1A). The size and expression of all mutant constructs was validated at the RNA and protein level. The expected protein was detected for all constructs lacking one or two regions and for the constructs MN1Δ1-4, MN1Δ3-7, and MN1Δ5-7 lacking three or more regions. The remaining constructs lacking three or more regions did not, however, yield detectable protein (Figure S1A–B).

Freshly isolated bone marrow cells were transduced with MN1 mutation constructs or control (CTL) vector and plated in CFC medium, and replating ability and proportion of transduced cells (GFP+) were measured. While GFP-positive cells were lost in CTL-transduced cells after the second replating, GFP-positive cells outgrew non-transduced cells for internal deletion constructs (strategy 1) and could be replated up to the fifth plating, with the exception of MN1Δ6, where no colonies grew after the fourth plating (Figure S2A–B). For progressive N-terminal deletions (strategy 2), only cells lacking the most N-terminal domain (MN1Δ1) immortalized bone marrow cells in vitro, and competitively outgrew non-transduced cells; deletion of larger MN1 N-terminal stretches resulted in loss of replating capacity (Figure S2C and D). Cumulative deletions from the C-terminus (strategy 3) could immortalize bone marrow cells up to MN1Δ3-7, in which only 317 N-terminal amino acids are retained (Figure S2E and F), including MN1Δ4-7 which showed colony replating ability despite protein being unable to be detected by Western blot (Figure S1). In summary, the N-terminus of MN1 is necessary and sufficient to immortalize bone marrow cells in vitro with select regions, such as amino acids 1008–1201 playing a significant role in in vitro immortalization.

The N-terminal domain of MN1 is required for its leukemogenic potential in vivo

MN1-transduced bone marrow cells were transplanted into lethally irradiated mice, and engraftment in peripheral blood was monitored monthly. Regardless of the mutation construct, mice showed at least minimal engraftment 4 weeks post-transplant (engraftment $\geq 1\%$). All internal deletion (strategy 1) constructs showed statistically significant higher engraftment than CTL mice with increasing engraftment over 16 weeks (Figure 1B). Progressive N-terminal deletion (strategy 2) constructs also showed engraftment at 4 weeks post-transplant, although engraftment levels did not significantly differ from control mice except for MN1Δ1, which showed higher early engraftment levels similar to full-length MN1. In addition, engraftment decreased over 16 weeks, suggesting that these constructs, including MN1Δ1, had defects in their proliferative and self-renewal capabilities and, thus, were unable to outcompete the co-transplanted normal bone marrow cells (Figure 1C and Table S3). Of the progressive C-terminal deletions (strategy 3), MN1Δ7 showed the highest engraftment levels, and MN1Δ6-7, MN1Δ5-7 and MN1Δ3-7 had significantly higher engraftment of transduced cells compared to CTL cells at 16 weeks (Figure 1D). The MN1 mutations that enhanced engraftment and proliferation in vivo also induced high WBC counts, anemia, and thrombocytopenia (Figures S3–S5, Tables S4–5).

All transplantation groups were fully characterized at time of sacrifice including bone marrow morphology with blast count, immunophenotype of GFP^{+} bone marrow cells, spleen weight and (for most constructs) secondary transplantations (Table S3). For mice succumbing to hematologic disease, the diagnosis is noted in Table S3 and supported by bone marrow morphology (Figure 1H). In summary, deletions including the first 221 N-terminal

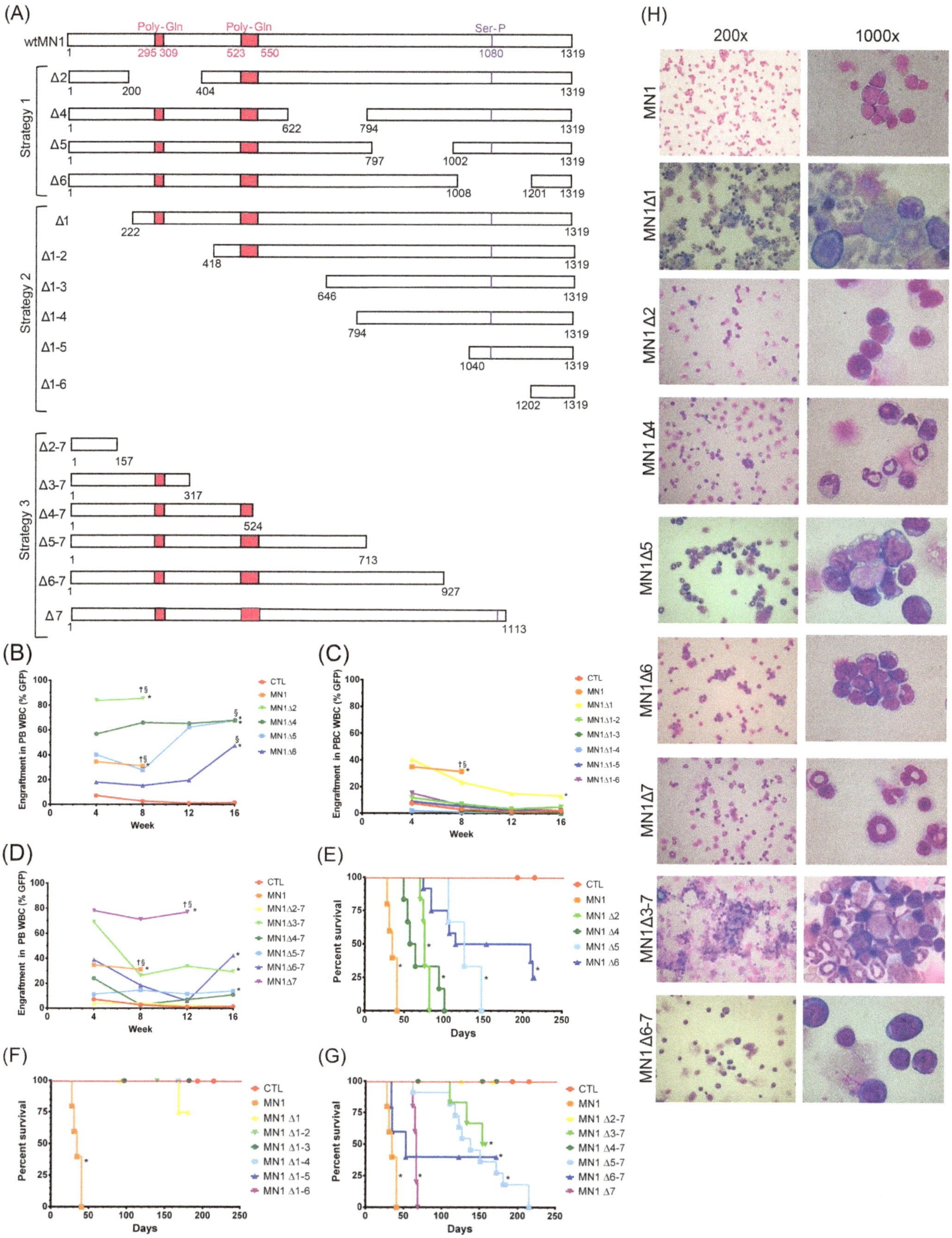
(A)
wtMN1
Poly-Gln
Poly-Gln
Ser-P
Strategy 1
Strategy 2
Strategy 3
(B)
Engraftment in PB WBC (% GFP)
Week
CTL
MN1
MN1Δ2
MN1Δ4
MN1Δ5
MN1Δ6
(C)
Engraftment in PBC WBC (% GFP)
Week
MN1Δ1
MN1Δ1-2
MN1Δ1-3
MN1Δ1-4
MN1Δ1-5
MN1Δ1-6
(D)
Engraftment in PB WBC (% GFP)
Week
MN1Δ2-7
MN1Δ3-7
MN1Δ4-7
MN1Δ5-7
MN1Δ6-7
MN1Δ7
(E)
Percent survival
Days
(F)
Percent survival
Days
(G)
Percent survival
Days
(H)
200x
1000x
MN1
MN1Δ1
MN1 Δ2
MN1 Δ4
MN1Δ5
MN1Δ6
MN1Δ7
MN1Δ3-7
MN1Δ6-7

Figure 1. The N-terminal region of MN1 is required for its leukemogenic potential. (A) MN1 mutation constructs for structure-function analysis. In strategy 1 distinct stretches of approximately 200 amino acids were deleted throughout wildtype MN1. In strategy 2, stretches of approximately 200 amino acids were cumulatively deleted starting from the MN1 N-terminus. In strategy 3, stretches of approximately 200 amino acids were cumulatively deleted starting from the MN1 C-terminus. (B–D) Percentage of transgene-positive white blood cells engrafting in peripheral blood of transplanted mice at 4-week intervals. P values are given for the comparison of the indicated construct with CTL-transduced cells. The average engraftment is shown. Number of analysed mice and standard error can be found in Table S1. (E-G) Survival of mice receiving transplants of cells transduced with (E) strategy 1, (F) strategy 2, and (G) strategy 3 MN1 deletions. P values are given for the comparison of the indicated construct with CTL-transduced cells. The number of analysed mice is detailed in Table S1. (H) Morphology of bone marrow cells at death of diseased mice. The cells were Wright-Giemsa stained. Images were visualised using a Nikon Eclipse 80i microscope (Nikon, Mississauga, ON, Canada) and a 20x/0.40 numerical aperture objective, or a 100x/1.25 numerical aperture objective and Nikon Immersion Oil (Nikon). A Nikon Coolpix 995 camera (Nikon) was used to capture images. § engraftment in peripheral blood at the indicated time point or at death in cases where a mouse died before that time point. † all mice were dead at this time point due to disease. * indicates $P<0.05$, ** indicates $P<0.001$.

amino acids prevented MN1-induced AML, except one MN1Δ1 mouse that died with low engraftment, low WBC count, and a non-elevated blast count (Figure 1F). Confocal microscopy of cells expressing MN1Δ1 showed the protein present in both the cytoplasm and the nucleus to a similar extent as MN1, suggesting that loss of this region did not impact the ability of the mutant to localize to the nucleus. (Figure S6). Deletion of domains 2, 5, 6, or 7 did not affect the ability of MN1 to induce AML, although their loss significantly prolonged disease latency (Figure 1E). Deletion of domain 4 resulted in a rapid disease onset with low blast count, most likely a myelproliferative disease (Figure 1E and G). Combined deletion of domains 6 and 7 (MN1Δ6–7) at the C-terminus resulted in AML with 60% penetrance (Figure 1G). Interestingly, despite showing nuclear localization of the protein by confocal microscopy (Figure S6), deletion of domains 5–7 (MN1Δ5–7) at the C-terminus in two independent experiments resulted in T-lymphoblastic leukemia (see below). The minimal portion of MN1 with biologic function was MN1Δ3-7, corresponding to the 317 amino acids at the N-terminus, which induced a myeloproliferative disease with long latency and 50% penetrance (Figure 1G). In summary, these data suggest that the N-terminus of MN1 is required and sufficient for its proliferation-enhancing function in vivo (see also Table 1).

The N-terminal region of MN1 is required to block megakaryocyte/erythroid differentiation

Peripheral blood from mice transplanted with MN1-transduced bone marrow cells was also assayed at 4-week intervals to determine the engraftment of red blood cells. The majority of mutants showed decreasing red blood cell engraftment over the 16-week period or the lifetime of the mouse. MN1Δ2 and MN1Δ4 mice had high engraftment levels at 4 weeks corresponding to high WBC engraftment. Only two constructs, MN1Δ1 and MN1Δ5, showed an increase in red blood cell engraftment over time, although the absolute number of red blood cells and hemoglobin did not increase in these mice (Figure 2A–C). When comparing the ratio of transgene positive RBC to WBC, MN1Δ1 and to a lesser extent MN1Δ5 were the only mutant constructs that showed a higher engraftment in red blood cells than white blood cells; a difference that increased over 16 weeks (Figure 2D–F). To assess the ability of MN1 deletion mutants to support megakaryocyte differentiation, we performed CFU-Mk assays of all internally-deleted (strategy 1) and select N- and C-terminally deleted (strategy 2 and 3) constructs. CTL cells, but not full-length MN1 cells, formed few, small CFU-Mk colonies. Similar to full-length MN1 cells, most MN1 deletion mutants were unable to form CFU-Mk colonies. However, N-terminally deleted (MN1Δ1) cells gave rise to 2 to 3-fold more colonies and larger colonies than control-transduced cells, sustained over two replatings (Figure 2G and H). A small number of colonies were also derived from MN1Δ6-transduced cells (Figure 2G). Together, these experiments suggest that the ability of MN1 to block erythroid-megakaryocyte differentiation can be localized to the N-terminus, with some contribution of domains 5 and 6 (see also Table 1).

The C-terminal region of MN1 is required to block myeloid differentiation

To assess the effect of MN1 deletions on resistance to ATRA, we transduced ND13 bone marrow cells, previously reported to immortalize cells in vitro [27], with all MN1 deletion mutants. ND13 control cells were sensitive to *in vitro* ATRA administration with an IC50 of 0.27 μM. ND13+MN1-transduced cells were highly resistant with an IC50 of 32.4 μM, while MN1-transduced cells were even more ATRA resistant with an IC50 beyond 100 μM. When distinct regions were internally deleted from MN1 (strategy1), loss of domains 2 or 4 had no effect on ATRA resistance (Figure 3A). However, loss of domain 5, 6, or 7 restored ATRA sensitivity of the cells (Figure 3B). Progressive N-terminal deletions (strategy 2) with 2 or more domains deleted from the N-terminus were sensitive to ATRA (Figure 3C and D). All constructs with cumulative deletions of the C-terminus (strategy 3) were sensitive to ATRA (Figure 3E and F), highlighting the importance of the most C-terminal 206 amino acids of MN1 for ATRA resistance. These data suggest that the MN1 C-terminus

Table 1. Role of MN1 regions in leukemia cell fate regulation.

Phenotype	Required Domain(s)	Dispensable Domain(s)	Deletions likely too large to have any effect
Proliferation/Self-Renewal	1	One of: 3, 4, 5, 6, 7	2-7, 1-2, 1-3,1-4, 1-5, 1-6
Myeloid Differentiation Block	2, 7	One of: 1, 4, 5, 6	
Megakaryocyte/Erythroid Differentiation Block	1	One of: 2, 4, 5, 6, 7, 3–7, 5–7	
ATRA resistance	5, 6, 7	One of: 1, 2, 4	
Lymphoid Differentiation Block	5–7	One of: 1, 2, 4	

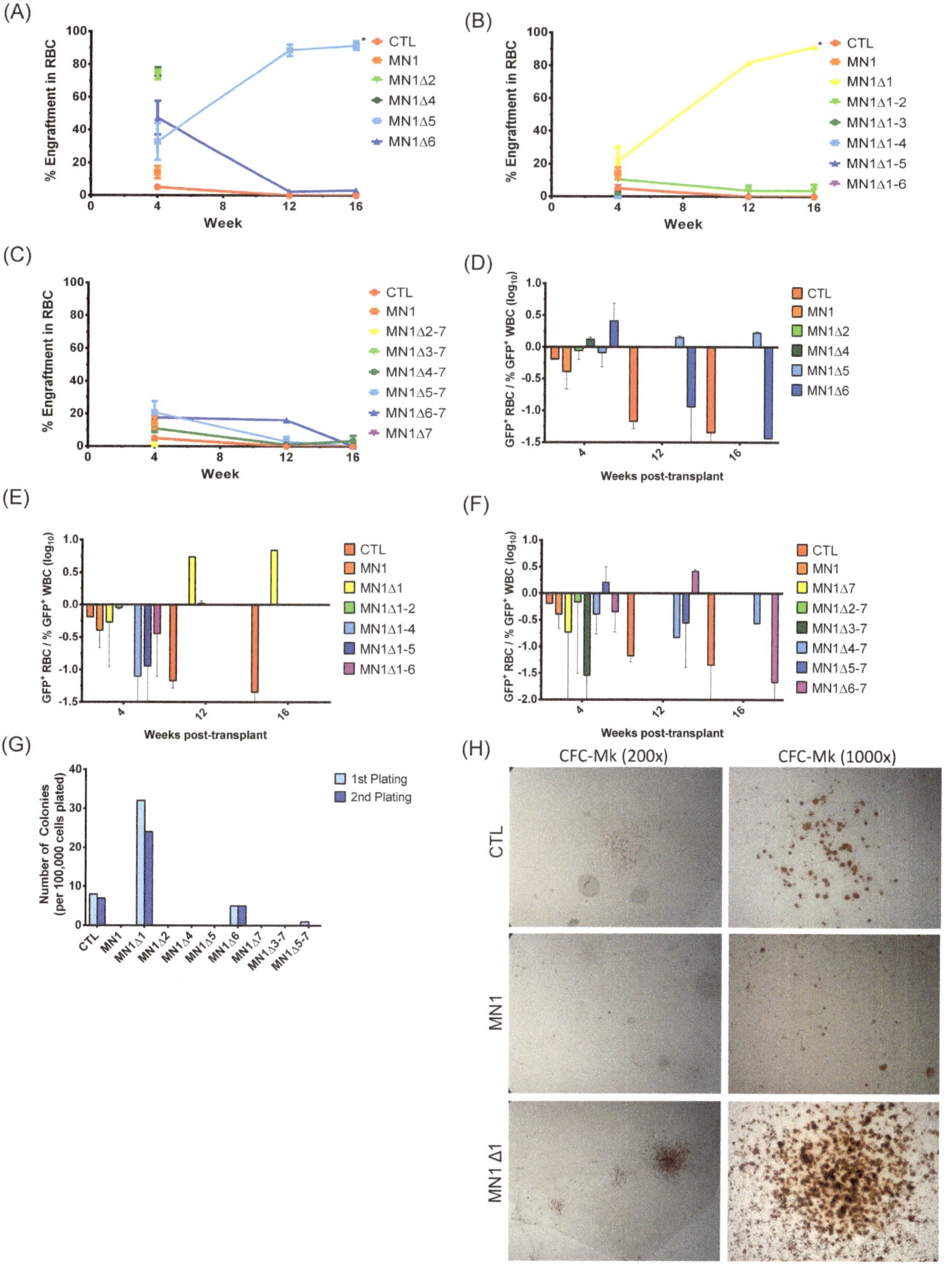
(A)
% Engraftment in RBC
Week
CTL
MN1
MN1Δ2
MN1Δ4
MN1Δ5
MN1Δ6
(B)
% Engraftment in RBC
Week
CTL
MN1
MN1Δ1
MN1Δ1-2
MN1Δ1-3
MN1Δ1-4
MN1Δ1-5
MN1Δ1-6
(C)
% Engraftment in RBC
Week
CTL
MN1
MN1Δ2-7
MN1Δ3-7
MN1Δ4-7
MN1Δ5-7
MN1Δ6-7
MN1Δ7
(D)
GFP+ RBC / % GFP+ WBC (log10)
Weeks post-transplant
CTL
MN1
MN1Δ2
MN1Δ4
MN1Δ5
MN1Δ6
(E)
GFP+ RBC / % GFP+ WBC (log10)
Weeks post-transplant
CTL
MN1
MN1Δ1
MN1Δ1-2
MN1Δ1-4
MN1Δ1-5
MN1Δ1-6
(F)
GFP+ RBC / % GFP+ WBC (log10)
Weeks post-transplant
CTL
MN1
MN1Δ7
MN1Δ2-7
MN1Δ3-7
MN1Δ4-7
MN1Δ5-7
MN1Δ6-7
(G)
Number of Colonies (per 100,000 cells plated)
1st Plating
2nd Plating
CTL MN1 MN1Δ1 MN1Δ2 MN1Δ4 MN1Δ5 MN1Δ6 MN1Δ7 MN1Δ3-7 MN1Δ5-7
(H)
CFC-Mk (200x)
CFC-Mk (1000x)
CTL
MN1
MN1 Δ1

Figure 2. The N-terminal region of MN1 is required to block megakaryocyte/erythroid differentiation. (A–C) Percentage of transgene positive red blood cells engrafting in peripheral blood of transplanted mice at 4-week intervals. P values are calculated for the comparison of the indicated construct with CTL-transduced cells. The number of analysed mice and standard error is detailed in Table S3. (D–F) Proportion of red blood cells (RBC) compared to white blood cells (WBC) expressing (D) strategy 1, (E) strategy 2, or (F) strategy 3 MN1 deletion constructs after transplantation. P values are calculated for the comparison of the indicated construct with CTL-transduced cells. The number of analysed mice and standard error is detailed in Table S3. (G) Megakaryocyte colony-forming ability of mouse bone marrow cells transduced with MN1 deletion constructs (mean ± SD, n = 4). (H) Micrographs of representative CFC-Mk slides at the end of the first plating of bone marrow cells transduced with CTL vector, full-length MN1 or MN1Δ1. Images were visualised using a Nikon Eclipse 80i microscope (Nikon, Mississauga, ON, Canada) and a 20x/0.40 numerical aperture objective, or a 100x/1.25 numerical aperture objective and Nikon Immersion Oil (Nikon). A Nikon Coolpix 995 camera (Nikon) was used to capture images. * indicates P<0.05.

plays an important role in regulating resistance to ATRA in MN1 cells, with the MN1 N-terminus (amino acids 222–418) being important for maintaining functionality of the MN1 protein.

We performed gene expression profiling on GFP-positive bulk MN1-, MN1Δ1- and MN1Δ7-transduced bone marrow cells, and normal $Gr1^+CD11b^+$ differentiated myeloid cells sorted from bone marrow. Unsupervised hierarchical clustering showed that bulk C-terminally deleted MN1 cells (MN1Δ7, with an average 26.9% $GFP^+/Gr1^+/CD11b^+$ population) clustered with $Gr1^+CD11b^+$ normal myeloid cells, which have been previously shown to have

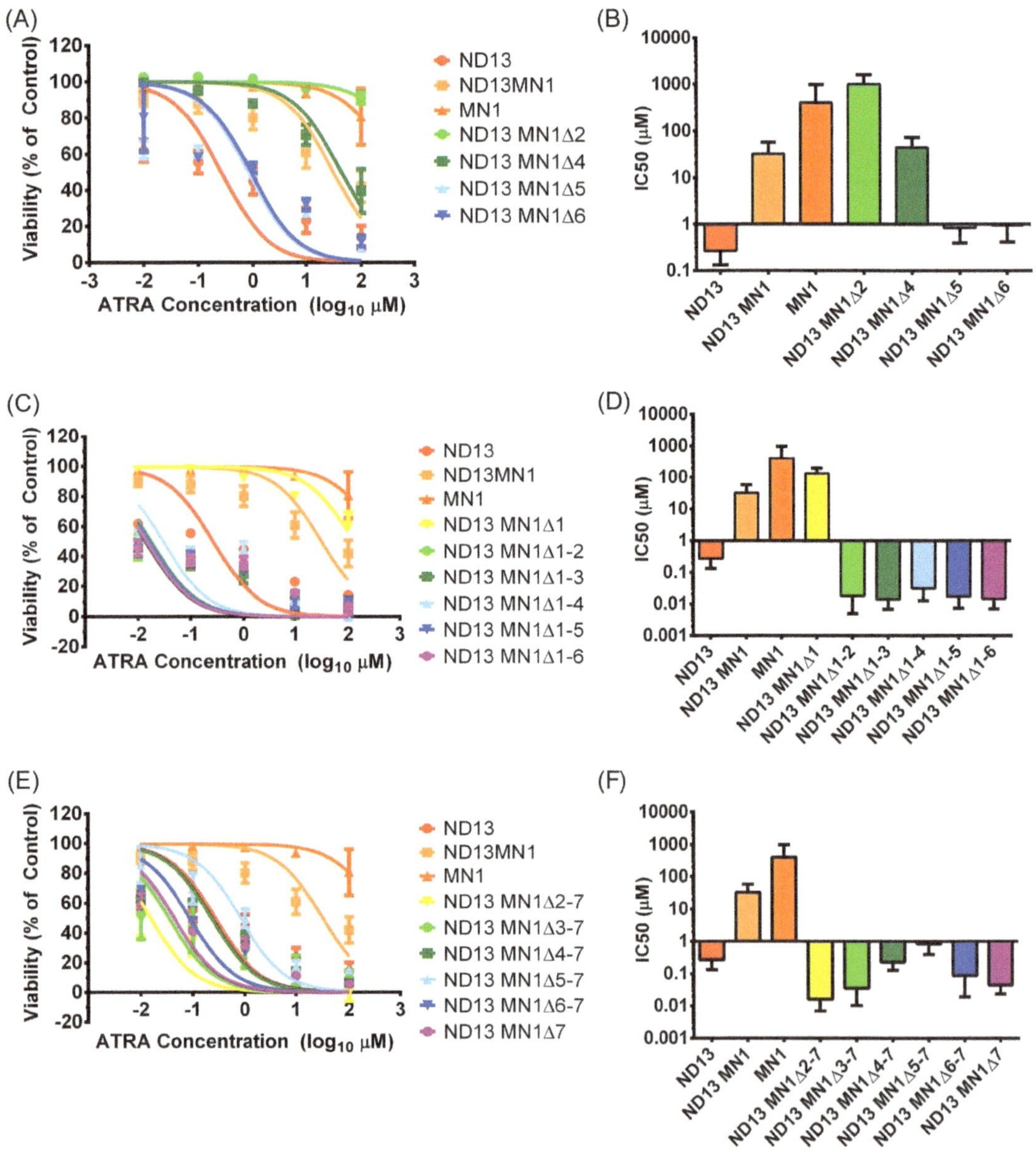

Figure 3. The C-terminal region of MN1 is required to block myeloid differentiation. (A–F) In vitro sensitivity to ATRA of ND13-immortalized cells that were transduced with MN1 deletion constructs. Dose-response curves are shown in the left panels (A, C, E) and IC50 values are shown in the right panels (B, D, F) for each deletion strategy (mean ± SD, n≥6).

low Mn1 expression [17]. Alternatively, N-terminally deleted MN1 cells (MN1Δ1, with an average 24.3% $GFP^{+}/Gr1^{+}/CD11b^{+}$ population) clustered with wildtype MN1 cells (Figure 4A). Comparison of the 60 most differentially expressed gene ontology gene sets between wildtype MN1 and MN1Δ1 or MN1Δ7 cells showed that those related to differentiation and metabolism were overrepresented in MN1Δ7 cells compared to MN1Δ1 cells (Figure 4B and Table S7). Conversely, gene sets related to signal transduction and cell structure were overrepresented in MN1Δ1 cells (Figure 4B and Table S8). The most differentially expressed genes in MN1Δ1 compared to MN1 cells were *HOXA9*, *HOXA10* and *MEIS2* (Table S9). These genes are among the most important genes driving self-renewal of HSCs, and their low expression in MN1Δ1 cells may explain their loss of leukemogenic potential. Several Krüppel-like factors were upregulated in MN1Δ1 cells, providing a link for their preferential erythroid differentiation. In MN1Δ7 cells 3 members of the eosinophil cationic protein (*Ecp* or *Ear1*, *2*, *3*) and eosinophil peroxidase were most differentially upregulated compared to MN1 cells (Table S10).

To compare the differentiation potential of cells transduced with different MN1 deletions, the immunophenotype of GFP positive cells in peripheral blood at week 4 post-transplant and in bone marrow at death was compared for all deletion constructs (Figures S7–S9). Expression of the progenitor cell marker cKit inversely correlated with those of the myeloid markers Gr1 and CD11b. Loss of the C-terminus and unexpectedly, also the loss of domain region 2, resulted in increased expression of myeloid markers Gr1 and CD11b, as well as mature neutrophils (MN1Δ7) and monocytic cells (MN1Δ2) besides blast cells in bone marrow smears of diseased mice (Figure 1H and Figures S7–S8). In summary, the C-terminal region is required to block myeloid differentiation and to induce resistance against ATRA, while domain 2 prevents myeloid differentiation but is dispensable for ATRA resistance (see also Table 1).

A 606 amino-acid C-terminal region of MN1 is required to prevent T-lymphoid differentiation

Combining deletion of the three most C-terminally located regions in MN1Δ5-7 resulted in delayed onset of leukemia with a median survival of 123 days (Figure 1G and Table S3). Interestingly, immunophenotypic analysis revealed CD4/CD8 double positive T cells within the GFP gate, and morphologic analysis showed blast cells in diseased mice in two independent experiments (Figure 5A–B), consistent with a diagnosis of T-lymphoblastic leukemia. Furthermore, these cells also induced T-ALL upon secondary transplantation (Figure 5C–D). Despite the differences in leukemic phenotype, MN1Δ5-7 was also shown to localise to the nucleus (Figure S6). In summary, these data suggest that the extended C-terminus of MN1 is required to block lymphoid differentiation and demonstrates the role of MN1 in regulating hematopoietic cell fate (see also Table 1 and Figure S9).

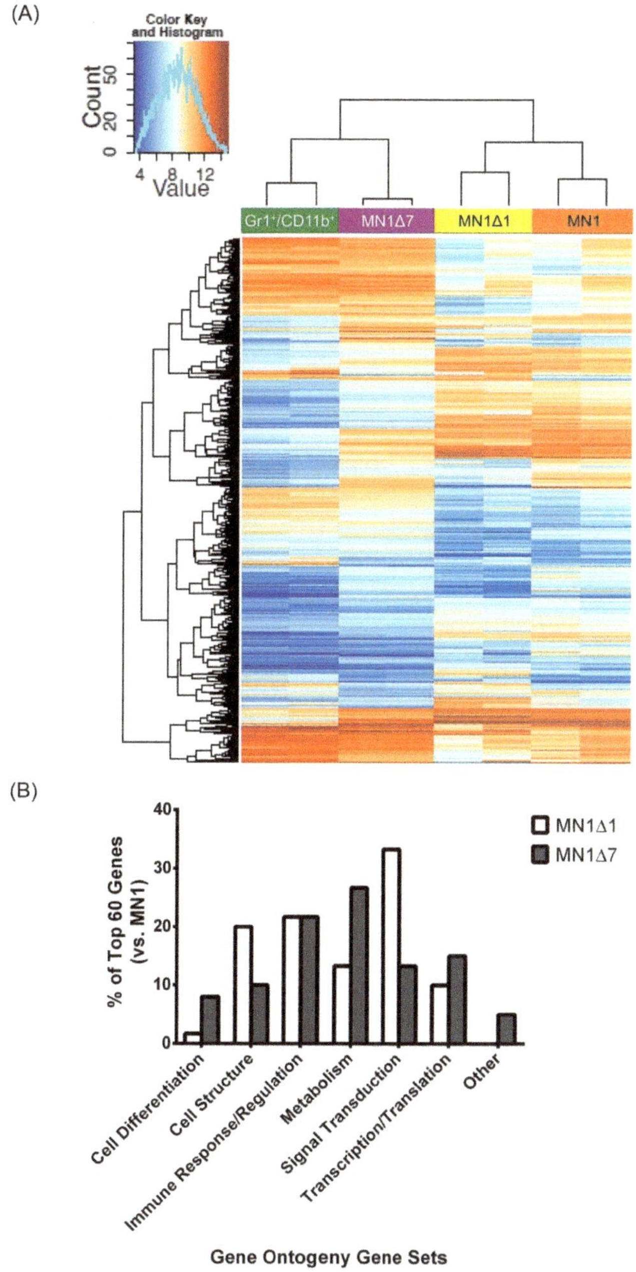

Figure 4. Hierarchical clustering of cells with N- and C-terminally deleted MN1. (A) Heat map of differentially regulated pathways for enhanced proliferation and blocked differentiation. (B) Comparison of top 60 enriched gene ontology gene sets for the comparison of MN1Δ1 and MN1Δ7 with wildtype MN1.

Discussion

In this study, we systematically determined the functional properties of MN1 deletion mutants to identify regions that encode the key leukemogenic functions of MN1. Our analyses demonstrate that a single gene can induce leukemia by a "double-hit", as the two functions promoting proliferation and inhibiting differentiation are encoded in structurally distinct regions. We also show that the myeloid or lymphoid lineage identity of leukemias can be determined by different mutations of the same oncogene, thus providing a potential explanation for the similar mutation spectrum in phenotypically distinct diseases like AML and T-ALL.

Deletion of the 221 most N-terminal amino acids (MN1Δ1) abolished the leukemogenicity of MN1 in vivo, as evidenced by decreased WBC engraftment in mice over time and failure to develop leukemia. However, the MN1Δ1 mutant provided both growth advantage and retention of ATRA resistance to bone marrow cells in vitro. We report the novel finding that MN1Δ1-transduced cells preferentially differentiated to the erythroid lineage in vivo and had an increased megakaryocyte differentiation

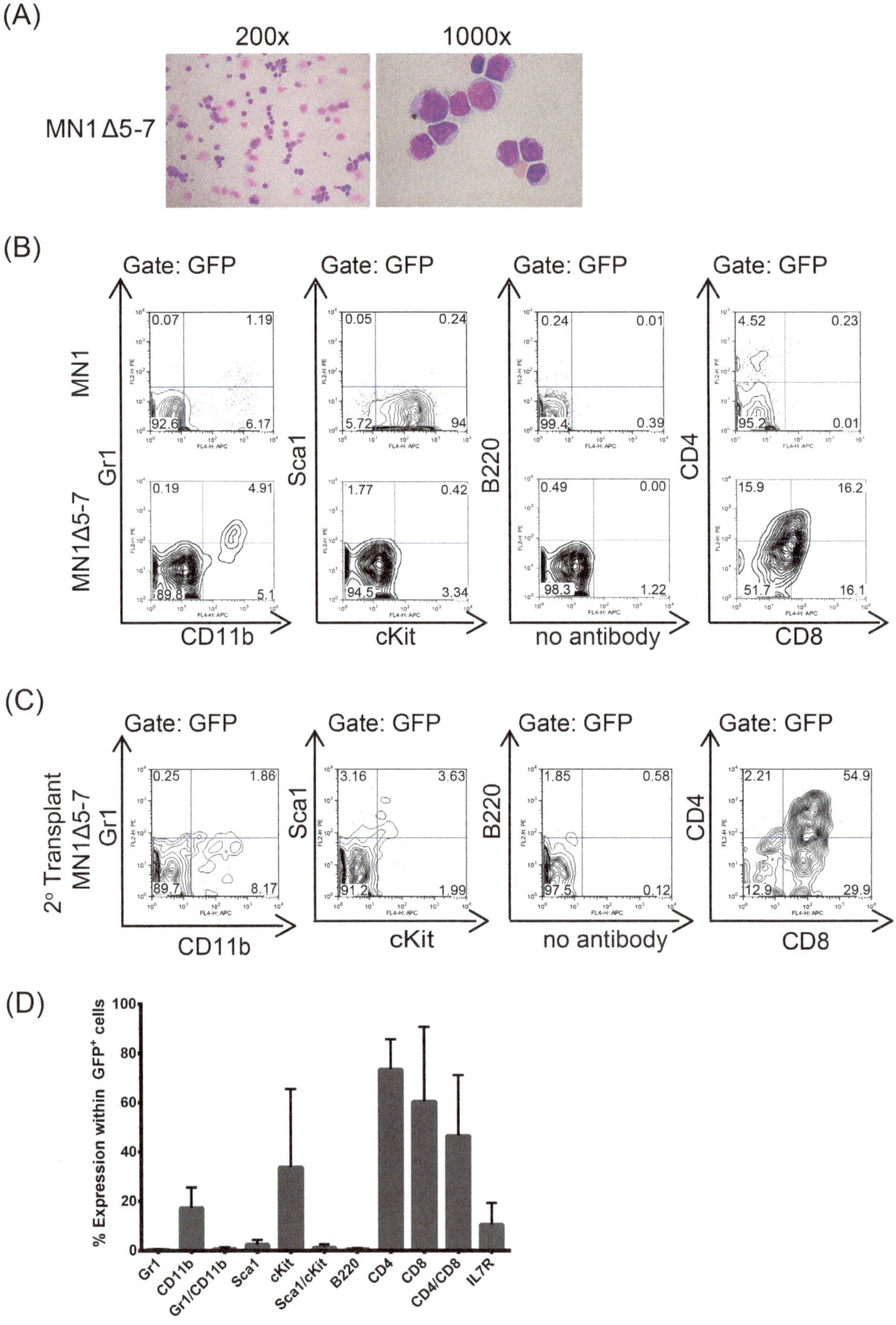
(A)
200x
1000x
MN1 Δ5-7
(B)
Gate: GFP
MN1
MN1Δ5-7
Gr1
CD11b
0.07
1.19
92.6
6.17
0.19
4.91
89.8
5.1
Sca1
cKit
0.05
0.24
5.72
94
1.77
0.42
94.5
3.34
B220
no antibody
0.24
0.01
99.4
0.39
0.49
0.00
98.3
1.22
CD4
CD8
4.52
0.23
95.2
0.01
15.9
16.2
51.7
16.1
(C)
2° Transplant MN1Δ5-7
Gate: GFP
Gr1
CD11b
0.25
1.86
89.7
8.17
Sca1
cKit
3.16
3.63
91.2
1.99
B220
no antibody
1.85
0.58
97.5
0.12
CD4
CD8
2.21
54.9
12.9
29.9
(D)
% Expression within GFP+ cells
100
80
60
40
20
0
Gr1
CD11b
Gr1/CD11b
Sca1
cKit
Sca1/cKit
B220
CD4
CD8
CD4/CD8
IL7R

Figure 5. A 606 amino-acid C-terminal portion of MN1 prevents T-lymphoid differentiation. (A) Morphology of bone marrow cells from MN1Δ5-7 mice at death, showing a shift in leukemia from AML, as seen in MN1 leukemia, to an ALL leukemia upon loss of the C-terminal domains 5–7. (B) Representative immunophenotype of GFP^+ MN1Δ5-7 bone marrow cells compared to wildtype MN1 bone marrow cells at death. (C) Representative immunophenotype of secondary transplants of GFP^+ MN1Δ5-7 bone marrow cells at death. (D) Average cell surface marker expression for secondary transplants of GFP^+ MN1Δ5-7 bone marrow cells at death (mean ± SEM, n = 3).

potential in vitro, suggesting that the most N-terminal sequence of MN1 is also critical in blocking megakaryocyte/erythroid differentiation (Figure 6). Consistent with the reduced proliferative ability of MN1Δ1 cells, expression levels of HOXA9, HOXA10, and MEIS2 were most differentially downregulated compared to full-length MN1. In addition, JUN and FOS, factors of the AP1 complex, were most upregulated together with Kruppel-like factors (KLF) 2, 3, 4 and 6, which play an important role in erythroid differentiation and bind DNA at CACCC motifs [40–43]. Interestingly, the CACCC motif has also been identified as a consensus motif for MN1 binding to DNA in an oligonucleotide selection assay [44,45].

Additional deletion of a region containing the first poly-Gln repeat (MN1Δ1-2) abolished any functional effect of MN1 in vitro and in vivo, despite the formation of protein. Conversely, the N-terminal sequence up to amino acid 317 (MN1Δ3-7) was sufficient to induce strong myeloproliferation with high WBC counts and large spleen with full myeloid differentiation potential, demonstrating that the MN1 N-terminus is driving proliferation in MN1 leukemia. We have previously shown that MN1 and MEIS1 share a high proportion of their regulatory chromatin sites and that MN1 leukemogenicity depends on MEIS1 [17]. Therefore, we speculate that the N-terminus is required for localization of MN1 to MEIS1 chromatin binding sites. In addition, van Wely *et al.* showed that MN1 interacts with P300 at amino acids 48 to 256, a region with considerable transcription activation function [44], the majority of which overlaps with domain 1. Future studies will be required to demonstrate if interaction between the MN1 N-terminus and P300 is required for the N-terminal functions promoting proliferation and blocking megakaryocyte/erythroid differentiation.

Several levels of evidence suggested that the MN1 C-terminus is required to inhibit myeloid differentiation (Table 1). First, loss of individual domains 5, 6, or 7 restored sensitivity to ATRA in vitro. Second, myeloid surface markers Gr1 and CD11b were most highly expressed in cells transduced with MN1Δ7 in vivo. In addition, gene expression profiling showed a close relationship of MN1Δ7 cells to differentiated myeloid cells, and more differentiation-related gene sets were upregulated in MN1Δ7 than in MN1Δ1 cells. Third, cumulative loss of domains 5, 6 and 7 resulted in loss of myeloid identity (see below). Lastly, cumulative deletion of domains 3 to 7 (MN1Δ3-7) resulted in a myeloproliferative disease with full differentiation potential to mature neutrophils (Table 1). These data suggest that the C-terminal regions (MN1Δ5, 6, 7) are the critical regions mediating resistance to ATRA-cytotoxicity, with some contribution from amino acids 222–418 (Figure 6). Recent work by Sharma et al. which showed that *Ccl9* and *Irf8* were upregulated in both MN1Δ7 cells and the MN1 model fused to the transcriptional activation domain VP16 (MN1VP16), suggesting that phenotypic similarities between the two models may be rooted in underlying gene expression patterns [46]. Van Wely et al. showed that MN1 binds to retinoic-acid

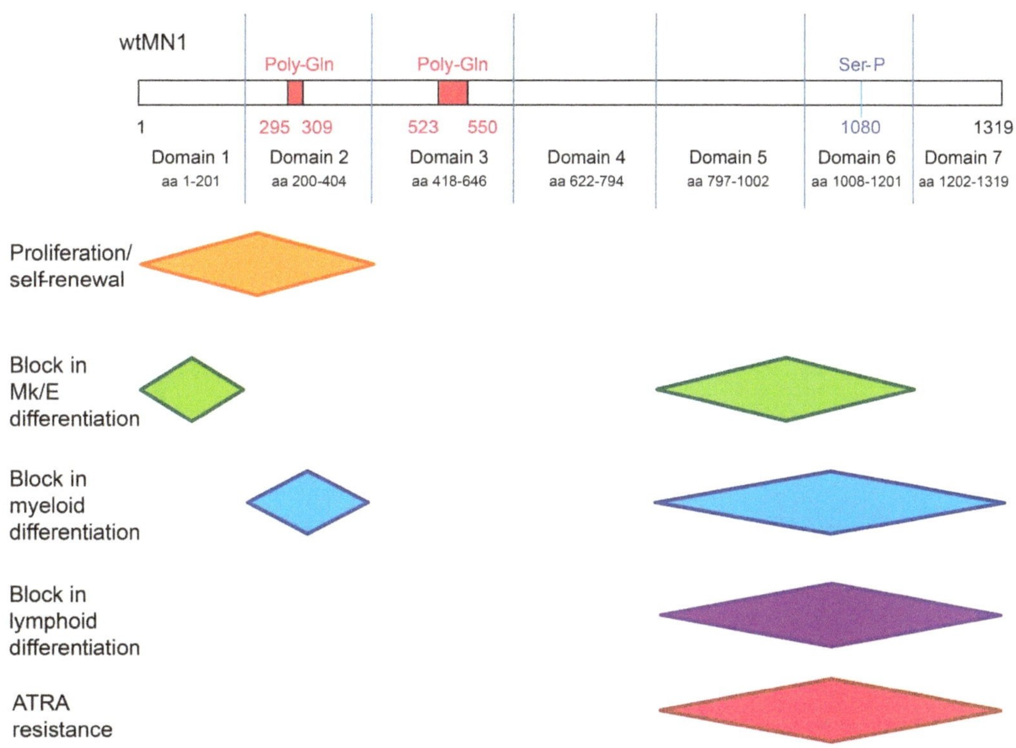

Figure 6. Functionally defined regions of MN1.

response elements by an oligonucleotide selection assay [44] and, combined with our data, we hypothesize that the MN1 C-terminus directs MN1 to retinoic acid response elements to regulate transcription. Although retroviral overexpression, as used in this study, is likely to lead to artificially high transcriptional expression of MN1 and the mutants, we found that AML patients with the highest MN1 expression had similar expression levels to our murine MN1-transduced cell lines with the lowest MN1 expression, suggesting that at least some of our cell lines are comparable to patient data (data not shown). In addition, previous studies have shown that MN1 induces resistance to ATRA-induced differentiation and cell death [22], and that high-level expression of MN1 predicts ATRA resistance in AML patients, suggesting its future use as a biomarker for ATRA treatment [22,47].

Deletion of a 606 amino acid fragment from the C-terminus reproducibly resulted in T-lymphoblastic leukemia with CD4- and CD8-double positive cells in mice. This suggests that the C-terminus of MN1 directs hematopoietic progenitor cells towards the myeloid lineage, but in its absence, allows differentiation towards the T cell lineage. Although this study cannot rule out that T-cell precursors may have been transduced by MN1Δ5-7, resulting in a bias or advantage towards lymphoid differentiation seen in the T-ALLs that developed, it is unlikely as findings were consistent in two independent experiments performed and supported by similar findings by an independent group [48]. Interestingly, mice lacking a portion of this 606 amino acid fragment, namely MN1Δ5 or MN1Δ7, developed AML. This suggests that amino acids 714–797 may be critical for myeloid differentiation, and it is only in their absence that lymphoid differentiation may occur. Kawagoe and Grosveld also described CD4/CD8 double positive T cell lymphomas in mice expressing the MN1/TEL fusion oncoprotein under the control of the AML1 promoter [49]. In this fusion protein, the 60 C-terminal amino acids of MN1 are lost due to the fusion to TEL [50]. As AML1 is also expressed in the T-lineage, these data suggest that overexpression of MN1 in T-progenitor cells can promote leukemogenesis, with Neumann and colleagues providing evidence of MN1 overexpression in T-lymphoblastic leukemias [51]. Taken together, we suggest that the C-terminus of MN1 encoded by amino acids 513–1319 (domains 5–7) instructs progenitor cells to the myeloid lineage and that in its absence progenitor cells can differentiate to the lymphoid lineage (Table 1).

During preparation of the present paper, one other group characterised functional MN1 regions, creating deletion constructs modelled off known MN1 protein domains in U937 cells [48]. Consistent with our data, Kandilci and colleagues reported decreased growth and colony-forming ability in vitro upon loss of the MN1 N-terminus. Kandilci *et al.* also showed that the loss of MN1 amino acids 570–1273 gave rise to T-cell lymphoma. This deleted region partially overlaps with our MN1Δ5-7 mutant, supporting the idea that the MN1 C-terminus promotes a myeloid-skew to MN1 leukemia. Finally, Kandilci *et al.* were also able to localise ATRA resistance to amino acids 18–458, but not 12–228, with their MN1-transduced U937 cells showing increased CD11b expression after 3 days of treatment. Interestingly, this region partially overlaps with domain 2 of our deletion mutants, providing support for our observation of increased CD11b expression in peripheral blood of animals transplanted with MN1Δ2. Kandilci *et al.* did not, however, report increased CD11b expression in C-terminal deletions, although this may be attributed to their most C-terminal deletion mutant retaining the 46 most C-terminal amino acids. It is possible that retention of these critical amino acids may have abrogated the differentiation effect seen in our complete deletions.

In summary, we characterized functional regions of the MN1 protein by a systematic mutation analysis and identified key regions that enhance proliferation and self-renewal, block myeloid, megakaryocytic/erythroid, and lymphoid differentiation, and induce resistance against ATRA. Our data support a critical function of MN1 as a key cell fate regulator in malignant hematopoiesis and provide a powerful new model for further dissection of the molecular events controlling transformation and the resulting leukemic phenotype.

Supporting Information

Figure S1 Expression levels of MN1 deletion constructs. (A) Western blots illustrating the expression and size of protein products of the MN1 deletion constructs compared to full-length MN1. The figure is a composite of multiple gels with each lane representing a single construct stained with either anti-HA or anti-β-actin antibody. (B) Gel electrophoresis with PCR products illustrating the relative size of the MN1 deletion constructs compared to full-length MN1. (C–E) Expression levels of MN1 deletion constructs measured by qRT-PCR. MN1 deletion constructs were transduced in cells immortalized by NUP98HOXD13 (ND13). Mean ± SD, n = 3.

Figure S2 Potential of MN1 variants to immortalize bone marrow cells in vitro. Left panels (A, C, E) show number of CFC colonies per plating in methylcellulose under myeloid cytokine conditions. 5-FU pretreated bone marrow cells were transduced with MN1 deletions and were plated after transduction without sorting of cells. Right panels (B, D, F) show percentage of GFP positive cells at the end of each round of plating.

Figure S3 White blood cell count in transplanted mice. (A–C) White blood cell count (WBC) in peripheral blood of mice at 4-week intervals after transplantation. MN1 mutation constructs were used from (A) Strategy 1, (B) Strategy 2, and (C) Strategy 3. P values are given for the comparison of the indicated construct with CTL. The average WBC count is shown. Number of analyzed mice and standard error can be found in Table S5. § WBC count in peripheral blood at the indicated time point or at death in cases where a mouse died before that time point. † indicates that all mice were dead at this time point due to disease. * indicates $P < 0.05$.

Figure S4 Red blood cell count in transplanted mice. (A–C) Red blood cell count (RBC) in peripheral blood of mice at 4 week intervals after transplantation. MN1 mutation constructs were used from (A) Strategy 1, (B) Strategy 2, and (C) Strategy 3. P values are given for the comparison of the indicated construct with CTL. The average RBC count is shown. Number of analyzed mice and standard error can be found in Table S5. § RBC count in peripheral blood at the indicated time point or at death in cases where a mouse died before that time point. † indicates that all mice were dead at this time point due to disease. * indicates $P < 0.05$.

Figure S5 Platelet count in transplanted mice. (A–C) Platelet count in peripheral blood of mice at 4 week intervals after transplantation. MN1 mutation constructs were used from (A) Strategy 1, (B) Strategy 2, and (C) Strategy 3. P values are given for the comparison of the indicated construct with CTL. The average platelet count is shown. Number of analyzed mice and standard deviation can be found in Table S5. § Platelet count in peripheral blood at the indicated time point or at death in cases where a mouse died before that time point. † indicates that all mice were dead at this time point due to disease. * indicates P<0.05.

Figure S6 Confocal microscopy of MN1-transduced cells. Representative confocal microscopy images of GP + E86 cells transduced with (A) negative control, (B) MN1 tagged with an HA-tag, (C) MN1Δ1 with an HA-tag, and (D) MN1Δ5–7 with an HA-tag stained with (i) DAPI or (ii) anti-HA and (iii) DAPI and anti-HA merged.

Figure S7 Immunophenotype of MN1-transduced cells in transplanted mice – stem and progenitor markers. Percentage of GFP-expressing cells and expression of ckit and Sca1 in GFP+ cells in peripheral blood at 4 weeks and in bone marrow at death of mice receiving transplants of MN1-transduced cells. (A) Strategy 1, (B) Strategy 2, and (C) Strategy 3 MN1 constructs. Mean ± SEM. The number of analyzed mice is provided in Table S6.

Figure S8 Immunophenotype of MN1-transduced cells in transplanted mice – myeloid markers. Expression of myeloid markers in GFP+ cells in peripheral blood at 4 weeks and in bone marrow at death of mice receiving transplants of MN1-transduced cells. (A) Strategy 1, (B) Strategy 2, and (C) Strategy 3 MN1 constructs. Mean ± SEM. The number of analyzed mice is provided in Table S6.

Figure S9 Immunophenotype of MN1-transduced cells in transplanted mice – T-cell markers. Expression of T-cell markers in GFP+ cells in peripheral blood at 4 weeks and in bone marrow at death of mice receiving transplants of MN1-transduced cells. (A) Strategy 1, (B) Strategy 2, and (C) Strategy 3 MN1 constructs. Mean ± SEM. The number of analyzed mice is provided in Table S6.

Table S1 MN1 deletion mutant primer sequences.

Table S2 MN1 qPCR primer sequences.

Table S3 Characterisation of mouse phenotype after transplantation with MN1 deletion constructs.

Table S4 *In vivo* engraftment of cells transduced with MN1 deletion constructs.

Table S5 Peripheral blood counts in mice receiving transplants of cells transduced with MN1 deletion constructs.

Table S6 Immunophenotype of GFP-positive cells in peripheral blood of mice receiving transplants of cells transduced with MN1 deletion constructs.

Table S7 Gene ontology gene sets enriched in MN1Δ7 cells compared to MN1 cells.

Table S8 Gene ontology gene sets enriched in MN1Δ1 cells compared to MN1 cells.

Table S9 Differentially Expressed Genes in MN1Δ1 cells compared to MN1 cells.

Table S10 Differentially Expressed Genes in MN1Δ7 cells compared to MN1 cells.

Acknowledgments

We thank Patty Rosten, Christy Brookes, Justin Smrz, the staff of the Flow Cytometry Facility of the Terry Fox Laboratory, and the staff of the Animal Resource Centre of the BC Cancer Agency, and the staff of the Imaging Facility at the Child and Family Research Institute for their excellent technical assistance.

Author Contributions

Conceived and designed the experiments: CKL RKH MH. Performed the experiments: CKL YM FK DTS BA EY PB A. Schwarzer A. Sharma GP ML GL SV SF APW MH. Analyzed the data: CKL MY FK DTS BA EY PB A. Schwarzer A. Sharma GP ML GL SV SF CJE AK APW MH. Contributed reagents/materials/analysis tools: CKL YM FK DTS BA EY PB A. Schwarzer A. Sharma GP ML GL SV SF APW MH. Wrote the paper: CKL RKH MH.

References

1. Gilliland DG (2001) Hematologic malignancies. Curr Opin Hematol 8: 189–191.
2. Cancer Genome Atlas Research N (2013) Genomic and epigenomic landscapes of adult de novo acute myeloid leukemia. N Engl J Med 368: 2059–2074.
3. Dick JE (2008) Stem cell concepts renew cancer research. Blood 112: 4793–4807.
4. Kirstetter P, Schuster MB, Bereshchenko O, Moore S, Dvinge H, et al. (2008) Modeling of C/EBPalpha mutant acute myeloid leukemia reveals a common expression signature of committed myeloid leukemia-initiating cells. Cancer Cell 13: 299–310.
5. Deshpande AJ, Cusan M, Rawat VP, Reuter H, Krause A, et al. (2006) Acute myeloid leukemia is propagated by a leukemic stem cell with lymphoid characteristics in a mouse model of CALM/AF10-positive leukemia. Cancer Cell 10: 363–374.
6. Somervaille TC, Cleary ML (2006) Identification and characterization of leukemia stem cells in murine MLL-AF9 acute myeloid leukemia. Cancer Cell 10: 257–268.
7. Goardon N, Marchi E, Atzberger A, Quek L, Schuh A, et al. (2011) Coexistence of LMPP-like and GMP-like leukemia stem cells in acute myeloid leukemia. Cancer Cell 19: 138–152.
8. Heuser M, Sly LM, Argiropoulos B, Kuchenbauer F, Lai C, et al. (2009) Modeling the functional heterogeneity of leukemia stem cells: role of STAT5 in leukemia stem cell self-renewal. Blood 114: 3983–3993.
9. Thol F, Damm F, Ludeking A, Winschel C, Wagner K, et al. (2011) Incidence and prognostic influence of DNMT3A mutations in acute myeloid leukemia. J Clin Oncol 29: 2889–2896.
10. Neumann M, Heesch S, Schlee C, Schwartz S, Gokbuget N, et al. (2013) Whole-exome sequencing in adult ETP-ALL reveals a high rate of DNMT3A mutations. Blood 121: 4749–4752.
11. Vannucchi AM, Lasho TL, Guglielmelli P, Biamonte F, Pardanani A, et al. (2013) Mutations and prognosis in primary myelofibrosis. Leukemia 27: 1861–1869.
12. Horton SJ, Jaques J, Woolthuis C, van Dijk J, Mesuraca M, et al. (2013) MLL-AF9-mediated immortalization of human hematopoietic cells along different lineages changes during ontogeny. Leukemia 27: 1116–1126.
13. Wei J, Wunderlich M, Fox C, Alvarez S, Cigudosa JC, et al. (2008) Microenvironment determines lineage fate in a human model of MLL-AF9 leukemia. Cancer Cell 13: 483–495.
14. Raaijmakers MH, Mukherjee S, Guo S, Zhang S, Kobayashi T, et al. (2010) Bone progenitor dysfunction induces myelodysplasia and secondary leukaemia. Nature 464: 852–857.

15. Morin RD, Johnson NA, Severson TM, Mungall AJ, An J, et al. (2010) Somatic mutations altering EZH2 (Tyr641) in follicular and diffuse large B-cell lymphomas of germinal-center origin. Nat Genet 42: 181–185.
16. Ernst T, Chase AJ, Score J, Hidalgo-Curtis CE, Bryant C, et al. (2010) Inactivating mutations of the histone methyltransferase gene EZH2 in myeloid disorders. Nat Genet 42: 722–726.
17. Heuser M, Yun H, Berg T, Yung E, Argiropoulos B, et al. (2011) Cell of origin in AML: susceptibility to MN1-induced transformation is regulated by the MEIS1/AbdB-like HOX protein complex. Cancer Cell 20: 39–52.
18. Kandilci A, Grosveld GC (2009) Reintroduction of CEBPA in MN1-overexpressing hematopoietic cells prevents their hyperproliferation and restores myeloid differentiation. Blood 114: 1596–1606.
19. Heuser M, Beutel G, Krauter J, Dohner K, von Neuhoff N, et al. (2006) High meningioma 1 (MN1) expression as a predictor for poor outcome in acute myeloid leukemia with normal cytogenetics. Blood 108: 3898–3905.
20. Carella C, Bonten J, Sirma S, Kranenburg TA, Terranova S, et al. (2007) MN1 overexpression is an important step in the development of inv(16) AML. Leukemia 21: 1679–1690.
21. Valk PJ, Verhaak RG, Beijen MA, Erpelinck CA, Barjesteh van Waalwijk van Doorn-Khosrovani S, et al. (2004) Prognostically useful gene-expression profiles in acute myeloid leukemia. N Engl J Med 350: 1617–1628.
22. Heuser M, Argiropoulos B, Kuchenbauer F, Yung E, Piper J, et al. (2007) MN1 overexpression induces acute myeloid leukemia in mice and predicts ATRA resistance in patients with AML. Blood 110: 1639–1647.
23. Langer C, Marcucci G, Holland KB, Radmacher MD, Maharry K, et al. (2009) Prognostic importance of MN1 transcript levels, and biologic insights from MN1-associated gene and microRNA expression signatures in cytogenetically normal acute myeloid leukemia: a cancer and leukemia group B study. J Clin Oncol 27: 3198–3204.
24. Schwind S, Marcucci G, Kohlschmidt J, Radmacher MD, Mrozek K, et al. (2011) Low expression of MN1 associates with better treatment response in older patients with de novo cytogenetically normal acute myeloid leukemia. Blood 118: 4188–4198.
25. Haferlach C, Kern W, Schindela S, Kohlmann A, Alpermann T, et al. (2011) Gene expression of BAALC, CDKN1B, ERG, and MN1 adds independent prognostic information to cytogenetics and molecular mutations in adult acute myeloid leukemia. Genes Chromosomes Cancer 51: 257–265.
26. Liu T, Jankovic D, Brault L, Ehret S, Baty F, et al. (2010) Functional characterization of high levels of meningioma 1 as collaborating oncogene in acute leukemia. Leukemia 24: 601–612.
27. Pineault N, Buske C, Feuring-Buske M, Abramovich C, Rosten P, et al. (2003) Induction of acute myeloid leukemia in mice by the human leukemia-specific fusion gene NUP98-HOXD13 in concert with Meis1. Blood 101: 4529–4538.
28. Schambach A, Wodrich H, Hildinger M, Bohne J, Krausslich HG, et al. (2000) Context dependence of different modules for posttranscriptional enhancement of gene expression from retroviral vectors. Mol Ther 2: 435–445.
29. Antonchuk J, Sauvageau G, Humphries RK (2002) HOXB4-induced expansion of adult hematopoietic stem cells ex vivo. Cell 109: 39–45.
30. Gurevich RM, Aplan PD, Humphries RK (2004) NUP98-topoisomerase I acute myeloid leukemia-associated fusion gene has potent leukemogenic activities independent of an engineered catalytic site mutation. Blood 104: 1127–1136.
31. Starczynowski DT, Kuchenbauer F, Argiropoulos B, Sung S, Morin R, et al. (2010) Identification of miR-145 and miR-146a as mediators of the 5q-syndrome phenotype. Nat Med 16: 49–58.
32. Heuser M, Yap DB, Leung M, de Algara TR, Tafech A, et al. (2009) Loss of MLL5 results in pleiotropic hematopoietic defects, reduced neutrophil immune function, and extreme sensitivity to DNA demethylation. Blood 113: 1432–1443.
33. Bruce MA, Butte MJ (2013) Real-time GPU-based 3D Deconvolution. Opt Express 21: 4766–4773.
34. Vonesch C, Unser M (2008) A fast thresholded landweber algorithm for wavelet-regularized multidimensional deconvolution. IEEE Trans Image Process 17: 539–549.
35. Gentleman RC, Carey VJ, Bates DM, Bolstad B, Dettling M, et al. (2004) Bioconductor: open software development for computational biology and bioinformatics. Genome Biol 5: R80.
36. Kauffmann A, Gentleman R, Huber W (2009) arrayQualityMetrics–a bioconductor package for quality assessment of microarray data. Bioinformatics 25: 415–416.
37. Gautier L, Cope L, Bolstad BM, Irizarry RA (2004) affy–analysis of Affymetrix GeneChip data at the probe level. Bioinformatics 20: 307–315.
38. Smyth G (2005) Limma: linear models for microarray data.; Gentleman R, Carey V, Dudoit S, Irizarry R, and Huber W., editor. New York: Springer.
39. Subramanian A, Tamayo P, Mootha VK, Mukherjee S, Ebert BL, et al. (2005) Gene set enrichment analysis: a knowledge-based approach for interpreting genome-wide expression profiles. Proc Natl Acad Sci U S A 102: 15545–15550.
40. Jacobs-Helber SM, Sawyer ST (2004) Jun N-terminal kinase promotes proliferation of immature erythroid cells and erythropoietin-dependent cell lines. Blood 104: 696–703.
41. Funnell AP, Norton LJ, Mak KS, Burdach J, Artuz CM, et al. (2012) The CACCC-binding protein KLF3/BKLF represses a subset of KLF1/EKLF target genes and is required for proper erythroid maturation in vivo. Mol Cell Biol 32: 3281–3292.
42. Kalra IS, Alam MM, Choudhary PK, Pace BS (2011) Kruppel-like Factor 4 activates HBG gene expression in primary erythroid cells. Br J Haematol 154: 248–259.
43. Marini MG, Porcu L, Asunis I, Loi MG, Ristaldi MS, et al. (2010) Regulation of the human HBA genes by KLF4 in erythroid cell lines. Br J Haematol 149: 748–758.
44. van Wely KH, Molijn AC, Buijs A, Meester-Smoor MA, Aarnoudse AJ, et al. (2003) The MN1 oncoprotein synergizes with coactivators RAC3 and p300 in RAR-RXR-mediated transcription. Oncogene 22: 699–709.
45. Meester-Smoor MA, Molijn AC, Zhao Y, Groen NA, Groffen CA, et al. (2007) The MN1 oncoprotein activates transcription of the IGFBP5 promoter through a CACCC-rich consensus sequence. J Mol Endocrinol 38: 113–125.
46. Sharma A YH, Jyotsana N, Chaturvedi A, Schwarzer A, Yung E, et al. (2014) Constitutive Irf8 expression inhibits AML by activation of repressed immune response signaling. Leukemia.
47. Burnett AK, Hills RK, Green C, Jenkinson S, Koo K, et al. (2010) The impact on outcome of the addition of all-trans retinoic acid to intensive chemotherapy in younger patients with nonacute promyelocytic acute myeloid leukemia: overall results and results in genotypic subgroups defined by mutations in NPM1, FLT3, and CEBPA. Blood 115: 948–956.
48. Kandilci A, Surtel J, Janke L, Neale G, Terranova S, et al. (2013) Mapping of MN1 sequences necessary for myeloid transformation. PLoS One 8: e61706.
49. Kawagoe H, Grosveld GC (2005) MN1-TEL myeloid oncoprotein expressed in multipotent progenitors perturbs both myeloid and lymphoid growth and causes T-lymphoid tumors in mice. Blood 106: 4278–4286.
50. Buijs A, Sherr S, van Baal S, van Bezouw S, van der Plas D, et al. (1995) Translocation (12;22) (p13;q11) in myeloproliferative disorders results in fusion of the ETS-like TEL gene on 12p13 to the MN1 gene on 22q11. Oncogene 10: 1511–1519.
51. Neumann M, Heesch S, Gokbuget N, Schwartz S, Schlee C, et al. (2012) Clinical and molecular characterization of early T-cell precursor leukemia: a high-risk subgroup in adult T-ALL with a high frequency of FLT3 mutations. Blood Cancer J 2: e55.

6

Effect of Omega-3 Fatty Acid Ethyl Esters on the Oxylipin Composition of Lipoproteins in Hypertriglyceridemic, Statin-Treated Subjects

John W. Newman[1,2], Theresa L. Pedersen[1], Verdayne R. Brandenburg[3], William S. Harris[4], Gregory C. Shearer[4,5,6,7]*

1 USDA, ARS, WHNRC, Obesity and Metabolism Research Unit, Davis, CA, United States of America, **2** Department of Nutrition, University of California Davis, Davis, CA, United States of America, **3** Family Medicine, Sanford School of Medicine, University of South Dakota, Sioux Falls, SD, United States of America, **4** Internal Medicine, Sanford School of Medicine, University of South Dakota, Sioux Falls, SD, United States of America, **5** Basic Biomedical Sciences, Sanford School of Medicine, University of South Dakota, Sioux Falls, SD, United States of America, **6** Cardiovascular Health Research Center, Sanford Research/USD, Sioux Falls, South Dakota, United States of America, **7** Department of Nutritional Sciences, The Pennsylvania State University, University Park, Pennsylvania, United States of America

Abstract

Background: Oxylipins mediate inflammation, vascular tension, and more. Their presence in lipoproteins could explain why lipoproteins mediate nearly identical activities.

Methods: To determine how oxylipins are distributed in the lipoproteins of hypertriglyceridemic subjects, and whether omega-3 fatty acids alter them in a manner consistent with improved cardiovascular health, we recruited 15 dyslipidemic subjects whose levels of low density lipoprotein cholesterol (LDL-C) were at goal but who remained hypertriglyceridemic (200–499 mg/dL). They were treated them with the indicated dose of 4 g/d omega-3 acid ethyl esters (P-OM3) for 8 weeks. Measured oxylipins included mid-chain alcohols (HETEs, HEPEs and HDoHEs), ketones (KETEs), epoxides (as EpETrEs, EpETEs, and EpDPEs).

Results: At baseline, arachidonate-oxylipins (HETEs, KETEs, and EpETrEs) were most abundant in plasma with the greatest fraction of total abundance (mean |95% CI|) being carried in high density lipoproteins (HDL); 42% |31, 57| followed by very low density lipoproteins (VLDL); 27% |20, 36|; and LDL 21% |16, 28|. EPA- and DHA-derived oxylipins constituted less than 11% of total. HDL carried alcohols and epoxides but VLDL was also rich in ketones. Treatment decreased AA-derived oxylipins across lipoprotein classes (−23% |−33, −12|, $p = 0.0003$), and expanded EPA−(322% |241, 422|, $p < 0.0001$) and DHA-derived oxylipins (123% |80, 176|, $p < 0.0001$).

Conclusions: Each lipoprotein class carries a unique oxylipin complement. P-OM3 treatment alters the oxylipin content of all classes, reducing pro-inflammatory and increasing anti-inflammatory species, consistent with the improved inflammatory and vascular status associated with the treatment.

Trial Registration: ClinicalTrials.gov NCT00959842

Editor: Giuseppe Danilo Norata, University of Milan, Italy

Funding: This study was funded by a grant from GlaxoSmithKline (LVZ113350), who also donated the study drug (Lovaza). This study was supported in part by USDA Agricultural Research Service intramural project 5306-51530-019-00D (JWN). All opinions expressed in this manuscript represent the views of the researchers and not necessarily those of the USDA. The USDA is an equal opportunity provider and employer. The funders had no role in study design, data collection and analysis, decision to publish, or preparation of the manuscript.

Competing Interests: JWN, TLP and VRB have nothing to disclose. This was an investigator-initiated study funded by GlaxoSmithKline. GlaxoSmithKline had no role in analysis or interpretation of the study results. GCS and WSH received speakership honoraria from GlaxoSmithKline while the trial was ongoing.

* Email: gcs13@psu.edu

Introduction

The control of LDL-C is effective in reducing cardiovascular disease (CVD; see list of abbreviations, File S3) [1–3], however other components of risk have yet to be effectively managed, including inflammation and impaired endothelial function. Fatty acids (FA) play an important role in these processes. Polyunsaturated FAs undergo modification into oxylipins, an important superclass of lipid mediators which includes the arachidonic acid (AA)-derived eicosanoids. These autacoids are primarily generated by one of three enzymatic pathways: cyclooxygenases (COXs) which generate the prostanoids and thromboids; lipoxygenases (LOXs) which generate leukotrienes, resolvins, hepoxilins and mid-chain alcohols; and cytochrome p450s (CYPs) which generate epoxides and omega-terminal alcohols [4].

Table 1. Demographics and treatment effects on vascular and metabolic characteristics (N = 15).

Y	Baseline[a]	Final[a]	Change from baseline Mean (95% CI)[b]	p-val
Demographics				
Age (yrs)	59 |46, 68|[c]	.	.	.
Female n (%)	5 (33%)	.	.	.
Vascular				
BMI	30.7 (28, 33)	30.6 (28, 33)	−0.03 (−0.44, 0.39)	0.89
BPM	72.6 (68, 77)	69.4 (65, 74)	−3.2 (0.017, −5.7)	0.68
Systolic	136 (130, 140)	136 (130, 140)	−0.1 (−6.2, 5.9)	0.96
Diastolic[L]	81.5 (77, 86)	80.3 (76, 85)	−1.5% (−4.7, 1.7)	0.32
Metabolism (non-lipid)				
Total Protein (gm/dL)[L, C]	7.29 (7.1, 7.5)	7.06 (6.9, 7.2)	−3.1% (−5.9, −0.16)	0.04
Glucose (mg/dL)[L, C]	106 (100, 110)	104 (98, 110)	−2.4% (−6.8, 2.2)	0.28
A1C (%) [L, C]	5.91 (5.6, 6.3)	5.99 (5.6, 6.4)	1.4% (−6.4, 9.9)	0.71
RBC Fatty acid composition (weight %)				
C18:2n6[L]	10.2 (9.3, 11.2)	9.8 (8.9, 10.7)	−4% (−8, 0)[d]	0.054
C18:3n6[L]	0.13 (0.12, 0.15)	0.12 (0.11, 0.14)	−16% (−41, 20)[d]	0.32
C18:3n3[L]	0.06 (0.04, 0.08)	0.05 (0.04, 0.07)	−6% (−16, 6)[d]	0.31
C20:3n6[L]	1.6 (1.3, 1.9)	1.4 (1.2, 1.6)	−13% (−19, −5)[d]	0.003
C20:4n6[L]	17 (17, 18)	15 (14, 16)	−13% (−15, −10)[d]	<0.0001
C20:5n3[L]	0.49 (0.41, 0.58)	1.90 (1.59, 2.27)	288% (214, 380)[d]	<0.0001
C22:6n3[L]	3.9 (3.5, 4.3)	6.4 (5.8, 7.1)	64% (50, 80)[d]	<0.0001
OMX-3[L]	4.4 (4.0, 4.9)	8.4 (7.5, 9.3)	90% (71, 112)[d]	<0.0001
Lipid/lipoprotein parameters				
Triglyceride (mg/dL)[C]	237 (200, 270)	187 (160, 220)	−49 (−81, −17)	0.005
Phospholipids (mg/dL)	307 (280, 330)	249 (220, 280)	−58 (−90, −26)	0.002
Cholesterol (mg/dL)[L, C]	174 (160, 190)	167 (160, 180)	−3.8% (−11, 3.7)	0.29
VLDL-C (mg/dL)[C]	47 (41, 54)	38 (31, 44)	−9.7 (−16, −3.2)	0.007
LDL-C (mg/dL)[C, L]	88 (78, 99)	90 (80, 100)	2.1% (−7.9, 13)	0.68
HDL-C (mg/dL)[C, L]	38 (33, 42)	39 (35, 44)	4.4% (−1.8, 11)	0.16
Chol/HDL (ratio)[C, L]	4.6 (4.1, 5.2)	4.3 (3.8, 4.8)	−7.8% (−14, −0.64)	0.04
TG/HDL (ratio)[C, L]	6.0 (4.6, 7.9)	4.5 (3.4, 5.9)	−21% (−38, −11)	0.004

[L]Log-transformed to satisfy test assumptions.
[C]from clinical lipid panel.
[a]Least squares mean (95% CI).
[b]adjusted for age and sex.
[c]Median |Inter-quartile range|.
[d]denotes a relative change from baseline value, not an absolute change in (weight %).

Oxylipins are potent mediators of inflammation and vascular function, and their potencies can vary by parent FA [5–7]. While most *in vivo* studies have focused on AA-metabolites, we have shown that the administration of prescription omega-3 fatty acids (P-OM3) can reduce the abundance of oxylipins derived from AA, while increasing the abundance of eicosapentaenoate- (EPA) and docosahexaenoate- (DHA) derived oxylipins [8,9]. Oxylipins are generally considered to act locally, however their presence in plasma suggests they act in an endocrine fashion as well. In rats, most oxylipins (>90% of those present in plasma) are found acylated in the glycerolipids of lipoproteins [10]. While the specific distribution of oxylipins within human lipoproteins has not been reported, in an animal model of chronic, inflammatory disease with dyslipidemia there is a shift of lipoprotein-oxylipin profiles in an inflammatory direction [11]. Further, the release of oxylipins by lipoprotein lipase from rat lipoproteins demonstrates they may be delivered to LpL-expressing tissues (adipose, heart, and skeletal muscle) esterified in circulating glycerolipids [10]. Oxylipins are known to be esterified in cellular phospholipids [12,13], suggesting that lipoprotein phospholipids may also carry oxylipins.

Given the effects of P-OM3 on oxylipin profiles [8] and their concurrent reduction of CVD risk, serum TG, inflammation, and improvement in vascular function, it is plausible omega-3 fatty acids produce these effects by altering the quantity and quality of lipoprotein-oxylipins. In the current study we examine the impact of P-OM3, in the context of a statin-induced, maximal reduction in levels of low density lipoprotein cholesterol (LDL-C). We compared lipoprotein oxylipin composition in a change-from-baseline design in order to 1) document the distribution of oxylipins among lipoproteins in humans and 2) measure the effect

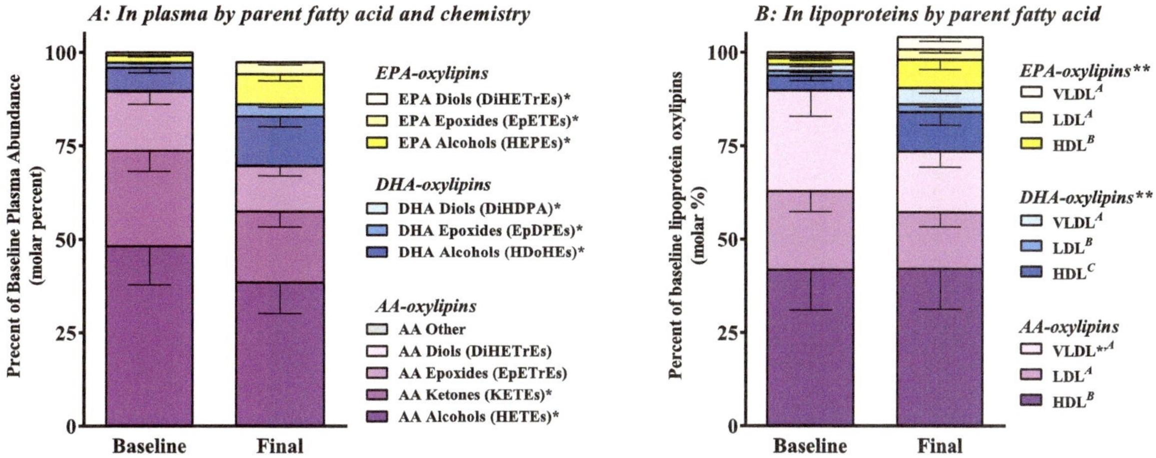

Figure 1. Distribution of oxylipins in plasma compartments. The distributions of oxylipins are expressed as a percent of the total baseline abundance before and after treatment. **A:** Oxylipins in plasma by parent fatty acid and chemistry, regardless of distribution in HDL, LDL, VLDL, or 'free'. A mixed-model ANOVA was used for each FA. **B:** Oxylipins in lipoprotein by parent fatty acid, regardless of chemistry. A mixed-model ANOVA was used for each FA pool. n = 14: LDL was not recovered for one subject, making total calculations impossible. *p<0.05, **p<0.0005 versus baseline. Letters (^{A,B,C}) indicate results of Tukey's HSD test for differences between lipoproteins. Those sharing a letter are not different.

of P-OM3 on the lipoprotein distribution of oxylipins, especially on certain pro- and anti-inflammatory, and on vasoactive oxylipins.

Methods

Participants & study location

The study was conducted by Sanford Research/USD in cooperation with physicians at Sanford Health. Our goal was to enroll subjects matching the inclusion/exclusion criteria used in the COMBOS trial [14] so our findings would reflect what occurred in that study. Accordingly, subjects on statin therapy with persistent hypertriglyceridemia were selected from the electronic medical records at Sanford Health and screened to ensure they met the COMBOS criteria (Figure S1 in File S1), then were contacted by letter and invited to participate. Responders were screened during a phone interview and, if qualifying, were sent to the study physician (VB) for a screening visit where clinical lipid and safety panels were drawn. Qualifying subjects returned one week later for a baseline visit after which they began P-OM3 therapy. They returned 63 days later for their final visit where compliance was assessed by pill count. Subjects were recruited from September 2009 to February 2010. The protocol was registered at clinicaltrials.gov (NCT00959842) and approved by the IRB at Sanford Research/USD and written informed consent was obtained prior to participation.

Study design

This was designed as a simple open-label, change-from-baseline study. Treatment was for 8 weeks with 4 g/day prescription omega-3 acid ethyl esters (P-OM3; Lovaza, GlaxoSmithKline). This dose provided 1,860 mg of EPA and 1,500 mg of DHA for a total of 3.4 g omega-3 FAs/day as acid ethyl esters for a total of 3.4 g omega-3 FAs/day. The dose is indicated in the USA for triglycerides >500 mg/dL and has variation on levels and purposing in other nations as well. Since P-OM3 affects the composition and concentration of the lipoproteins themselves (most notably VLDL), the oxylipin concentration was normalized to lipoprotein phospholipid in order to highlight how each lipoprotein's composition was affected. Our objectives were to 1) characterize lipoprotein-oxylipin at baseline and generally characterize the inflammatory and vascular activities; 2) demonstrate the effect of P-OM3 therapy on the per phospholipid (PL) concentration of omega-3 oxylipins (EPA & DHA derived) and omega-6 oxylipins (AA derived) in HDL, LDL and VLDL as well as plasma. We also tested whether P-OM3 treatment: 3) increased the abundance of CYP-epoxygenase oxylipins over LOX oxylipins; 4) changed the abundance of oxylipins within the CYP-epxoygenase pathway as measured by the epoxide/diol ratio at each measured FA-double bond position; and 5) changed the abundance of oxylipins within the LOX pathway as measured by the mid-chain alcohol/ketone ratio at each measured FA-double bond position. Our interest was to investigate the plausibility of lipid mediators in mediating effects, not interventional efficacy. Thus, we operated under IND-exemption and specifically did not analyze by "intent-to-treat." We measured the octadecanoic oxylipins (LA- and αLA-derived), but report these results in supplemental documents (since this study focused on AA-, EPA- and DHA-derived oxylipins.

Plasma lipids

Plasma samples for lipoprotein composition were frozen in 20% sucrose. A single overnight spin recovered VLDL in a PBS fraction above the sucrose, and LDL in the sucrose gradient. HDL was further fractionated using FPLC on a Sepharose 6 10/300 GL column (GE Lifesciences, Upsala Sweden) [15]. Cholesterol, phospholipids, triglycerides and total proteins were measured using standard colorimetric assays, SDS-PAGE was used as a quality control [16].

Fatty acids

The fatty acid composition of each lipoprotein fraction was measured as previously reported [17].

Oxylipins

The esterified oxylipin composition of each lipoprotein fraction was determined as previously described for plasma [18].

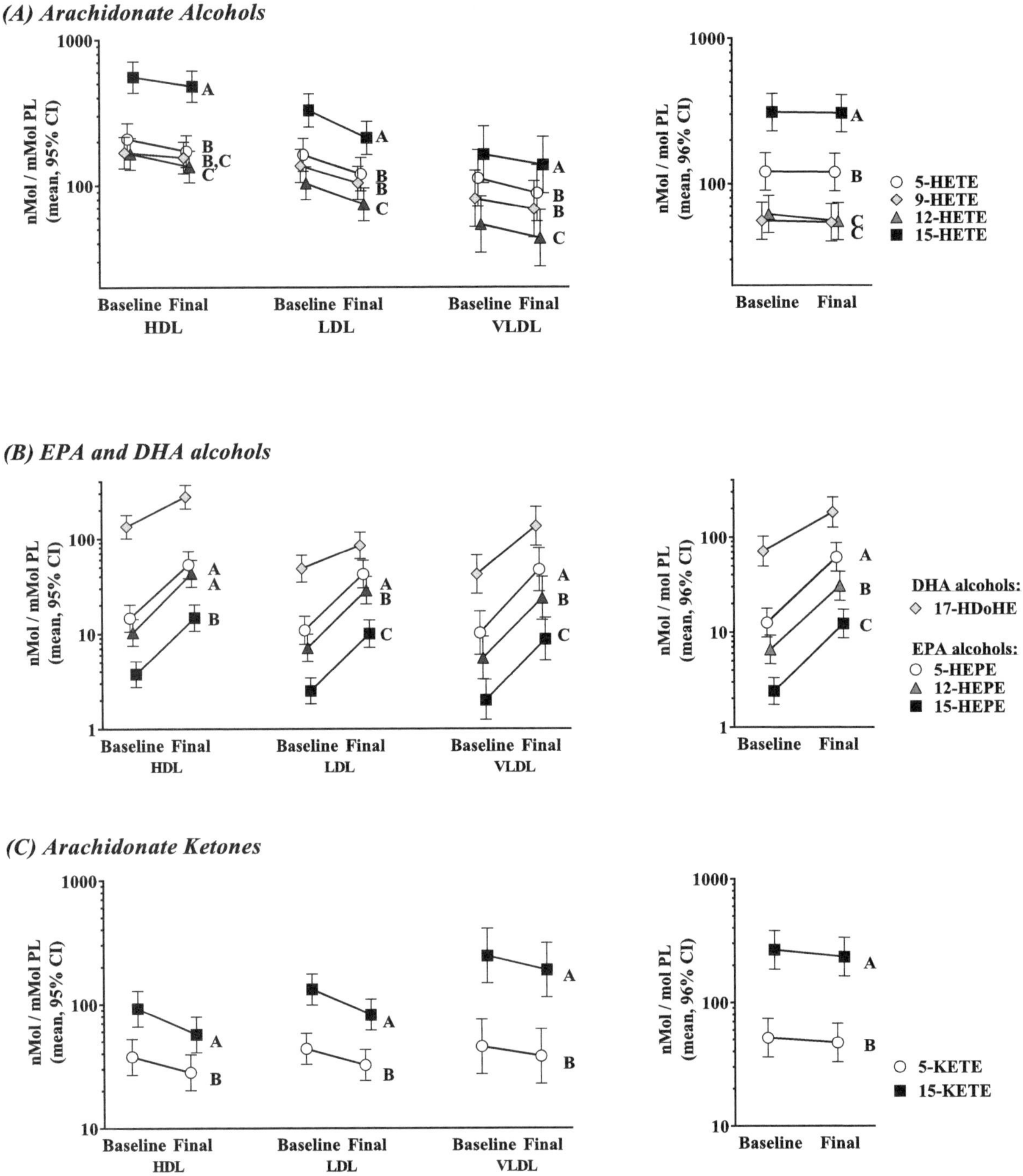

Figure 2. Distribution of fatty acid alcohols and ketones. The per-phospholipid concentration of mid-chain alcohols as AA-derived HETEs (**A**), EPA-derived HEPEs (**B**), DHA-derived HDoHEs (**B**) and AA-derived ketones (**C**) are shown in lipoproteins and plasma. Regioisomers are shaped and shaded by our best estimate of homologous double-bond positions across all figures. HETEs are mainly products of LOX, but are also products of CYP and autooxidation. KETEs are the HETE-dehydrogenase product of HETEs. Values for EPA and DHA ketones were not available. The effect of P-OM3 adjusted for age and sex was uniform regardless of regioisomer. The mean adjusted effects are shown graphically in Figure S2 in File S1; A mixed model ANOVA was used to test for differences on ln[nM oxylipin/mM PL]. The least-squares mean [95% CI] are shown. Tukey's HSD test was used for post hoc differences between regioisomer levels, and regioisomers sharing a letter are not different. Since no interactions were significant, the term was dropped and the parameter estimate was used to calculate a mean difference [95% CI]. Note that since the test was on log-transformed data, the effect is a proportional one (*i.e.* percent change). Note the log scale of the *y*-axis. Note that EPA and DHA oxylipins are shown on the same graphs for brevity, but constitute separate ANOVA tests. [a]9-HETE is an autooxidative product and is not formed by LOX.

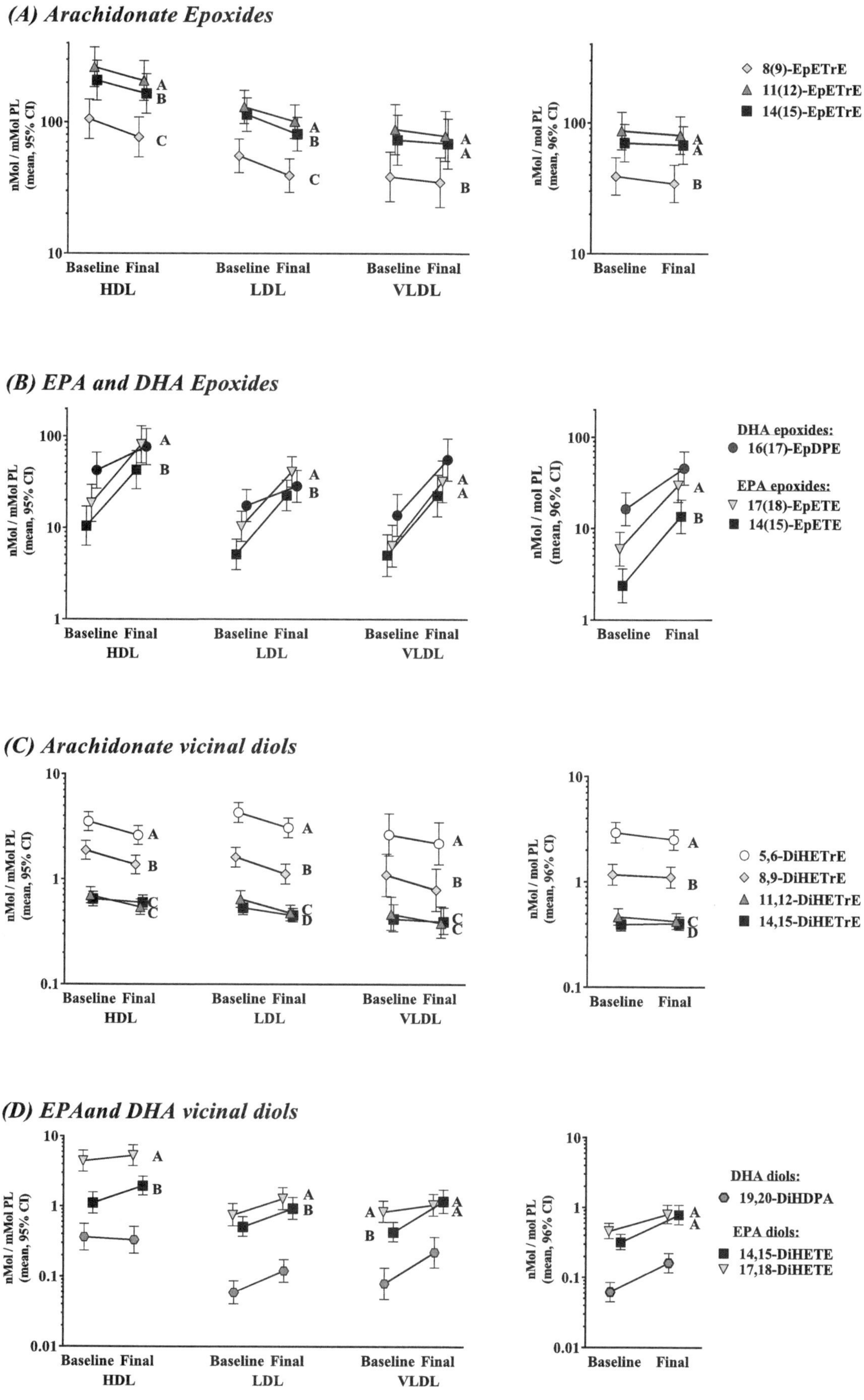
(A) Arachidonate Epoxides
nMol / mMol PL (mean, 95% CI)
nMol / mol PL (mean, 96% CI)
Baseline Final
HDL
LDL
VLDL
8(9)-EpETrE
11(12)-EpETrE
14(15)-EpETrE
(B) EPA and DHA Epoxides
DHA epoxides:
16(17)-EpDPE
EPA epoxides:
17(18)-EpETE
14(15)-EpETE
(C) Arachidonate vicinal diols
5,6-DiHETrE
8,9-DiHETrE
11,12-DiHETrE
14,15-DiHETrE
(D) EPAand DHA vicinal diols
DHA diols:
19,20-DiHDPA
EPA diols:
14,15-DiHETE
17,18-DiHETE

Figure 3. Distribution of fatty acids epoxides and vicinal diols. The per-phospholipid concentrations of epoxides as AA-derived EpETrEs (**A**), EPA-derived EpETEs (**B**), DHA-derived EpDPEs (**B**) AA-derived DiHETrEs (**C**), EPA-derived Di HETEs (**D**), and DHA-derived DiHDPAs (**D**) are shown in lipoproteins and plasma. Regioisomers are color coded by our best estimate of homologous double-bond positions across all figures. Epoxides are products of CYP-epoxygenase and can also be generated via autooxidation. Vicinal diols are the unique products of soluble epoxide hydrolase on epoxides. The effect of P-OM3 adjusted for age and sex was uniform regardless of regioisomer. The mean adjusted effects are shown graphically in Figure S2 in File S1; A mixed model ANOVA was used to test for differences on ln[nM oxylipin/mM PL]. The least-squares mean [95% CI] are shown. Tukey's HSD test was used for post hoc differences between regioisomer levels, and regioisomers sharing a letter are not different. Since no interactions were significant, the term was dropped and the parameter estimate was used to calculate a mean effect [95% CI]. Note that since the test was on log-transformed data, the effect is a proportional one (*i.e.* percent change). Note the log scale of the *y*-axis. Note that EPA and DHA oxylipins are shown on the same graph for brevity, but constitute separate ANOVA tests.

Statistical methods

Differences were assessed using mixed model ANOVAs adjusting for age and sex since these are known to affect lipoprotein outcomes. A natural logarithmic transformation was used to stabilize the variance and reduce skewness. Geometric means and 95% confidence intervals for baseline and follow-up were calculated for each treatment group. True effect size after accounting for age and sex are derived from the indicator parameter estimate and its standard error. Since logarithmic transformations were used, the effects are best understood as proportional, or percent, changes. If the interaction p-value was less than 0.2, the interaction was maintained in the model, otherwise it was dropped in order to obtain a pooled estimate of the treatment effect. JMP Pro 9.0.2 was used for statistical tests except where specified as using GraphPad Prism 6.01.

Results

Participant flow, baseline characteristics & blood lipids

A diagram representing subject flow is given in Figure S1 in File S1. Compliance was high, with 93% (91, 95) of pills administered taken on average; no subjects took less than 80%. In comparison to the COMBOS trial's active group, subjects in our study had lower serum TGs (282 *vs.* 237) and HDL-C (47 *vs.* 38) respectively [14] (Table 1). P-OM3 decreased plasma triglycerides by 49 (81, 17) mg/dL, VLDL-cholesterol by 9.7 mg/dL, and plasma phospholipids by 58 (90, 26) mg/dL. While oxylipins are incorporated into the PL, TG, and CE components of lipoproteins, those with 20+ carbons (eicosanoids and docosanoids) are primarily found in PL [13]. No survey has yet investigated oxylipin distribution among lipoprotein-lipids, however adjusting the data by fractional PL concentration resulted in the largest reduction in Aikake's corrected information criteria (AICc) for every oxylipin and lipoprotein fraction. Thus, oxylipins were normalized to PL using a molecular weight of 784 mg/mmol. The octadecanoids presented in Table S1 in File S2 should be interpreted cautiously since, based on unpublished findings in rodent models, we believe they are also prevalent in triglyceride and cholesterol esters. Adjustments for sex and age were rarely significant.

Plasma oxylipin distribution

Plasma oxylipins at baseline were primarily represented by AA-alcohols (HETEs), secondly by AA-ketones (KETEs), thirdly by AA-epoxides (EpETrEs), and then by EPA- and DHA-oxylipins (Figure 1). Since the change in AA-alcohols, AA-Ketones, and AA-epoxides was the same ($p_{interaction} = 0.93$), the pooled estimate for reduction in AA-oxylipins was −23% |−33, −12|, $p = 0.0003$. Vicinal diols and other AA-oxylipins (not visible) followed the same trend however we did not formally test them since their lower abundance meant different variance. EPA pools were likewise uniformly expanded by 322% |241, 422|, $p < 0.0001$, and DHA pools by 123% |80, 176|, $p < 0.0001$; (EPA $p_{interaction} = 0.70$ and DHA $p_{interaction} = 0.71$). Treatment with P-OM3 reduced both the total and proportional abundance of AA-oxylipins, and increased the amount of EPA- and DHA-oxylipins.

Similar patterns emerged when oxylipins were analyzed by lipoprotein. Since the change in AA-oxylipins in HDL appeared to be distinct from that of VLDL ($p_{interaction\ Visit\ \times\ HDL} = 0.07$), we estimated the changes separately for each lipoprotein pool of AA-oxylipins. AA-oxylipins did not decrease in HDL 0% |−20, +17|, $p_{unadjusted} = 0.97$, or in LDL −18% |−42, +2|, $p_{unadjusted} = 0.11$, however they did decrease in VLDL by −15% |−28, −3|, $p_{unadjusted} = 0.02$. EPA and DHA lipoprotein oxylipin pools were uniformly increased allowing for pooled estimates. EPA oxylipins increased by 308% |203, 450|, $p < 0.0001$, and DHA increased by 125% |68, 203|, $p < 0.0001$, regardless of lipoprotein. The complete set of oxylipins including regioisomers can be found in Table S1 in File S2.

Fatty-acid alcohols & ketones at baseline

The per-phospholipid concentration (nM oxylipin/mM PL) of AA, EPA and DHA mid-chain alcohols (HETEs, HEPEs, and HDoHEs respectively) at the baseline and final visits in HDL, LDL and VLDL are represented in Figure 2 and compared to plasma. P-OM3 did not affect the abundance of the regioisomers relative to each other (*e.g.* 5-HEPE to 15-HEPE). As previously reported [8], 15-HETE and 5-HETE were most abundant in plasma, but in lipoproteins 5-HETE was about as abundant as 9-HETE, an oxylipin that is not produced enzymatically and thought to be strictly an autooxidation product [19]. HDL contained the most HETEs per mole phospholipid and appears to represent the largest HETE pool in plasma. Among omega-3 alcohols, the DHA-derived 17-HDoHE was nearly as abundant as some HETEs in HDL and VLDL, but not in LDL. EPA- and DHA-alcohols both reflected the trend seen with HETEs, being most abundant in HDL followed by LDL then VLDL.

Mid-chain alcohols can be converted to ketones by HETE-dehydrogenase [20]. AA-ketones (KETEs) were present in each lipoprotein class in reverse order as alcohols, with VLDL>LDL>HDL (Figure 2).

Fatty acid epoxides & vicinal diols at baseline

Fatty acid epoxides are produced by CYP-epoxygenases, but can also be autooxidatively generated. With the exception of the 5(6)-EpETrE, they are hydrolyzed by soluble epoxide hydrolase to produce vicinal diols. Epoxides were present at much higher levels than diols and were most abundant in HDL followed by LDL and VLDL. 14(15)- and 11(12)-EpETrE were the most abundant epoxides followed by the 8(9)-EpETrE (Figure 3). The DHA-derived 16(17)-EpDPE was the next most abundant, followed by EPA-epoxides. Among vicinal diols, the most abundant AA-diol was the 5,6-DiHETrE, decreasing in abundance with progression toward the ω-terminus, in reverse order as epoxide abundances.

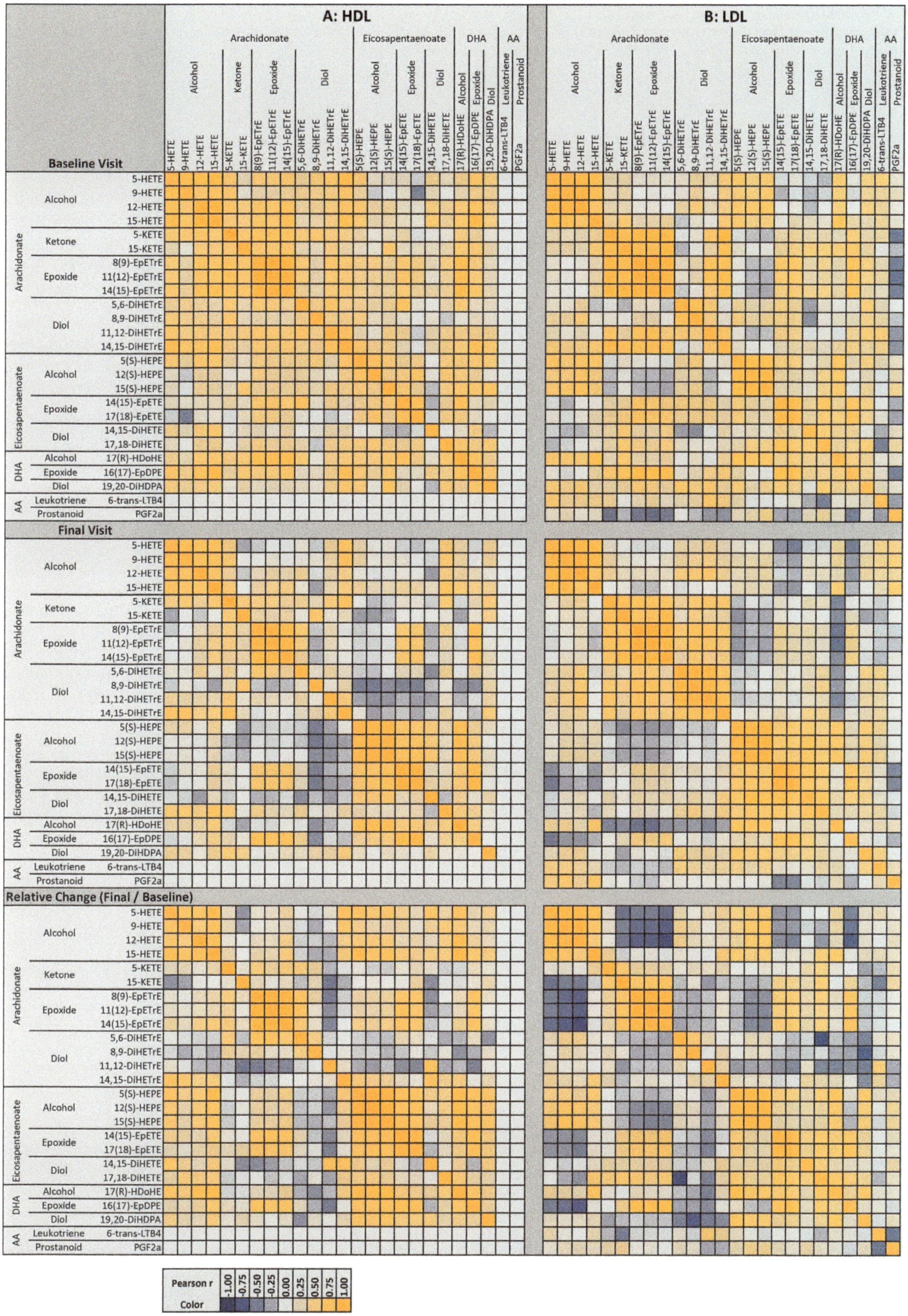
A: HDL
B: LDL
Arachidonate
Eicosapentaenoate
DHA
AA
Alcohol
Ketone
Epoxide
Diol
Leukotriene
Prostanoid
5-HETE
9-HETE
12-HETE
15-HETE
5-KETE
15-KETE
8(9)-EpETrE
11(12)-EpETrE
14(15)-EpETrE
5,6-DiHETrE
8,9-DiHETrE
11,12-DiHETrE
14,15-DiHETrE
5(S)-HEPE
12(S)-HEPE
15(S)-HEPE
14(15)-EpETE
17(18)-EpETE
14,15-DiHETE
17,18-DiHETE
17(R)-HDoHE
16(17)-EpDPE
19,20-DiHDPA
6-trans-LTB4
PGF2a
Baseline Visit
Final Visit
Relative Change (Final / Baseline)
Pearson r
Color
-1.00
-0.75
-0.50
-0.25
0.00
0.25
0.50
0.75
1.00

Figure 4. Correlation Heat Map for HDL and LDL. The Pearson correlation coefficient (r) among lipoprotein-oxylipins for HDL (**A**) and LDL (**B**) is shown before treatment **(top)**, after treatment **(middle)** as correlation of nM oxylipin/mM PL along with the change in oxylipins due to treatment **(bottom)** expressed as ln(nM oxylipin$_{final}$/mM PL$_{final}$)/ln(nM oxylipin$_{baseline}$/mM PL$_{baseline}$).

EPA diols were as, or more, abundant as AA-diols in many cases; the DHA-diol 19,20-DiHDPA was the least abundant.

Treatment effects

The effect of P-OM3 treatment on lipoprotein and plasma oxylipins are summarized by chemical class and parent fatty acid in Figure S2 in File S1.

With one exception (VLDL-EPA-diols) the effect of treatment within fatty-acid and chemical class was the same, regardless of regioisomer. For both lipoproteins and plasma, there was a large increase in EPA and DHA oxylipins. EPA-alcohols and epoxides were increased from 300–400% of control, roughly equivalent to the increase in red blood cell EPA. EPA-diols were not increased to the same extent as EPA-alcohols or EPA-epoxides, and in HDL, DHA-diols were not increased at all. DHA-alcohols and -epoxides were increased in LDL and HDL to between 150% and 210% of baseline, however among VLDL this was 320% (157, 652) and 404% (207, 790) for alcohols and epoxides respectively, meaning DHA-epoxides were present in VLDL beyond the simple increase in RBC-DHA abundance. The effect of treatment among EPA and DHA-diols was more complex. DHA-diols in HDL were not increased at all by treatment, however in LDL they were increased by about the same amount as RBC DHA. In VLDL, DHA-diols were increased even more so. EPA-diols were increased less than the increase in RBC-EPA. In VLDL, an increase occurred in only one of the two regioisomers measured (17,18-DiHETE). P-OM3 also lowered AA oxylipins, particularly in HDL and LDL.

Correlation of oxylipins with their parent (precursor) fatty acids by lipoprotein class

By demonstrating the association of oxylipins with their parent fatty acids, we help establish how amenable oxylipins are to precursor availability. Even at the baseline visit, EPA alcohols and epoxides were strongly related to erythrocyte EPA content, and this association persisted after treatment (Table S2 in File S2). DHA showed some similarities to EPA in association with DHA-oxylipins, however this dependence was reduced after treatment.

Loss of correlation among oxylipin species by lipoprotein class

The Pearson correlation matrices before and after P-OM3 treatment are presented in Figures 4 and 5. These matrices are useful in describing the independence of oxylipins species. At their baseline visit, the median |inter-quartile range| correlation among plasma oxylipins was 0.59 |0.39, 0.72|, a relatively strong interdependence of oxylipins, irrespective of parent FA or chemistry class. HDL and LDL oxylipins (Figure 4) were more independent; LDL oxylipins were the most independent ($r = 0.32$ |0.09, 0.55|), with nearly as much independence among HDL oxylipins, 0.44 |0.25, 0.59|. VLDL were the most interdependent, with strong correlations ($r = 0.85$ |0.77, 0.91| among nearly every oxylipin (Figure 5). P-OM3 treatment disrupted these interdependencies, demonstrated also by a shift in the distribution of correlation coefficients (Figure S3 in File S1). The effect was most pronounced among VLDL oxylipins, in which the correlations dropped by 0.52 to 0.33 |0.11, 0.66|, meaning oxylipins were less dependent one another and therefore reflective of more than one latent factor. In a similar manner, the median correlation also dropped among HDL and plasma oxylipins, to 020 |−0.03, 0.49| and 0.34 |0.11, 0.61| respectively, but dropped more moderately in LDL, by 0.08 to 0.24 |0.01, 0.49|.

Comparison of LOX versus CYP pathway metabolites

The products of two major fatty-acid oxygenation pathways are prominently represented in the data; LOX and CYP. A formal means to test whether P-OM3 affects the relative activities is to test the effect of treatment on the ratio of epoxides to alcohols by lipoprotein and by modification position; for instance, an increase in the 11(12)-EpETrE to 12-HETE ratio can be interpreted as increased CYP-epoxygenase pathway activity relative to the 12-LOX pathway.

Among AA metabolites, the relative abundance of epoxides to alcohols was dependent upon the position of the modification and the lipoprotein ($p_{interaction} = 0.002$). Specifically, there was no difference between plasma and any lipoproteins at the 11/12 position, however the abundance of 14(15)-EpETrE relative to 15-HETE was uniquely low in plasma compared to that in lipoproteins.

Among the metabolites of EPA, no differences in plasma and lipoproteins were present, however unlike AA metabolites, epoxides were overall more abundant than alcohols and so the pooled epoxide: alcohol ratio in lipoproteins was 2.62 (2.05, 3.35) compared to 0.77 (0.87, 0.93) for AA. This suggests that some biological process key to the appearance of epoxides in lipoproteins favors EPA, whereas AA is favored in producing alcohols. While EPA-epoxides were more abundant than alcohols at the "same" double bond (*i.e.* ω–*x* double bond; see Figure S4 in File S1) compared to AA-epoxides, further examination of this phenomenon revealed that the structural consistency was the number of vicinal double bonds; like the 14(15)-EpETE, which was the only epoxide:alcohol measured in the EPA-oxylipin family, the AA-derived 11(12)-EpETrE has 2 vicinal double bonds and also outnumbers alcohols (Figure S4 in File S1). Among other FAs, alcohols outnumbered epoxides (*i.e.* the ratio <1). Treatment had no effect on the ratio for any FA family.

Intra-pathway precursor/product ratios

As with comparisons of different pathways, within-pathway effects can be estimated using product:precursor ratios. Here, effects on the CYP-epoxygenase pathway was measured using the diol:epoxide ratio (Figure S5 in File S1) and effects on the LOX pathway as ketone:alcohol ratios (Figure S5 in File S1). Treatment had no effect on arachidonate diol:epoxide ratios, which were especially low at the 14/15 and the 11/12 position. Treatment increased the diol:epoxide ratio at the 14,15 position of EPA by 84% |48, 130| and by 152% |101, 217| at the 17,18 position. Further, AA-epoxides were most abundant in HDL compared to plasma and other lipoproteins; among EPA-epoxides it was either the same (14/15 position) or reduced (17/18 position).

The distribution of alcohols and ketones among lipoproteins was more complex than with CYP pathway products and treatment had no effect. Among metabolites at the 5 position, HDL had the highest relative abundance of alcohols, followed by LDL then VLDL and plasma. Metabolites at the 15 position were more varied among lipoproteins, with HDL having a higher relative

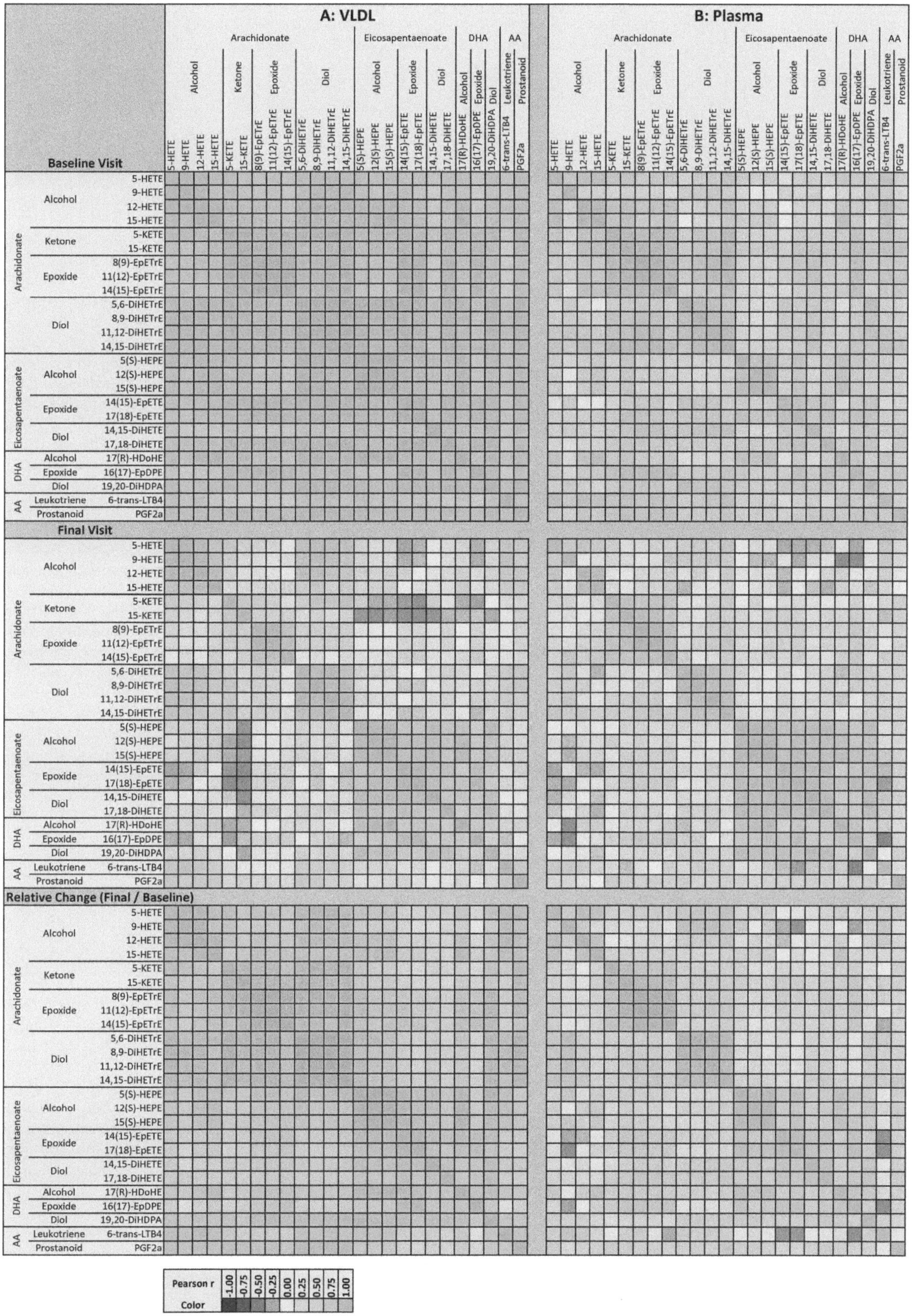
A: VLDL
B: Plasma
Arachidonate
Eicosapentaenoate
DHA
AA
Alcohol
Ketone
Epoxide
Diol
Leukotriene
Prostanoid
5-HETE
9-HETE
12-HETE
15-HETE
5-KETE
15-KETE
8(9)-EpETrE
11(12)-EpETrE
14(15)-EpETrE
5,6-DiHETrE
8,9-DiHETrE
11,12-DiHETrE
14,15-DiHETrE
5(S)-HEPE
12(S)-HEPE
15(S)-HEPE
14(15)-EpETE
17(18)-EpETE
14,15-DiHETE
17,18-DiHETE
17(R)-HDoHE
16(17)-EpDPE
19,20-DiHDPA
6-trans-LTB4
PGF2a
Baseline Visit
Final Visit
Relative Change (Final / Baseline)
Pearson r
Color
-1.00
-0.75
-0.50
-0.25
0.00
0.25
0.50
0.75
1.00

Figure 5. Correlation Heat Map for VLDL and whole plasma-oxylipins. The Pearson correlation coefficient (r) among lipoprotein-oxylipins for VLDL (**A**) and whole plasma oxylipins (**B**) is shown before treatment **(top)**, after treatment **(middle)** as correlation of nM oxylipin/mM PL along with the change in oxylipins due to treatment **(bottom)** expressed as ln(nM $oxylipin_{final}$/mM PL_{final})/ln(nM $oxylipin_{baseline}$/mM $PL_{baseline}$).

abundance of alcohols, followed by LDL, then plasma, then VLDL, in which ketones actually outnumbered alcohols.

Discussion

The transport of oxylipins by lipoproteins has profound mechanistic implications since it reveals a non-local source of lipid mediators that could exert an effect on tissues. Here we used a targeted lipidomic investigation of lipoprotein oxylipins to demonstrate abundant, pro-inflammatory oxylipins in lipoproteins at baseline. Based on the general activity of the various oxylipins, we also demonstrate redistribution toward a less inflammatory profile in response to treatment with omega-3 FAs. Notably, this was observed in subjects with LDL-C at NCEP goals and whose LDL-C was unaffected by P-OM3.

This is the first lipidomic characterization of human lipoprotein-oxylipins. At baseline, VLDL, LDL, and HDL each have unique, characteristic oxylipins. Among LOX pathway products, HDL is enriched in mid-chain alcohols while VLDL is enriched in ketones. These lipoproteins could thus deliver LOX metabolites [10,21] to their tissue targets, bypassing the local requirement for LOX activity. If true, it has implications for transcellular biosynthesis of 5-LOX metabolites such as leukotrienes and ketones. Similar activity has been noted [22] however a role for lipoproteins in delivering intermediates has not. The different composition of VLDL compared to HDL indicates each fraction would deliver different intermediates, and so have different actions: by delivering mid-chain alcohols, HDL could bypass the specific requirement for 5-LOX activity; however by delivering ketones, VLDL could additionally bypass the requirement for HETE-dehydrogenase and directly activate the OXE-receptor (*i.e.* TG1019, R527 and hGPCR48) [23]. Among LOX pathways, 5-LOX is known for its pro-inflammatory effects and 5-HETE, the AA product, is inflammatory and pro-atherogenic [24]. The same may not be true of its EPA homolog 5-HEPE, which has insulin sensitizing properties in animal models [25]. The difference in activities illustrates one means by which increasing the abundance of EPA oxylipins could have beneficial effects, especially when doing so at the expense of the AA homolog. The bioactivities of other LOX pathways are more difficult to summarize because their effects are less consistently pro- or anti-inflammatory. 12-LOX is generally considered pro-inflammatory, with activities such as mediation of endoplasmic reticulum stress and IL-12 secretion in adipocytes by 12-HETE (a 12-LOX product) [26], it may also have beneficial effects [27]. Unfortunately, a more pragmatic reason such comparisons can't be made is that in most cases only AA-metabolites have been studied. This makes it difficult to predict the effect of increasing EPA and DHA homologs.

A second major pathway covered is the CYP-epoxygenase pathway, whose fatty acid epoxides have potent vaso-protective activities, including protection from both septic [28] and hypertensive vascular diseases [29]. Fatty acid epoxides act on resistance vessels to produce an endothelial hyperpolarizing effect [30], and EC_{50} estimates are available in the same model for AA-, EPA- and DHA-epoxides [31,32]. These studies offer a means to estimate the impact of P-OM3 treatment. Table 2 shows the hypothetical vasodilatory capacity of each lipoprotein, indicating that the benefit of P-OM3 treatment on measured epoxides is uniquely increased in VLDL. Imputing values and activities to unmeasured regioisomers (Table S3 in File S2) based on biochemical relationships observed in prior work [33] yields similar results. The former, empirical approach (Table 2) indicates an increased vasodilatory capacity among VLDL-epoxides, despite a 20% decrease in serum TG (*i.e.* VLDL). The imputed approach indicates increases in HDL and LDL, but again, the largest increase is in VLDL. Vasorelaxation is impaired in subjects with well controlled LDL-C and persistent hypertriglyceridemia [34], and VLDL contribute to the impairment [35]. Omega-3 FAs do not affect blood pressure in normotensive subjects, but induce a 7 mm Hg decrease in mean arterial when blood pressure is carefully measured (*i.e.* 24-hour ambulatory monitoring) in Stage 1 hypertensives [36]. More generally, they improve endothelial function in conjunction with lower serum TG [37,38]. Given the correspondence between the effects of epoxides on vasodilation and the effects of omega-3 FAs on blood pressure, VLDL-epoxides seem a plausible explanation for this effect, but without specifically enquiring the VLDL-oxylipin pool, this relationship might not appear in plasma and be missed.

The global impact of P-OM3 treatment on lipoprotein-oxylipins is indicated by the decreased interdependencies. Greater interdependency, by definition, means less independence among oxylipin associated signaling pathways, and consequently a constrained system. At baseline, oxylipins within each lipoprotein class were very interdependent as indicated by high correlations, most extremely so among VLDL, but also among HDL, LDL and plasma in whole. While a major effect of P-OM3 was to increase nearly every omega-3 oxylipin regardless of lipoprotein class, P-OM3 also reduced the covariance of lipoprotein-oxylipins as well. Correlations within chemistry and parent fatty acid groupings remained strong after treatment, however correlation between oxylipins of different chemistry or parent FAs were weakened, indicating increasing flexibility of the system's bioactivity. Increased independence was most notable among VLDL- and HDL-oxylipins, and less so among LDL-oxylipins. Since the subjects here are already treated to near optimal LDL-C levels, it is unknown whether this is a natural feature of LDL, or a consequence of statin therapy. Surprisingly, only EPA abundance was strongly related to the observed abundance of EPA derived oxylipins, suggesting that factors other than simple precursor abundance are also responsible for the presence of oxylipins.

P-OM3 induced changes consistent with reduced inflammatory stress and a more flexible response to new stressors but the well known destinations of the lipoproteins themselves must also inform analyses since the destinations of lipoprotein-oxylipins reflect their parent lipoprotein. Thus, a complete understanding will require leveraging knowledge of oxylipin biology with that of lipoprotein-lipid trafficking. Most simplistically, this means hypothesizing directional transport of VLDL-oxylipins to peripheral tissues *via* lipoprotein lipase or receptor-mediated uptake, implying the myocardium, skeletal muscle and adipose are the primary recipients of VLDL-oxylipins. Conversely, for HDL it means peripheral acquisition of oxylipins from tissues by PL and cholesterol uptake followed by reverse transport to hepatocytes. Such an approach would go far in explaining the high abundance of pro-inflammatory oxylipins in HDL, a lipoprotein well known for its vaso-protective, anti-inflammatory effects: given HDL

Table 2. Estimation of changes in lipoprotein-epoxide bioactivity.[a]

	Net potency for vasodilation[b]							
	HDL		LDL		VLDL		Plasma	
	Bs	Final	Bs	Final	Bs	Final	Bs	Final
Net AA [32]	0.99	0.77	0.52	0.38	0.34	0.31	0.33	0.31
Net EPA [32]	0.09	0.37	0.05	0.19	0.03	0.15	0.03	0.13
Net DHA [31]	0.07	0.14	0.03	0.05	0.02	0.10	0.03	0.08
Total	1.15	1.27	0.59	0.62	0.40	0.56	0.39	0.52
Percent-change		+11%		+4%		+42%		+34%

[a]unmeasured epoxides not included in calculation. Number of unmeasured epoxides: AA = 1, EPA = 3, DHA = 6. A table accounting for bioactivities of unmeasured epoxides by imputation is included in Table S3 in File S2.
[b]Net potency measured as Σ -EC_{50}×$[Epoxide]_{measured}$ as reported by Ye *et al* & Zhang *et al.*
Note: potencies are measured in nM^2/mM PL. Abbreviation: Bs – Baseline.

removal of oxylipins from peripheral tissues, the higher levels of HDL-HETEs and HDL-HODEs are consistent with more removal from peripheral tissues, and so provide a basis for the anti-inflammatory effect of HDL. Prior evidence in VLDL-oxylipins are consistent. The release of oxylipins from VLDL by LpL combined with the effect of lipolysis products on endothelial inflammation [21] support the use of lipoprotein lipid trafficking as a guide [10]. Further, unique bioactivities of lipoprotein lipolysis products by various LpL-family lipase/lipoprotein combinations on PPARs [39–42] suggest further study of each lipid pool (*i.e.* PL, cholesterol, TG, *etc.*) would increase the fidelity of findings.

Limitations

This was a change from baseline study, meaning that we did not control for regression-to-the-mean effects by use of a placebo group. We attempted to control for this effect by requiring two prior high TG samples and a qualifying plasma sample with high TGs. In the COMBOS trial, TG in the placebo group was 3.5% lower after treatment, compared to a 49% decrease with active treatment in this study, suggesting the regression to the mean effect is small for lipoprotein lipids. While regression-to-the-mean effect sizes for oxylipins are unknown, prior studies indicate they are small however we cannot rule this out. As products of polyunsaturated fatty acids, it is possible that saturation of fatty acids in the acceptor lipid pools limits the impact of P-OM3, especially on EPA- and DHA-oxylipins.

Conclusion

The oxylipin composition of each lipoprotein is unique, dependent on parent fatty acid and generating enzymatic pathways. Omega-3 fatty acids reduce pro-inflammatory species (*i.e.* HETEs) and increase anti-inflammatory species (*i.e.* EpETEs). These findings demonstrate a plausible mechanism for reducing cardiovascular risk by modulating lipoprotein-oxylipins.

Supporting Information

Checklist S1 Trend checklist.

File S1 Supporting figures.

File S2 Supporting tables.

File S3 Supplemental list of abbreviations.

Protocol S1 Study protocol.

Acknowledgments

All opinions expressed in this manuscript represent the views of the researchers and not necessarily those of the USDA. The USDA is an equal opportunity provider and employer.

Author Contributions

Conceived and designed the experiments: GCS JWN. Performed the experiments: JWN TLP VRB WSH GCS. Analyzed the data: JWN TLP GCS. Contributed reagents/materials/analysis tools: JWN TLP GCS. Wrote the paper: GCS JWN.

References

1. (2001) Executive Summary of The Third Report of The National Cholesterol Education Program (NCEP) Expert Panel on Detection, Evaluation, And Treatment of High Blood Cholesterol In Adults (Adult Treatment Panel III). JAMA 285: 2486–2497.
2. Grundy SM, Cleeman JI, Merz CN, Brewer HB Jr, Clark LT, et al. (2004) Implications of recent clinical trials for the National Cholesterol Education Program Adult Treatment Panel III guidelines. Circulation 110: 227–239.
3. Perk J, De Backer G, Gohlke H, Graham I, Reiner Z, et al. (2012) European Guidelines on cardiovascular disease prevention in clinical practice (version 2012): The Fifth Joint Task Force of the European Society of Cardiology and Other Societies on Cardiovascular Disease Prevention in Clinical Practice (constituted by representatives of nine societies and by invited experts). Atherosclerosis.
4. Buczynski MW, Dumlao DS, Dennis EA (2009) Thematic Review Series: Proteomics. An integrated omics analysis of eicosanoid biology. J Lipid Res 50: 1015–1038.
5. Westphal C, Konkel A, Schunck WH (2011) CYP-eicosanoids—a new link between omega-3 fatty acids and cardiac disease? Prostaglandins Other Lipid Mediat 96: 99–108.
6. Serhan CN (2002) Lipoxins and aspirin-triggered 15-epi-lipoxin biosynthesis: an update and role in anti-inflammation and pro-resolution. Prostaglandins Other Lipid Mediat 68–69: 433–455.
7. Mozaffarian D, Wu JH (2011) Omega-3 fatty acids and cardiovascular disease: effects on risk factors, molecular pathways, and clinical events. J Am Coll Cardiol 58: 2047–2067.
8. Keenan AH, Pedersen TL, Fillaus K, Larson MK, Shearer GC, et al. (2012) Basal omega-3 fatty acid status affects fatty acid and oxylipin responses to high-dose n3-HUFA in healthy volunteers. J Lipid Res.
9. Shearer GC, Harris WS, Pedersen TL, Newman JW (2010) Detection of omega-3 oxylipins in human plasma and response to treatment with omega-3 acid ethyl esters. J Lipid Res 51: 2074–2081.
10. Shearer GC, Newman JW (2008) Lipoprotein lipase releases esterified oxylipins from very low-density lipoproteins. Prostaglandins Leukot Essent Fatty Acids 79: 215–222.
11. Newman JW, Kaysen GA, Hammock BD, Shearer GC (2007) Proteinuria increases oxylipid concentrations in VLDL and HDL but not LDL particles in the rat. J Lipid Res 48: 1792–1800.
12. Stenson WF, Parker CW (1979) 12-L-hydroxy-5,8,10,14-eicosatetraenoic acid, a chemotactic fatty acid, is incorporated into neutrophil phospholipids and triglyceride. Prostaglandins 18: 285–292.
13. Fang X, Weintraub NL, Stoll LL, Spector AA (1999) Epoxyeicosatrienoic acids increase intracellular calcium concentration in vascular smooth muscle cells. Hypertension 34: 1242–1246.
14. Davidson MH, Stein EA, Bays HE, Maki KC, Doyle RT, et al. (2007) Efficacy and tolerability of adding prescription omega-3 fatty acids 4 g/d to simvastatin 40 mg/d in hypertriglyceridemic patients: an 8-week, randomized, double-blind, placebo-controlled study. Clin Ther 29: 1354–1367.
15. Innis-Whitehouse W, Li X, Brown WV, Le NA (1998) An efficient chromatographic system for lipoprotein fractionation using whole plasma. J Lipid Res 39: 679–690.
16. Shearer GC, Newman JW, Hammock BD, Kaysen GA (2005) Graded effects of proteinuria on HDL structure in nephrotic rats. J Am Soc Nephrol 16: 1309–1319.
17. Shearer GC, Chen J, Chen Y, Harris WS (2009) Myocardial infarction does not affect fatty-acid profiles in rats. Prostaglandins Leukot Essent Fatty Acids 81: 411–416.
18. Gladine C, Newman JW, Durand T, Pedersen TL, Galano JM, et al. (2014) Lipid profiling following intake of the omega 3 fatty acid DHA identifies the peroxidized metabolites F4-neuroprostanes as the best predictors of atherosclerosis prevention. PLoS One 9: e89393.
19. Mallat Z, Nakamura T, Ohan J, Leseche G, Tedgui A, et al. (1999) The relationship of hydroxyeicosatetraenoic acids and F2-isoprostanes to plaque instability in human carotid atherosclerosis. J Clin Invest 103: 421–427.
20. Erlemann KR, Rokach J, Powell WS (2004) Oxidative stress stimulates the synthesis of the eosinophil chemoattractant 5-oxo-6,8,11,14-eicosatetraenoic acid by inflammatory cells. J Biol Chem 279: 40376–40384.
21. Wang L, Gill R, Pedersen TL, Higgins LJ, Newman JW, et al. (2009) Triglyceride-rich lipoprotein lipolysis releases neutral and oxidized FFAs that induce endothelial cell inflammation. J Lipid Res 50: 204–213.
22. Zarini S, Gijon MA, Ransome AE, Murphy RC, Sala A (2009) Transcellular biosynthesis of cysteinyl leukotrienes in vivo during mouse peritoneal inflammation. Proc Natl Acad Sci U S A 106: 8296–8301.
23. Grant GE, Rokach J, Powell WS (2009) 5-Oxo-ETE and the OXE receptor. Prostaglandins Other Lipid Mediat 89: 98–104.
24. Whatling C, McPheat W, Herslof M (2007) The potential link between atherosclerosis and the 5-lipoxygenase pathway: investigational agents with new implications for the cardiovascular field. Expert Opin Investig Drugs 16: 1879–1893.
25. Kogure R, Toyama K, Hiyamuta S, Kojima I, Takeda S (2011) 5-Hydroxy-eicosapentaenoic acid is an endogenous GPR119 agonist and enhances glucose-dependent insulin secretion. Biochem Biophys Res Commun 416: 58–63.
26. Cole BK, Kuhn NS, Green-Mitchell SM, Leone KA, Raab RM, et al. (2012) 12/15-Lipoxygenase signaling in the endoplasmic reticulum stress response. Am J Physiol Endocrinol Metab 302: E654–665.
27. Wittwer J, Hersberger M (2007) The two faces of the 15-lipoxygenase in atherosclerosis. Prostaglandins Leukot Essent Fatty Acids 77: 67–77.
28. Schmelzer KR, Kubala L, Newman JW, Kim IH, Eiserich JP, et al. (2005) Soluble epoxide hydrolase is a therapeutic target for acute inflammation. Proc Natl Acad Sci U S A 102: 9772–9777.
29. Neckar J, Kopkan L, Huskova Z, Kolar F, Papousek F, et al. (2012) Inhibition of soluble epoxide hydrolase by cis-4-[4-(3-adamantan-1-ylureido)cyclohexyl-oxy]-benzoic acid exhibits antihypertensive and cardioprotective actions in transgenic rats with angiotensin II-dependent hypertension. Clin Sci (Lond) 122: 513–525.
30. Larsen BT, Zhang DX, Gutterman DD (2007) Epoxyeicosatrienoic acids, TRP channels, and intracellular Ca2+ in the vasculature: an endothelium-derived endothelium-hyperpolarizing factor? Arterioscler Thromb Vasc Biol 27: 2496–2498.
31. Ye D, Zhang D, Oltman C, Dellsperger K, Lee HC, et al. (2002) Cytochrome p-450 epoxygenase metabolites of docosahexaenoate potently dilate coronary arterioles by activating large-conductance calcium-activated potassium channels. J Pharmacol Exp Ther 303: 768–776.
32. Zhang Y, Oltman CL, Lu T, Lee HC, Dellsperger KC, et al. (2001) EET homologs potently dilate coronary microvessels and activate BK(Ca) channels. Am J Physiol Heart Circ Physiol 280: H2430–2440.
33. Newman JW, Hammock BD (2001) Optimized thiol derivatizing reagent for the mass spectral analysis of disubstituted epoxy fatty acids. J Chromatogr A 925: 223–240.
34. Lewis TV, Dart AM, Chin-Dusting JP (1999) Endothelium-dependent relaxation by acetylcholine is impaired in hypertriglyceridemic humans with normal levels of plasma LDL cholesterol. J Am Coll Cardiol 33: 805–812.
35. Norata GD, Pirillo A, Callegari E, Hamsten A, Catapano AL, et al. (2003) Gene expression and intracellular pathways involved in endothelial dysfunction induced by VLDL and oxidised VLDL. Cardiovasc Res 59: 169–180.
36. Prisco D, Paniccia R, Bandinelli B, Filippini M, Francalanci I, et al. (1998) Effect of medium-term supplementation with a moderate dose of n-3 polyunsaturated fatty acids on blood pressure in mild hypertensive patients. Thromb Res 91: 105–112.
37. Mori TA, Watts GF, Burke V, Hilme E, Puddey IB, et al. (2000) Differential effects of eicosapentaenoic acid and docosahexaenoic acid on vascular reactivity of the forearm microcirculation in hyperlipidemic, overweight men. Circulation 102: 1264–1269.
38. Goodfellow J, Bellamy MF, Ramsey MW, Jones CJ, Lewis MJ (2000) Dietary supplementation with marine omega-3 fatty acids improve systemic large artery endothelial function in subjects with hypercholesterolemia. J Am Coll Cardiol 35: 265–270.
39. Ziouzenkova O, Perrey S, Asatryan L, Hwang J, MacNaul KL, et al. (2003) Lipolysis of triglyceride-rich lipoproteins generates PPAR ligands: evidence for an antiinflammatory role for lipoprotein lipase. Proc Natl Acad Sci U S A 100: 2730–2735.
40. Ruby MA, Goldenson B, Orasanu G, Johnston TP, Plutzky J, et al. (2010) VLDL hydrolysis by LPL activates PPAR-alpha through generation of unbound fatty acids. J Lipid Res 51: 2275–2281.
41. Brown JD, Oligino E, Rader DJ, Saghatelian A, Plutzky J (2011) VLDL hydrolysis by hepatic lipase regulates PPARdelta transcriptional responses. PLoS One 6: e21209.
42. Ahmed W, Orasanu G, Nehra V, Asatryan L, Rader DJ, et al. (2006) High-density lipoprotein hydrolysis by endothelial lipase activates PPARalpha: a candidate mechanism for high-density lipoprotein-mediated repression of leukocyte adhesion. Circ Res 98: 490–498.

7

Inhibition of Platelet Activation and Thrombus Formation by Adenosine and Inosine: Studies on Their Relative Contribution and Molecular Modeling

Eduardo Fuentes[1,2]*, Jaime Pereira[3], Diego Mezzano[3], Marcelo Alarcón[1,2], Julio Caballero[4], Iván Palomo[1,2]*

1 Department of Clinical Biochemistry and Immunohematology, Faculty of Health Sciences, Interdisciplinary Excellence Research Program on Healthy Aging (PIEI-ES), Universidad de Talca, Talca, Chile, **2** Centro de Estudios en Alimentos Procesados (CEAP), CONICYT-Regional, Gore Maule, Talca, Chile, **3** Department of Hematology-Oncology, School of Medicine, Pontificia Universidad Católica de Chile, Santiago, Chile, **4** Center for Bioinformatics and Molecular Simulations, Faculty of Engineering in Bioinformatics, Universidad de Talca, Talca, Chile

Abstract

Background: The inhibitory effect of adenosine on platelet aggregation is abrogated after the addition of adenosine-deaminase. Inosine is a naturally occurring nucleoside degraded from adenosine.

Objectives: The mechanisms of antiplatelet action of adenosine and inosine *in vitro* and *in vivo*, and their differential biological effects by molecular modeling were investigated.

Results: Adenosine (0.5, 1 and 2 mmol/L) inhibited phosphatidylserine exposure from 52±4% in the control group to 44±4 ($p<0.05$), 29±2 ($p<0.01$) and 20±3% ($p<0.001$). P-selectin expression in the presence of adenosine 0.5, 1 and 2 mmol/L was inhibited from 32±4 to 27±2 ($p<0.05$), 14±3 ($p<0.01$) and 9±3% ($p<0.001$), respectively. At the concentrations tested, only inosine to 4 mmol/L had effect on platelet P-selectin expression ($p<0.05$). Adenosine and inosine inhibited platelet aggregation and ATP release stimulated by ADP and collagen. Adenosine and inosine reduced collagen-induced platelet adhesion and aggregate formation under flow. At the same concentrations adenosine inhibited platelet aggregation, decreased the levels of sCD40L and increased intraplatelet cAMP. In addition, SQ22536 (an adenylate cyclase inhibitor) and ZM241385 (a potent adenosine receptor A_{2A} antagonist) attenuated the effect of adenosine on platelet aggregation induced by ADP and intraplatelet level of cAMP. Adenosine and inosine significantly inhibited thrombosis formation *in vivo* (62±2% occlusion at 60 min [n = 6, $p<0.01$] and 72±1.9% occlusion at 60 min, [n = 6, $p<0.05$], respectively) compared with the control (98±2% occlusion at 60 min, n = 6). A_{2A} is the adenosine receptor present in platelets; it is known that inosine is not an A_{2A} ligand. Docking of adenosine and inosine inside A_{2A} showed that the main difference is the formation by adenosine of an additional hydrogen bond between the NH_2 of the adenine group and the residues Asn253 in H6 and Glu169 in EL2 of the A_{2A} receptor.

Conclusion: Therefore, adenosine and inosine may represent novel agents lowering the risk of arterial thrombosis.

Editor: James P. Brody, Irvine, United States of America

Funding: This work was funded by the CONICYT REGIONAL / GORE MAULE / CEAP / R09I2001, Interdisciplinary Excellence Research Program on Healthy Aging (PIEI-ES), and supported by grant no. 1130216 (I. P., M. G., R. M., M. A., J. C.) from Fondecyt, Chile. The funders had no role in study design, data collection and analysis, decision to publish, or preparation of the manuscript.

Competing Interests: The authors have declared that no competing interests exist.

* Email: ipalomo@utalca.cl (IP); edfuentes@utalca.cl (EF)

Introduction

Cardiovascular diseases (CVD) (i.e., acute myocardial infarction, cerebrovascular disease and peripheral arterial thrombosis) have increased significantly in recent years [1,2]. The major and independent risk factors for CVD are cigarette smoking, elevated blood pressure, elevated serum total cholesterol and diabetes, among others [3,4]. Platelet hyper-aggregability is associated with risk factors for CVD [5]. Thus platelets from patients with type 1 and type 2 diabetes exhibit enhanced platelet aggregation activity early [6,7].

Platelet accumulation at vascular injury sites is the primary event in arterial thrombosis and its activation is a critical component of atherothrombosis [8]. Patients with unstable complex lesions had a fivefold higher expression of platelet activation than patients with stable angina, indicating an intense thrombogenic potential [9]. Also platelets could be directly involved in the unstable plaque through the production and release of pro-inflammatory molecules, including a variety of cytokines, such as TGF-β, IL-1β and sCD40L, among others [10,11].

Antiplatelet therapy has been used for a long time in an effort to prevent, as well as to treat, thrombotic diseases [12–14]. The multiple pathways of platelet activation limit the effect of specific receptor/pathway inhibitors, resulting in limited clinical efficacy [15,16]. In this way, the best-known inhibitor and turn off signaling in platelet activation is cyclic adenosine monophosphate (cAMP) [17,18].

Adenosine is a key endogenous molecule that regulates tissue function by activating four G-protein-coupled adenosine receptors: A_1, A_{2A}, A_{2B} and A_3. Both A_2 adenosine receptors, A_{2A} and A_{2B}, are coupled to G_s, leading to stimulation of adenylyl cyclase and consequent elevation of cAMP [19]. Adenosine is also recognized as one of the most important endogenous molecules able to prevent tissue injury in ischemia-reperfusion [20]. Inosine is another endogenous purine nucleoside, which is formed during the breakdown of adenosine by adenosine deaminase [21]. Inosine potently inhibited the production of the proinflammatory cytokines (TNF-α, IL-1 and IL-12) and its effect was partially reversed by blockade of adenosine A_1 and A_2 receptors [22].

Given the high structural similitude between adenosine and inosine, the main aim of this work was to investigate the relative contribution of these two molecules on platelet activation and thrombus formation. Furthermore, we performed docking experiments on the adenosine receptor A_{2A} in order to explain their differential biological effects at a molecular level.

Materials and Methods

Animal research

This study was carried out under recommendations according to the Guide for the Care and Use of Laboratory Animals of the National Institutes of Health. The protocol was approved by the Committee on the Ethics of Animal Experiments of the Universidad de Talca. All efforts were made to minimize suffering.

Reagents and antibodies

The agonist adenosine 5′- diphosphate bis (ADP), acetylsalicylic acid (ASA), rose bengal, adenosine, inosine and prostaglandin E_1 (PGE_1) were from Sigma-Aldrich (St. Louis, Missouri/MO, U.S.A), while the collagen was obtained from Hormon-Chemie (Munich, Germany). Calcein-AM, bovine serum albumin (BSA), SQ22536 (adenylate cyclase inhibitor) and ZM241385 (adenosine receptor A_{2A} antagonist) were obtained from Sigma-Aldrich (St. Louis, Missouri/MO, USA), whereas Luciferase luciferin reagent was obtained from Chrono-Log corp (Havertown, PA) and microfluidic chambers were from Bioflux (Fluxion, San Francisco, California, USA). Annexin V FITC Apoptosis KIT and antibodies (anti-CD62P-PE and anti-CD61-FITC) were obtained from BD Pharmingen (BD Biosciences, San Diego, CA, USA).

Preparation of human platelet suspensions

After receiving written informed consent from all volunteers, venous blood samples (blood volume of 30 mL was extracted from each volunteer) were taken from six young healthy volunteers (range 20–30 years). The samples were placed in 3.2% citrate tubes (9:1 v/v) by phlebotomy with vacuum tube system (Becton Dickinson Vacutainer Systems, Franklin Lakes, NJ, USA). The protocol was authorized by the ethics committee of the Universidad de Talca in accordance with the Declaration of Helsinki (approved by the 18th World Medical Assembly in Helsinki, Finland, 1964). Samples obtained from each volunteer were processed independently for each assay and centrifuged at 240 *g* for 10 min to obtain platelet-rich plasma (PRP). Following this, two-thirds of PRP was removed and centrifuged (10 min at 650 *g*). The pellet was then washed with HEPES-Tyrode's buffer containing PGE_1 (120 nmol/L). Washed platelets were prepared in HEPES-Tyrode's buffer at a concentration of 200×10^9 platelets/L (Bayer Advia 60 Hematology System, Tarrytown, NY, USA). Platelets were kept at 4°C during all the isolation steps after blood samples were taken.

Flow cytometry analysis for phosphatidylserine externalization and P-selectin exposure

Loss of platelet membrane phopholipid asymmetry with externalization of phosphatidylserine (PS) and P-selectin expression on platelets were determined by flow cytometry [23]. To 480 μL of citrated whole blood, collagen 1.5 μg/mL and ADP 8 μmol/L (final concentrations) were added for 10 min at 37°C, with stirring at 240 *g*. In each experiment, previous to the addition of platelet agonists, the sample was incubated with saline, adenosine (0.5 to 2 mmol/L) or inosine (1 to 4 mmol/L) for 10 min at room temperature. To determine phosphatidylserine externalization, 50 μL of PRP obtained of sample was diluted with 150 μL of binding buffer (10 mmol/L Hepes, 150 mmol/L NaCl, 5.0 mmol/L KCl, 1.0 mmol/L $MgCl_2$, 2.0 mmol/L $CaCl_2$, pH 7.4) and incubated for 25 min in the dark with 0.6 μg/mL (final concentration) of annexin V-FITC and anti-CD61-PE. To determine platelet P-selectin expression, 50 μL of sample was mixed with saturated concentrations of anti-CD62P-PE and anti-CD61-FITC and incubated for 25 min in the dark. Then, red cells were lysed using FACS lysing solution for 15 min. Samples were then centrifuged and washed for analysis. The samples were acquired and analyzed in Accuri C6 flow cytometer (BD, Biosciences, USA).

Platelet populations were gated on cell size using forward scatter (FSC) vs side scatter (SSC) and CD61 positivity to distinguish them from electronic noise. The light scatter and fluorescence channels were set at logarithmic gain and 5,000 events per sample analyzed. Fluorescence intensities of differentially stained populations were expressed as mean channel value using the cSampler Software (BD Biosciences, USA). All measurements were performed from six separate platelet donors.

Measurement of platelet secretion and aggregation

Platelet ATP secretion and aggregation were monitored by light transmission according to Born and Cross [24], using a lumi-aggregometer (Chrono-Log, Havertown, PA, USA). Briefly, 480 μL of PRP in the reaction vessel was pre-incubated with 20 μL of saline, PGE_1 (0.02 mmol/L), adenosine (0.5 to 2 mmol/L) or inosine (1 to 4 mmol/L). After 3 min of incubation, 20 μL of agonist (ADP 8 μmol/L or collagen 1.5 μg/mL) was added to initiate platelet aggregation, which was measured for 6 min. To determine platelet ATP secretion 50 μL of luciferin/luciferase was added within 2 min before stimulation. Platelet ATP secretion and aggregation (maximal amplitude [%]) were determined by software AGGRO/LINK (Chrono-Log, Havertown, PA, USA). Inhibition of the maximal platelet secretion and aggregation was expressed as a percentage with respect to control (saline). The concentration required to inhibit platelet secretion and aggregation by 50% (IC_{50}) was calculated from the dose-response curves. All measurements were performed from six separate platelet donors.

Platelet adhesion and aggregation under controlled flow

Experiments under flow were performed in a BioFlux 200 flow system (Fluxion, San Francisco, California, USA) with high shear plates (48 wells, 0–20 dyne/cm^2). Using manual mode in the

BioFlux software, the microfluidic chambers were coated for 1 hour with 20 μL of collagen 200 μg/mL at a wall shear rate of 200 s^{-1}.

The plaque coating was allowed to dry at room temperature for one hour. The channels were perfused with phosphate-buffered saline (PBS) for 10 min at room temperature at wall shear rate of 200 s^{-1} to remove the interface. Then, the channels were blocked with BSA 5% for 10 min at room temperature at wall shear rate of 200 s^{-1}. Whole blood anticoagulated with sodium citrate was labeled with calcein-AM (4 μmol/L) and incubated at room temperature with saline, PGE_1 (0.02 mmol/L), adenosine (0.5 to 2 mmol/L) or inosine (1 to 4 mmol/L). After one hour of incubation, the blood was added to the inlet of the well and chambers were perfused for 10 min at room temperature a wall shear rate of 1000 s^{-1}. The plates were mounted on the stage of an inverted fluorescence microscope (TE200, NIKON, Japan) [25].

Platelet deposition was observed and recorded in real-time (30 frames per min) with a CCD camera (QICAM, QIMaging, Surrey, BC, Canada). Bright field and fluorescence microscopy for real-time visualization of platelet adhesion and aggregation in flowing blood was used. For each flow experiment, fluorescence images were analyzed off-stage by quantifying the area covered by platelets with the ImageJ software (version 1.26t, NIH, USA). In each field, the area covered by platelets was quantified. All measurements were performed from six separate platelet donors.

Effect of ZM241385 and SQ22536 on antiplatelet activity

To investigate whether platelet antiaggregant activity of adenosine and inosine was mediated by stimulation of adenosine receptor A_{2A}/adenylyl cyclase pathway, PRP (480 μL at 200×10^9 platelets/L) was pretreated with SQ22536 (250 μmol/L) or ZM241385 (30 μmol/L) for 3 min. Then, the same PRP was preincubated with 20 μL of adenosine (2 mmol/L) or inosine (4 mmol/L) for 3 min prior to the addition of ADP 8 μmol/L. Platelets were first exposed to ZM241385 or SQ22536 and then ADP was used as controls. All measurements were performed from six separate platelet donors.

Measurement of cAMP levels in platelets

The effect of adenosine (0.5 to 2 mmol/L) or inosine (1 to 4 mmol/L) on platelet levels of cAMP was evaluated in PRP samples (500 μL) following 5 min incubation without stirring. Reactions were stopped with 150 μL of ice-cold 10% trichloroacetic acid. Precipitated proteins were removed by centrifugation at 2.000 *g* for 15 min at 4°C. Following addition of 150 μL of HCl 1 mol/L, the supernatant was submitted to 6 ether extractions v/v and lyophilized. Samples were stored at −70°C until assay. Before determination, the powder was dissolved in 200 μL of PBS, pH 6.2. cAMP Direct Immunoassay Kit (BioVision Research Products, Mountain View, CA, USA) was employed. All measurements were performed from six separate platelet donors.

Molecular Docking

Docking was performed using Glide [26], which is contained in Maestro software (Maestro, Version 9.0, Schrödinger, LLC, New York, NY, 2007). Glide docking uses a series of hierarchical filters to find the best possible ligand binding locations in a previously built receptor grid space. The filters include a systematic search approach, which samples the positional, conformational, and orientational space of the ligand before evaluating the energy interactions between the ligand and the protein.

The coordinates of the adenosine receptor A_{2A} were extracted from the X-ray crystal structure of human $A_{2A}R$ with adenosine bound (accession code in Protein Data Bank (PDB): 2YDO). The structures of adenosine and inosine were sketched with Maestro software. The extra-precision (XP) module of Glide was used. A grid box of 30Å × 30Å × 30Å was first centered on the center of mass of the adenosine in PDB 2YDO. Default docking parameters were used [27]. The docking hierarchy began with the systematic conformational expansion of the ligand followed by placement in the receptor site. Then minimization of the ligand in the field of the receptor was carried out using the OPLS-AA [28] force field with a distance-dependent dielectric of 2.0. Afterward, the lowest energy poses were subjected to a Monte Carlo procedure that samples the nearby torsional minima. The best pose for a given ligand was determined by the Emodel score, while different compounds were ranked using GlideScore [29]. The docking poses for both ligands were analyzed by examining their relative total energy score. The more energetically favorable conformations were selected as the best poses.

Thrombus formation in murine model

All studies were approved by the committee on animal care and conform to the Guide for the care and use of Laboratory Animals of Universidad de Talca. The Thrombosis in mice was performed by photochemical injury using a modification of the model described by Przyklenk and Whittaker [30]. For murine model we used the same mice species (C57BL/6) and gender (male) for both in control and experimental groups. Briefly, mice (12–16 weeks old) were anesthetized with a combination of tribromoethanol (270 mg/kg) and xylazine (13 mg/kg), before anesthetizing the animals; the mice were carefully handled to minimize stress and quickly anesthetized. Twenty-four hours prior to surgery, systolic blood pressure was measured using a noninvasive blood pressure meter (BP-98A, Softron Co. Ltd., Tokyo, Japan) in awake mice and during thrombosis. Throughout the procedure, animals were kept on a heating pad maintained at 37°C. After the administration of anesthesia, the mice were placed in the supine position and the mesentery was exposed by central incision in the abdomen, permitting visualization of thrombus development in mesenteric artery. The mice were injected with rose bengal through tail vein injection in a volume of 0.1 mL at a concentration of 50 mg/kg. Just after injection, a 1.5-mW green light laser (532 nm) was applied to the desired site of mesenteric artery and blood flow was monitored for 60 min. Stable occlusion was defined as a blood flow of 0 mL/min for 3 min. Saline (control group, n = 6), ASA (200 mg/kg, n = 6), adenosine (200 mg/kg, n = 6) or inosine (200 mg/kg, n = 6) was administered intraperitoneally 30 min before experiment. After laser exposure, the image of the injury generated of the injured vessel was recorded with a charge-coupled device camera (Optronics, Goleta, CA). The recorded video image was digitized and then analyzed with ImageJ software (version 1.26t, NIH, USA) [31]. In control experiments, neither injection of rose bengal without green laser or without rose bengal with green laser, resulted in any alterations in blood flow (data not shown).

Measurement of sCD40L levels

Soluble CD40 ligand (sCD40L) was determined using a Human sCD40-Ligand Quantikine kit (R & D systems, Minneapolis, MN). Briefly, washed platelets (200×10^9 platelets/L) were pretreated with saline, ASA (0.3 mmol/L), adenosine (0.5 to 2 mmol/L) or inosine (1 to 4 mmol/L) for 15 min at 37°C and then stimulated by thrombin (2 U/mL) for 45 min at 37°C. Finally, the supernatants were collected following centrifugation at 11.000 *g* for 10 min at 4°C and stored at −70°C prior to sCD40L measurements by ELISA as described earlier [32]. All measurements were performed from six separate platelet donors.

Statistical analysis

Data were analyzed using SPSS version 17.0 (SPSS, Inc., Chicago, Illinois. and expressed as mean ± standard error of mean (SEM). Six or more independent experiments were performed for the different assays. Results were expressed as percent inhibition or as percentage of control (as 100%). Fifty-percent inhibitory concentration (IC_{50}) of adenosine or inosine against agonist-induced platelet function was calculated from the dose-response curves. Differences between groups were analyzed by Student's t-test or one-way analysis of variance (ANOVA) using Tukey's post-hoc test. P values <0.05 were considered significant.

Results

In vitro findings antiplatelet effects

Effects of adenosine and inosine on platelet activation events. The antiplatelet effects of adenosine and inosine were explored by testing their activity on different activation-dependent events in human platelets. Activated platelets expose PS, which is a key phenomenon for generating a burst of thrombin essential for thrombus growth. Collagen/ADP-induced externalization of PS assessed by annexin-V binding in the presence of adenosine 0.5, 1 and 2 mmol/L was inhibited from 52±4% in the control group to 44±4% ($p<0.05$), 29±2 ($p<0.01$), and 20±3% ($p<0.001$), respectively. Whereas collagen/ADP-induced externalization of PS assessed by annexin-V binding was only slightly inhibited by 4 mmol/L of inosine ($p<0.05$) (Figure 1A). The influence of adenosine (0.5 to 2 mmol/L) and inosine (1 to 4 mmol/L) on P-selectin expression by human platelet after stimulation of ADP/collagen in citrated whole blood was measured by flow cytometry. P-selectin expression in the presence of adenosine 0.5, 1 and 2 mmol/L was inhibited from 32±4 to 27±2 ($p<0.05$), 14±3 ($p<0.01$) and 9±3% ($p<0.001$), respectively. At the concentrations tested, inosine only to 4 mmol/L has effect on platelet P-selectin expression ($p<0.05$) (Figure 1B).

Effects of adenosine and inosine on platelet ATP secretion and aggregation. The effects of adenosine and inosine on platelet ATP secretion induced by ADP and collagen are shown in Figure 2A. Adenosine inhibited ADP-induced ATP secretion with

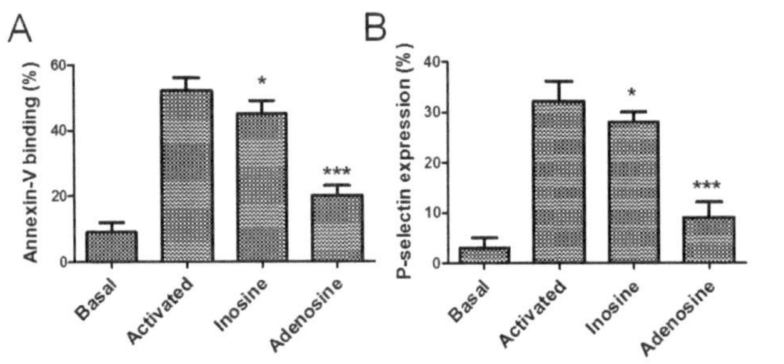

Figure 1. Effects of adenosine and inosine on platelet activation. Blood sample was incubated with saline, adenosine (2 mmol/L) or inosine (4 mmol/L) for 10 min, prior to measuring human platelet activation induced by agonists (collagen/ADP). Phosphatidylserine externalization (n = 9 experiments, panel A) and P-selectin expression (n = 6 experiments, panel B) were determined by flow cytometry. The basal bar represents the fluorescence in unstimulated sample. The graph depicts the mean ± SEM, *p<0.05 and ***p<0.001. The results presented are from 6 separate volunteers (each donors performed as single triplicates).

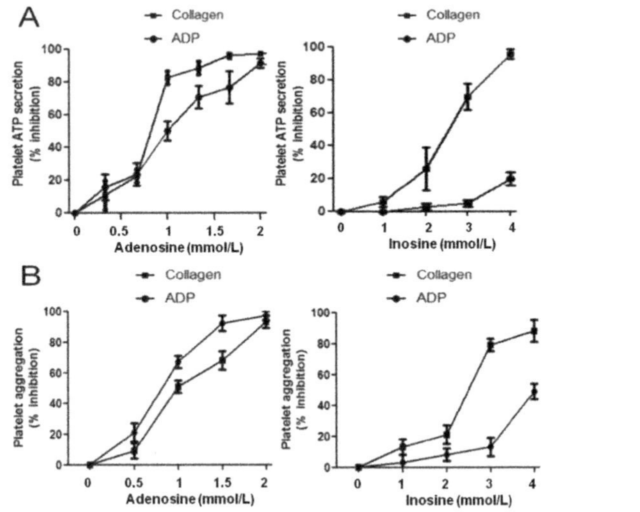

Figure 2. Effects of adenosine and inosine on ADP (8 µmol/L), collagen (1.5 µg/mL), induced platelet ATP secretion (A) and aggregation (B). PRP was pre-incubated with saline (control), adenosine (0.5 to 2 mmol/L) or inosine (1 to 4 mmol/L). After 3 min of incubation, 20 µL of agonist (ADP 8 µmol/L or collagen 1.5 µg/mL) was added to initiate platelet aggregation, which was measured for 6 min. The inhibition of the maximal platelet ATP secretion and aggregation were expressed as a percentage with respect to control (mean ± SEM; n = 6). The results presented are from 6 separate volunteers (each donors performed as single triplicates).

a 50% inhibitory concentration (IC_{50}) of 0.96 mmol/L. Similarly, the IC_{50} concentration for adenosine on collagen-induced platelet ATP-secretion was about 0.78 mmol/L. Moreover, inosine effectively inhibited the collagen-induced platelet ATP secretion with an IC_{50} of 2.3 mmol/L.

The effects of adenosine and inosine on ADP- and collagen-induced platelet aggregation are shown in Figure 2B. Adenosine effectively reduced ADP-induced platelet aggregation with an IC_{50} of 0.53 mmol/L. Similarly; adenosine suppressed collagen-induced platelet aggregation with an IC_{50} of 0.87 mmol/L. Moreover, inosine effectively inhibited collagen-induced platelet aggregation with an IC_{50} of 2.38 mmol/L. In addition, inosine showed only a mild inhibitory effect (46±5%, $p<0.05$) over ADP-induced platelet aggregation at a concentration of 4 mmol/L.

Adenosine and inosine impair platelet adhesion on immobilized collagen under flow conditions. The effects of adenosine and inosine on platelet adhesion/aggregation to immobilized collagen under arterial flow conditions are shown in Figure 3. After perfusion of citrate-anticoagulated blood over collagen coated plaque surfaces at 37°C with a wall shear rate of $1000\ s^{-1}$ for 10 min, rapid platelet adhesion and aggregate formation were observed (Figure 3A). Adenosine (0.5 to 2 mmol/L) and inosine (1 to 4 mmol/L) concentration-dependently reduced collagen-induced platelet adhesion and aggregate formation under controlled flow. As shown in Figure 3B, platelet adhesion and aggregate formation under controlled flow in presence of adenosine 0.5, 1 and 2 mmol/L was inhibited from 60±8 to 24±4 ($p<0.001$), 17±6 ($p<0.001$) and 3±2% ($p<0.001$), respectively. Similarly, in presence of inosine 1, 2 and 4 mmol/L platelet adhesion and aggregate formation under controlled flow was inhibited from 60±8 to 42±5 ($p<0.01$), 24±4 ($p<0.001$) and 12±4% ($p<0.001$), respectively.

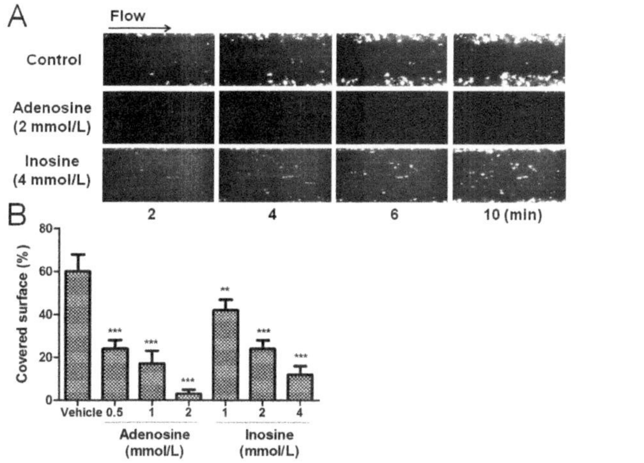

Figure 3. Effects of adenosine and inosine on collagen-induced platelet adhesion and aggregation under arterial flow conditions. Panel A shows the time-lapse of 10 min at 10 dyne/cm^2. Panel B shows the surface covered by platelets expressed as the percentage of the total surface observed, values are mean ± SEM; n = 6. **$p<0.01$ and ***$p<0.001$. The results presented are from 6 separate volunteers (each donors performed as single triplicates).

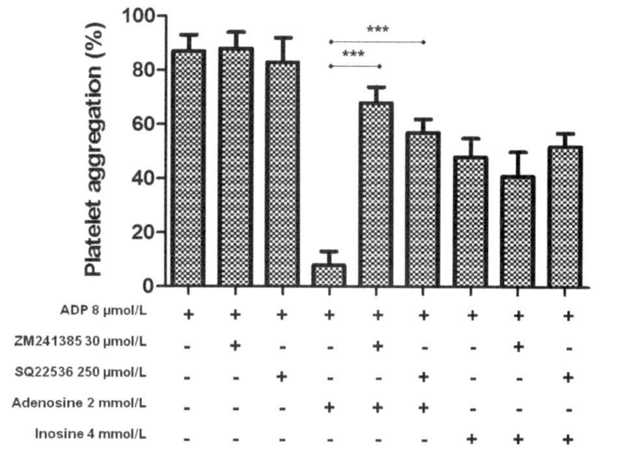

Figure 4. Effect of adenosine receptor A_{2A} antagonist (ZM241385) and adenylyl cyclase inhibitor (SQ22536) on ADP-induced platelet aggregation. PRP suspension was incubated with ADP, adenosine or inosine plus ADP or pretreated with SQ22536 or ZM241385 for 3 min, followed by addition of adenosine or inosine and ADP. The graph depicts the mean ± SEM of n = 6 experiments. ***$p<0.001$. The results presented are from 6 separate volunteers (each donors performed as single triplicates).

Mechanisms involved

Effect of ZM241385 and SQ22536 on ADP-induced platelet aggregation. We tested whether ZM241385 and SQ22536 could reverse the inhibitory effect of adenosine and inosine on platelet aggregation induced by ADP. As shown in Figure 4, ZM241385 (30 µmol/L) and SQ22536 (250 µmol/L) attenuated the inhibitory effect of adenosine against ADP-induced platelet aggregation from 8±5 to 68±6 and 57±5%, respectively ($p<0.001$). In addition, we found that SQ22536 attenuated an increase of intraplatelet levels of cAMP by adenosine from 29±2 to 9±1 pmol/10^8 platelets ($p<0.05$). On the contrary, ZM241385 and SQ22536 did not have any effect on the platelet antiaggregant activity of inosine (1 to 4 mmol/L). ZM241385 and SQ22536 alone did not exert any effect on ADP-induced platelet aggregation and with no statistical differences between them.

Effects of adenosine and inosine on intraplatelet levels of cAMP. We investigated whether the effects of adenosine and inosine on platelet function were mediated by changes in platelet cAMP levels. As shown in Figure 5, levels of cAMP in resting platelets were significantly lower compared with PGE_1 (0.02 mmol/L)-treated platelets ($p<0.001$). At the same concentrations adenosine significantly inhibits platelet aggregation and concentration-dependently (0.5 to 2 mmol/L) increased the intraplatelet levels of cAMP ($p<0.001$). On the other hand, inosine (1 to 4 mmol/L) did not show any effect on intraplatelet levels of cAMP.

Molecular docking. Figure 6 shows the alignment of the cocrystallized adenosine structure versus the docked structures for adenosine and inosine. According to this figure, the docked adenosine structure fitted in an optimal way with the adenosine in the crystal structure, and the inosine had the same orientation inside the adenosine receptor A_{2A} binding pocket. Both compounds contain a ribose group that extends deep into the ligand-binding pocket where it has hydrogen bond (HB) interactions with the residues Ser277 and His278 in H7. In addition, both compounds have a π-stacking interaction with Phe168 in extracellular loop 2 (EL2).

Adenosine forms an additional HB between the NH_2 of the adenine group and the residues Asn253 in H6 and Glu169 in EL2

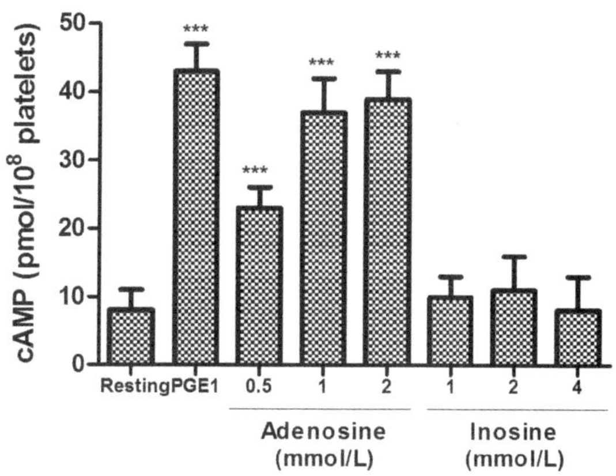

Figure 5. Effects of adenosine and inosine on intraplatelet levels of cAMP. Platelets were incubated with PGE_1 (0.02 mmol/L, positive control), adenosine (0.5 to 2 mmol/L) or inosine (1 to 4 mmol/L) for measurement of cAMP formations as described in *Materials and methods.* ***$p<0.001$ as compared with resting platelets (n = 6). The results presented are from 6 separate volunteers (each donors performed as single triplicates).

of the adenosine receptor A_{2A}, whereas the hypoxanthine group of inosine cannot establish these interactions. The role of Glu169 in ligand binding has been identified previously in the literature [33], suggesting that it is either directly or indirectly involved in the molecular recognition of both adenosine agonists and antagonists [33].

In vivo assessment of the antithrombotic potential

Effect on arterial thrombus formation *in vivo*. To study arterial thrombus development in mesenteric artery, anesthetized animals received saline, ASA, adenosine or inosine at a dose of

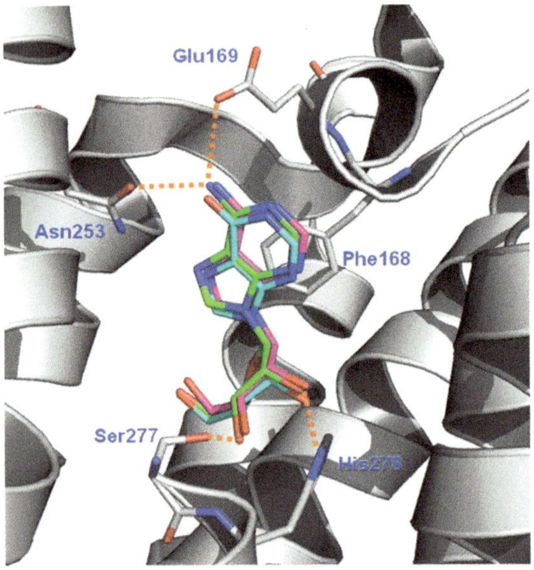

A_{2A}:	164:	VACLFEDVVPM	248:	PLHIINCF
A_{2B}:	169:	VKCLFENVVPM	249:	PVHAVNCV
A_1:	167:	IKCEFEKVISM	249:	PLHILNCI
A_3:	164:	LSCQFVSVMRM	245:	PLSIINCI

Figure 6. Molecular modeling of adenosine and inosine on adenosine receptor A2A. (top) Molecular conformations of adenosine (green) and inosine (cyan) obtained using docking inside adenosine receptor A2A binding pocket are represented. The X-ray reference structure of adenosine is represented in purple (PDB code: 2YDO). A comparison between the conformations reflects that inosine and adenosine adopt the same binding orientation inside adenosine receptor A2A (bottom). Alignment of the A_{2A} motifs that contain residues Glu169 and Asn253 with A_{2B}, A_1, and A_3.

200 mg/kg body weight by intraperitoneal injection. The effect of adenosine and inosine on arterial thrombus formation was examined and is shown in Figure 7A. Both adenosine and inosine showed a different kinetic inhibition on arterial thrombus formation (Figure 7B). The thrombotic vessel occlusion at 60 min was inhibited from 98±2 to 30±1.8% (n = 6, $p<0.001$) by pretreatment with ASA. Similarly, adenosine and inosine significantly inhibited arterial occlusion. Administration of adenosine showed a significant reduction in occlusion extent compared with the negative control at 60 min (62±2 vs 98±2%, respectively, n = 6) ($p<0.01$). On the other hand, inosine exhibited a minor effect on occlusion size reduction from 98±2 to 72±1.9% (n = 6, $p<0.05$) (Figure 7C).

Additional anti-inflammatory properties

Effect on the levels of sCD40L. As platelets are considered the major source of sCD40L in blood, we examined the effect of adenosine and inosine on the release of sCD40L. As observed in Figure 8, we found that adenosine (0.5 to 2 mmol/L) concentration-dependently reduced thrombin-induced sCD40L released from platelets ($p<0.001$). Adenosine exhibited a similar effect as ASA on sCD40L release. Moreover, inosine has a residual effect only at 4 mmol/L over sCD40L released from platelet ($p<0.05$).

Discussion

In this study, we have demonstrated that adenosine and inosine display *in vitro* and *in vivo* antiplatelet activities and reduce platelet release of atherosclerotic-related inflammatory mediator (sCD40L). This inhibitory effect of adenosine and inosine was demonstrated with the use of different agonists (ADP and collagen) and this inhibition was directly proportional to the concentrations used.

Adenosine is a natural product and endogenous nucleoside with antiplatelet activity [34–36]. Adenosine through G-protein linked receptors activate adenylate cyclase and increase cellular cAMP levels, showing inhibition of platelet function [37,38]. Studies have established that the inhibitory effect of adenosine on platelet aggregation disappears after the addition of adenosine-deaminase [39,40], and converts the purine nucleoside into inosine [41]. However, our results show that inosine possesses antiplatelet activity *in vitro* by significantly inhibiting platelet function (activation, secretion, aggregation and adhesion), releasing sCD40L and for the first time we have demonstrated prevention of thrombus growth *in vivo*. In addition, another study has established that inosine markedly inhibited platelet activation *in vitro* and *in vivo*, as well as cerebral ischemia [42].

Platelet-derived P-selectin seems to contribute to atherosclerotic lesion development and arterial thrombogenesis by forming large stable platelet-leukocyte aggregates [43]. Our results show that adenosine and inosine inhibited P-selectin expression on human platelets induced by ADP/collagen. In this sense, adenosine and inosine could inhibit platelet-leukocyte conjugate formation [44]. It has been shown that the increase of cAMP levels regulates P-selectin expression via activation of PKA [38,45]. In fact, we have recently demonstrated that an increase in intraplatelet cAMP by adenosine markedly increases the phosphorylation of PKA in human platelets [46].

When platelets adhere to collagen, a ligand-binding–induced signal is generated, leading to platelet spreading that render adherent platelets resistant to shear forces at the site of vascular damage [47]. Interestingly, we found that under conditions of arterial shear, adenosine and inosine significantly reduced platelet adhesion and aggregation to collagen as compared with the negative control.

In the last decade several lines of evidence have supported the notion that the secretion of platelet pro-inflammatory molecules (sCD40L, RANTES, sP-selectin, among others) plays a pathogenic role in both the onset and progression of the atherosclerotic process as well as in thrombotic occlusion of the vessels [48,49]. Platelets interact with monocytes via a CD40-CD40L-mediated pathway that causes their adherence to the inflamed endothelial layer [50]. Thus, high levels of sCD40L have been associated with platelet activation, suggesting a prognostic marker in patients with advanced atherosclerosis [51]. This study demonstrates for the first time that adenosine and inosine, among its antiplatelet activities, decreases the inflammatory component of activated platelets, by reducing the release of sCD40L.

In this study, ZM241385 (adenosine receptor A_{2A} antagonist) and SQ22536 (adenylyl cyclase inhibitor) were able to attenuate the effect of adenosine on ADP-induced platelet aggregation, but failed to affect the platelet aggregation induced by ADP [52]. These findings suggest that inhibition of platelet aggregation by adenosine is mediated by the stimulation of adenosine receptor A_{2A}/adenylate cyclase with increased intraplatelet cAMP concentrations. Adenosine increased cAMP levels and significantly inhibited platelet aggregation stimulated by ADP and collagen. Two recent observations may explain these findings showing that intraplatelet cAMP levels downregulate P2Y1R expression [53] and contribute to maintaining GPVI in a monomeric form on resting platelets [54]. Thus, adenosine through elevation of cAMP suppresses the sCD40L release due to the inhibition of adenylyl cyclase inhibition [46,55]. However, ZM241385 and SQ22536

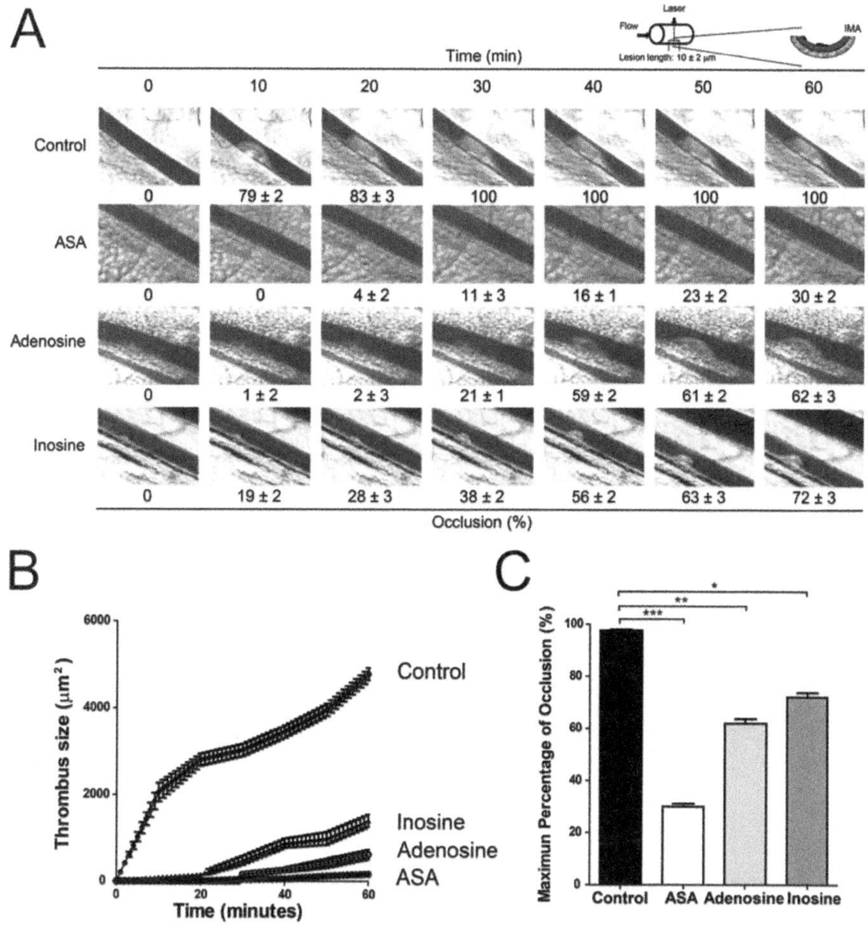

Figure 7. Adenosine and inosine inhibited arterial thrombosis formation. Panel A shows thrombus formation after laser irradiation in the saline control group (n = 6); ASA (acetylsalicylic acid) (200 mg/kg, n = 6); adenosine (200 mg/kg, n = 6) and inosine (200 mg/kg, n = 6). The figures below each photograph represent the percentages of occlusions caused by thrombus formation. Panel B shows the time course changes of thrombus size (μm²). Panel C shows maximum percentage of occlusion at 60 min after laser irradiation. For panels A and C the percentages of occlusions were calculated using the percentage of a certain area where the occlusion is greater. The graph depicts the mean± SEM of n = 6 experiments. *p<0.05, **p<0.01 and ***p<0.001.

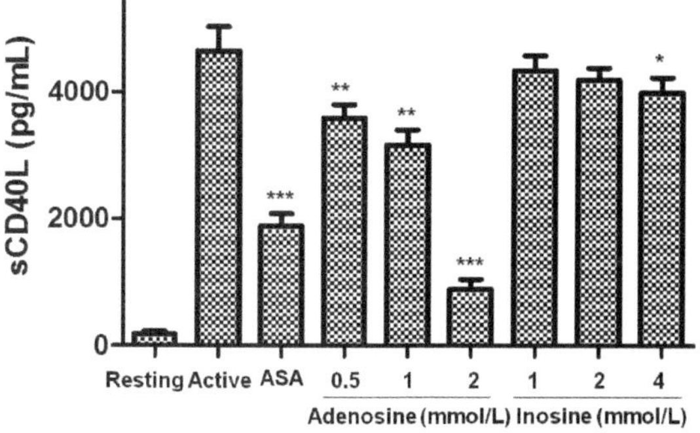

Figure 8. Effect of adenosine and inosine on release of sCD40L from platelets. Washed platelets were incubated with saline, adenosine, inosine or ASA (acetylsalicylic acid) and then stimulated with thrombin. The graph depicts the mean± SEM of n = 6 experiments. *p<0.05, **p<0.01 and ***p<0.001 as compared with the active (saline and then stimulated with thrombin). The results presented are from 6 separate volunteers (each donors performed as single triplicates).

were not able to attenuate the effect of inosine on ADP-induced platelet aggregation. Thus inosine by intraplatelet signaling pathways inhibits platelet function (phospholipase C activation rather than PKC) [42]. In this sense, different mechanisms may underlie the antiplatelet activity of adenosine and inosine. In fact, different biological functions of both nucleosides have also been demonstrated [56].

Previously, it has been suggested that adenosine is a natural ligand for the four receptors of the family (A_1, A_{2A}, A_{2B} and A_3), while inosine is only a weak agonist for the A_1 and A_3 adenosine receptors [57]. In addition, A_{2A} and A_{2B} receptors are naturally expressed in platelets [58,59]. The adenosine receptor A_{2A} has a structure consisting of seven transmembrane helices (H1–H7). The binding modes of adenosine and other adenosine receptor A_{2A} agonists have been reported recently [60]. Despite the high structural similitude and antiplatelet activity between adenosine and inosine, the latter is ineffective at adenosine receptor A_{2A} [60]. We performed docking experiments in order to explain this paradigm at a molecular level. The main difference is that adenosine forms an additional HB between the NH_2 of the adenine group and the residues Asn253 in H6 and Glu169 in EL2 of the adenosine receptor A_{2A}, whereas the hypoxanthine group of inosine cannot create these interactions, therefore losing its activity on the receptor and without an effect on cAMP levels.

In Figure 6 we have also included the alignment of the adenosine receptor A_{2A} sequence motifs that include the $A_{2A}R$ residues Glu169 and Asn253 to explain why inosine is not an adenosine receptor A2A ligand, but it is at least a weak agonist for A_1 and A_3 adenosine receptors. We can see that Asn253 is conserved in all the adenosine receptors. However, the FED motif in adenosine receptor A2A that contains Glu169 is different in other adenosine receptors. The FED motif is optimal for including adenine, but not optimal for including hypoxanthine. The phenylalanine forms the pi-pi stacking with the purine ring, glutamate forms the HB interaction with NH_2 of adenine, and aspartate is at the entrance of the pocket (it could be involved in the attraction of the ligand). The phenylalanine is conserved in all the adenosine receptors. However, the glutamate is not conserved in the A_3 receptor. Since there is no glutamate in the A_3 receptor, the negative density of the carbonyl oxygens in the hypoxanthine does not perceive a negative charge that prevents its binding. On the other hand, the aspartate at the entrance is mutated by asparagine in the A_{2B} receptor (a neutral amino acid), and by a lysine in the A_1 receptor (positively charged amino acid). The lysine could contribute to the attraction of the hypoxanthine ring (due to the negative density of hypoxanthine). Summarizing, the changes in FED motif in A_1 and A_3 receptors could explain why inosine is at least a weak agonist for these receptors, but there is no evidence that A_1 and A_3 receptors are in platelets.

Platelet aggregation plays a key role in the pathogenesis of arterial thrombosis [61]. Therefore, inhibition of platelet aggregation by drugs has been used extensively for the prevention of thromboembolic events especially in patients with acute coronary syndromes. In this study, using a murine model of real-time thrombus formation [62], we demonstrated that adenosine and inosine significantly reduced thrombus growth *in vivo* although to a lesser extent than the effect observed with aspirin.

Conclusion

Our data supports the notion that the mechanisms underlying antiplatelet activity resulting from the interaction adenosine-adenosine receptor A_{2A} seem to be related to a substantial increase in platelet cAMP levels with inhibition of P-selectin expression, sCD40L release and downregulated downstream signaling pathways of ADP and collagen receptors. On the other hand, although inosine does not seem to interact with platelet receptors it was capable of significantly inhibiting platelet adhesion and aggregation under flow and thrombus growth *in vivo*.

Author Contributions

Conceived and designed the experiments: EF MA JC JP IP. Performed the experiments: EF MA JC. Analyzed the data: JP DM IP. Contributed reagents/materials/analysis tools: IP JP. Contributed to the writing of the manuscript: EF JP IP.

References

1. Palomo GI, Icaza NG, Mujica EV, Nunez FL, Leiva ME, et al. (2007) Prevalence of cardiovascular risk factors in adult from Talca, Chile. Rev Med Chil 135: 904–912.
2. Bautista LE, Orostegui M, Vera LM, Prada GE, Orozco LC, et al. (2006) Prevalence and impact of cardiovascular risk factors in Bucaramanga, Colombia: results from the Countrywide Integrated Noncommunicable Disease Intervention Programme (CINDI/CARMEN) baseline survey. Eur J Cardiovasc Prev Rehabil 13: 769–775.
3. Grundy SM, Pasternak R, Greenland P, Smith S Jr, Fuster V (1999) Assessment of cardiovascular risk by use of multiple-risk-factor assessment equations: a statement for healthcare professionals from the American Heart Association and the American College of Cardiology. Circulation 100: 1481–1492.
4. Mujica V, Urzua A, Leiva E, Diaz N, Moore-Carrasco R, et al. (2010) Intervention with education and exercise reverses the metabolic syndrome in adults. J Am Soc Hypertens 4: 148–153.
5. Willoughby S, Holmes A, Loscalzo J (2002) Platelets and cardiovascular disease. Eur J Cardiovasc Nurs 1: 273–288.
6. Sagel J, Colwell JA, Crook L, Laimins M (1975) Increased platelet aggregation in early diabetus mellitus. Ann Intern Med 82: 733–738.
7. Palomo I, Moore-Carrasco R, Alarcon M, Rojas A, Espana F, et al. (2010) Pathophysiology of the proatherothrombotic state in the metabolic syndrome. Front Biosci (Schol Ed) 2: 194–208.
8. Ruggeri ZM (1997) Mechanisms initiating platelet thrombus formation. Thromb Haemost 78: 611–616.
9. Chakhtoura EY, Shamoon FE, Haft JI, Obiedzinski GR, Cohen AJ, et al. (2000) Comparison of platelet activation in unstable and stable angina pectoris and correlation with coronary angiographic findings. Am J Cardiol 86: 835–839.
10. Galliera E, Corsi MM, Banfi G (2012) Platelet rich plasma therapy: inflammatory molecules involved in tissue healing. J Biol Regul Homeost Agents 26: 35S–42S.
11. Fuentes QE, Fuentes QF, Andres V, Pello OM, de Mora JF, et al. (2013) Role of platelets as mediators that link inflammation and thrombosis in atherosclerosis. Platelets 24: 255–262.
12. Collins B, Hollidge C (2003) Antithrombotic drug market. Nat Rev Drug Discov 2: 11–12.
13. Palomo I, Toro C, Alarcon M (2008) The role of platelets in the pathophysiology of atherosclerosis (Review). Mol Med Rep 1: 179–184.
14. Ji X and Hou M (2011) Novel agents for anti-platelet therapy. J Hematol Oncol 4: 44.
15. Patrono C, Baigent C, Hirsh J, Roth G (2008) Antiplatelet drugs: American College of Chest Physicians Evidence-Based Clinical Practice Guidelines (8th Edition). Chest 133: 199S–233S.
16. Tantry US, Etherington A, Bliden KP, Gurbel PA (2006) Antiplatelet therapy: current strategies and future trends. Future Cardiol 2: 343–366.
17. Lerea KM, Glomset JA, Krebs EG (1987) Agents that elevate cAMP levels in platelets decrease thrombin binding. J Biol Chem 262: 282–288.
18. Lerea KM, Glomset JA (1987) Agents that elevate the concentration of cAMP in platelets inhibit the formation of a NaDodSO4-resistant complex between thrombin and a 40-kDa protein. Proc Natl Acad Sci U S A 84: 5620–5624.
19. Fredholm BB, AP IJ, Jacobson KA, Klotz KN, Linden J (2001) International Union of Pharmacology. XXV. Nomenclature and classification of adenosine receptors. Pharmacol Rev 53: 527–552.
20. Hasko G, Linden J, Cronstein B, Pacher P (2008) Adenosine receptors: therapeutic aspects for inflammatory and immune diseases. Nat Rev Drug Discov 7: 759–770.
21. Cristalli G, Costanzi S, Lambertucci C, Lupidi G, Vittori S, et al. (2001) Adenosine deaminase: functional implications and different classes of inhibitors. Med Res Rev 21: 105–128.
22. Hasko G, Kuhel DG, Nemeth ZH, Mabley JG, Stachlewitz RF, et al. (2000) Inosine inhibits inflammatory cytokine production by a posttranscriptional mechanism and protects against endotoxin-induced shock. J Immunol 164: 1013–1019.
23. Ritchie JL, Alexander HD, Rea IM (2000) Flow cytometry analysis of platelet P-selectin expression in whole blood–methodological considerations. Clin Lab Haematol 22: 359–363.
24. Born GV, Cross MJ (1963) The Aggregation of Blood Platelets. J Physiol 168: 178–195.
25. Conant CG, Schwartz MA, Nevill T, Ionescu-Zanetti C (2009) Platelet adhesion and aggregation under flow using microfluidic flow cells. J Vis Exp.
26. Friesner R, Banks J, Murphy R, Halgren T, Klicic J, et al. (2004) Glide: a new approach for rapid, accurate docking and scoring. 1. Method and assessment of docking accuracy. Journal of Medicinal Chemistry 47: 1739–1749.
27. Munoz C, Adasme F, Alzate-Morales JH, Vergara-Jaque A, Kniess T, et al. (2012) Study of differences in the VEGFR2 inhibitory activities between semaxanib and SU5205 using 3D-QSAR, docking, and molecular dynamics simulations. J Mol Graph Model 32: 39–48.
28. Jorgensen W, Maxwell D, Tirado-Rives J (1996) Development and testing of the OPLS all-atom force field on conformational energetics and properties of organic liquids. Journal of the American Chemical Society 118: 11225–11236.
29. Eldridge MD, Murray CW, Auton TR, Paolini GV, Mee RP (1997) Empirical scoring functions: I. The development of a fast empirical scoring function to estimate the binding affinity of ligands in receptor complexes. J Comput Aided Mol Des 11: 425–445.
30. Przyklenk K, Whittaker P (2007) Adaptation of a photochemical method to initiate recurrent platelet-mediated thrombosis in small animals. Lasers Med Sci 22: 42–45.
31. Abramoff MD, Magalhaes PJ, Ram SJ (2004) Image Processing with ImageJ. Biophotonics International 11: 36–42.

32. Antczak AJ, Singh N, Gay SR, Worth RG (2010) IgG-complex stimulated platelets: a source of sCD40L and RANTES in initiation of inflammatory cascade. Cell Immunol 263: 129–133.
33. Kim J, Jiang Q, Glashofer M, Yehle S, Wess J, et al. (1996) Glutamate residues in the second extracellular loop of the human A2a adenosine receptor are required for ligand recognition. Mol Pharmacol 49: 683–691.
34. Fuentes E, Castro R, Astudillo L, Carrasco G, Alarcón M, et al. (2012) Bioassay-Guided Isolation and HPLC Determination of Bioactive Compound That Relate to the Antiplatelet Activity (Adhesion, Secretion, and Aggregation) from Solanum lycopersicum. Evidence-Based Complementary and Alternative Medicine: 1–10.
35. Wang J, Huang ZG, Cao H, Wang YT, Hui P, et al. (2008) Screening of anti-platelet aggregation agents from Panax notoginseng using human platelet extraction and HPLC-DAD-ESI-MS/MS. J Sep Sci 31: 1173–1180.
36. Fuentes E, Castro R, Astudillo L, Carrasco G, Alarcon M, et al. (2012) Bioassay-Guided Isolation and HPLC Determination of Bioactive Compound That Relate to the Antiplatelet Activity (Adhesion, Secretion, and Aggregation) from Solanum lycopersicum. Evid Based Complement Alternat Med 2012: 147031.
37. Anfossi G, Russo I, Massucco P, Mattiello L, Cavalot F, et al. (2002) Adenosine increases human platelet levels of cGMP through nitric oxide: possible role in its antiaggregating effect. Thromb Res 105: 71–78.
38. Minamino T, Kitakaze M, Asanuma H, Tomiyama Y, Shiraga M, et al. (1998) Endogenous adenosine inhibits P-selectin-dependent formation of coronary thromboemboli during hypoperfusion in dogs. J Clin Invest 101: 1643–1653.
39. Altman R, Rouvier J, Weisenberger H (1985) Identification of platelet inhibitor present in the melon (Cucurbitacea cucumis melo). Thromb Haemost 53: 312–313.
40. Dutta-Roy AK, Crosbie L, Gordon MJ (2001) Effects of tomato extract on human platelet aggregation in vitro. Platelets 12: 218–227.
41. Hasko G, Sitkovsky MV, Szabo C (2004) Immunomodulatory and neuroprotective effects of inosine. Trends Pharmacol Sci 25: 152–157.
42. Hsiao G, Lin KH, Chang Y, Chen TL, Tzu NH, et al. (2005) Protective mechanisms of inosine in platelet activation and cerebral ischemic damage. Arterioscler Thromb Vasc Biol 25: 1998–2004.
43. Burger PC, Wagner DD (2003) Platelet P-selectin facilitates atherosclerotic lesion development. Blood 101: 2661–2666.
44. Storey RF, Judge HM, Wilcox RG, Heptinstall S (2002) Inhibition of ADP-induced P-selectin expression and platelet-leukocyte conjugate formation by clopidogrel and the P2Y12 receptor antagonist AR-C69931MX but not aspirin. Thromb Haemost 88: 488–494.
45. Libersan D, Rousseau G, Merhi Y (2003) Differential regulation of P-selectin expression by protein kinase A and protein kinase G in thrombin-stimulated human platelets. Thromb Haemost 89: 310–317.
46. Fuentes E, Badimon L, Caballero J, Padro T, Vilahur G, et al. (2013) Protective mechanisms of adenosine 5′-monophosphate in platelet activation and thrombus formation. Thromb Haemost 111.
47. Inoue O, Suzuki-Inoue K, Dean WL, Frampton J, Watson SP (2003) Integrin alpha2beta1 mediates outside-in regulation of platelet spreading on collagen through activation of Src kinases and PLCgamma2. J Cell Biol 160: 769–780.
48. Aukrust P, Muller F, Ueland T, Berget T, Aaser E, et al. (1999) Enhanced levels of soluble and membrane-bound CD40 ligand in patients with unstable angina. Possible reflection of T lymphocyte and platelet involvement in the pathogenesis of acute coronary syndromes. Circulation 100: 614–620.
49. Wagner DD, Burger PC (2003) Platelets in inflammation and thrombosis. Arterioscler Thromb Vasc Biol 23: 2131–2137.
50. Harding SA, Sommerfield AJ, Sarma J, Twomey PJ, Newby DE, et al. (2004) Increased CD40 ligand and platelet-monocyte aggregates in patients with type 1 diabetes mellitus. Atherosclerosis 176: 321–325.
51. Setianto BY, Hartopo AB, Gharini PP, Anggrahini DW, Irawan B (2010) Circulating soluble CD40 ligand mediates the interaction between neutrophils and platelets in acute coronary syndrome. Heart Vessels 25: 282–287.
52. Daniel JL, Dangelmaier C, Jin J, Kim YB, Kunapuli SP (1999) Role of intracellular signaling events in ADP-induced platelet aggregation. Thromb Haemost 82: 1322–1326.
53. Yang D, Chen H, Koupenova M, Carroll SH, Eliades A, et al. (2010) A new role for the A2b adenosine receptor in regulating platelet function. J Thromb Haemost 8: 817–827.
54. Loyau S, Dumont B, Ollivier V, Boulaftali Y, Feldman L, et al. (2012) Platelet glycoprotein VI dimerization, an active process inducing receptor competence, is an indicator of platelet reactivity. Arterioscler Thromb Vasc Biol 32: 778–785.
55. Enomoto Y, Adachi S, Doi T, Natsume H, Kato K, et al. (2011) cAMP regulates ADP-induced HSP27 phosphorylation in human platelets. Int J Mol Med 27: 695–700.
56. Hoffmeister HM, Betz R, Fiechtner H, Seipel L (1987) Myocardial and circulatory effects of inosine. Cardiovasc Res 21: 65–71.
57. Fredholm BB, Irenius E, Kull B, Schulte G (2001) Comparison of the potency of adenosine as an agonist at human adenosine receptors expressed in Chinese hamster ovary cells. Biochem Pharmacol 61: 443–448.
58. Zhao Z, Makaritsis K, Francis CE, Gavras H, Ravid K (2000) A role for the A3 adenosine receptor in determining tissue levels of cAMP and blood pressure: studies in knock-out mice. Biochim Biophys Acta 1500: 280–290.
59. Johnston-Cox HA, Ravid K (2011) Adenosine and blood platelets. Purinergic Signal 7: 357–365.
60. Lebon G, Warne T, Edwards PC, Bennett K, Langmead CJ, et al. (2011) Agonist-bound adenosine A2A receptor structures reveal common features of GPCR activation. Nature 474: 521–525.
61. Barrett NE, Holbrook L, Jones S, Kaiser WJ, Moraes LA, et al. (2008) Future innovations in anti-platelet therapies. Br J Pharmacol 154: 918–939.
62. Fukuoka T, Hattori K, Maruyama H, Hirayama M, Tanahashi N (2012) Laser-induced thrombus formation in mouse brain microvasculature: effect of clopidogrel. J Thromb Thrombolysis 34: 193–198.

Chronic Glucocorticoid Exposure-Induced Epididymal Adiposity Is Associated with Mitochondrial Dysfunction in White Adipose Tissue of Male C57BL/6J Mice

Jie Yu[1,2], Bing Yu[1,2], Jun He[1,2], Ping Zheng[1,2], Xiangbing Mao[1,2], Guoquan Han[1,3], Daiwen Chen[1,2]*

1 Animal Nutrition Institute, Sichuan Agricultural University, Chengdu, 611130, People's Republic of China, **2** Key Laboratory for Animal Disease-Resistance Nutrition of China Ministry of Education, Sichuan Agricultural University, Chengdu, 611130, People's Republic of China, **3** College of Food Science, Sichuan Agricultural University, Ya'an, 625014, People's Republic of China

Abstract

Prolonged and excessive glucocorticoids (GC) exposure resulted from Cushing's syndrome or GC therapy develops central obesity. Moreover, mitochondria are crucial in adipose energy homeostasis. Thus, we tested the hypothesis that mitochondrial dysfunction may contribute to chronic GC exposure-induced epididymal adiposity in the present study. A total of thirty-six 5-week-old male C57BL/6J mice (~20 g) were administrated with 100 μg/ml corticosterone (CORT) or vehicle through drinking water for 4 weeks. Chronic CORT exposure mildly decreased body weight without altering food and water intake in mice. The epididymal fat accumulation was increased, but adipocyte size was decreased by CORT. CORT also increased plasma CORT, insulin, leptin, and fibroblast growth factor 21 concentrations as measured by RIA or ELISA. Interestingly, CORT increased plasma levels of triacylglycerols and nonesterified fatty acids, and up-regulated the expression of both lipolytic and lipogenic genes as determined by real-time RT-PCR. Furthermore, CORT impaired mitochondrial biogenesis and oxidative function in epididymal WAT. The reactive oxygen species production was increased and the activities of anti-oxidative enzymes were reduced by CORT treatment as well. Taken together, these findings reveal that chronic CORT administration-induced epididymal adiposity is, at least in part, associated with mitochondrial dysfunction in mouse epididymal white adipose tissue.

Editor: Marià Alemany, Faculty of Biology, Spain

Funding: This work was supported by Key Project (13ZA0261) from Sichuan Department of Education (JY) and Program for Changjiang Scholars and Innovative Research Team in University (IRT0555-5) from Ministry of Education of China (DC). The funders had no role in study design, data collection and analysis, decision to publish, or preparation of the manuscript.

Competing Interests: The authors have declared that no competing interests exist.

* Email: dwchen@sicau.edu.cn

Introduction

Glucocorticoids (GC) are adrenal cortex-secreted steroid hormones stimulated upon hypothalamic-pituitary-adrenal (HPA) axis activation due to endocrine disorder and/or stress [1–3]. Patients with chronic exposure to excess GC, either resulted from Cushing's syndrome or receiving GC therapy for the purposes of anti-inflammatory and/or immunosuppression, develop numerous metabolic changes including obesity, fatty liver, dyslipidemia, and glucose intolerance [4–6]. Obesity is part of metabolic syndrome and shares with a number of other diseases common pathogenic origins like inflammation [7]. Hypercortisolemia-induced obesity is characterized by central adiposity caused by distributing fat accumulation from subcutaneous adipose tissue to the metabolically more active visceral fat [8,9]. In addition, mice selectively expressing the glucocorticoid-activating enzyme, 11 β-hydroxysteroid dehydrogenase type 1 (11βHSD1), in adipose tissue shows central obesity phenotype [10], whereas the suppression of 11βHSD1 attenuates adipogenesis [11]. Though the lipogenic effect of GC has been well defined in the past decades, GC are also widely known to stimulate lipolysis through activating hormone sensitive lipase (HSL) and mobilizing nonesterified fatty acids (NEFA) to β-oxidation as "stress" hormones [12–14]. Most recently, it has been documented that GC simultaneously increase both lipolysis and adipogenesis through separate pathways [15]. The dual roles of GC in lipid metabolism, apparently, make the process through which GC exposure induces adiposity more elusive.

Mitochondria are double-membrane organelles that produce the majority of cellular ATP and reactive oxygen species (ROS) mediated by the mitochondrial-specific proteins [16,17]. White adipocyte mitochondria support the anaplerotic generation of metabolic intermediates for fatty acid synthesis[18]. Decreased mitochondrial density and oxidative phosphorylation activity in white adipocytes have been shown in both rodent and human obesity [19–21]. Likewise, reduced mitochondrial DNA (mtDNA) copy number directly correlates with increased lipogenesis in white adipose tissue (WAT) [22]. Furthermore, enhanced mitochondrial biogenesis increases the fatty acids oxidation and decreases the susceptibility of high-fat diet-induced obesity [23,24]. Thus, mitochondria play prominent role in WAT lipid homeostasis.

The objective of the present study was to test the hypothesis that impaired mitochondrial functions may contribute to chronic GC exposure-induced epididymal adiposity.

Materials and Methods

Ethics statement

All animal-related procedures were approved by Sichuan Agricultural University Institutional Animal Care and Use Committee (M2012-07-08). All surgery was performed under isoflurane anesthesia, and all efforts were made to minimize suffering.

Animals, housing, and treatment

Thirty-six 5-week-old male C57BL/6J mice (~20 g) that are originally purchased from Jackson Laboratory (Bar Harbor, ME, USA) were obtained from Sichuan Academy of Medical Sciences (Chengdu, Sichuan, China). Mice were group-housed (3 mice/cage) in standard polycarbonate cages at 21±2°C on timed 12-h dark, 12-h light cycles and had free access to standard rodent chow and tap water. After 1-week acclimation, animals were assigned into 2 treatments by body weight. According to previous report [25], 100 μg/ml of CORT (Sigma-Aldrich, St. Louis, MO, USA) was dissolved in ethanol, and then diluted in tap water to a final ethanol concentration of 1% (v/v). Mice were provided with drinking water containing 100 μg/ml CORT or 1% (v/v) ethanol solution alone (vehicle). During the experimental period, *ad libitum* diet remained available.

Animals were weighed weekly. After 4-week of the treatment, mice were anaesthetized and sacrificed. Blood was collected and centrifuged at 3000 g for 15 min at 4°C. Plasma samples were stored at −20°C for future measurements. Epididymal, retroperitoneal and inguinal subcutaneous WAT depots were dissected and weighed as previously described [26]. The tissue samples were frozen and stored at −80°C for further analysis.

Histological analysis

The collected epididymal WAT was fixed in formalin solution, dehydrated, paraffin-embedded, and sectioned. Sections (10 μm thick) were stained with hematoxylin and eosin, then examined and photographed under Olympus Microscope Digital Camera DP21 (Olympus China, LTD., Beijing, China). Adipocyte sizes were measured for at least 200 individual cells per mice with Image J software (National Institutes of Health, Bethesda, MD, USA).

Hormone and biochemical measurements

Plasma CORT concentrations were measured using a commercial radioimmunoassay (RIA) kit from MP Biomedicals Inc. (Solon, OH, USA). Plasma insulin, leptin contents were determined with specific mouse enzyme-linked immunosorbent assay (ELISA) kits (Millipore, Billerica, MA, USA). For plasma fibroblast growth factor 21 (FGF21), ELISA kit (BioVendor, Candler, NC, USA) was applied to measure the concentrations. All measurements were performed according to respective manufacturer's instructions.

The concentrations of triglyceride, NEFA and malondialdehyde (MDA) were measured using commercial assays (Jiancheng Institute of Bioengineering, Nanjing, Jiangsu, China) as described previously [27]. The activities of superoxide dismutase (EC Number: 1.15.1.1), gluthathione peroxidase (EC Number: 1.11.1.9) and catalase (EC Number: 1.11.1.6) were measured using specific commercial kits (Nanjing Jiancheng Institute of Bioengineering, Nanjing, China) according to the provided instructions, respectively.

DNA and RNA extraction

Total RNA from frozen adipose tissues was extracted using TRI reagent (Takara, Dalian, China) and further purified with Qiagen RNeasy Mini kit (Qiagen, Valencia, CA, USA) [27]. Total DNA was isolated from epididymal WAT using a DNAiso Reagent (Takara). Concentration and integrity of the extracted RNA were determined with an Agilent 2100 Bioanalyzer (Santa Clara, CA, USA).

Quantitative real-time PCR

Quantitative Real-time PCR was conducted as previous report [28,29]. Briefly, the cDNA was synthesized from 1 μg total RNA using random primers and reverse transcriptase (Takara). Real-time quantitative PCRs were performed using Power SYBR Green PCR master mix (Applied Biosystems, Foster City, CA, USA) on an Applied Biosystems 7900HT real-time PCR system. The conditions for these PCRs were 40 cycles of 95°C for 15 sec and 60°C for 1 min. The real-time PCR of each sample were performed in duplicate. The data were analyzed using 18S rRNA as the internal control with the cycle threshold ($2^{-\Delta\Delta CT}$) method, as recommended by Applied Biosystems. Based on the Ct values, adipose expression of 18S rRNA was not affected by CORT treatment. The mtDNA analysis was performed as described [30], mtDNA was amplified using primers specific for the mitochondrial cytochrome b (Cyt B) gene and normalized to genomic DNA by amplification of the large ribosomal protein p 0 (36B4). All primers used in this study are shown in Table 1.

Mitochondrial biogenesis methods

Citrate synthase (EC Number: 2.3.3.1) activity in isolated mitochondria preparations of epididymal WAT was measured with spectrophotometer using citrate synthase kit (Sigma-Aldrich) following manufacturer's instructions. NAD^+ and NADH levels in isolated mitochondria preparations were determined using the NAD/NADH assay kit purchased from BioAssay Systems (Hayward, CA, USA). Mitochondria were isolated using the Qproteome Mitochondria Isolation Kit (Qiagen).

Statistical analysis

All statistical analyses were performed using SAS statistical packages (SAS Institute, Cary, NC, USA). Unpaired *t* test were applied to evaluate the comparisons between two groups. Data are presented as the mean ± SEM. Differences at $P<0.05$ are considered significant.

Results

Chronic CORT mildly decreases body weight

We treated adult mice with 100 μg/ml of CORT through drinking water for 4 weeks to determine the effect of chronic CORT exposure on body weight change in mice. Mice in CORT group lost weight after the first week of treatment, but this did not reach statistical significance ($P>0.05$, Fig. 1). In the subsequent weeks, CORT-treated animals were smaller than vehicle-treated controls, but there is no significance ($P>0.05$, Fig. 1). CORT exposure slightly decreased the daily food intake (5.30±0.33 g vs 4.46±0.28 g, $P>0.05$). No significant change in daily drinking water intake was observed after CORT treatment (6.95±0.43 ml vs 7.13±0.15 ml, $P>0.05$).

Table 1. Primer sequences used in this study.

Gene	Sequence (5′-3′)	Accession No.	Amplicon size (bp)
CytB	F: TGAGGGGGCTTCTCAGTAGA	NC_005089	118
	R: CTGTTTCGTGGAGGAAGAGG		
36B4	F: TGCCACACTCCATCATCAAT	NM_007475	240
	R: CGAAGAGACCGAATCCCATA		
PGC-1α	F: AATGCAGCGGTCTTAGCACT	NM_008904	193
	R: GTGTGAGGAGGGTCATCGTT		
NRF-1	F: CCACGTTGGATGAGTACACG	NM_001164226	120
	R: GCACCACATTCTCCAAAGGT		
CytC	F: CCAAATCTCCACGGTCTGTT	NM_007808	100
	R: TATCCTCTCCCCAGGTGATG		
IDH3α	F: GAGGTTTTGCTGGTGGTGTT	NM_029573	155
	R: TCCTCCTGGTCCTTGAATTG		
SIRT1	F: AGTTCCAGCCGTCTCTGTGT	NM_019812	198
	R: CTCCACGAACAGCTTCACAA		
PPARγ	F: CCCTGGCAAAGCATTTGTAT	NM_001127330	225
	R: GAAACTGGCACCCTTGAAAA		
CPT-1α	F: CCAGGCTACAGTGGGACATT	NM_013495	100
	R: AAGGAATGCAGGTCCACATC		
HSL	F: TGCTCTTCTTCGAGGGTGAT	NM_010719	183
	R: TCTCGTTGCGTTTGTAGTGC		
ATGL	F: TATCCGGTGGATGAAAGAGC	NM_001163689	112
	R: CAGTTCCACCTGCTCAGACA		
FAS	F: CCCTTGATGAAGAGGGATCA	NM_007988	115
	R: ACTCCACAGGTGGGAACAAG		
m18S rRNA	F: ACCGCGGTTCTATTTTGTTG	NR_003278	181
	R: TCGTCTTCGAAACTCCGACT		

Chronic CORT exposure increases epididymal fat accumulation, but decreases adipocyte size

The body composition of CORT-treated mice was subsequently analyzed to determine the relative amounts of WAT. CORT exposure significantly increased epididymal WAT mass ($P<0.05$, Fig. 2A), but did not alter retroperitoneal WAT (0.154±0.012 g vs 0.149±0.007 g, $P>0.05$) and inguinal WAT (0.287±0.048 g vs 0.267±0.043 g, $P>0.05$) weight compared with controls. Moreover, epididymal WAT made up a significantly larger proportion of their total body weight when compared to control mice ($P<0.05$, Fig. 2B). Interestingly, in the histological analysis, CORT-treated mice had significantly smaller adipocytes in their epididymal WAT compared with vehicle-treated animals ($P<0.05$, Fig. 2C and 2D), suggesting that the increased epididymal WAT mass is resulted from adipocyte hyperplasia.

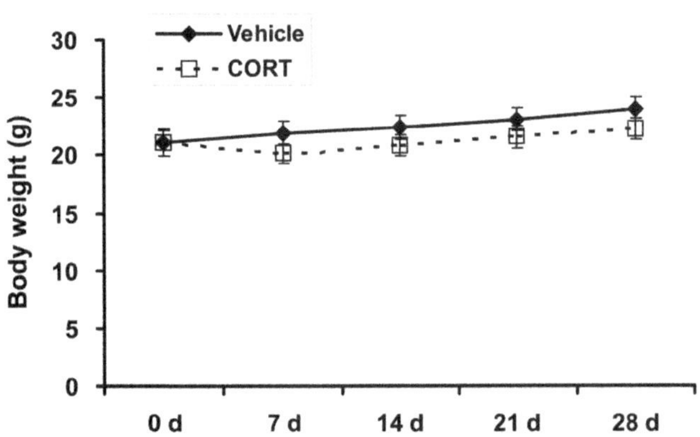

Figure 1. Effect of CORT on body weight of mice. Total body weight of mice treated with 100 µg/ml corticosterone (CORT) or vehicle during the experimental period. Data are expressed as group means ± SEM (n = 6 by group). * $P<0.05$ compared with vehicle.

Chronic CORT exposure changes plasma hormone levels and lipid profile

To determine the circulating levels of hormones included in the regulation of lipid metabolism, plasma concentrations of CORT, insulin, leptin, and FGF21 were measured. Meanwhile, plasma triacylglycerols and NEFA levels were tested to determine the blood lipid profile. As expected, chronic CORT exposure induced significant increase in plasma CORT concentration compared with the control group ($P<0.05$, Table 2). CORT also significantly increased plasma concentrations of insulin, leptin and FGF21 when compared to control mice ($P<0.05$, Table 2). CORT group showed significantly higher triacylglycerols and NEFA levels compared with the vehicle group ($P<0.05$, Table 2).

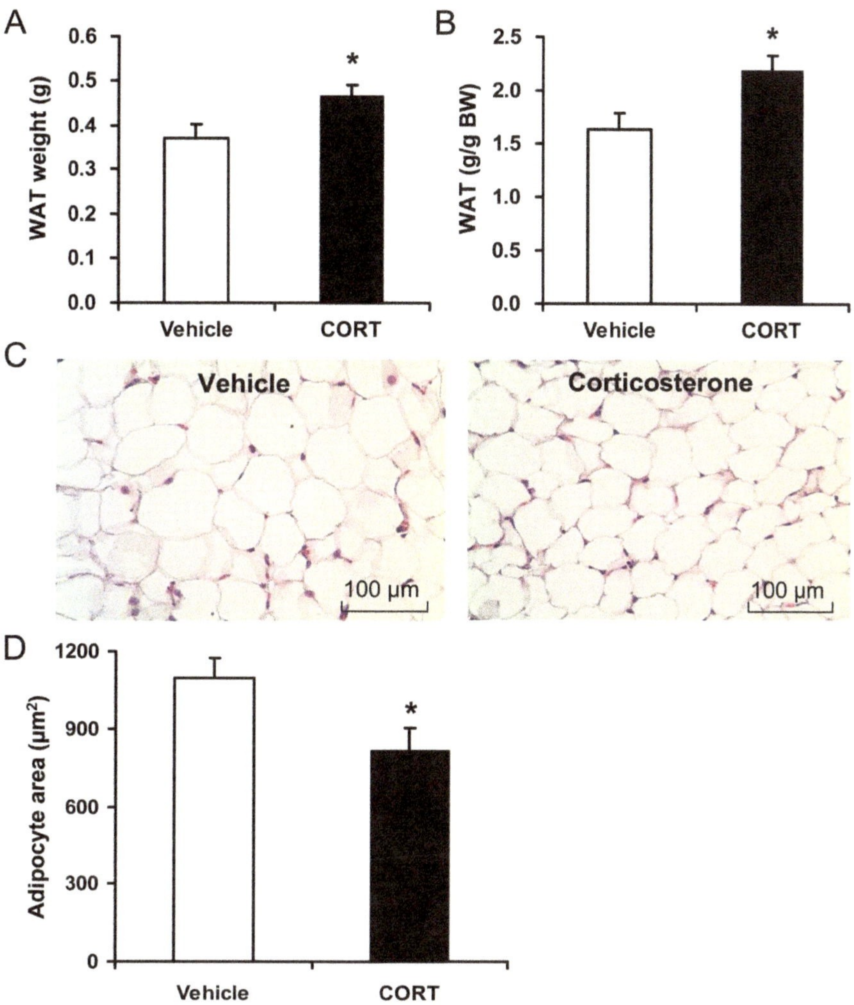

Figure 2. Effect of CORT on epididymal WAT weight and adipocyte size of mice. (**A**) Weight of epididymal white adipose tissue (WAT) and (**B**) relative contribution of epididymal WAT to total body weight in mice treated with 100 μg/ml corticosterone (CORT) or vehicle for 4 weeks. (**C**) Paraffin sections of epididymal WAT of mice treated with CORT or vehicle were stained with hematoxylin and eosin. Scale bar: 100 μm. (**D**) The average adipocyte cell area of epididymal fat in mice treated with CORT or vehicle. Data are expressed as group means ± SEM (n = 6 by group). * $P < 0.05$ compared with vehicle.

Table 2. Effect of CORT on plasma hormone levels and lipid profile of mice.

	Vehicle	CORT
Corticosterone (ng/ml)	23.0±2.5	195.1±16.6*
Insulin (ng/ml)	1.52±0.21	7.49±0.15*
Leptin (ng/ml)	1.61±0.06	7.37±0.90*
FGF21 (pg/ml)	165.0±8.7	355.1±14.0*
Triacylglycerols (mM)	0.58±0.16	1.20±0.16*
NEFA (μM)	449.1±70.7	686.4±77.7*

Plasma concentrations of corticosterone, insulin, leptin, fibroblast growth factor 21 (FGF21), triacylglycerols and nonesterified fatty acids (NEFA) in mice treated with 100 μg/ml CORT or vehicle for 4 weeks.

Data are expressed as group means ± SEM (n = 6 by group).

* $P<0.05$ compared with vehicle.

Chronic CORT exposure alters the expression of lipolysis and lipogenesis-related genes in epididymal WAT

We next determined the effects of chronic CORT exposure on the expression of genes related to lipolysis and lipogenesis. The expression of hormone-sensitive lipase *(HSL)* in epididymal WAT was significantly increased by CORT treatment ($P<0.05$, Fig. 3A). CORT also increased another lipolysis-related adipose triglyceride lipase *(ATGL)* expression in epididymal WAT compared with the control group ($P<0.05$, Fig. 3A). Interestingly, the mRNA expression of fatty acid synthase *(FAS)* and peroxisome proliferators-activated receptor γ *(PPARγ)*, the well known adipogenesis-related genes, were also increased 5.8 and 2.0 folds after 4-week CORT treatment, respectively ($P<0.05$, Fig. 3B).

Chronic CORT exposure impairs mitochondrial biogenesis and functions in epididymal WAT

To determine the effects of chronic CORT exposure on mitochondrial biogenesis and functions, we measured mtDNA amount, mitochondrial gene expression, mitochondrial enzymatic activity, and NAD^+ metabolism in epididymal WAT. The abundance of mtDNA in CORT-treated mice was significantly less than that in vehicle-treated controls ($P<0.05$, Fig. 4A). The mRNA levels of mitochondrial genes responsible for mitochondrial biogenesis and functions, including sirtuin 1 *(SIRT1)*, PPARγ coactivator 1α *(PGC1α)*, nuclear respiratory factor-1 *(NRF-1)*, cytochrome c *(CytC)*, carnitine palmitoyltransferase 1α *(CPT1α)* and isocitrate dehydrogenase 3α *(IDH3α)* were significantly decreased by CORT treatment when compared with control mice ($P<0.05$, Fig. 4B). Furthermore, CORT exposure induced a ~40% decrease in citrate synthase activity ($P<0.05$, Fig. 4C). Though NADH level was not changed (data not shown), NAD^+ level tended to be reduced ($P=0.09$, Fig. 4D), and in turn intracellular NAD^+/NADH ratio was remarkably decreased by CORT compared with vehicle ($P<0.05$, Fig. 4E).

Chronic CORT exposure decreases ROS defense system in epididymal WAT

We further measured the concentration of MDA and the activities of three major anti-oxidative enzymes (superoxide dismutase, gluthathione peroxidase and catalase) in epididymal WAT to determine the effects of chronic CORT exposure on ROS defense system. CORT group showed significantly higher MDA levels compared with controls ($P<0.05$, Fig. 5A), indicating more lipid peroxide accumulated in epididymal WAT of CORT-treated mice. Meanwhile, CORT treatment significantly decreased the activities of superoxide dismutase, gluthathione peroxidase and catalase in epididymal WAT of CORT-consumed mice when compared with vehicle-treated animals ($P<0.05$, Fig. 5B, 5C and 5D).

Discussion

The metabolic syndrome presented in the patients suffering from either chronic endogenous hypercortisolism or exogenous GCs treatment contributes to the greater risk of cardiovascular diseases, diabetes and obesity, and reduces the life quality [5,31]. In this study, our intriguing findings showed that chronic administration of CORT, the principal GC in mouse, through drinking water increases epididymal WAT amount without body weight gain, decreases epididymal adipocyte sizes, increases the expression of both lipogenic and lipolytic genes, impairs mitochondrial biogenesis, functions and antioxidant process when compared with control mice. Considering the crucial role of mitochondria in energy homeostasis, therefore, we have supposed that the epididymal adiposity appears during chronic GC exposure might be associated with GC-induced mitochondrial dysfunction.

Recent study has developed a potential model of the metabolic syndrome resulted from chronic CORT treatment [25]. This mouse model was applied in the present study to investigate the metabolic outcomes of mice under chronic CORT exposure. The CORT-treated mice averagely received 713 μg/d of CORT through drinking water according to the calculation from water intake. This oral dose is comparable with other studies conducted with subcutaneous GC pellets in male mice and female rats [32,33]. As expected, plasma concentrations of CORT, insulin, leptin and FGF21 were elevated in mice treated with CORT. Although single plasma CORT levels give little information, previous studies using similar approach have demonstrated the hormone availability and endocrine physiology [25,34]. Therefore, mouse exposed to CORT through drinking water could be a suitable model for human hypercortisolemia.

Surprisingly, we did not find rapid increases in body weight caused by chronic CORT treatment as previously published work [25]. However, as shown by numerous reports [8,15,25,35–37], increased intra-abdominal rather than subcutaneous WAT together with elevated plasma triacylglycerols and NEFA levels in CORT-treated mice were also observed in this study, pointing to a sarcopenic phenotype. Active GC contributes to the sarcopenia, since excess GC induce hypoandrogenism and insulin resistance, both of which tend to decrease protein retention and

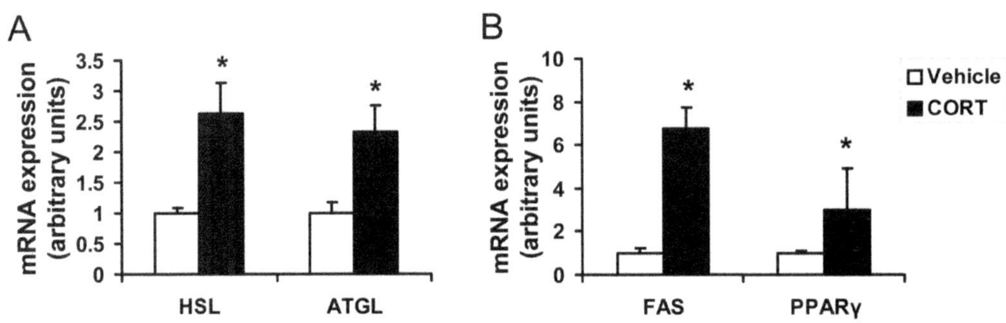

Figure 3. Effect of CORT on expressions of lipolytic and lipogenic genes in epididymal WAT of mice. (**A**) Relative expression of lipolysis-related genes, and (**B**) lipogenesis-related genes in epididymal white adipose tissue (WAT) of mice treated with 100 μg/ml CORT or vehicle for 4 weeks. Data are expressed as group means ± SEM (n = 6 by group). All the mRNA expression data are normalized to the house keeping gene (18S rRNA). * $P<0.05$ compared with vehicle.

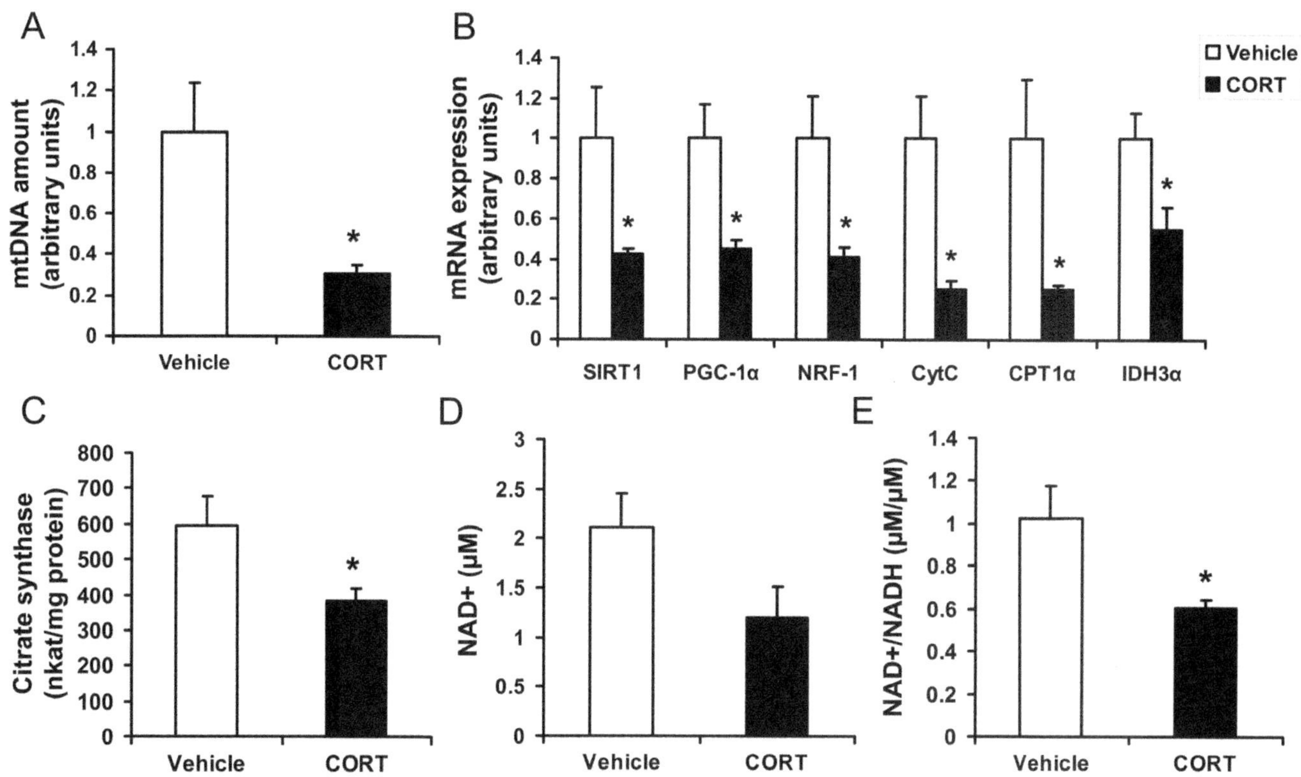

Figure 4. Effect of CORT on mitochondrial biogenesis and function in epididymal WAT of mice. (**A**) Relative abundance of mitochondrial DNA (mtDNA), (**B**) relative mRNA levels of mitochondrial genes responsible for mitochondrial biogenesis and function, (**C**) activity of citrate synthase (CS), (**D**) NAD^+ levels, and (**E**) NAD^+/NADH ratio in epididymal white adipose tissue (WAT) of mice treated with 100 μg/ml CORT or vehicle for 4 weeks. Data are expressed as group means ± SEM (n = 6 by group). All the mRNA expression data are normalized to the house keeping gene (18S rRNA), mtDNA is the relative amount to genomic DNA * $P<0.05$ compared with vehicle.

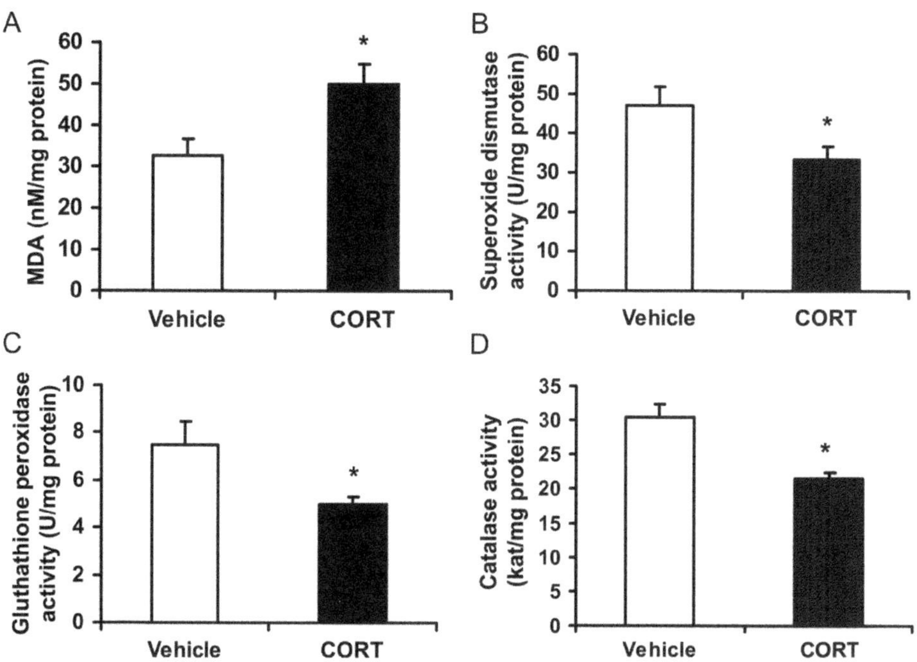

Figure 5. Effect of CORT on ROS defense system in epididymal WAT of mice. (**A**) Concentration of malondialdehyde (MDA), and activities of (**B**) superoxide dismutase, (**C**) gluthathione peroxidase, and (**D**) catalase in epididymal white adipose tissue (WAT) of mice treated with 100 μg/ml CORT or vehicle for 4 weeks. Data are expressed as group means ± SEM (n = 6 by group). * $P<0.05$ compared with vehicle.

induce loss of minerals from bone, muscle and other tissues [38,39]. It's suggested that CORT-induced sacopenia leads to the relative increase in WAT at the expense of the rest of the body in the present study.

Another surprising finding in our study is that chronic CORT exposure reduced epididymal adipocyte size despite increased epididymal WAT weight. For exploring the mechanism underlying this phenomenon, the expression of genes related to lipolysis and lipogenesis were subsequently measured. In agreement with several recent studies [15,40], we showed the up-regulation of these gene expression by chronic CORT exposure. A number of studies have also demonstrated either adipolytic or adipogenic effect of GC *in vivo* and *in vitrio*, depending on GC type, concentration, and duration [10,41–44]. However, GC are most likely acting as a lipolytic or lipogenic factor through separate pathways. Lipolysis and lipogenesis are putatively concomitant in epididymal WAT under GC administration, and like our data, GC prefer to stimulate epididymal adipocyte hyperplasia rather than hypertrophy to induce central obesity.

Chronic CORT induces epididymal fat enlargement, and mitochondrial defects cause adiposity [45], but the relevant point is the linkage between these manifestations. Previous studies reported the present of glucocorticoid receptor (GR) and glucocorticoid response elements (GREs) in mitochondria [46,47], suggesting glucocorticoids are able to directly act in mitochondria, and then regulate the energy metabolism, since mitochondria play key actors in global energy modulation [45]. Our results suggest that CORT impairs mitochondrial biogenesis and oxidative function in epididymal fat. In line with our data, a most recent report using rat pheochromocytoma PC12 cells has shown excessive glucocorticoid increases protein carbonylation, inhibits activities of mitochondrial complex I and superoxide dismutase [48]. Similarly, decreased activities of anti-oxidative enzymes and increased ROS levels were also observed in our CORT-treated epididymal WAT of mice, suggesting the failure of ROS defense system, which, on the other hand, is also an evidence of mitochondrial dysfunction [49]. Adipose tissue is peculiar in its defence systems, namely 11βHSD1, corticosteroid receptor regulation, and corticosteroid-binding globulin (CBG). Through the systems, GC action and availability could be modulated in adipose tissue [50], which make the mechanism by which CORT induces epididymal adiposity more complicated. However, it's clear that glucocorticoids elicit metabolic syndrome through alteration of ROS, damage to mitochondria, ER stress. Mitochondrial dysfunction also leads to abnormal lipid accumulation and the deterioration of the differentiation process [51]. These findings suggest that mitochondrial dysfunction contribute to CORT-induced epididymal adiposity, but the exact mechanism still warrants further investigation.

In conclusion, the present results indicate that chronic CORT administration induces epididymal adiposity and adipocyte hyperplasia. This is, at least in part, associate with mitochondrial dysfunction in epididymal WAT. Our work offers a potential explanation for the underlying mechanism of metabolic complications of excess glucocorticoid.

Acknowledgments

We are grateful to Ying Yao and Yu Chen for technical assistance with gene expression analysis.

Author Contributions

Conceived and designed the experiments: JY DC. Performed the experiments: JY BY JH PZ XM. Analyzed the data: JY BY JH PZ. Contributed reagents/materials/analysis tools: XM GH. Wrote the paper: JY DC.

References

1. Anagnostis P, Athyros VG, Tziomalos K, Karagiannis A, Mikhailidis DP (2009) Clinical review: The pathogenetic role of cortisol in the metabolic syndrome: a hypothesis. J Clin Endocrinol Metab 94: 2692–2701.
2. Liu D, Diorio J, Tannenbaum B, Caldji C, Francis D, et al. (1997) Maternal care, hippocampal glucocorticoid receptors, and hypothalamic-pituitary-adrenal responses to stress. Science 277: 1659–1662.
3. Davies NA, Gillett A, McAlpine C, Seabrook L, Baxter G, et al. (2013) The effect of ACTH upon faecal glucocorticoid excretion in the koala. J Endocrinol.
4. Buttgereit F, Burmester GR, Lipworth BJ (2005) Optimised glucocorticoid therapy: the sharpening of an old spear. Lancet 365: 801–803.
5. Arnaldi G, Angeli A, Atkinson AB, Bertagna X, Cavagnini F, et al. (2003) Diagnosis and complications of Cushing's syndrome: a consensus statement. J Clin Endocrinol Metab 88: 5593–5602.
6. Minami I, Tateno T, Yoshimoto T, Doi M, Izumiyama H, et al. (2006) Subclinical Cushings disease with amelioration of metabolic comorbidities after removal of pituitary tumor. Intern Med 45: 1231–1235.
7. Alemany M (2013) Relationship between energy dense diets and white adipose tissue inflammation in metabolic syndrome. Nutr Res 33: 1–11.
8. Mayo-Smith W, Hayes CW, Biller BM, Klibanski A, Rosenthal H, et al. (1989) Body fat distribution measured with CT: correlations in healthy subjects, patients with anorexia nervosa, and patients with Cushing syndrome. Radiology 170: 515–518.
9. Galitzky J, Bouloumie A (2013) Human visceral-fat-specific glucocorticoid tuning of adipogenesis. Cell Metab 18: 3–5.
10. Masuzaki H, Paterson J, Shinyama H, Morton NM, Mullins JJ, et al. (2001) A transgenic model of visceral obesity and the metabolic syndrome. Science 294: 2166–2170.
11. Liu Y, Park F, Pietrusz JL, Jia G, Singh RJ, et al. (2008) Suppression of 11beta-hydroxysteroid dehydrogenase type 1 with RNA interference substantially attenuates 3T3-L1 adipogenesis. Physiol Genomics 32: 343–351.
12. Slavin BG, Ong JM, Kern PA (1994) Hormonal regulation of hormone-sensitive lipase activity and mRNA levels in isolated rat adipocytes. J Lipid Res 35: 1535–1541.
13. Divertie GD, Jensen MD, Miles JM (1991) Stimulation of lipolysis in humans by physiological hypercortisolemia. Diabetes 40: 1228–1232.
14. Djurhuus CB, Gravholt CH, Nielsen S, Mengel A, Christiansen JS, et al. (2002) Effects of cortisol on lipolysis and regional interstitial glycerol levels in humans. Am J Physiol Endocrinol Metab 283: E172–177.
15. Campbell JE, Peckett AJ, D'Souza A M, Hawke TJ, Riddell MC (2011) Adipogenic and lipolytic effects of chronic glucocorticoid exposure. Am J Physiol Cell Physiol 300: C198–209.
16. Patti ME, Corvera S (2010) The role of mitochondria in the pathogenesis of type 2 diabetes. Endocr Rev 31: 364–395.
17. Starkov AA (2008) The role of mitochondria in reactive oxygen species metabolism and signaling. Ann N Y Acad Sci 1147: 37–52.
18. Owen OE, Kalhan SC, Hanson RW (2002) The key role of anaplerosis and cataplerosis for citric acid cycle function. J Biol Chem 277: 30409–30412.
19. Wilson-Fritch L, Nicoloro S, Chouinard M, Lazar MA, Chui PC, et al. (2004) Mitochondrial remodeling in adipose tissue associated with obesity and treatment with rosiglitazone. J Clin Invest 114: 1281–1289.
20. Rong JX, Qiu Y, Hansen MK, Zhu L, Zhang V, et al. (2007) Adipose mitochondrial biogenesis is suppressed in db/db and high-fat diet-fed mice and improved by rosiglitazone. Diabetes 56: 1751–1760.
21. Okamoto Y, Higashiyama H, Rong JX, McVey MJ, Kinoshita M, et al. (2007) Comparison of mitochondrial and macrophage content between subcutaneous and visceral fat in db/db mice. Exp Mol Pathol 83: 73–83.
22. Kaaman M, Sparks LM, van Harmelen V, Smith SR, Sjolin E, et al. (2007) Strong association between mitochondrial DNA copy number and lipogenesis in human white adipose tissue. Diabetologia 50: 2526–2533.
23. Tedesco L, Valerio A, Cervino C, Cardile A, Pagano C, et al. (2008) Cannabinoid type 1 receptor blockade promotes mitochondrial biogenesis through endothelial nitric oxide synthase expression in white adipocytes. Diabetes 57: 2028–2036.
24. Nishino N, Tamori Y, Tateya S, Kawaguchi T, Shibakusa T, et al. (2008) FSP27 contributes to efficient energy storage in murine white adipocytes by promoting the formation of unilocular lipid droplets. J Clin Invest 118: 2808–2821.
25. Karatsoreos IN, Bhagat SM, Bowles NP, Weil ZM, Pfaff DW, et al. (2010) Endocrine and physiological changes in response to chronic corticosterone: a potential model of the metabolic syndrome in mouse. Endocrinology 151: 2117–2127.

26. Seale P, Conroe HM, Estall J, Kajimura S, Frontini A, et al. (2011) Prdm16 determines the thermogenic program of subcutaneous white adipose tissue in mice. J Clin Invest 121: 96–105.
27. Liu J, Chen D, Yao Y, Yu B, Mao X, et al. (2012) Intrauterine growth retardation increases the susceptibility of pigs to high-fat diet-induced mitochondrial dysfunction in skeletal muscle. PLoS One 7: e34835.
28. Yu J, Zhao L, Wang A, Eleswarapu S, Ge X, et al. (2012) Growth hormone stimulates transcription of the fibroblast growth factor 21 gene in the liver through the signal transducer and activator of transcription 5. Endocrinology 153: 750–758.
29. Yu J, Yu B, Jiang H, Chen D (2012) Conjugated linoleic acid induces hepatic expression of fibroblast growth factor 21 through PPAR-alpha. Br J Nutr 107: 461–465.
30. D'Antona G, Ragni M, Cardile A, Tedesco L, Dossena M, et al. (2010) Branched-chain amino acid supplementation promotes survival and supports cardiac and skeletal muscle mitochondrial biogenesis in middle-aged mice. Cell Metab 12: 362–372.
31. Grundy SM, Brewer HB Jr, Cleeman JI, Smith SC Jr, Lenfant C (2004) Definition of metabolic syndrome: Report of the National Heart, Lung, and Blood Institute/American Heart Association conference on scientific issues related to definition. Circulation 109: 433–438.
32. Murray F, Smith DW, Hutson PH (2008) Chronic low dose corticosterone exposure decreased hippocampal cell proliferation, volume and induced anxiety and depression like behaviours in mice. Eur J Pharmacol 583: 115–127.
33. Rees SL, Panesar S, Steiner M, Fleming AS (2004) The effects of adrenalectomy and corticosterone replacement on maternal behavior in the postpartum rat. Horm Behav 46: 411–419.
34. Cassano AE, White JR, Penraat KA, Wilson CD, Rasmussen S, et al. (2012) Anatomic, hematologic, and biochemical features of C57BL/6NCrl mice maintained on chronic oral corticosterone. Comp Med 62: 348–360.
35. Stewart PM (2005) Tissue-specific Cushing's syndrome uncovers a new target in treating the metabolic syndrome—11beta-hydroxysteroid dehydrogenase type 1. Clin Med 5: 142–146.
36. Stewart PM (2003) Tissue-specific Cushing's syndrome, 11beta-hydroxysteroid dehydrogenases and the redefinition of corticosteroid hormone action. Eur J Endocrinol 149: 163–168.
37. Schuff KG (2003) Issues in the diagnosis of Cushing's syndrome for the primary care physician. Prim Care 30: 791–799.
38. Hassan-Smith Z, Morgan S, Sherlock M, Bujalska I, Tomlinson J, et al. (2014) 11β-hydroxysteroid dehydrogenase type 1 and age-associated muscle weakness in mice: implications for human ageing. The Lancet 383: S53.
39. Pezaro C, Mukherji D, Tunariu N, Cassidy A, Omlin A, et al. (2013) Sarcopenia and change in body composition following maximal androgen suppression with abiraterone in men with castration-resistant prostate cancer. British journal of cancer 109: 325–331.
40. Lee MJ, Fried SK (2012) Glucocorticoids antagonize tumor necrosis factor-alpha-stimulated lipolysis and resistance to the antilipolytic effect of insulin in human adipocytes. Am J Physiol Endocrinol Metab 303: E1126–1133.
41. Berdanier CD (1989) Role of glucocorticoids in the regulation of lipogenesis. FASEB J 3: 2179–2183.
42. Gathercole LL, Morgan SA, Bujalska IJ, Hauton D, Stewart PM, et al. (2011) Regulation of lipogenesis by glucocorticoids and insulin in human adipose tissue. PLoS One 6: e26223.
43. Xu C, He J, Jiang H, Zu L, Zhai W, et al. (2009) Direct effect of glucocorticoids on lipolysis in adipocytes. Mol Endocrinol 23: 1161–1170.
44. Lundgren M, Buren J, Lindgren P, Myrnas T, Ruge T, et al. (2008) Sex- and depot-specific lipolysis regulation in human adipocytes: interplay between adrenergic stimulation and glucocorticoids. Horm Metab Res 40: 854–860.
45. Nunnari J, Suomalainen A (2012) Mitochondria: in sickness and in health. Cell 148: 1145–1159.
46. Demonacos C, Djordjevic-Markovic R, Tsawdaroglou N, Sekeris CE (1995) The mitochondrion as a primary site of action of glucocorticoids: the interaction of the glucocorticoid receptor with mitochondrial DNA sequences showing partial similarity to the nuclear glucocorticoid responsive elements. J Steroid Biochem Mol Biol 55: 43–55.
47. Tsiriyotis C, Spandidos DA, Sekeris CE (1997) The mitochondrion as a primary site of action of glucocorticoids: mitochondrial nucleotide sequences, showing similarity to hormone response elements, confer dexamethasone inducibility to chimaeric genes transfected in LATK- cells. Biochem Biophys Res Commun 235: 349–354.
48. Tang VM, Young AH, Tan H, Beasley C, Wang JF (2013) Glucocorticoids increase protein carbonylation and mitochondrial dysfunction. Horm Metab Res 45: 709–715.
49. Murphy MP (2013) Mitochondrial dysfunction indirectly elevates ROS production by the endoplasmic reticulum. Cell Metab 18: 145–146.
50. Wang M (2005) The role of glucocorticoid action in the pathophysiology of the metabolic syndrome. Nutr Metab 2: 1–14.
51. Lu RH, Ji H, Chang ZG, Su SS, Yang GS (2010) Mitochondrial development and the influence of its dysfunction during rat adipocyte differentiation. Mol Biol Rep 37: 2173–2182.

Cerebral Artery Alpha-1 AR Subtypes: High Altitude Long-Term Acclimatization Responses

Ravi Goyal[1,2]*, Dipali Goyal[1,2], Nina Chu[1,2], Jonathan Van Wickle[1,2], Lawrence D. Longo[1,2]

1 Center for Perinatal Biology, Department of Basic Sciences, School of Medicine, Loma Linda University, Loma Linda, California, United States of America, **2** Epigenuity LLC, Loma Linda, California, United States of America

Abstract

In response to hypoxia and other stress, the sympathetic (adrenergic) nervous system regulates arterial contractility and blood flow, partly through differential activities of the alpha1 (α_1) - adrenergic receptor (AR) subtypes (α1A-, α1B-, and α1D-AR). Thus, we tested the hypothesis that with acclimatization to long-term hypoxia (LTH), contractility of middle cerebral arteries (MCA) is regulated by changes in expression and activation of the specific α_1-AR subtypes. We conducted experiments in MCA from adult normoxic sheep maintained near sea level (300 m) and those exposed to LTH (110 days at 3801 m). Following acclimatization to LTH, ovine MCA showed a 20% reduction ($n = 5$; $P<0.05$) in the maximum tension achieved by 10^{-5} M phenylephrine (PHE). LTH-acclimatized cerebral arteries also demonstrated a statistically significant ($P<0.05$) inhibition of PHE-induced contractility in the presence of specific α1-AR subtype antagonists. Importantly, compared to normoxic vessels, there was significantly greater ($P<0.05$) α1B-AR subtype mRNA and protein levels in LTH acclimatized MCA. Also, our results demonstrate that extracellular regulated kinase 1 and 2 (ERK1/2)-mediated negative feedback regulation of PHE-induced contractility is modulated by α1B-AR subtype. Overall, in ovine MCA, LTH produces profound effects on α1-AR subtype expression and function.

Editor: Xiongwen Chen, Temple University, United States of America

Funding: The studies were supported by United States Public Health Service Grant PO1 HD031226 to LDL. The funders had no role in study design, data collection and analysis, decision to publish, or preparation of the manuscript.

Competing Interests: On behalf of all the authors employed by Epigenuity LLC.

* Email: rgoyal@llu.edu

Introduction

Acute hypoxia leads to a significant increase in cerebral blood flow [1]. However, with successful acclimatization to hypoxia, the cerebral blood flow returns to the values similar to individuals at sea-level [2,3]. Associated changes with the normal acclimatization response include: hypercapnia, polycythemia, high hemoglobin concentration, and angiogenesis. These changes are crucial to maintain normal blood flow normal with adequate tissue oxygenation [4]. Dysregulation of the normal acclimatization responses can lead to acute or chronic mountain sickness, high altitude cerebral edema, chronic migraine headache, and other high altitude-associated disorders [5–8]. To study the cellular/sub-cellular mechanisms responsible for successful acclimatization, we exposed adult sheep to LTH (~110 days) at an altitude of 3801 m. In previous studies, at this altitude, we have reported that the arterial PO_2 fell by 40% and cardiac output decreased 14% [9,10]. Of note, in the LTH animal the distribution of the reduced cardiac output was altered so that blood flow to the brain was maintained at near normal levels [2,3].

Thus, to maintain cerebral blood flow despite a steady-state decrease in cardiac output, the basal cerebrovascular resistance probably decreases in response to acclimatization to LTH. One possible contribution to a decrease in cerebrovascular resistance could be a shift in the structure and/or composition of the cerebral arteries favoring larger diameters and reduced hydraulic resistance. Inconsistent with this possibility, LTH had no significant effects on average artery wall thicknesses or water content [11].

Another mechanism that could potentially contribute to the LTH associated decreased cerebrovascular resistance is that of decreased vascular tone. Responses to exogenous nitric oxide (vasodilator) released from s-nitroso-N-acetylpenicillamine, however, does not differ significantly in normoxic and LTH sheep MCA [3]. Similarly, LTH had no significant effect on vasodilator responses to the calcium ionophore A23187 or shear-stress-induced nitric oxide release in fetal MCA [3]. Thus, based on our previous studies, clearly the reduced cerebrovascular resistance characteristic of LTH acclimatization must involve other mechanisms.

Another important influence on cerebrovascular resistance under stress is the release of vasoactive neurohormones from perivascular nerves. The largest neural component of the cerebral vasculature is adrenergic in nature [12–15], and this serves an important role in regulating cerebral arterial contractility and blood flow [13,16]. Importantly, the role of adrenergic regulation increases substantially during stress, and plays an important role in maintaining cerebral blood flow [17]. Also, acclimatized sheep have significantly higher basal norepinephrine and epinephrine levels compared to sea-level controls [11]. Paradoxically, despite these increased catecholamine levels, we observed ~20% reduction in contractile responses to nor-epinephrine in LTH acclima-

Table 1. Pharmacological Agents Used in the Present Study.

Full Name	Abbreviation	Conc. Molar	Target	Company	Cat #
PHE HCl	PHE	10^{-5}	A1-AR antagonist	Sigma	P-6126
2-([2,6-Dimethoxyphenoxyethyl]a-minomethyl)-1,4-benzodioxane hydrochloride	WB	10^{-7}	α1A-AR antagonist	Sigma	B-018
chlor-ethyl-clonidine	CEC	10^{-5}	α1B-AR antagonist	Sigma	B-003
8-(2-[4-(2-Methoxyphenyl)-1-piperazinyl]ethyl)-8-azaspiro(4.5)decane-7,9-dione	BMY	10^{-7}	α1D-AR antagonist	Sigma	B-134
	PD98059	2×10^{-5}	ERK inhibitor	Sigma	P-215
Y-27632 dihydrochloride	Y27632	10^{-5}	Rho-Kinase inhibitor	Tocris	1254
2-[1-(3-(Amidinothio)propyl)-1H-indol-3-yl]-3-(1-methylindol-3-yl)maleimide methanesulfonate	Ro31-8220	10^{-5}	Pan-PKC inhibitor	Enzo Life Sciences	EL-283
2,2′,3,3′,4,4′-Hexahydroxy-1,1′ -biphenyl-6,6′ -dimethanol-dimethyl ether	HBDDE	5×10^{-5}	PKCα+PKCγ inhibitor	Enzo Life Sciences	EL-273
4,5-bis[(4-Fluorophenyl)amino]phthalimide	DAPH-7	4×10^{-6}	PKCβ inhibitor	Enzo Life Sciences	EL-387
N-Myristoyl-Glu-Ala-Val-Ser-Leu-Lys-Pro-Thr	Myristoylated PKC eV-2	10^{-5}	PKCε inhibitor	Biomol Life Sciences	P-223

tized sheep cerebral arteries [11]. To explore the mechanisms of these findings, we examined α1-AR densities on the sea-level normoxic control and LTH acclimatized arteries. With LTH acclimatization, we observed a 66% and 61% reduction in α1-AR density in sheep common carotid and MCA, respectively [18].

Radio-ligand binding and molecular cloning in several species have demonstrated that the α1-AR family has three structurally distinct subtypes (α1A-, α1B-, α1D-), which are widely expressed in tissues including cerebral arteries, and have differing amino acid sequences and pharmacological properties [19]. Several reviews have considered these in detail [20–22]. Although the three α_1-adrenoceptor subtypes have been reported in various cell types, little is known about their expression, physiological functions, or downstream pathways in MCA. We have shown that in adult ovine cerebral arteries all three α1-AR subtypes are present [12]. Unknown, however, is the extent to which these subtypes are modulated as a consequence of LTH. Thus, we tested the hypothesis that LTH acclimatization of cerebral arterial contractility is regulated by changes in expression and/or activation of α_1-AR subtypes (α_{1A}-, α_{1B}-, and α_{1D}-AR). The present study provides a deeper understanding of cerebral arterial contractility, and provides insights into the LTH regulation of α1-AR expression.

Methods

Experimental animals and tissues

All experimental procedures were performed within the regulations of the Animal Welfare Act, the National Institutes of Health Guide for the Care and Use of Laboratory Animals, and were approved by the Animal Care and Use Committee of Loma Linda University. Sheep were obtained from Nebeker Ranch (Lancaster, CA), as previously described [12,23]. For these studies, we used MCA from ~2 years old ewes that either had been maintained near sea level (300 m) or those acclimatized to high altitude (3,801 m, 12,470 ft; Barcroft Laboratory, White Mountain Research Station, Bishop, CA) for ~110 days immediately before the studies.

For every experiment, 4 to 5 sheep were used from each experimental group. A total of 30 normoxic controls and 30 LTH sheep were used for completion of the present study. Following LTH exposure, animals maintained at high altitude were transported to the Center for Perinatal Biology, Loma Linda University. Upon their arrival at the Center, we placed a tracheal catheter in the sheep through which N_2 flowed at a rate adjusted to maintain its PaO_2 at ~60 Torr, similar to the value at high altitude [24]. All studies were conducted within 48 hours of placing the tracheal catheter. At the time of study, ewes were euthanized with an overdose of the proprietary solution, Euthasol

Table 2. Inhibitory concentration for 50% reduction in PHE contractile responses (IC_{50}) and Dissociation constants (-K_B) values of α_1-AR subtypes inhibitors for phenylephrine-induced contractility in ovine middle cerebral arteries.

Receptor-Drug	K_B (M)	IC_{50} - Values
α1A – WB (10^{-7} M)	1.1×10^{-8}	6.9±0.1
α1B – CEC (10^{-5} M)	5.3×10^{-10}	7.3±0.1
α1D – BMY (10^{-7} M)	6.7×10^{-9}	6.5±0.1

Table 3. Primers used in the present study.

Gene Name	Accession No.	Forward Primer	Reverse Primer	Amplicon Length (Base Pairs)
ADRA1A	XM_004004166.1	TGCACTCGGTCACACACTAC	TGACTTGTCGGTCTTGAGGC	492
ADRA1B	XM_004009542.1	GAAGAAGACCACGGGGGAAG	AGAAGGGCAGAACGGTGAAG	411
ADRA1D	XM_004014355.1	CAACGTGCTGGTCATCCTCT	ATAGCCTGCCTCCTCTGTGA	424
18S	AY753190.1	GCTCGCTCCTCTCCTACTTG	GATCGGCCCGAGGTTATCTA	190
GAPDH	NM_001190390.1	GAGCGAGATCCTGCCAACAT	GAAGTCGCAGGAGACAACCT	624
ACTB	NM_001009784.1	ATGCTTCTAGGCGGACTGTT	CGAAGACAGGAGCAGTGGAG	248

(pentobarbital sodium 100 mg/Kg and phenytoin sodium 10 mg/Kg; Virbac, Ft. Worth, Tx). The brains were removed, following which we obtained the MCA for further analysis. We performed studies in isolated vessels cleaned of adipose and connective tissue. To avoid the complications of endothelial-mediated effects, we carefully removed the endothelium by inserting a small wire three times, as described previously [12,23–26]. Removal of endothelium was examined functionally by stimulating the arterial segments with 122 mM KCl and at the plateau of the response, 100 μM acetylcholine was applied [24,27]. Failure of acetylcholine to relax the arterial segment was taken as a confirmation of the removal of endothelium. On application of acetylcholine, if the arterial segment relaxed, it was discarded from the study. We used the vessels immediately for the experiments. Table 1 presents the specific pharmacological agents used in the present study.

Measurement of middle cerebral artery contractility

We have described this technique in several reports [12,23,24,28–30]. MCA were dissected free from parenchyma and cut into 5 mm long rings in ice-cold modified Krebs-Henseleit (K–H) solution at 4–5°C containing in mM: 120 NaCl; 4.8 KCl; 1.2 K_2HPO_4; 25 $NaHCO_3$; 1.2 $MgCl_2$; 2.5 $CaCl_2$; 10 glucose. The arterial rings were suspended in organ baths (Radnoti Glass Instruments, Inc. Monrovia, CA) that contained 10 ml of modified K-H buffer maintained at 37°C and aerated with 95% O_2 and 5% CO_2 (pH = 7.4). Isometric force was recorded using low compliance force transducers (Radnoti Glass Instruments, Inc) with analogue to digital data collection systems and software (Powerlab 16/30/Chart 5.5 AD Instruments, Colorado Springs, CO). At the beginning of each experiment, vessels were equilibrated without tension for one hour. In view of our previous findings, following stabilization the optimum resting tension was 0.7 gram (g), as at this tension the contractility response to 122 mM KCl was maximal. The contractile response to 122 mM KCl was used to normalize for the variation in smooth muscle mass in each arterial ring [12,23]. For all vessels, we evaluated the contractile response for tension by measuring the maximum peak height, and expressing it in both absolute terms and as percentage K_{max} (a measure of "efficacy"), and calculated pD_2 (the negative logarithm of the EC_{50}, or half-maximal concentration for PHE (a selective α_1-AR agonist), and an index of tissue "sensitivity" or "potency").

The Role of α_1-AR subtype blockers

Three pharmacologically distinct α_1-AR subtypes can be distinguished with pharmacological agents [12,19]. The α_{1A}-AR is selectively inhibited by WB [2-([2,6-Dimethoxyphenoxyethyl]aminomethyl)-1,4-benzodioxane hydrochloride] [31], the α_{1B}-AR subtype is selectively inhibited by CEC (chlor-ethyl-clonidine) [32], and BMY [8-(2-[4-(2-Methoxyphenyl)-1-piperazinyl]ethyl)-8-azaspiro(4.5)decane-7,9-dione] selectively inhibits the α_{1D}-AR subtype [33]. Each of these antagonists is well characterized with known inhibitory concentration to reduce 50% of PHE response (IC_{50}) for vascular adrenergic receptors. First, using a given concentration of PHE (10^{-9} to 10^{-2} M) PHE, we performed a dose-response curve. Then following washout (~5 min) and 40 min re-equilibration, we repeated the PHE dose-response in the presence of the α_1-AR subtype blockers (concentrations are given in Table-1). To examine the role of α1-adrenergic receptor

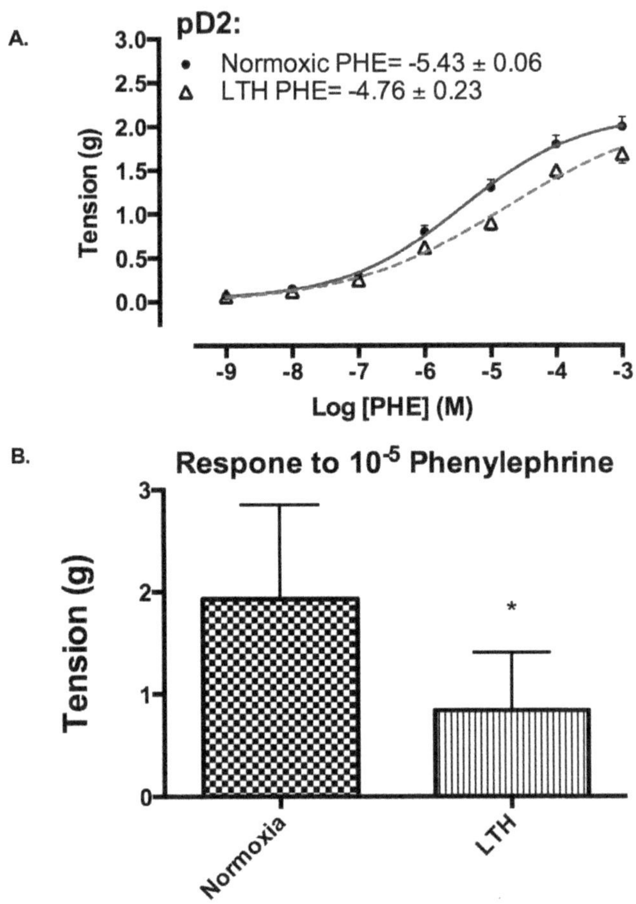

Figure 1. Phenylephrine (PHE) responses in normoxic and LTH ovine MCA. *(A)* Dose-response curves in response to PHE under normoxic (●, solid line) and LTH (Δ, dashed line) conditions. *(B)* Tension (g) at EC_{50} in normoxic and LTH sheep MCA. n = 5 sheep in each group. Values are means ± standard error of means. *Denotes P = <0.05.

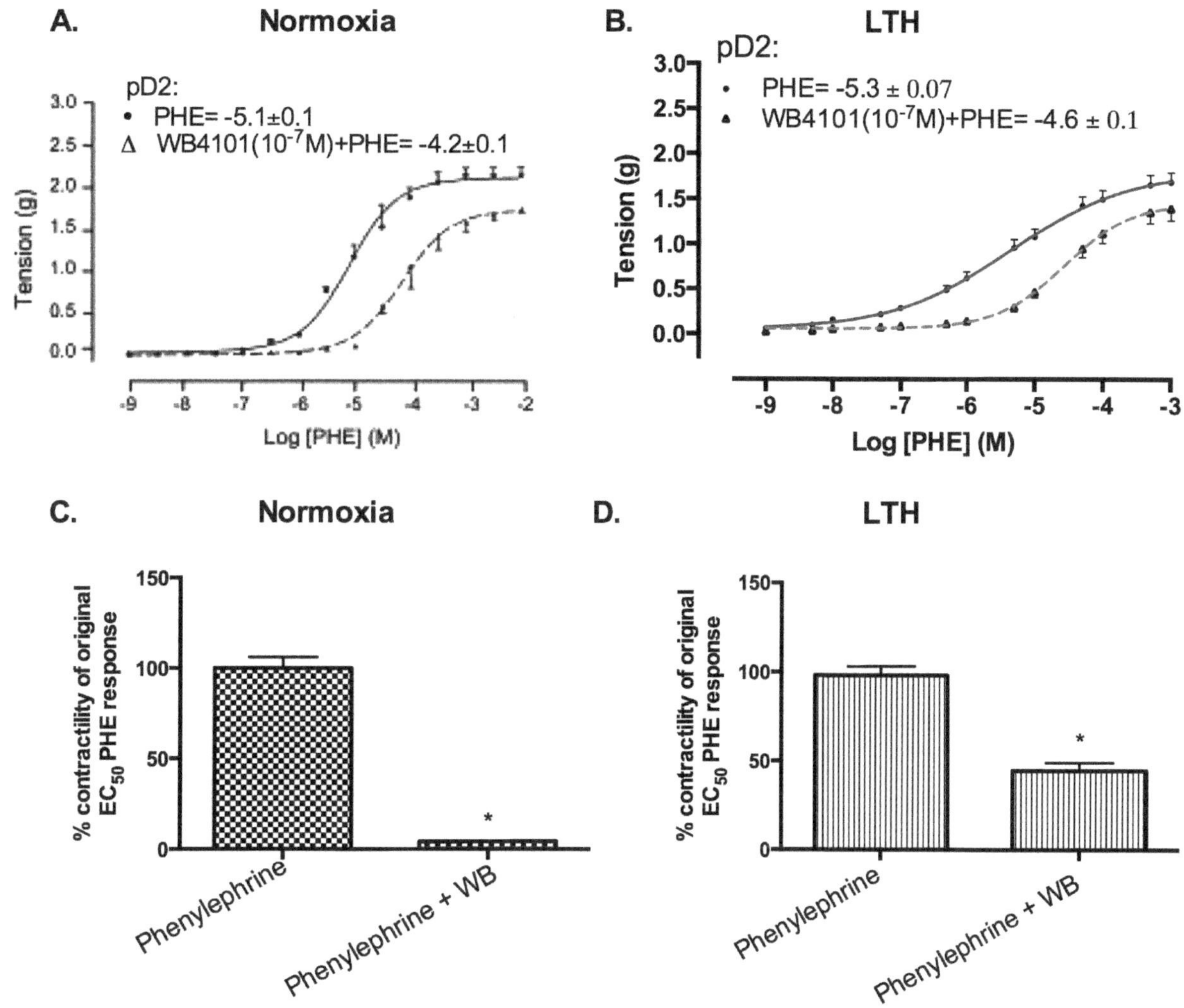

Figure 2. PHE responses in presence and absence of α1A-AR subtype antagonist (10^{-7} M WB) in normoxic and LTH ovine MCA. (A) Dose-response curves in normoxic MCA. Vascular tensions (g) for MCA in response to PHE alone (●, solid line), and in the presence of 10^{-7} M WB (Δ, dashed line).(B) Dose-response curves in LTH MCA. (C) Tension (g) at EC50 in normoxic sheep MCA. (D) Tension (g) at EC50 in LTH sheep MCA. n = 5 sheep in each group. Values are means ± standard error of means. *Denotes P = <0.05.

subtypes, the antagonists were administered 20 min before the application of PHE. For each agent, we determined the IC_{50} and dissociation constant K_B (Table 2).

Immunoblot of α_1-AR subtypes

As noted, ovine MCA were cleaned of adventitia and the endothelium was denuded in a phosphate-free balanced salt solution (BSS) of the following composition (mM): 126 NaCl; 5 KCl; 10 HEPES; 1 $MgCl_2$; 2 $CaCl_2$; 10 glucose; pH 7.4 (adjusted with NaOH). The arteries were homogenized with a tissue grinder in ice-cold cell lysis buffer (Cell Signaling Technology, Danvers, MA), as described previously [12]. Protein concentrations were measured using a protein assay kit (Bio-Rad Laboratories, Hercules, CA) and bovine serum albumin (BSA) was used as a reference protein standard. Mini Trans-Blot Electrophoretic Transfer Cell system (Bio-Rad Laboratories) was used to transfer proteins from the gel to a nitrocellulose membrane at 100 V for 3 h. We then performed an overnight incubation of subtype specific primary antibodies (1:500 dilution) for α1A-, α1B-, and α1D-AR (Santa Cruz Biotechnology, Santa Cruz, CA). We used α-actin as an internal control for equal protein loading, as well as the blocking peptide for each subtype specific antibody as a negative control (Santa Cruz Biotechnology). The membrane was then incubated in chemiluminescence luminol reagent (Pierce, Rockford, IL) for 1 min, and the protein band was detected using Alpha Innotech Chemiluminescent imaging system (San Leandro, CA).

Real Time PCR Analysis of mRNA Expression

To examine the extent to which LTH induced changes in α1-AR subtype mRNA expression, we examined the expression levels of the three subtypes by real-time PCR. We designed primers with the use of Primer 3 web-based software (http://frodo.wi.mit.edu/primer3/). These primers (Table 3) were synthesized by Integrated DNA technologies (Coralville, CA). We isolated and quantified RNA by Allprep DNA/RNA Mini Kit, according to the manufacturer's instructions (Qiagen Inc, Valencia, CA Cat # 80204). To check for RNA quality and quantity, isolated mRNA

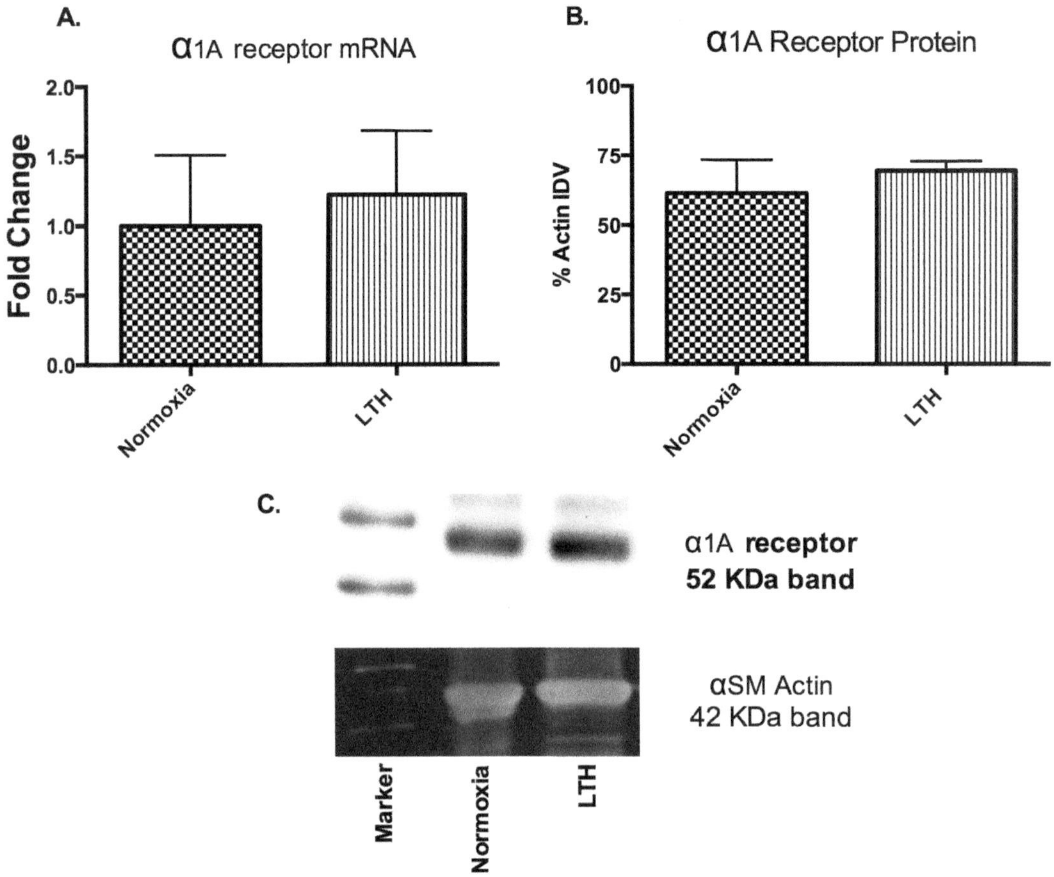

Figure 3. α1A AR expression. (A) Relative mRNA levels in normoxic and LTH cerebral arteries by real-time PCR. (B) Relative α1-AR antigen levels detected by western immunoblot analysis. IDV - Integrated Density Value. n = 5 sheep in each group. Values are means ± standard error of means. *Denotes P = <0.05. Fold change was relative to 18 s Ribosomal RNA.

was analyzed using a NanoDrop 1000 Spectrophotometer (Thermofisher Scientific, Waltham, MA) at 260/280 wavelength UV rays, and a 260/280 ratio of 1.8 to 2 was accepted for quantification with real-time PCR. RNA integrity was analyzed on 1% agarose gel (Figure S2). Samples with clear 28 s and 18 s bands were included in further analysis. The mRNA was treated with genomic DNA wipeout buffer, and then reverse transcribed using Quantitect cDNA synthesis kit (Qiagen, Valencia, CA). Relative expression was normalized to 18S RNA, and fold-changes were calculated using the ΔΔCt method with normalization of individual PCR efficiencies [34]. GAPDH and Beta Actin also were examined as controls (Figure S1A & S1B). Samples (n = 4 from each group) were analyzed on the Roche LightCycler 1.5 (Roche, Indianapolis, IN).

Statistical analysis

All values were calculated as means ± standard error of mean (SEM). In all cases, *n* values refer to the number of animals for a particular study in each experimental group. For testing differences between two groups, we used a simple unpaired Student's t-test. Where applicable, we used analysis of variance with repeated measures (Prism, GraphPad Software, La Jolla, CA). A *P*-value of <0.05 was considered significant.

Results

Changes in PHE response with LTH acclimatization

With LTH acclimatization, we observed a right-shift of the PHE dose-response curve (Figure 1A). The EC_{50} for PHE was $\sim 10^{-5}$ M in both oxygenation groups. Also, the maximum tension achieved in MCA by 10^{-5} M PHE was reduced significantly in the LTH exposed arteries as compared to the normoxic control (Figure 1B).

Role of α_{1A}-AR subtypes in cerebrovascular contraction

In both normoxic and LTH ovine MCA (5 animals in each group), the α1A-AR subtype antagonist (WB) reduced the PHE-induced contractility (Figure 2A & B). In normoxic animals, in the presence of α1A-AR antagonist (WB4101, 10^{-7} M) the receptor sensitivity for PHE was reduced ~20% (pD2 increased from −5.1±0.1 to −4.2±0.1). In LTH MCA, however, the α1A-AR antagonist reduced the receptor sensitivity for PHE only ~15% (pD2 increased from −5.3±0.1 to −4.5±0.06). Importantly, in normoxic cerebral arteries 10^{-7} M WB reduced 10^{-5} M (EC_{50}) PHE-induced contractile response ~90% (Figure 2C). While, in LTH acclimatized arteries, the 10^{-7} M of WB only reduced the 10^{-5} M PHE-induced contractile responses ~50% (Figure 2D). Thus, it appears that the role of α1A-AR subtype is reduced in PHE-induced contractility.

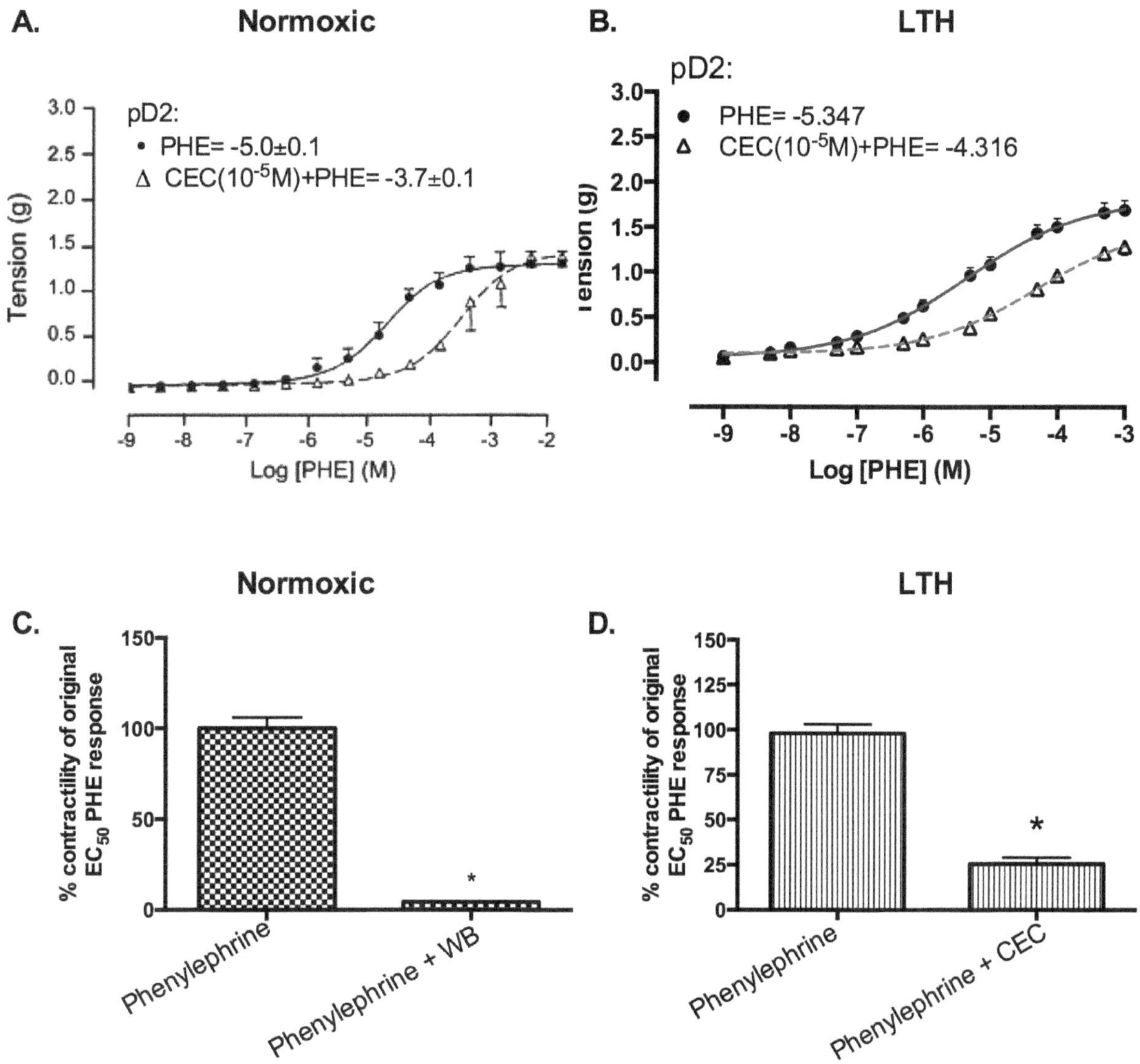

Figure 4. PHE responses in presence and absence of α1B-AR subtype antagonist (10^{-5} M CEC) in normoxic and LTH ovine MCA. (A) Dose-response curves in normoxic MCA. Vascular tensions (g) for MCA in response to PHE alone (●, solid line), and in the presence of 10^{-5} M CEC (Δ, dashed line).(B) Dose-response curves in LTH MCA. (C) Tension (g) at EC50 in normoxic sheep MCA. (D) Tension (g) at EC50 in LTH sheep MCA. n = 5 sheep in each group. Values are means ± standard error of means. *Denotes P = <0.05.

α_{1A}-AR expression

The reduced role of α1-AR subtype in PHE-induced contractility may be a consequence of reduced expression. Therefore, we examined mRNA and protein levels of the α1A-AR subtype. Neither mRNA and nor protein levels of α1A-AR subtype expression were changed with LTH (Figure 3A, B, & C).

Role of α_{1B}-AR subtypes in cerebrovascular contraction

As seen in Figure 4A & B, selective α1B-AR antagonist (10^{-5} M CEC) reduced the receptor PHE sensitivity ~26% (pD2 increased from −5.0±0.1 to −3.7±0.1) and 19% (pD2 increased from −5.3±0.1 to −4.3±0.1) in normoxic and LTH MCA, respectively. Additionally, 10^{-5} M of CEC, reduced the 10^{-5} M PHE induced contractility ~85% and ~74% in normoxic and LTH MCA, respectively (Figure 4C & 4D). Thus, LTH resulted in a significant reduction in the role of the α1B-AR subtype in PHE-induced contractility.

α_{1B}-AR expression

As noted above, the reduced role of the α1B-AR subtype in PHE-induced contractility may be a consequence of reduced expression. Thus, we examined the α1B-AR mRNA and protein levels. Surprisingly, both mRNA and protein levels of α1B-AR subtype increased significantly with LTH acclimatization (Figure 5A, B, & C).

Role of α_{1D}-AR subtypes in cerebrovascular contraction

Next, we examined the role of α1D-AR in PHE-induced contractile responses. As demonstrated in Figure 6A, in normoxic MCA, the α1D-AR antagonist (BMY) produced a significant ~95% reduction in 10^{-5} PHE-induced contractile response. In contrast, in the MCA from LTH acclimatized animals, α1D-AR antagonist reduced the 10^{-5} M PHE-induced contractile response only ~9% (Figure 6B). Importantly, the changes in PHE receptor sensitivity in the presence of α1D-AR antagonist were ~24% (pD2

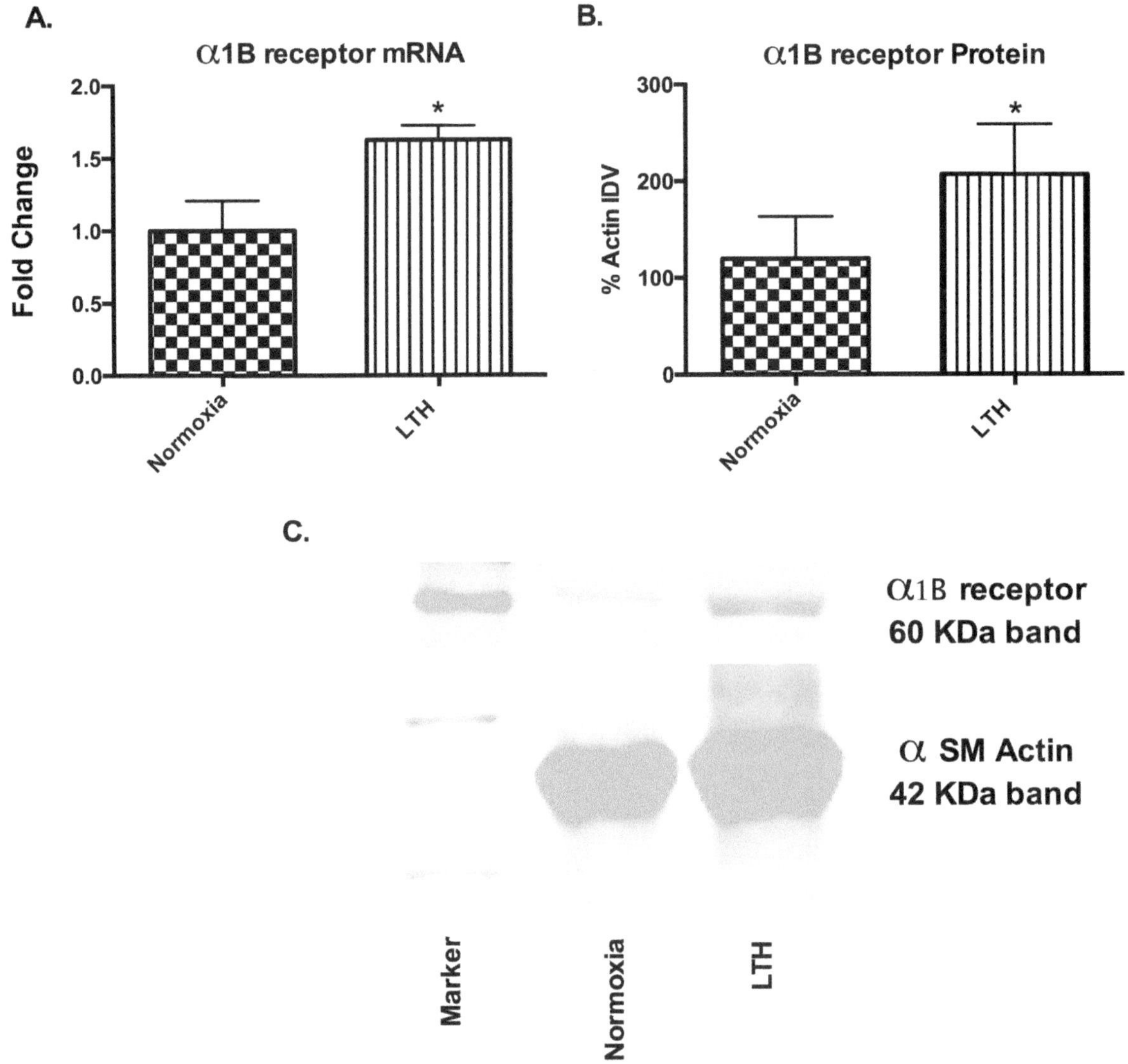

Figure 5. α1B AR expression. (A) Relative mRNA levels in normoxic and LTH cerebral arteries by real-time PCR. (B) Relative α1-AR antigen levels detected by western immunoblot analysis. IDV - Integrated Density Value. n = 5 sheep in each group. Values are means ± standard error of means. *Denotes P = <0.05. Fold change was relative to 18 s Ribosomal RNA.

increased from −5.2±0.1 to −4±0.1) and ~−3% (pD2 increased from −5.3±0.1 to −5.5±0.05) in normoxic and LTH MCA, respectively, and as with α1A-AR subtype contractility was reduced to a much lesser extent in LTH, compared to normoxic vessels (Figure 6C & 6D).

α_{1D}-AR expression

Similar to the reduced role of α1D-AR subtype in contractile responses, while we observed no change in α1D-AR mRNA levels (Figure 7A) there was a ~30% decrease in its protein levels (Figure 7B & C).

LTH-induced changes in contractile responses did not co-relate with the changes in receptor expression. Thus, LTH may be regulating the α1-AR mediated contractile responses by downstream signal transduction pathways. A major mechanism through which α1-AR regulates contractile responses is through protein kinase C (PKC).

LTH and role of PKC in PHE-mediated contractility

Figure 8 demonstrates the relative role of PKC and several of its isoforms in the two experimental groups. As evident, with LTH exposure, MCA demonstrated a significant increase in PKC antagonist-mediated inhibition of PHE induced contractility. The major PKC isoforms appear to be PKC α, β and γ.

LTH and role of Extracellular Regulated Kinases 1 and 2 (ERK1/2) in PHE-mediated contractility

Previously, we have demonstrated that ERK1/2 act as negative regulators of PKC-induced contractile responses [23]. Therefore, we examined the role of ERK1/2 in PHE-induced MCA contractility under conditions of LTH. In response to the ERK1/2 antagonist (2×10^{-4} PD98059), we observed a significant increase in PHE-induced contractility in both normoxic and LTH arteries (Figure 9). However, ERK1/2 inhibition produced significantly less increase in the PHE-induced contractile responses in MCA from LTH acclimatized animals. To elucidate further the

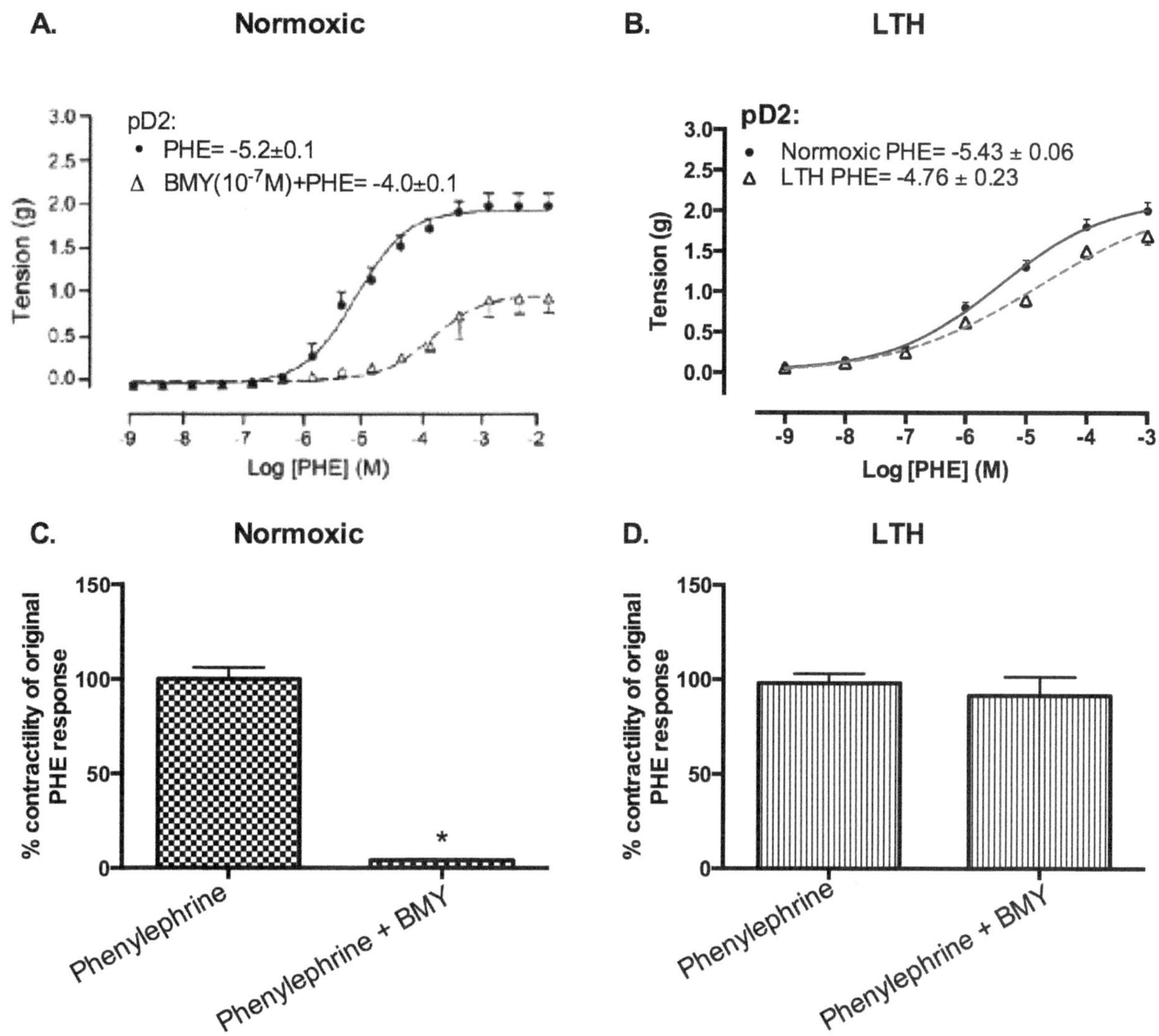

Figure 6. PHE responses in presence and absence of α1D-AR subtype antagonist (10^{-7} M BMY) in normoxic and LTH ovine MCA. (A) Dose-response curves in normoxic MCA. Vascular tensions (g) for MCA in response to PHE alone (●, solid line), and in the presence of 10^{-7} M BMY (Δ, dashed line).(B) Dose-response curves in LTH MCA. ((C) Tension (g) at EC50 in normoxic sheep MCA. (D) Tension (g) at EC50 in LTH sheep MCA. n = 5 sheep in each group. Values are means ± standard error of means. *Denotes P = <0.05.

specific α1-AR subtypes mediating ERK activation, we examined the PHE-induced contractile responses in the presence of ERK inhibitor (2×10^{-5} PD98059) in presence of specific α1-AR antagonists. As seen in Figure 9, inhibition of α1B-AR subtype abolishes the ERK-mediated negative regulation of PHE contractility in the normoxic vessel, while decreasing it significantly in LTH. Of importance, inhibition of α1A- and α1D-AR receptors failed to abolish the ERK-mediated negative regulation of PHE-induced MCA contractility.

LTH and role of Rho kinase in PHE-mediated contractility

As seen in Figure 10, upon application of a Rho kinase inhibitor (10^{-5} Y-27632), we observed essentially a complete inhibition of PHE-induced contractility in both normoxic and LTH acclimatized MCA. No significant differences were observed in the presence of the several α1-AR subtype inhibitors.

Discussion

The present report is an extension of our previous studies on the mechanisms by which the cerebral vasculature acclimatizes to LTH. Previously, we have demonstrated that in response to such acclimatization, cerebral blood flow is maintained to levels similar to those in a normoxic animal [2,3]. Importantly, an inability to maintain normal cerebral blood flow may lead to life threatening disorders such as high-altitude associated cerebral edema and other cerebral manifestations of acute/chronic mountain sickness. Also, in the LTH acclimatized sheep, we have observed a significant increase in norepinephrine (NE) levels and a ~20% reduction in NE-induced MCA contractile responses compared to normoxic controls [11]. The catecholamine NE can act on α1, α2, and/or β1 receptors; however, we have shown that MCA contract in response to NE via stimulation of α1-AR [12,30]. Also, the α2-AR are chiefly pre-junctional in MCA and do not appear to regulate NE-mediated contractile responses [35].

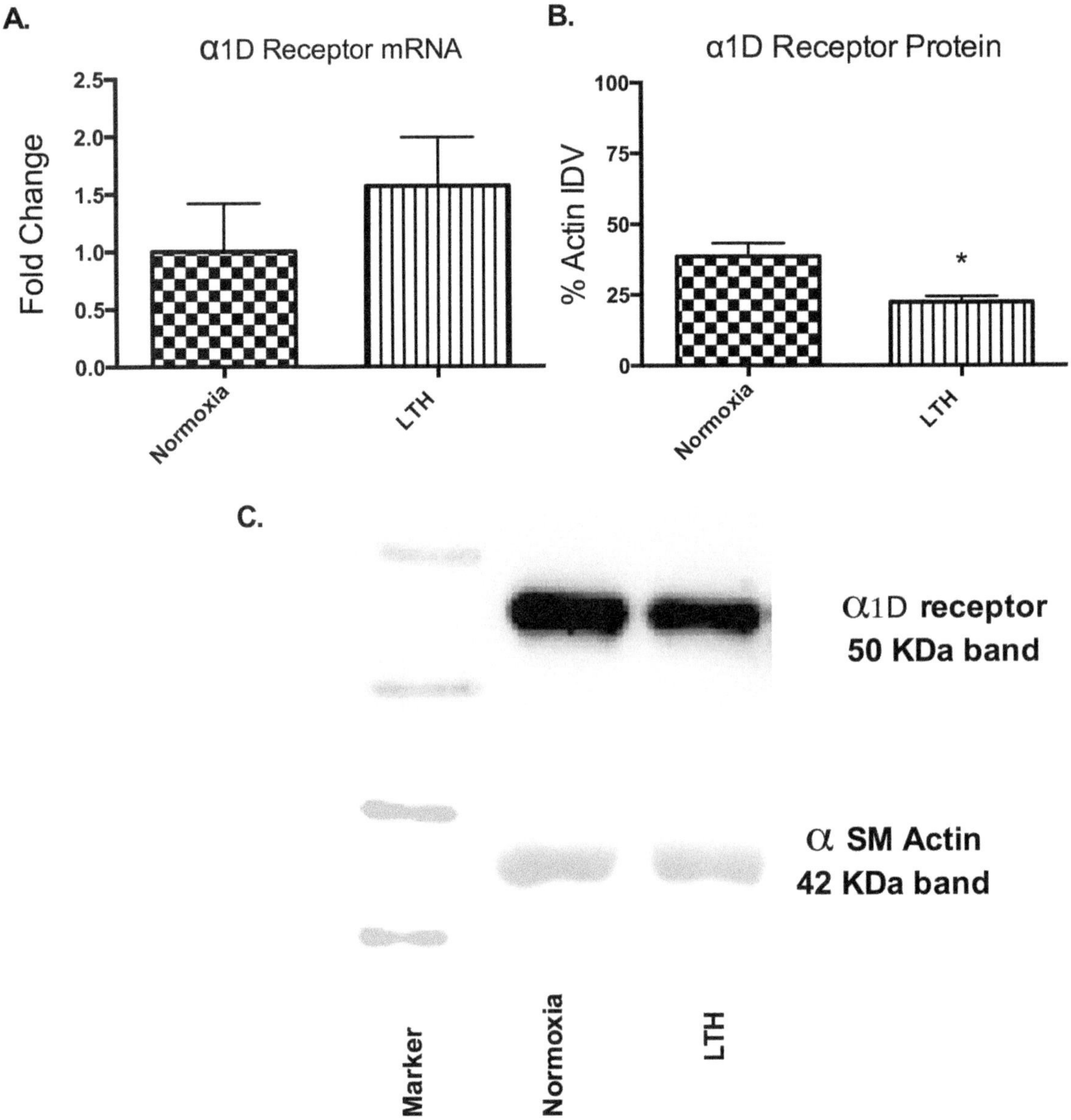

Figure 7. α1D AR expression. (A) Relative mRNA levels in normoxic and LTH cerebral arteries by real-time PCR. (B) Relative α1-AR antigen levels detected by western immunoblot analysis. IDV - Integrated Density Value. n = 5 sheep in each group. Values are means ± standard error of means. *Denotes P = <0.05. Fold change was relative to 18 s Ribosomal RNA.

In the present study, by use of α1-AR specific agonist (PHE) and subtype antagonists, we examined the role of LTH in mediating the regulation of specific α1-AR subtypes. In LTH acclimatized cerebral arteries, PHE-induced contractile responses were reduced to a similar extent (~20%), as compared to norepinephrine [11]. Nonetheless, based on our previous [18] and the present study, the sensitivity of α1-AR is reduced with LTH acclimatization (Figure 1). Importantly, in the present study, we observed a significantly lower role of α1A-AR subtype in PHE-induced contractile responses, as compared to their normoxic counterpart (Figure 2). We observed no reduction in α1a-AR mRNA or protein expression (Figure 3). Therefore, it appears that the reduction in the role of α1-AR in PHE-induced contractile responses may be downstream at the second messenger level or may be negated by some counter-regulatory mechanisms such as nitric oxide pathway. Another explanation for this may be that receptors are being internalized. In a similar manner, LTH acclimatization reduced the role of α1B-AR in PHE-induced MCA contractile responses (Figure 4), despite a significant increase in both the α1B-AR mRNA and protein levels (Figure 5). A clear rationale for the inverse relationships observed is not known. In addition, we observed a significantly reduced role of α1D-AR in PHE-induced contractile responses in LTH acclimatized arteries. This was associated with a significant reduction in α1D-AR protein expression, despite no significant change in mRNA levels. This suggests a post-transcriptional regulation of α1D-AR subtype protein expression. Apparently changes in the expression of α1-AR as well as the PHE-induced contractile responses due to LTH acclimatization suggest changes in the downstream signaling pathways. As is well known, the three α_1-

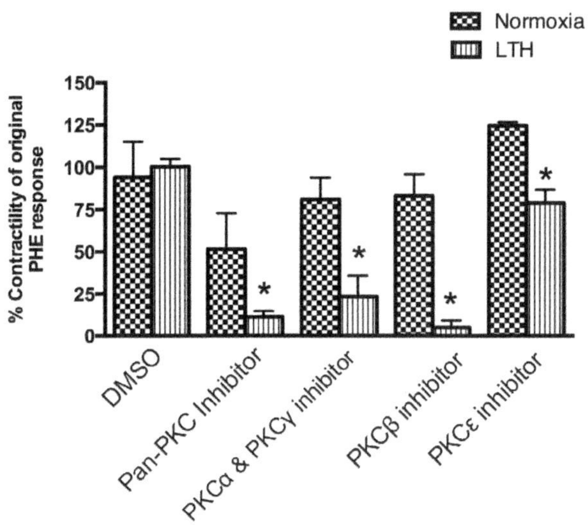

Figure 8. PHE responses in the presence of PKC inhibitors. DMSO - Dimethyl sulfoxide was used as vehicle for PKC inhibitors. Pan-PKC inhibitors -10^{-5} M Ro31-8220; PKCα and γ inhibitor -5×10^{-5} M HBDDE, PKCβ inhibitor -4×10^{-6} M DAPH7, and PKC epsilon -10^{-5} Myristoylated PKC eV1-2 inhibitor. n = 5 sheep in each group. Values are means ± standard error of means. *Denotes P = <0.05.

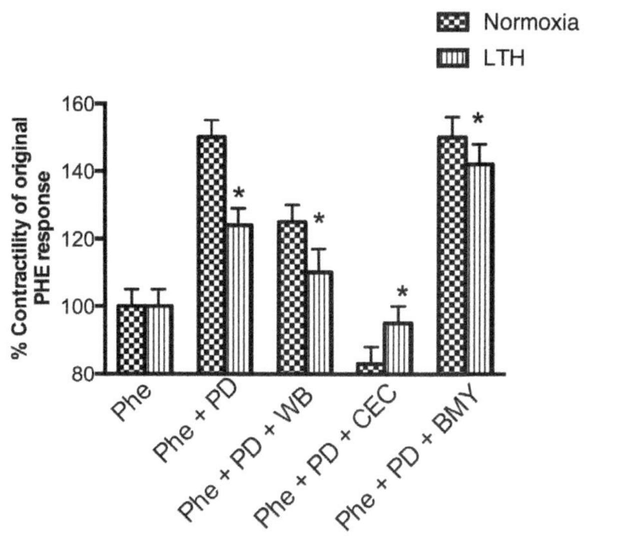

Figure 9. PHE responses in the presence of ERK inhibitors in normoxic (A) and LTH (B) ovine MCA. Specific α1-AR antagonists and ERK inhibitor was added 20 minutes before adding PHE. PHE -10^{-5} PHE; ERK inhibitor - PD98059 -2×10^{-5} PD; WB - α1-AR subtype antagonist -10^{-7} M WB-4101; CEC - α1B-AR subtype antagonist – 10^{-5} M chlor-ethyl-clonidine; BMY - α1D-AR subtype antagonist – 10^{-7} M BMY-7378. n = 5 sheep in each group. Values are means ± standard error of means. *Denotes P = <0.05.

AR subtypes, members of $G_q/_{11}$ protein coupled receptors, activate PLC-β to hydrolyze phosphatidylinositol 4,5,bisphosphate to form inositol 1,4,5, tri-phosphate [Ins(1,4,5)P_3] and di-acyl glyerol (DAG). Ins(1,4,5)P_3 acts on its receptors in the sarcoplasmic reticulum to trigger calcium release and other calcium dependent contractility pathways. DAG with and without calcium activates the several PKC isoforms. Previously, we have demonstrated that LTH leads to a 44% reduction in Ins(1,4,5)P3 release by NE-induced α1-AR activation [18]. In the present study, we show that LTH is also associated with an increased involvement of PKC in α1-AR induced contractility. Of note, LTH is known to suppress calcium-dependent mechanisms and increase reliance of calcium-sensitization mechanisms [24,36].

We also have shown that ERK1/2 negatively regulate PKC-induced contractility and play a major role in calcium-sensitization pathway [23]. In the present study, we also demonstrate that PHE-induced contractility is increased significantly by inhibition of ERK phosphorylation (Figure 10). Inhibition of α1B-AR, did not produce an increase in PHE-induced contractility by ERK inhibitors. This finding suggests that PHE activates α1B-AR which (may be via PKC) activates ERK, which in-turn negatively regulates arterial contractility. Another important pathway, which can be activated by PKC is of Rho kinase [37]. Of note, inhibition of Rho kinase by Y-27632, completely inhibited PHE-induced contractile responses in both normoxic and LTH acclimatized sheep MCA. This is in agreement with a previous study demonstrating a significant inhibition of PHE-induced contractile response in rat-tail artery [38]. Thus, it appears that Rho kinase is critically involved in PHE-induced cerebral arterial contractility.

The role of specific α_1-AR subtypes in the regulation of cerebrovascular tone and cerebral blood flow in response to LTH acclimatization is not well understood. A normal acclimatization response is associated with an increase in hematocrit, hemoglobin concentration, and capillary density along with normal cerebral blood flow. However, the regulatory pathways maintaining normal (as in sea-level control) cerebral blood flow despite reduced cardiac output are not completely understood. In recent years, studies have demonstrated that adrenergic system assumes an important role in the maintenance of the cerebral blood flow. Moreover, unlike other systemic circulatory beds, large arteries have been shown to play a crucial role in the regulation and maintenance of CBF [39]. During increased flow demand, there is a significant pressure gradient from carotid to cerebral arteries [40]. Additionally, other studies suggest that much of the change in systemic pressure results in dilation/contraction of the large arteries that supply the brain [41]. These studies underscore the importance of middle cerebral artery in the regulation of CBF, and suggest that failure of middle cerebral artery to effectively regulate the pressure of the blood reaching delicate intracerebral and plial arteries may

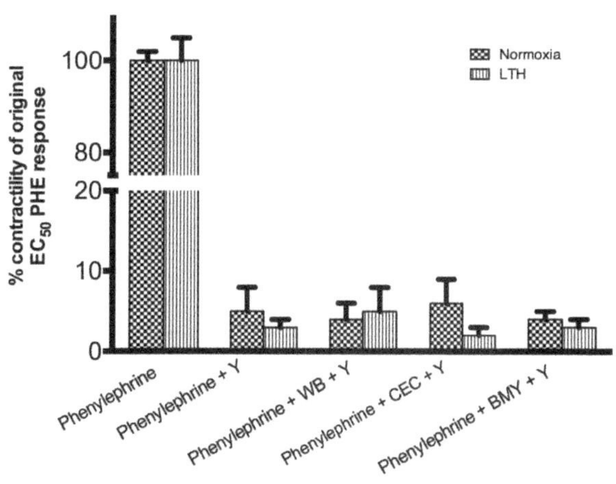

Figure 10. PHE responses in the presence of rho kinase inhibitor (10^{-5} M Y-27632) and specific α1-AR subtypes antagonists. n = 5 sheep in each group. Values are means ± standard error of means. *Denotes P = <0.05.

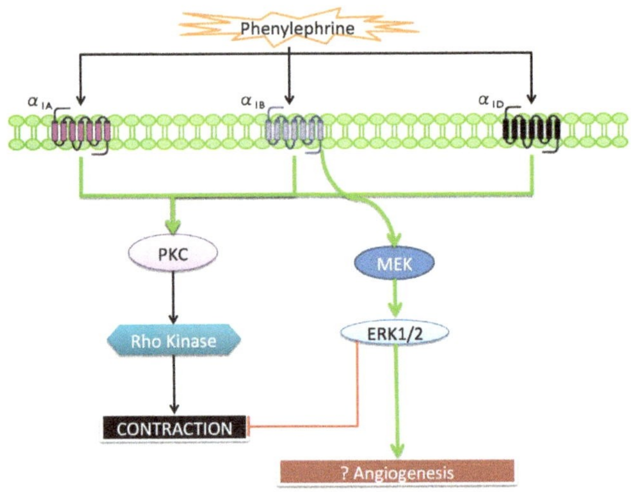

Figure 11. Proposed signal transduction pathways for specific α_1-AR subtype-mediated MCA contraction in MCA.

lead to their rupture with hemorrhage. This is of vital importance, as the α_1-AR subtypes play a role in regulation of large cerebral arteries. Quite obviously, we yet have much to learn about α_1-AR subtypes and their changing role with LTH acclimatization. A caveat of these studies concerns the relative selectivity of the purported pharmacologic agonist/antagonists for the several α_1-AR subtypes, as there may be some limited interaction with other adrenergic and non adrenergic receptors. Nonetheless, in previous studies, these agents have been demonstrated to be quite selective antagonists for α_1-AR subtypes [12,19,31–33].

Perspective and Significance

The present study extends our understanding of the ovine adrenergic system in the contractility of MCA and ultimately regulation of the cerebral blood flow. It is a logical extension of our previous findings and illustrates a small facet of this complexity. The findings provide details regarding LTH-induced acclimatization in expression and functions of the α_1-AR subtypes, as well as their coupling to downstream pathways. For a mechanistic overview, Figure 11 presents a schema based on our present understanding of the role of specific α_1-AR subtype-mediated mechanisms in ovine MCA. An important take home message of the present study is LTH-induced increase in α1B-AR expression and their role in ERK activation. Nonetheless, this study makes apparent the complexity of intracellular signaling pathways and raises a number of important questions. For instance, by what mechanisms does LTH increase α1B-AR expression? What is the functional significance of increase in α_{1B}- AR with LTH? To what extent is α1B-AR-mediated ERK activation responsible for vascular growth and/or other gene expression? What other signaling pathways are involved in α_1-AR-mediated contractile responses in adult ovine MCA? Also of importance, how can we explain the paradox of decreased PHE-induced contractility despite an increase or no change in α1-AR subtype levels? This suggests acclimatization to LTH may be associated with changes in the plasma membrane receptor localization or internalization, or changes in the other signal transduction pathways. Insight into these pathways and physiologic mechanisms may prove to be of great clinical value in developing therapeutic interventions to prevent and/or ameliorate the sequelae of functional dysregulation of cerebral blood flow at high altitude and other conditions associated with LTH exposure.

Supporting Information

Figure S1 Relative mRNA levels (A) Glyceraldehyde 3-Phosphate Dehydrogenase and (B) Beta Actin in normoxic and LTH cerebral arteries by real-time PCR. n = 5 sheep in each group. Values are means ± standard error of means. *Denotes P = <0.05. Fold change was relative to 18 s Ribosomal RNA. GAPDH - Glyceraldehyde 3- Phosphate Dehydrogenase; ACTB - Beta Actin.

Figure S2 Picture of RNA integrity gel demonstrating two distinct bands of 28 s and 18 s RNA bands. Samples 1 to 5 represents RNA isolated from normoxic cerebral arteries, whereas samples 6 to 10 represents those from LTH acclimatized sheep.

Author Contributions

Conceived and designed the experiments: RG LDL. Performed the experiments: RG DG NC JVW. Analyzed the data: RG. Contributed reagents/materials/analysis tools: RG LDL. Contributed to the writing of the manuscript: RG LDL.

References

1. Peeters LL, Sheldon RE, Jones MD, Makowski EL, Meschia G (1979) Blood flow to fetal organs as a function of arterial oxygen content. Am J Obstet Gynecol 135: 637–646.
2. Kitanaka T, Gilbert RD, Longo LD (1989) Maternal responses to long-term hypoxemia in sheep. Am J Physiol 256: R1340–R1347.
3. Longo LD, Hull AD, Long DM, Pearce WJ (1993) Cerebrovascular adaptations to high-altitude hypoxemia in fetal and adult sheep. Am J Physiol 264: R65–R72.
4. West JB (2012) High-altitude medicine. Am J Respir Crit Care Med 186: 1229–1237.
5. Brown JK, Purvis RJ, Forfar JO, Cockburn F (1974) Neurological aspects of perinatal asphyxia. 16: 567–580.
6. Longo LD, Packianathan S (1997) Hypoxia-ischaemia and the developing brain: hypotheses regarding the pathophysiology of fetal-neonatal brain damage. 104: 652–662.
7. Mulligan JC, Painter MJ, O'Donoghue PA, MacDonald HM, Allan AC et al. (1980) Neonatal asphyxia. II. Neonatal mortality and long-term sequelae. The Journal of pediatrics 96: 903–907.
8. Nelson KB (2003) Can we prevent cerebral palsy? 349: 1765–1769.
9. Onishi J, Kamitomo M, Stiffel VM, Gilbert RD (2003) Effects of long-term high-altitude hypoxia on myocardial protein kinase A activity and troponin I isoforms in fetal and nonpregnant sheep. J Soc Gynecol Investig 10: 189–193.
10. Kamitomo M, Longo LD, Gilbert RD (1994) Cardiac function in fetal sheep during two weeks of hypoxemia. 266: R1778–R1785.
11. Longo LD, Pearce WJ (1998) High altitude, hypoxic-induced modulation of noradrenergic-mediated responses in fetal and adult cerebral arteries. Comp Biochem Physiol, Part A Mol Integr Physiol 119: 683–694.
12. Goyal R, Mittal A, Chu N, Zhang L, Longo LD (2010) alpha(1)-Adrenergic receptor subtype function in fetal and adult cerebral arteries. Am J Physiol Heart Circ Physiol 298: H1797–H1806.
13. Bevan JA, Bevan RD (1984) Patterns of alpha-adrenoceptor regulation of the vasculature. Blood Vessels 21: 110–116.
14. McCalden TA (1981) Sympathetic control of the cerebral circulation. J Auton Pharmacol 1: 421–431.
15. Edvinsson L (1982) Vascular autonomic nerves and corresponding receptors in brain vessels. Pathol Biol 30: 261–268.
16. Purkayastha S, Saxena A, Eubank WL, Hoxha B, Raven PB (2013) Œ±1-Adrenergic receptor control of the cerebral vasculature in humans at rest and during exercise. Exp Physiol 98: 451–461.
17. Ter LM, van DJMC, Elting JWJ, Staal MJ, Absalom AR (2013) Sympathetic regulation of cerebral blood flow in humans: a review. Br J Anaesth 111: 361–367.

18. Ueno N, Zhao Y, Zhang L, Longo LD (1997) High altitude-induced changes in alpha1-adrenergic receptors and Ins(1,4,5)P3 responses in cerebral arteries. Am J Physiol 272: R669–R674.
19. Minneman KP, Esbenshade TA (1994) Alpha 1-adrenergic receptor subtypes. Annu Rev Pharmacol Toxicol 34: 117–133.
20. Docherty JR (1998) Subtypes of functional alpha1- and alpha2-adrenoceptors. European Journal of Pharmacology 361: 1–15.
21. Guimarães S, Moura D (2001) Vascular adrenoceptors: an update. Pharmacol Rev 53: 319–356.
22. Graham RM, Perez DM, Hwa J, Piascik MT (1996) Alpha1-adrenergic receptor subtypes: molecular structure, function, and signaling. Circulation Research 78: 737–749.
23. Goyal R, Mittal A, Chu N, Shi L, Zhang L et al. (2009) Maturation and the role of PKC-mediated contractility in ovine cerebral arteries. Am J Physiol Heart Circ Physiol 297: H2242–H2252.
24. Goyal R, Mittal A, Chu N, Arthur RA, Zhang L et al. (2010) Maturation and long-term hypoxia-induced acclimatization responses in PKC-mediated signaling pathways in ovine cerebral arterial contractility. Am J Physiol Regul Integr Comp Physiol 299: R1377–R1386.
25. Goyal R, Longo LD (2014) Acclimatization to Long-Term Hypoxia: Gene Expression in Ovine Carotid Arteries. Physiol Genomics.
26. Goyal R, Van WJ, Goyal D, Matei N, Longo LD (2013) Antenatal Maternal Long-Term Hypoxia: Acclimatization Responses with Altered Gene Expression in Ovine Fetal Carotid Arteries. PLoS ONE 8: e82200.
27. Greenberg B, Kishiyama S (1993) Endothelium-dependent and -independent responses to severe hypoxia in rat pulmonary artery. Am J Physiol 265: H1712–H1720.
28. Goyal R, Creel KD, Chavis E, Smith GD, Longo LD et al. (2008) Maturation of intracellular calcium homeostasis in sheep pulmonary arterial smooth muscle cells. Am J Physiol Lung Cell Mol Physiol 295: L905–L914.
29. Long W, Zhang L, Longo LD (2000) Cerebral artery KATP- and KCa-channel activity and contractility: changes with development. Am J Physiol Regul Integr Comp Physiol 279: R2004–R2014.
30. Longo LD, Ueno N, Zhao Y, Zhang L, Pearce WJ (1996) NE-induced contraction, alpha 1-adrenergic receptors, and Ins(1,4,5)P3 responses in cerebral arteries. Am J Physiol 270: H915–H923.
31. Morrow AL, Creese I (1986) Characterization of alpha 1-adrenergic receptor subtypes in rat brain: a reevaluation of [3H]WB4104 and [3H]prazosin binding. Mol Pharmacol 29: 321–330.
32. Minneman KP, Han C, Abel PW (1988) Comparison of alpha 1-adrenergic receptor subtypes distinguished by chlorethylclonidine and WB 4101. Mol Pharmacol 33: 509–514.
33. Goetz AS, King HK, Ward SD, True TA, Rimele TJ et al. (1995) BMY 7378 is a selective antagonist of the D subtype of alpha 1-adrenoceptors. European Journal of Pharmacology 272: R5–R6.
34. Ramakers C, Ruijter JM, Deprez RHL, Moorman AFM (2003) Assumption-free analysis of quantitative real-time polymerase chain reaction (PCR) data. Neurosci Lett 339: 62–66.
35. Bishai JM, Penninga L, Nijland R, Meulenaar R, Gheorghe CP et al. (2002) Pre- and postjunctional alpha(2)-adrenergic receptors in fetal and adult ovine cerebral arteries. Am J Physiol Regul Integr Comp Physiol 282: R1654–R1662.
36. Robertson TP, Aaronson PI, Ward JPT (2003) Ca2+ sensitization during sustained hypoxic pulmonary vasoconstriction is endothelium dependent. Am J Physiol Lung Cell Mol Physiol 284: L1121–L1126.
37. Kandabashi T, Shimokawa H, Miyata K, Kunihiro I, Eto Y et al. (2003) Evidence for protein kinase C-mediated activation of Rho-kinase in a porcine model of coronary artery spasm. Arteriosclerosis, Thrombosis, and Vascular Biology 23: 2209–2214.
38. Tsai MH, Jiang MJ (2006) Rho-kinase-mediated regulation of receptor-agonist-stimulated smooth muscle contraction. Pflugers Arch 453: 223–232.
39. Heistad DD, Marcus ML, Abboud FM (1978) Role of large arteries in regulation of cerebral blood flow in dogs. J Clin Invest 62: 761–768.
40. Dieckhoff D, Kanzow E (1969) On the location of the flow resistance in the cerebral circulation. Pflugers Archiv: European journal of physiology 310: 75–85.
41. Kontos HA, Wei EP, Navari RM, Levasseur JE, Rosenblum WI et al. (1978) Responses of cerebral arteries and arterioles to acute hypotension and hypertension. Am J Physiol 234: H371–H383.

Nitric Oxide Transport in Normal Human Thoracic Aorta: Effects of Hemodynamics and Nitric Oxide Scavengers

Xiao Liu[1], Zhenze Wang[1], Ping Zhao[1], Zhanming Fan[2], Anqiang Sun[1], Fan Zhan[1], Yubo Fan[1]*, Xiaoyan Deng[1]*

1 Key Laboratory for Biomechanics and Mechanobiology of the Ministry of Education, School of Biological Science and Medical Engineering, Beihang University, Beijing, China, **2** Radiologic Department, Beijing Anzhen Hospital, Capital Medical University, Beijing, China

Abstract

Despite the crucial role of nitric oxide (NO) in the homeostasis of the vasculature, little quantitative information exists concerning NO transport and distribution in medium and large-sized arteries where atherosclerosis and aneurysm occur and hemodynamics is complex. We hypothesized that local hemodynamics in arteries may govern NO transport and affect the distribution of NO in the arteries, hence playing an important role in the localization of vascular diseases. To substantiate this hypothesis, we presented a lumen/wall model of the human aorta based on its MRI images to simulate the production, transport and consumption of NO in the arterial lumen and within the aortic wall. The results demonstrated that the distribution of NO in the aorta was quite uneven with remarkably reduced NO bioavailability in regions of disturbed flow, and local hemodynamics could affect NO distribution mainly via flow dependent NO production rate of endothelium. In addition, erythrocytes in the blood could moderately modulate NO concentration in the aorta, especially at the endothelial surface. However, the reaction of NO within the wall could only slightly affect NO concentration on the luminal surface, but strongly reduce NO concentration within the aortic wall. A strong positive correlation was revealed between wall shear stress and NO concentration, which was affected by local hemodynamics and NO reaction rate. In conclusion, the distribution of NO in the aorta may be determined by local hemodynamics and modulated differently by NO scavengers in the lumen and within the wall.

Editor: David Jourd'heuil, Albany Medical College, United States of America

Funding: This work is supported by Grants-in-Aid from the National Natural Science Research Foundation of China (No. 31200703, 11332003, 61190123, 11202016, 11421202, http://www.nsfc.gov.cn), Specialized Research Fund for the Doctoral Program of Higher Education (20121102120038, http://www.cutech.edu.cn), the National Key Technology R&D Program (2012BAI18B02, http://www.most.gov.cn/), the 111 Project (B13003, http://www.moe.edu.cn/) and Beijing Natural Science Foundation (7132086, http://www.bjnsf.org/). The funders had no role in study design, data collection and analysis, decision to publish, or preparation of the manuscript.

Competing Interests: The authors have declared that no competing interests exist.

* Email: yubofan@buaa.edu.cn (YF); dengxy1953@buaa.edu.cn (XD)

Introduction

Nitric oxide (NO) secreted by vascular endothelium is a pivotal regulator in vascular homeostasis, and the change in its bioavailability has been proposed as a major mechanism of endothelial dysfunction and a crucial modulator of vascular diseases such as atherosclerosis and arterial aneurysm [1,2]. The hallmark of endothelial dysfunction is the impaired shear stress-dependent vasodilation mediated by NO [1]. In addition to causing smooth muscle relaxation, endothelial NO possesses many cardiovascular protective functions [3]. It can reduce endothelial permeability and thus suppress the influx of lipoproteins into the vascular wall. Besides, NO can also inhibit the oxidation of low density lipoproteins, prevent leukocytes from adhesion to the endothelium and hence migration into the vascular wall, and inhibit the proliferation/migration of vascular smooth muscle cells. Moreover, NO may inhibit platelet aggregation and adhesion to the vascular walls, hence preventing thrombosis.

To perform these versatile physiological functions, NO must be transported from the site of synthesis to its target, which is a complex process in the vasculature. The major NO-producing source in the vascular system is considered to be located at the vascular endothelium and its production rate is modulated by wall shear stress (the frictional force induced by the movement of blood on the endothelial cells) [4,5]. Once produced, endothelium-derived NO can be transported in two directions: one towards the lumen of the blood vessel and the other towards the vascular wall. In the lumen of the blood vessel, NO would be transported with the blood flow through convection and be consumed and degraded by numerous reactions, such as oxidation into nitrite, reaction with thiol group containing biomolecules to produce S-nitrosothiols, and formation of a complex with hemoglobin (Hb) [6]. Among these reactions, the most important one is the consumption by Hb that has a very high reaction rate. In the vascular wall, NO diffuses to its primary target, the adjacent smooth muscle cells, to modulate smooth muscle relaxation and vasodilation. In addition, NO in the vascular wall would also react with hemoproteins such as hemoglobin, myoglobin and cytoglobin [7,8]. Especially, it was demonstrated that cytoglobins expressed in the fibroblasts and smooth muscle cells in the vascular wall would contribute to NO dioxygenation and behave as an important NO sink [8].

To model and analyze NO transport and reaction in the vascular system, a number of theoretical studies have been performed. However, most of the studies were focused on arterioles where atherosclerosis and aneurysm seldom develop [9–11]. Until now, little quantitative information exists concerning NO transport and distribution in medium and large-sized arteries where atherosclerosis and arterial aneurysm occur. Different from the arterioles, blood flow rate in the arteries is relatively high. Therefore, the convection term of NO transport may play an important role. Fadel et al [12] and Plata et al [13] theoretically investigated the production and transport of endothelial NO using a parallel plate flow model and found that the convective transport of NO had an important impact on NO distribution. Very different from the simple flow patterns in the arterioles, the blood flow patterns in the vascular disease regions such as the inner walls of curved arterial segments and the outer walls of arterial bifurcations are much more complex, and possesses flow separation and recirculation with sharp spatial variations in wall shear stress [14,15]. Therefore, it is obvious that the complex hemodynamics in the arteries may affect the transport of NO and lead to non-uniform distribution of NO on the endothelium and in the arterial wall. We therefore hypothesized that locally impaired transport of NO and the non-uniformly distributed NO concentration may play an important role in the initialization and development of the localized vascular diseases such as atherosclerosis and arterial aneurysm. To verify this hypothesis, we numerically simulated the blood flow and the transport of NO in a lumen/wall model of a human aorta constructed based on MRI images under different hemodynamic conditions. In the numerical study, NO production rate at the blood-vessel wall interface was assumed to depend on wall shear stress and the effects of NO consumption rate in both arterial lumen and wall on NO concentration distribution were investigated.

Methods

Ethics Statement

The volunteer gave written, informed consent to this study that approved by the Ethical Committee of Peking University First Hospital and carried out in accordance with the regulation of the hospital.

MR imaging and 3-D geometrical reconstruction

The geometrical model of the aortic lumen was created from images acquired from a healthy male volunteer, which was described in detail previously [16,17]. The aortic wall was created with the thickness of the three supra-aortic vessels and thoracic aorta as 0.8 mm and 1.2 mm, respectively [18].

Numerical approaches

Governing equations

Fluid Dynamics

Due to the very low transmural fluid velocity and high NO diffusivity in the arterial wall, the convective term of NO can be neglected [19]. Therefore, the aortic wall was assumed as solid wall without fluid transport and so that flow simulation was only carried out in the aortic lumen.

(a) Lumen

The flow simulation in the aortic lumen was based on the three-dimensional incompressible Navier-Stokes and continuity equations:

$$\rho(\mathbf{u}_l \cdot \nabla)\mathbf{u}_l = -\nabla p_l + \nabla \cdot \boldsymbol{\tau} \quad (1)$$

$$\nabla \cdot \mathbf{u}_l = 0 \quad (2)$$

where $\mathbf{u}_l$ and p_l represent, respectively, the fluid velocity vector and the pressure. ρ is the density of blood ($\rho = 1050\ kg/m^3$). $\boldsymbol{\tau}$ is the stress tensor [20]

$$\boldsymbol{\tau} = 2\eta(\dot{\gamma})\mathbf{S} \quad (3)$$

where $\mathbf{S}$ and $\dot{\gamma}$ are the rate of deformation tensor and the shear rate, respectively. $\dot{\gamma}$ is related to the second invariant of $\mathbf{S}$. η represents the viscosity of the blood, which is a function of $\dot{\gamma}$. For the non-Newtonian blood flow simulation, the Carreau model is used to calculate the blood viscosity

$$\eta(\dot{\gamma}) = \eta_\infty + (\eta_0 - \eta_\infty)\left[1 + (\lambda\dot{\gamma})^2\right]^{\frac{n-1}{2}} \quad (4)$$

where $\eta_\infty = 3.45 \times 10^{-3}$ kg/(m s), $\eta_0 = 5.6 \times 10^{-2}$ kg/(m s), $n = 0.3568$, $\lambda = 3.313$ s [20].

Solute Dynamics

(b) Lumen

The mass transport of NO in the flowing blood can be described by the following steady advection-diffusion-reaction equation

$$D_l \Delta c_l - \mathbf{u}_l \cdot \nabla c_l - \dot{V}_l = 0 \quad (5)$$

where c_l is the concentration of NO, D_l is the diffusion coefficient of NO in blood and taken as $3.3 \times 10^{-9}\ \mathrm{m^2 s^{-1}}$ and $\dot{V}_l$ denotes NO consumed by reactions [10]. In the present study, the reaction term includes the oxidation by oxygen and the consumption by erythrocytes which are described by pseudo-second-order and first order reaction, respectively.

$$\dot{V}_l = k_{oxygen} c_l^2 + k_{ery} c_l \quad (6)$$

where k_{oxygen} is the pseudo-second-order reaction rate ($7.56 \times 10^{-6}\ \mathrm{nM^{-1}\,s^{-1}}$) [13]. k_{ery} is the first order reaction rate for NO consumption by RBCs in the lumen. k_{ery} was taken to be 2.3 $\mathrm{s^{-1}}$ to 230 $\mathrm{s^{-1}}$, which was calculated from the effective second-order rate constant between NO and the RBC-encapsulated hemoglobin (from $10^3\ \mathrm{M^{-1}\,s^{-1}}$ to $10^5\ \mathrm{M^{-1}\,s^{-1}}$) [21,22], with the assumption that the hemoglobin concentration in blood was 2.3 mM [23]. For a reference model, k_{ery} was taken to be 23 $\mathrm{s^{-1}}$.

(c) Endothelium

The NO production rate at the endothelium (R_{NO}) is a critical parameter in the computational simulation of NO transport. A number of experimental studies measured the oxidation products of NO and estimated the NO production rate at the endothelium [11,24]. However, due to the differences in experimental protocols, the reported data varied in a very wide range (from 0.035 to 68 μM/s) [11,24]. To investigate the effect of wall shear stress dependent NO production rate on the transport of NO, two separate models were compared. The reference one is the hyperbolic model which is based on the experimental measurements by Andrews et al [25] as described by:

$$R_{NO-\text{hyp}} = R_{basal} + R_{\max}\frac{|\tau_w|}{|\tau_w| + a} \quad (7)$$

where $R_{basal} = 2.13$ nMs^{-1}, $R_{max} = 457.5$ nMs^{-1} and $a = 3.5$ Pa.

The second is assumed to have a R_{NO} that was linearly dependent on WSS as described by [26]:

$$R_{NO-\text{linear}} = R_{ref}\frac{|\tau_w|}{\tau_{ref}} \quad (8)$$

where $R_{ref} = 150$ μM s^{-1}, $\tau_{ref} = 2.4$ Pa.

(d) Arterial wall

The transport of NO in the arterial wall was modeled by the following equation

$$D_w \Delta c_w - \dot{V}_w = 0 \quad (9)$$

where c_w is the concentration of NO in the arterial wall, D_w is the diffusivity of NO in arterial wall (8.48×10^{-10} m^{2}s^{-1}) and $\dot{V}_w$ is the reaction of NO [27]. The reaction is treated as a first-order rate expression, which is given by [28]

$$\dot{V}_w = k_w c_w \quad (10)$$

where k_w is the consumption rate constant, which was assumed to be 0.01 s^{-1} and 0.1 s^{-1}, respectively to investigate the role of wall consumption on the NO transport and distribution [28]. For the reference model, k_w was assumed as 0.01 s^{-1}.

Boundary conditions Flow transport equations (Eqs 1~2) are subject to the following boundary conditions:

BC-A: For the reference model, at each of the 3 aortic arch branches, 5% of flow volume was allowed to be ejected [17]. Studies demonstrated that the flow volume division at the outlets of the aorta can significantly affect hemodynamics in the aorta [29]. To investigate the effect of different flow volume division on NO transport, we also carried out simulations with flow volume at brachiocephalic artery, left common carotid artery and left subclavian artery as 13.4%, 10.6% and 12.0%, respectively [29].

BC-B: For the reference model, a flat inlet flow velocity profile was used assuming the time-average $Re = 790$ (velocity is 0.1 *m/s*) [17]. Blood flow rate (hence, Re) in the aorta varies dramatically from a resting state to a state of a strenuous exercise. Therefore, to verify the effect of hemodynamics on NO transport, we also carried out simulations at Re = 1185(one and a half of the reference one) and 1580 (twice of the reference one).

The boundary conditions for the mass transport equations (Eqs (5) and (9)) are as follows:

BC-1: The inflow concentration of NO (c_O) at the inlet is assumed to be 0 nM.

BC-2: The continuity of NO concentration is maintained and the mass flux across the endothelium is assumed to be the product of the endothelium NO production rate and the thickness of the endothelium. That is

$$c_l = c_w \quad (11)$$

$$\mathbf{N}_l \cdot \mathbf{n}_l - \mathbf{N}_w \cdot \mathbf{n}_l = R_{NO} T \quad (12)$$

$$\mathbf{N}_l = -D_l \nabla c_l + c_l \mathbf{u}_l;\ \mathbf{N}_w = -D_w \nabla c_w + c_w \mathbf{u}_w \quad (13)$$

where $\mathbf{N}_l \cdot \mathbf{n}_l$ is the flux of NO from the endothelium into the arterial wall, $-\mathbf{N}_w \cdot \mathbf{n}_l$ is the flux of NO from the endothelium into the lumen, T is the thickness of endothelium, which is assumed to be 2 μm and R_{NO} is the NO production rate.

BC-3: For other boundaries, the concentration gradient in the boundary normal direction is assumed to be zero.

Mesh grid A hexahedral mesh was produced using blocking and O-grid techniques with high quality hexahedral cells near the wall to capture the steep variation in mass transport within a thin fluid layer adjacent to the vessel wall (Fig. 1). In order to assure that the results were mesh-independent, the grid-adaptation technique was used, which refined the grid based on the geometric and numerical solution data. Mesh independence was considered to be achieved when the averaged difference in NO concentration between two successive simulations was less than 4%. Mesh independence was reached at 402,556 hexahedral cells for aortic wall and 813,060 hexahedral cells for aortic lumen, respectively.

Computation procedures The numerical calculations were carried out using a validated finite volume-based algorithm Fluent (Ansys. Inc. USA) with a user-defined C-like function (UDF). The UDF was used to solve the mass transport equations and validated by the results from Liu et al [19].

Statistical Analysis To quantitatively investigate the correlation between WSS and NO concentration at the endothelium, we computed the Spearman rank correlation coefficient (*r*) between them for all the simulation cases using MATLAB (The MathWorks, Natick, MA, USA).

Results

Hemodynamics may govern the non-uniform NO distribution in the aorta

Figure 2a shows the streamline and the distribution of wall shear stress (WSS) of the reference model. As shown in the figure with streamline, the blood flow takes a form of swirling flow from the ascending aorta to the aortic arch and separates from the mainstream forming disturbed flow patterns at the entry area of the three supra-aortic vessels (Regions A, D, E) and the distal end of the aortic arch (Region B). In these disturbed flow regions, WSS is relatively low. Particularly, the lowest WSS areas are located at regions A and B. Another low WSS region is located at the ascending aorta (Region C).

Figure 2b illustrates NO distribution at the lumen/wall interface and at the media/adventitia interface ($NO_{med\text{-}adv}$). At the lumen/wall interface, NO distributions at both the lumen-side and wall-side of the endothelium are analyzed. The luminal surface concentration (NO_{end}) characterizes the effects of NO convection and consumption in the lumen while the wall-side concentration ($NO_{sub\text{-}end}$) provides information of NO bioavailability in the subendothelial layer. As shown in the figure, the distribution of NO_{end} is quite similar to that of WSS, which is very uneven in the aorta. In the ascending aorta NO_{end} along the inner wall is relatively lower than that along the outer wall. In contrast, in the descending aorta NO_{end} along the inner wall is relatively higher. Similar to WSS, NO_{end} at disturbed flow regions A and B is

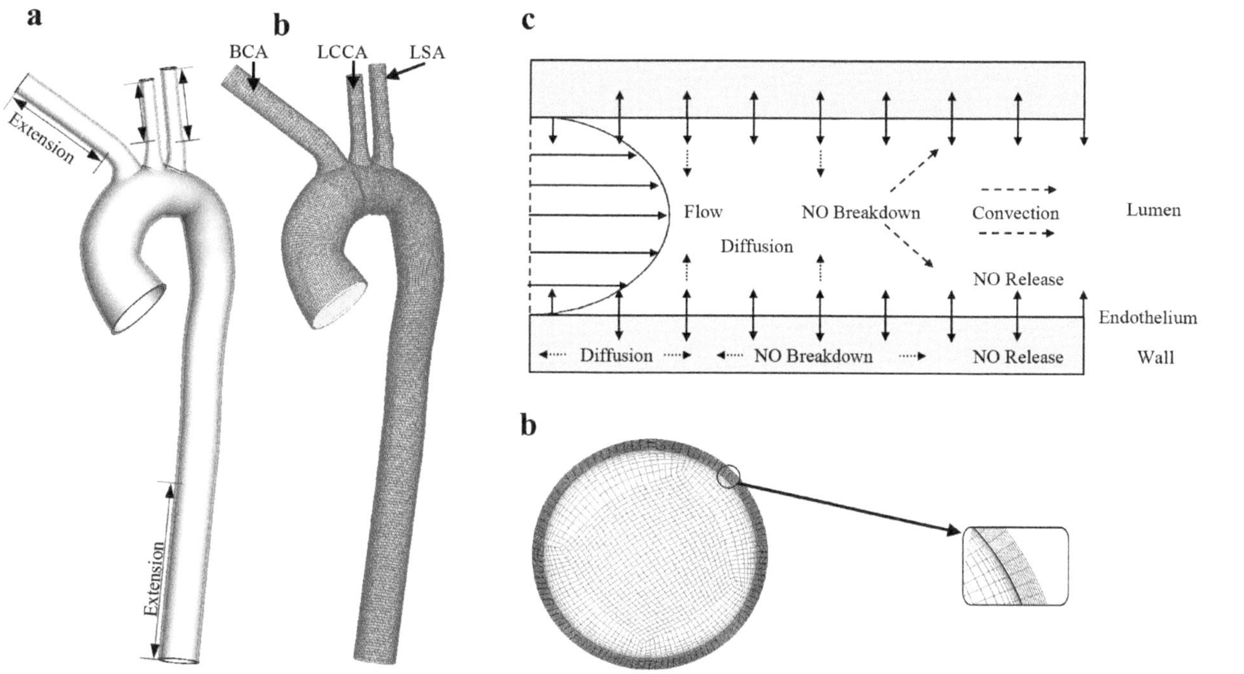

Figure 1. Illustration of the computational models. (a) Geometrical model of the investigated thoracic aorta with straight flow extensions to minimize the influence from outlet boundary conditions. (b) Computational meshes of the thoracic aorta. A structured hexahedral mesh was used with high quality hexahedral cells near the wall to capture the steep variation in NO transport within a thin fluid layer adjacent to the vessel wall. BCA (brachiocephalic artery), LCCA (left common carotid artery), LSA (left subclavian artery). (c) Schematic representation of the mathematical model. Wall shear stress dependent NO release at the endothelium was transported into arterial lumen and wall where physical (diffusion and convection), and biological (consumption) processes were undertaken.

the lowest. When compared to $NO_{sub\text{-}end}$, NO_{end} is relatively lower due to the convection and consumption in the lumen, but their distributions strongly resemble. The consumption reaction in the aortic wall may significantly reduce NO bioavailability, leading to $NO_{med\text{-}adv}$ more than ten times lower than $NO_{sub\text{-}end}$.

To better present NO transport process across the aortic wall, NO distributions in six representative slices along the longitudinal direction of the centerline of aorta are shown in figure 2c. It is clear that NO concentration in the aorta wall is non-uniform and it is relatively low in the inner wall. Specifically, NO concentration in the inner wall of the distal end of the aortic arch (slice D) is almost ten times lower than that in the outer wall.

As shown in Fig. 3a–b, generally speaking, the increase in Re causes an increase in both WSS and NO concentration, and the increase in the latter is according with that in the former from place to place. However, the increase rate of WSS is more than that of NO concentration, especially in the inner wall of the aorta. Moreover, as shown on figure 3, the increase rate of WSS and NO is quite uneven in the aorta. For instance, when compared to the reference model, WSS and NO_{end} for Re = 1185 increases approximate 50% in most regions of the aorta, but more than 100% at region D.

As demonstrated in Fig. 3c, when compared to the reference model, both WSS and NO is significantly reduced in the descending aorta due to the decrease in flow volume and greatly increases in the three supra-aortic vessels. In addition, the differences in NO concentration and WSS between the present model and the reference one are closely similar, which indicates that hemodynamics in the lumen of aorta can directly affect NO distribution in the aorta.

It is well documented that the NO production rate of the vascular endothelium depends on hemodynamics, specifically wall shear stress. We therefore calculated NO transport with other product rate that is linearly dependent on WSS (Eq. (8) in the section of method). As demonstrated in Fig. 3d, when compared to the reference simulation based on $R_{NO\text{-}hyp}$ in Eq. (7), due to the much higher NO production rate, NO concentration obtained for $R_{NO\text{-}linear}$ is much higher. For the two models, as illustrated in Fig. 2(b) and Fig. 3d, NO concentration is relatively low at regions A, B, C. However, close comparison finds that the distributions of NO_{end} and $NO_{sub\text{-}end}$ with $R_{NO\text{-}linear}$ are more similar to the distribution of WSS than those with $R_{NO\text{-}hyp}$. These results indicate that the magnitude and the form of NO production model have a great influence on the concentration distribution of NO in the aorta.

The consumption rate of NO in the lumen modulates NO distribution in the aorta

NO transported to the arterial lumen would be consumed by numerous reactions, especially by hemoglobin in erythrocytes at very high rate. To investigate the effects of the consumption rate of NO in the lumen on NO transport, simulations were carried out for several values of NO consumption rate by erythrocytes (k_{ery}). As is evident from Fig. 4a–b, the distribution of NO concentration in the aorta is very uneven for different k_{ery} and in all the cases the transport of NO is significantly hindered in the disturbed flow regions (Regions A and B), which further indicates hemodynamics plays an important role in the distribution of NO in the aorta. In addition, as shown in Fig. 4a–b, as k_{ery} increases, NO concentration at both the lumen/wall interface and the media/adventitia interface reduce remarkably, indicating that erythrocyte is an effective NO scavenger in the blood that modulates NO concentration in the arterial lumen and wall. More specifically,

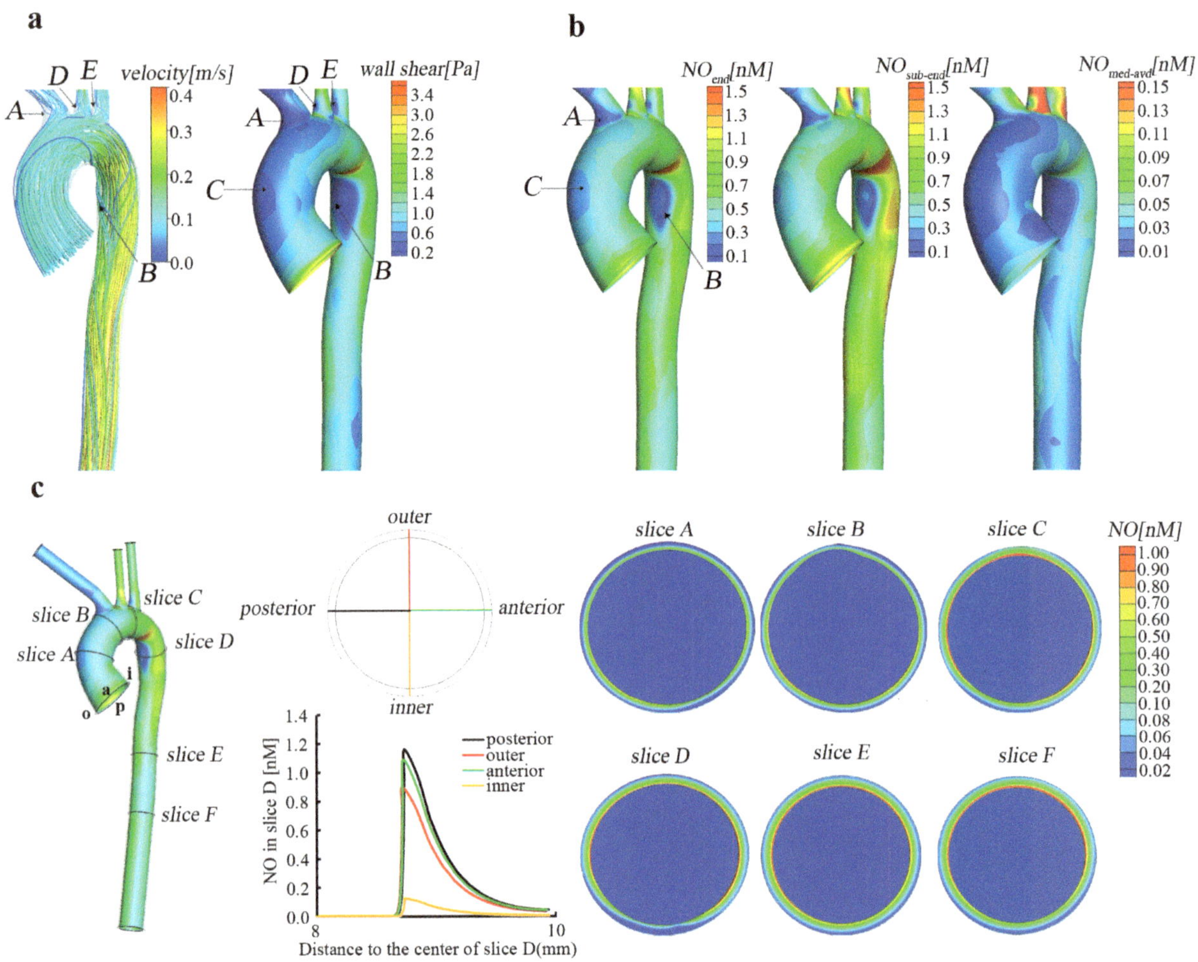

Figure 2. Uneven distributions of wall shear stress and NO in the aorta. (a) The streamline shows a swirling flow pattern and the wall shear stress is relatively low in the disturbed flow regions (A, B, D, and E). (b) The distributions of NO concentration at the endothelial surface towards lumen (NO_{end}) and wall ($NO_{sub\text{-}end}$), and at the media/adventitia interface ($NO_{med\text{-}adv}$) are very uneven and relatively low in the disturbed flow regions. (c) NO distributions of 6 representative slices in the aorta are used to show the NO distributions in the aortic lumen and wall. The model is with a contour plot of NO_{end}. a, p, o, i marked on the model is anterior, posterior, outer and inner wall of the aorta. The distributions of NO at slice D in the four directions is shown quite uneven.

k_{ery} may have a more significant influence on NO concentration at the endothelial surface than in the arterial wall. When compared to the reference model with $k_{ery} = 23\ s^{-1}$, for the case with $k_{ery} = 2.3\ s^{-1}$, NO concentration increases approximately 250% at the endothelial surface (NO_{end}) but only about 150% at the sub endothelial region ($NO_{sub\text{-}end}$) and the media/adventitia interface ($NO_{med\text{-}adv}$), and NO_{end} is a bit higher than $NO_{sub\text{-}end}$. However, for the case with $k_{ery} = 230\ s^{-1}$, NO_{end} decreases sharply approximately 75%, and quite lower than $NO_{sub\text{-}end}$ that decreases only 45%.

The reaction of NO in the wall strongly affects NO concentration in the aortic wall

NO diffusing into the vascular wall would be scavenged by smooth muscle cells and react with some hemoproteins. The measured reaction rate (k_w) is quite different and affected by the physiological condition [30]. To investigate the effects of consumption in the arterial wall on NO transport and distribution, simulations with $k_w = 0.1\ s^{-1}$ were carried out and compared with the reference model with $k_w = 0.01\ s^{-1}$. As shown in the Figure 4c, the increase in k_w has almost no effect on NO_{end} but greatly reduces NO concentration in the aortic wall ($NO_{sub\text{-}end}$ and $NO_{med\text{-}adv}$). For almost all the area of the aorta, the percentage difference in NO_{end} is only about 2%. However, the percentage difference in $NO_{sub\text{-}end}$ is about 40% at the thoracic aorta and approximately 20% at the three supra-aortic vessels. The increase in k_w decreases $NO_{med\text{-}adv}$ almost three orders of magnitude. These results indicate that the reaction of NO in the wall has strong effects on NO concentration in the aortic wall but no effects on the NO at the endothelial surface of towards the lumen.

Positive correlation between WSS and NO concentration at lumen/wall interface

Figures 5a–b show the relationship between wall shear stress and NO concentration at both the lumen-side and wall-side of the endothelium under different hemodynamics and reaction conditions. The figures were constructed by plotting the value of NO concentration against that of wall shear stress at each mesh node of the lumen/wall interface. It is evident that there is a relationship between WSS and NO concentration and NO concentration increases with increasing WSS. When WSS values are reduced to zero, NO concentration is close to zero. The results also

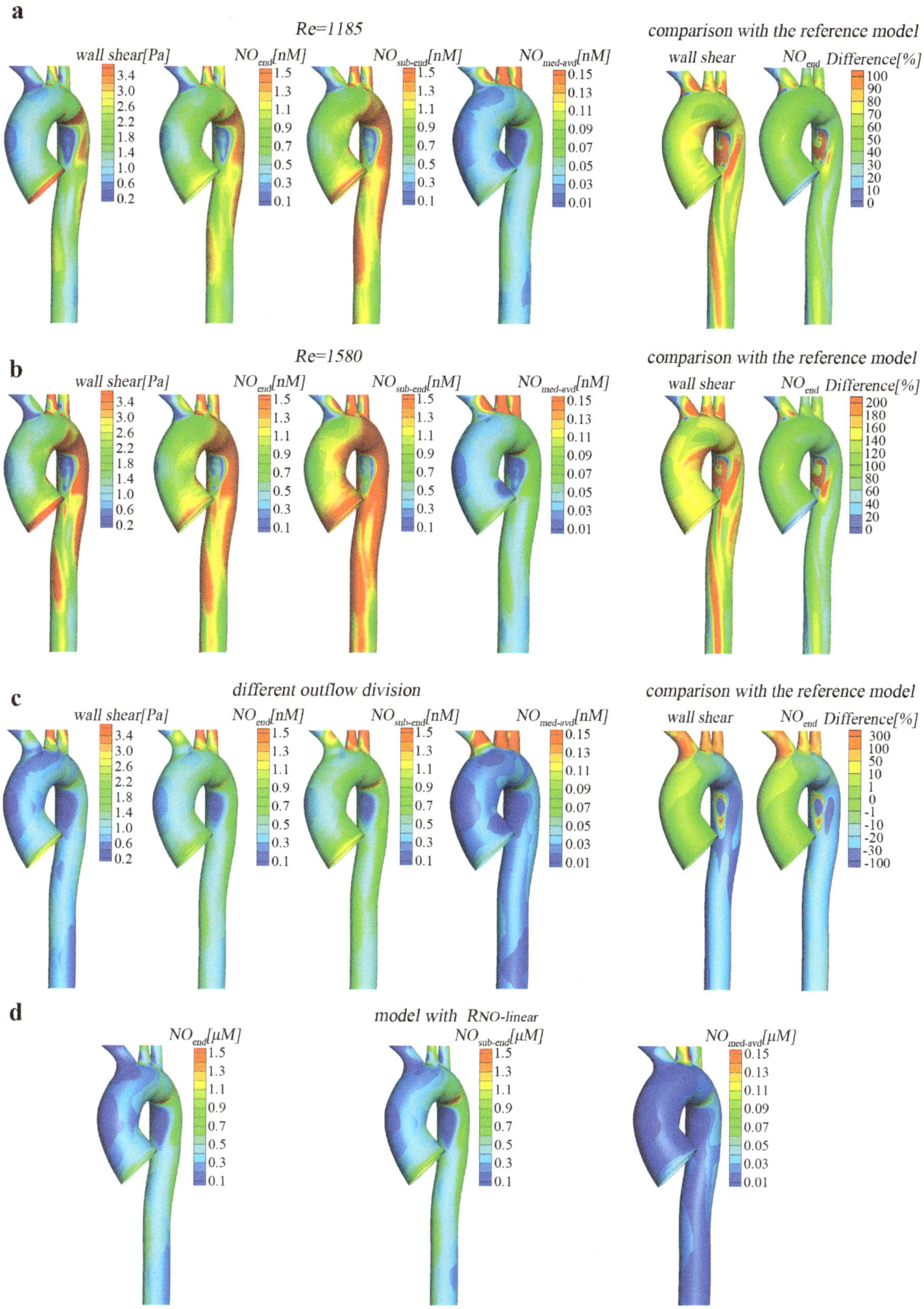

Figure 3. Changes in hemodynamics and shear dependent NO production rate affect the NO distribution in the aorta. (a–b) Comparison of the WSS and NO distribution between the reference simulation and the one at Re = 1185(one and a half of the reference one) and the one at Re = 1580 (twice of the reference one). Percentage difference = $(NO-NO_{reference})/NO_{reference}$. (c) Effects of different flow volume division at the outlets of the aorta. (d) The distributions of NO concentration for the NO production release model of $R_{NO\text{-}linear}$.

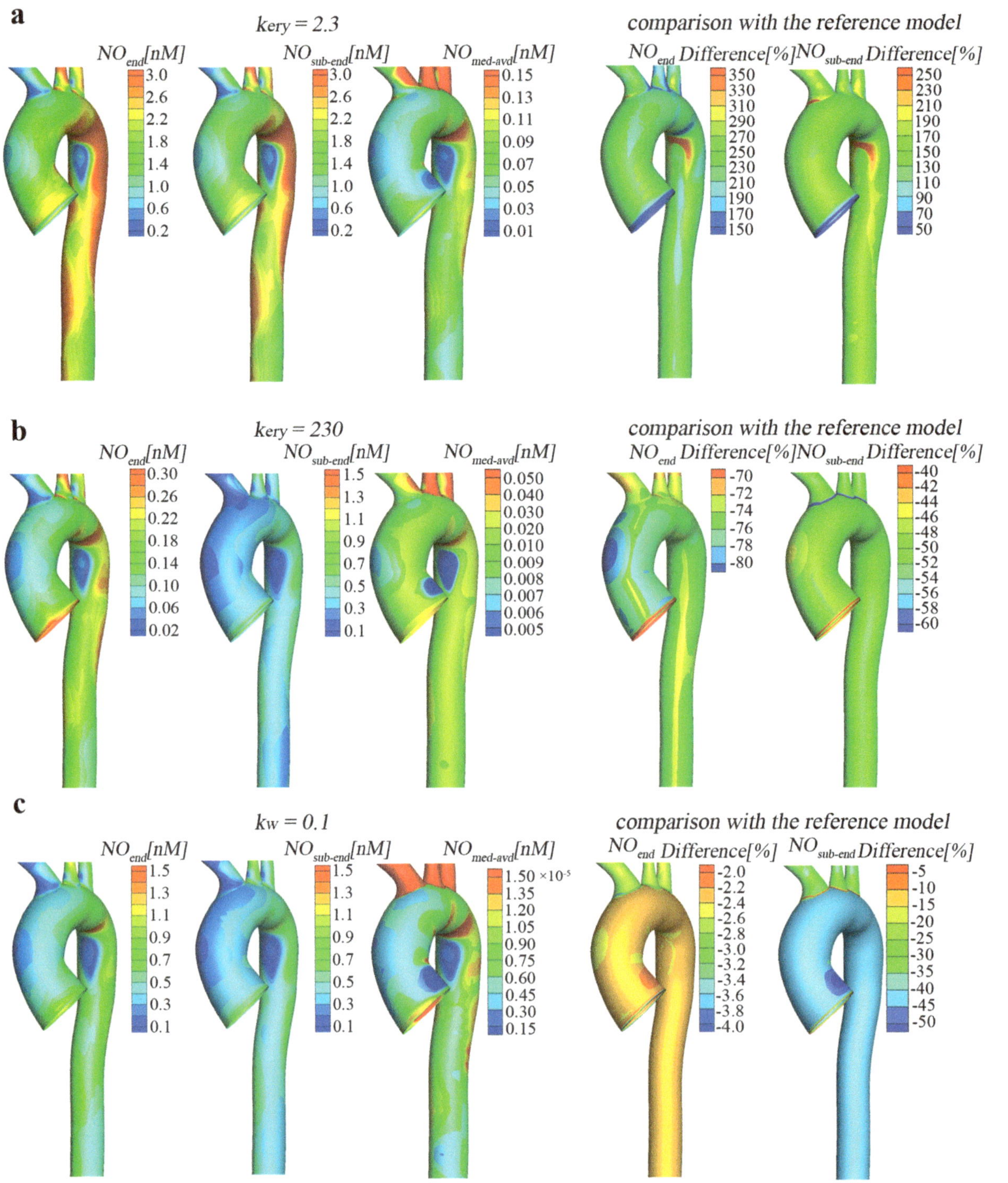

Figure 4. Effect of NO scavengers on the NO transport. The consumption rate of NO by erythrocytes (k_{ery}) in the lumen modulates NO distributions in the aorta. (a–b) Comparison of the NO distribution between the reference simulation and the one at $k_{ery} = 2.3$ (one tenth of the reference one) and at $k_{ery} = 230$ (ten times of the reference one). (c) Effects of the consumption rate of NO in the aortic wall $k_w = 0.1$ (ten times of the reference one). k_w strongly impacts the NO concentration in the aortic wall but slightly affects that at the surface of the endothelium to the lumen (NO_{end}).

demonstrate that profiles of the relationship between NO concentration and WSS for cases with Re = 1185, Re = 1580 and different flow volume division at outlets are overlapped, which indicates that the profile is almost independent on hemodynamics for the same NO production rate model. However, the profile of the relationship is significantly modulated by the production rate of NO and the consumption rate of NO in the lumen, and that between $NO_{sub\text{-}end}$ and WSS is further affected by the reaction rate of NO in the wall.

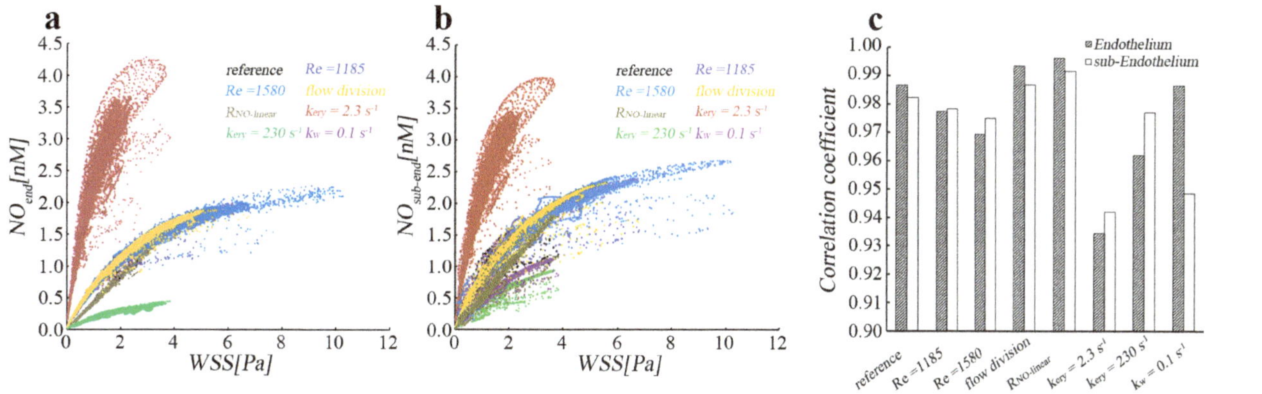

Figure 5. Positive correlation between wall shear stress (WSS) and NO concentration. (a–b) The relationship between WSS and NO concentration at the endothelial surface towards lumen (NO_{end}) and wall ($NO_{sub\text{-}end}$). The unit of NO concentration for $R_{NO\text{-}linear}$ is μM. (c) The spearman rank correlation coefficient between WSS and NO concentration.

Figure 5c illustrates the spearman rank correlation coefficient (r) between WSS and NO concentration. r is more than 0.93 for all the simulation cases, which indicates that a strong positive correlation exists between WSS and NO concentration. Moreover, the figure also shows that the correlation coefficient is affected by both hemodynamics and NO reaction rate in both arterial lumen and wall. For instance, when Reynolds number increases, r for both NO_{end} and $NO_{sub\text{-}end}$ may decrease and r becomes smaller for NO_{end} than for $NO_{sub\text{-}end}$. In addition, when k_{ery} is too low or too high, the consumption rate of NO in the lumen (k_{ery}) may decrease r. The reaction rate of NO in the wall may not affect r for NO_{end} but may greatly reduce r for $NO_{sub\text{-}end}$, when r_w increases. These results indicate that WSS is a key factor that determines the local concentration of NO, and it is modulated by other factors, such as k_{ery} and k_w.

Discussion

It is well documented that nitric oxide may have numerous cardiovascular protective properties [1], [3]. In the present study, we hypothesized that hemodynamics in the arteries may govern NO transport and lead to non-uniform distribution of NO in the arteries, hence playing an important role in the localization of vascular diseases such as atherosclerosis and arterial aneurysm. To substantiate this hypothesis, we numerically simulated the blood flow and NO transport in a lumen/wall model of a human aorta. Our results demonstrated that NO distributed unevenly in the aorta and reduced remarkably in disturbed flow regions (Fig. 2). By setting different flow boundary conditions such as the inlet blood flow rate (hence Re) and the outlet flow rate division, NO distribution in the aorta may be altered significantly (Fig. 3), indicating that alterations in hemodynamics such as exercise or stenosis may directly affect NO transport. Since NO production rate is WSS-dependent, hemodynamics may affect NO distribution mainly via shear dependent product rate (Fig. 3). Moreover, the erythrocyte in the lumen was an effective NO scavenger that modulated NO concentration in both the arterial lumen and wall, especially at the endothelial surface towards the lumen (Fig. 4). However, the reaction of NO in the wall had little effects on the luminal NO concentration, but could significantly affect NO concentration within the aortic wall (Fig. 4). The statistical analysis demonstrated that a strong positive correlation existed between WSS and NO concentration, and was affected by hemodynamics and NO reaction rate (Fig. 5).

Similar to the previous findings in the aorta, blood flow takes a form of swirling flow, but in some particular regions flow disturbance occurs [29,31]. Our results showed that in these disturbed flow regions, NO concentration on the endothelium and within the arterial wall were significantly reduced. For instance, NO concentration in the inner wall of the distal end of the aortic arch where flow disturbance occurs was almost ten times lower than that in the outer wall. The reduced NO bioavailability was largely due to the low NO production rate because of low WSS there. Several experimental studies demonstrated that endothelial nitric oxide synthase (eNOS) in the atheroma-prone regions with flow disturbance was either absent or significantly lower than that in normal flow regions [32,33]. It has been documented that when compared with those atherosclerosis-free regions, the atherosclerotic segments of the arteries has a remarkably reduced NO release production rate [34]. The reduced NO concentration in the disturbed flow regions might lead to atherogenesis by enhancing leucocyte adhesion to the endothelium and modifying low-density lipoproteins in the arterial wall [35,36]. In addition, mice model studies demonstrated that the deficiency in endothelial nitric oxide synthase would accelerate the development of atherosclerosis and induce spontaneous aortic aneurysm and dissection [37].

The present study investigated the effect of NO production rate on NO transport using two different models, one is hyperbolic model, and the other is linear model. The former may be more physiological than the latter, since NO concentration on the endothelium obtained with the former is several nM, which is the same order of magnitude measured on the endothelial cells and in dog coronary sinus [38,39]. Moreover, the results obtained revealed that the magnitude and the form of NO production rate have a great influence on the concentration distribution of NO in the aorta, indicating that abnormal NO production rate of dysfunctional endothelial cells may lead to the development of atherosclerosis. This theoretical finding may give an explanation to the experimental findings by others [40,41]. For instance, animal model studies demonstrated that increase in NO production by treatment with L-arginine, the precursor of nitric oxide, inhibited atherosclerotic lesion formation [40]. On the contrary, inhibition of NO production through L-arginine analogues such L-nitroarginine methylester (L-NAME) could significantly accelerate atherosclerotic lesion development [41].

Nitric oxide released from endothelial cells into blood reacts with several molecules. The reaction of NO with hemoglobin, which has a rapid reaction rate, accounts for several pathologies such as pulmonary and systemic hypertension, sickle-cell disease [42]. Our results showed that that ten time increase in NO consumption rate by erythrocytes only leads to 75% decrease in NO concentration on the endothelium and less than 50% decrease within the aortic wall, indicating that erythrocyte may not be a very strong modulator of NO in the aorta and it affects NO bioavailability on the endothelial surface more than that within the arterial wall. This phenomenon is different from the findings observed on the arterioles, in which hemoglobin is shown to be a strong NO scavenger [11]. The discrepancy might mostly be attributed to the relatively high blood flow velocity in the aorta, which may lead to a very thin concentration boundary layer near the aortic wall (see Figure 2c) and hence reduce the regulatory effect of the hemoglobin. The results may partly explain the phenomenon that atherosclerosis does not occur more preferentially in subjects with sickle-cell disease [43].

NO diffusing into the adjacent smooth muscle cells activates soluble guanylate cyclase (sGC), which catalyzes the formation of cyclic guanosine monophosphate (cGMP), leading to smooth muscle relaxation and vasodilation. It has been reported that NO concentration required to activate sGC varies in a wide range (100 pM–5 nM) [30]. The present study demonstrated that if k_w (the NO consumption rate constant in the arterial wall) was assumed to be 0.01 s^{-1}, the predicted NO concentration may be sufficiently high to activate sGC. However, if k_w increased ten times, NO concentration in the wall may decrease by approximately three orders of magnitude so that unable to activate sGC. These results indicate that the consumption rate of NO in the wall may be a very important factor that regulates NO concentration in the aortic wall. In fact, both human and animal model studies have demonstrated that augmented NO scavengers such as reactive oxygen species in atherosclerotic vessels may remarkably degrade NO in the arterial wall and hence accelerate atherosclerosis [44].

Flow-induced wall shear stress (WSS) has been recognized as one of the most important haemodynamic factors in the localization of vascular diseases [2,15]. Nevertheless, the underlying mechanism is still not very clear. WSS can modulate the biological function of the endothelium both via regulating the mechanotransduction of the endothelial cells and affecting the local concentration of chemicals/agonists at the endothelial surface [45–47]. As indicated in the present study, a strong positive correlation exists between WSS and NO concentration, which implies that WSS may also affect the endothelial biology through controlling NO concentration. The notion can be partly supported by some recent studies demonstrating that similar to WSS, flow-dependent mass transfer may also trigger endothelial cell signaling cascades [48].

In the present study, the blood flow was assumed steady and the compliance and motion of the aorta was neglected, which may affect the accuracy of our prediction on the absolute value of NO concentration. However, it can still shed some light on the general tendency of NO distribution in the aorta, since it is demonstrated that the compliance of the aortic wall and the pulsation of blood flow have a little effects on the distribution of WSS and exogenous macromolecules and micromolecules in the aorta [17,19,49]. Another limitation of the present study is that the RBC free plasma layer on the endothelial cells was not included in the modeling. Due to the much lower NO reaction rate in the RBC-free plasma layer, the influence of RBCs on NO transport in the aorta may be diminished by the existence of the layer. Therefore, the overall NO concentration predicted on the arterial wall may be underestimated. However, the NO distribution in the aorta may not be changed significantly by the simplification, since it was found that the layer had little effects on the distribution of NO in an idealized model of stenosed artery [19]. In addition, it should be pointed out that flow shear stress could regulate eNOS activity hence NO production through both transcriptional mechanism within seconds or minutes and posttranscriptional one within hours or days [50,51]. As the flow in the arteries in vivo is pulsatile, which would lead to dramatic changes in WSS on cells in a short time, the NO production in vivo might be the combining results of the two mechanisms. Under steady flow condition, both the two mechanisms would lead to a rapid increase in NO production rate at relatively low WSS, but at relatively high WSS, the transcriptional mechanism would cause more NO production [25,52]. The main NO production rate model (eq. 7) used in the present study was based on experimental measurements obtained within minutes, which may result from the transcriptional regulation of eNOS and hence may lead to overestimated production rate at relatively high WSS. Therefore, the distributions of NO at regions with high WSS may be somewhat overestimated. However, the NO distribution at low WSS region, which was the most concerned region, may be reasonable. Moreover, considering the great variance of NO production rate, we also calculated the NO transport using linear model (eq. 8, Figure 3d) which is almost three larger orders of magnitude than the hyperbolic model. The results of the two models were consistent, which indicated that despite the concentration value simulated might be not very accurate, the distribution would be reliable and have biological significance. To assess accurately the NO concentration value, NO production rate in response to different physiological flow conditions needs to be further measured and used in simulations.

Conclusions

Local hemodynamics may govern NO transport in the aorta. Disturbed flow in certain areas of the aorta could remarkably reduce NO bioavailability that may play an important role in the localization of vascular diseases such as atherosclerosis and arterial aneurysm. In addition, NO bioavailability in the aorta was modulated differently by the NO scavengers in the arterial lumen and in the arterial wall. NO bioavailability in the wall was very strongly affected by NO scavengers in the arterial wall, which implied that elimination of some of the scavengers may be an efficient approach to increase NO bioavailability and thus alleviate vascular disease.

Author Contributions

Conceived and designed the experiments: XYD YBF. Performed the experiments: XL ZZW. Analyzed the data: XL PZ ZMF YBF XYD. Contributed reagents/materials/analysis tools: XL AQS FZ. Contributed to the writing of the manuscript: XL XYD.

References

1. Davignon J, Ganz P (2004) Role of endothelial dysfunction in atherosclerosis. Circulation 109: III27–32.
2. Lasheras JC (2007) The biomechanics of arterial aneurysms. Annual Review of Fluid Mechanics 39: 293–319.
3. Napoli C, de Nigris F, Williams-Ignarro S, Pignalosa O, Sica V, et al. (2006) Nitric oxide and atherosclerosis: an update. Nitric Oxide 15: 265–279.
4. Moncada S, Palmer RM, Higgs EA (1991) Nitric oxide: physiology, pathophysiology, and pharmacology. Pharmacol Rev 43: 109–142.
5. Chen K, Pittman RN, Popel AS (2008) Nitric oxide in the vasculature: where does it come from and where does it go? A quantitative perspective. Antioxid Redox Signal 10: 1185–1198.

6. Jin RC, Loscalzo J (2010) Vascular Nitric Oxide: Formation and Function. J Blood Med 2010: 147–162.
7. Grisham MB, Jourd'Heuil D, Wink DA (1999) Nitric oxide. I. Physiological chemistry of nitric oxide and its metabolites:implications in inflammation. Am J Physiol 276: G315–321.
8. Halligan KE, Jourd'heuil FL, Jourd'heuil D (2009) Cytoglobin Is Expressed in the Vasculature and Regulates Cell Respiration and Proliferation via Nitric Oxide Dioxygenation. Journal of Biological Chemistry 284: 8539–8547.
9. Chen X, Jaron D, Barbee KA, Buerk DG (2006) The influence of radial RBC distribution, blood velocity profiles, and glycocalyx on coupled NO/O_2 transport. J Appl Physiol 100: 482–492.
10. Lancaster JR, Jr. (1994) Simulation of the diffusion and reaction of endogenously produced nitric oxide. Proc Natl Acad Sci U S A 91: 8137–8141.
11. Tsoukias NM (2008) Nitric oxide bioavailability in the microcirculation: insights from mathematical models. Microcirculation 15: 813–834.
12. Fadel AA, Barbee KA, Jaron D (2009) A computational model of nitric oxide production and transport in a parallel plate flow chamber. Ann Biomed Eng 37: 943–954.
13. Plata AM, Sherwin SJ, Krams R (2010) Endothelial nitric oxide production and transport in flow chambers: The importance of convection. Ann Biomed Eng 38: 2805–2816.
14. Cooke JP (2004) Flow, NO, and atherogenesis (vol 100, pg 768, 2003). Proc Natl Acad Sci U S A 101: 18262–18262.
15. Chiu JJ, Chien S (2011) Effects of disturbed flow on vascular endothelium: pathophysiological basis and clinical perspectives. Physiol Rev 91: 327–387.
16. Liu X, Pu F, Fan Y, Deng X, Li D, et al. (2009) A numerical study on the flow of blood and the transport of LDL in the human aorta: the physiological significance of the helical flow in the aortic arch. Am J Physiol Heart Circ Physiol 297: H163–170.
17. Liu X, Fan Y, Deng X (2010) Effect of spiral flow on the transport of oxygen in the aorta: a numerical study. Ann Biomed Eng 38: 917–926.
18. El Aidi H, Mani V, Weinshelbaum KB, Aguiar SH, Taniguchi H, et al. (2009) Cross-sectional, prospective study of MRI reproducibility in the assessment of plaque burden of the carotid arteries and aorta. Nat Clin Pract Cardiovasc Med 6: 219–228.
19. Liu X, Fan Y, Xu XY, Deng X (2012) Nitric oxide transport in an axisymmetric stenosis. J R Soc Interface 9: 2468–2478.
20. Cho YI, Kensey KR (1991) Effects of the non-Newtonian viscosity of blood on flows in a diseased arterial vessel. Part 1: Steady flows. Biorheology 28: 241–262.
21. Azarov I, Huang KT, Basu S, Gladwin MT, Hogg N, et al. (2005) Nitric oxide scavenging by red blood cells as a function of hematocrit and oxygenation. J Biol Chem 280: 39024–39032.
22. Liao JC, Hein TW, Vaughn MW, Huang KT, Kuo L (1999) Intravascular flow decreases erythrocyte consumption of nitric oxide. Proc Natl Acad Sci U S A 96: 8757–8761.
23. Vaughn MW, Kuo L, Liao JC (1998) Effective diffusion distance of nitric oxide in the microcirculation. Am J Physiol 274: H1705–1714.
24. Chen K, Popel AS (2006) Theoretical analysis of biochemical pathways of nitric oxide release from vascular endothelial cells. Free Radic Biol Med 41: 668–680.
25. Andrews AM, Jaron D, Buerk DG, Kirby PL, Barbee KA (2010) Direct, real-time measurement of shear stress-induced nitric oxide produced from endothelial cells in vitro. Nitric Oxide 23: 335–342.
26. Chen X, Buerk DG, Barbee KA, Kirby P, Jaron D (2011) 3D network model of NO transport in tissue. Med Biol Eng Comput 49: 633–647.
27. Liu X, Srinivasan P, Collard E, Grajdeanu P, Zweier JL, et al. (2008) Nitric oxide diffusion rate is reduced in the aortic wall. Biophys J 94: 1880–1889.
28. Vaughn MW, Kuo L, Liao JC (1998) Estimation of nitric oxide production and reaction rates in tissue by use of a mathematical model. Am J Physiol 274: H2163–2176.
29. Gallo D, De Santis G, Negri F, Tresoldi D, Ponzini R, et al. (2012) On the use of in vivo measured flow rates as boundary conditions for image-based hemodynamic models of the human aorta: implications for indicators of abnormal flow. Ann Biomed Eng 40: 729–741.
30. Hall CN, Garthwaite J (2009) What is the real physiological NO concentration in vivo? Nitric Oxide 21: 92–103.
31. Morbiducci U, Ponzini R, Rizzo G, Cadioli M, Esposito A, et al. (2011) Mechanistic insight into the physiological relevance of helical blood flow in the human aorta: an in vivo study. Biomechanics and Modeling in Mechanobiology 10: 339–355.
32. Cheng C, van Haperen R, de Waard M, van Damme LC, Tempel D, et al. (2005) Shear stress affects the intracellular distribution of eNOS: direct demonstration by a novel in vivo technique. Blood 106: 3691–3698.
33. de Nigris F, Lerman LO, Ignarro SW, Sica G, Lerman A, et al. (2004) Beneficial effects of antioxidants and L-arginine on oxidation-sensitive gene expression and endothelial NO synthase activity at sites of disturbed shear stress (vol 100, pg 1420, 2003). Proc Natl Acad Sci U S A 101: 18262–18262.
34. Oemar BS, Tschudi MR, Godoy N, Brovkovich V, Malinski T, et al. (1998) Reduced endothelial nitric oxide synthase expression and production in human atherosclerosis. Circulation 97: 2494–2498.
35. Cicha I, Goppelt-Struebe M, Yilmaz A, Daniel WG, Garlichs CD (2008) Endothelial dysfunction and monocyte recruitment in cells exposed to non-uniform shear stress. Clin Hemorheol Microcirc 39: 113–119.
36. Hsiai TK, Hwang J, Barr ML, Correa A, Hamilton R, et al. (2007) Hemodynamics influences vascular peroxynitrite formation: Implication for low-density lipoprotein apo-B-100 nitration. Free Radical Biology and Medicine 42: 519–529.
37. Kuhlencordt PJ, Gyurko R, Han F, Scherrer-Crosbie M, Aretz TH, et al. (2001) Accelerated atherosclerosis, aortic aneurysm formation, and ischemic heart disease in apolipoprotein E/endothelial nitric oxide synthase double-knockout mice. Circulation 104: 448–454.
38. Neishi Y, Mochizuki S, Miyasaka T, Kawamoto T, Kume T, et al. (2005) Evaluation of bioavailability of nitric oxide in coronary circulation by direct measurement of plasma nitric oxide concentration. Proc Natl Acad Sci U S A 102: 11456–11461.
39. Jiang S, Cheng R, Wang X, Xue T, Liu Y, et al. (2013) Real-time electrical detection of nitric oxide in biological systems with sub-nanomolar sensitivity. Nat Commun 4: 2225.
40. Aji W, Ravalli S, Szabolcs M, Jiang XC, Sciacca RR, et al. (1997) L-arginine prevents xanthoma development and inhibits atherosclerosis in LDL receptor knockout mice. Circulation 95: 430–437.
41. Kauser K, da Cunha V, Fitch R, Mallari C, Rubanyi GM (2000) Role of endogenous nitric oxide in progression of atherosclerosis in apolipoprotein E-deficient mice. Am J Physiol Heart Circ Physiol 278: H1679–1685.
42. Reiter CD, Wang X, Tanus-Santos JE, Hogg N, Cannon RO, 3rd, et al. (2002) Cell-free hemoglobin limits nitric oxide bioavailability in sickle-cell disease. Nat Med 8: 1383–1389.
43. Wang H, Luo W, Wang J, Guo C, Wolffe SL, et al. (2013) Paradoxical protection from atherosclerosis and thrombosis in a mouse model of sickle cell disease. Br J Haematol 162: 120–129.
44. Stocker R, Keaney JF, Jr. (2004) Role of oxidative modifications in atherosclerosis. Physiol Rev 84: 1381–1478.
45. Choi HW, Ferrara KW, Barakat AI (2007) Modulation of ATP/ADP concentration at the endothelial surface by shear stress: Effect of flow recirculation. Ann Biomed Eng 35: 505–516.
46. Davies PF (1995) Flow-mediated endothelial mechanotransduction. Physiol Rev 75: 519–560.
47. Plank MJ, Wall DJN, David T (2006) Atherosclerosis and calcium signalling in endothelial cells. Progress in Biophysics & Molecular Biology 91: 287–313.
48. Vandrangi P, Sosa M, Shyy JYJ, Rodgers VGJ (2012) Flow-Dependent Mass Transfer May Trigger Endothelial Signaling Cascades. Plos One 7.
49. Lantz J, Renner J, Karlsson M (2011) Wall Shear Stress in a Subject Specific Human Aorta - Influence of Fluid-Structure Interaction. International Journal of Applied Mechanics 3: 759–778.
50. Balligand JL, Feron O, Dessy C (2009) eNOS activation by physical forces: from short-term regulation of contraction to chronic remodeling of cardiovascular tissues. Physiol Rev 89: 481–534.
51. Boo YC, Jo H (2003) Flow-dependent regulation of endothelial nitric oxide synthase: role of protein kinases. Am J Physiol Cell Physiol 285: C499–508.
52. Kuchan MJ, Frangos JA (1994) Role of calcium and calmodulin in flow-induced nitric oxide production in endothelial cells. Am J Physiol 266: C628–636.

11

CD161$^+$ MAIT Cells Are Severely Reduced in Peripheral Blood and Lymph Nodes of HIV-Infected Individuals Independently of Disease Progression

Johanna Maria Eberhard[1,4,⁹], Philip Hartjen[1,2,4,⁹], Silke Kummer[1,4], Reinhold E. Schmidt[5,8], Maximilian Bockhorn[3], Clara Lehmann[6], Ashwin Balagopal[7], Joachim Hauber[4,8], Jan van Lunzen[1,4,8*,⁹], Julian Schulze zur Wiesch[1,4,8⁹]

1 Infectious Diseases Unit, Department of Medicine, University Medical Center Hamburg-Eppendorf, Hamburg, Germany, **2** Department of Oral and Maxillofacial Surgery, University Medical Center Hamburg-Eppendorf, Hamburg, Germany, **3** Department of General Surgery, University Medical Center Hamburg-Eppendorf, Hamburg, Germany, **4** Heinrich Pette Institute - Leibniz Institute for Experimental Virology, Hamburg, Germany, **5** Department of Immunology and Rheumatology, Hannover Medical School, Hanover, Germany, **6** Department of Internal Medicine I, University Hospital of Cologne, Cologne, Germany, **7** School of Medicine, Johns Hopkins University, Baltimore, Maryland, United States of America, **8** German Center for Infection Research (DZIF), partner site Hamburg and Hannover, Hamburg and Hannover, Germany

Abstract

Mucosal-associated invariant T (MAIT) cells are characterized by the combined expression of the semi-invariant T cell receptor (TCR) Vα7.2, the lectin receptor CD161, as well as IL-18R, and play an important role in antibacterial host defense of the gut. The current study characterized CD161$^+$ MAIT and CD161$^-$TCRVα7.2$^+$ T cell subsets within a large cohort of HIV patients with emphasis on patients with slow disease progression and elite controllers. Mononuclear cells from blood and lymph node samples as well as plasma from 63 patients and 26 healthy donors were analyzed by multicolor flow cytometry and ELISA for IL-18, sCD14 and sCD163. Additionally, MAIT cells were analyzed after *in vitro* stimulation with different cytokines and/or fixed *E.coli*. Reduced numbers of CD161$^+$ MAIT cells during HIV infection were detectable in the blood and lymph nodes of all patient groups, including elite controllers. CD161$^+$ MAIT cell numbers did not recover even after successful antiretroviral treatment. The loss of CD161$^+$ MAIT cells was correlated with higher levels of MAIT cell activation; an increased frequency of the CD161$^-$TCRVα7.2$^+$T cell subset in HIV infection was observed. *In vitro* stimulation of MAIT cells with IL-18 and IL-12, IL-7 and fixed *E.coli* also resulted in a rapid and additive reduction of the MAIT cell frequency defined by CD161, IL-18R and CCR6. In summary, the irreversible reduction of the CD161$^+$ MAIT cell subset seems to be an early event in HIV infection that is independent of later stages of the disease. This loss appears to be at least partially due to the distinctive vulnerability of MAIT cells to the pronounced stimulation by microbial products and cytokines during HIV-infection.

Editor: R. Keith Reeves, Beth Israel Deaconess Medical Center, Harvard Medical School, United States of America

Funding: This work was supported by the Werner Otto Stiftung, the German Research Agency (SFB841 project A6; JSzW), the DZIF (German Center for Infection Research; RES, JH, JvL, JSzW) and the ECHAM (European Cohort HIV Ageing and Metabolic liver disease; JvL, JME). The funders had no role in study design, data collection and analysis, decision to publish, or preparation of the manuscript.

Competing Interests: The authors have declared that no competing interests exist.

* Email: v.lunzen@uke.de

⁹ These authors contributed equally to this work.

Introduction

Chronic untreated HIV infection is characterized by general immune activation, immune dysregulation, high T cell turnover and a gradual decline of CD4$^+$ T cells through infection and bystander activation induced apoptotic death [1]. The transloca-tion of microbial products from the gastrointestinal (GI) tract to portal and systemic circulation has been proposed as a major driver of the generalized chronic immune activation that is associated with HIV disease progression [2].

A recently described T cell subset with limited receptor diversity and high abundance in mucosal tissues has been shown to recognize microbial products. These cells, termed mucosal-associated invariant T (MAIT) cells, can be identified by the surface expression of CD161 and the invariant TCRVα7.2 segment [1]. In general, MAIT cell responses are restricted by the conserved MHC-related-molecule-1 (MR1) that presents riboflavin precursors derived from bacteria and yeasts predominantly in the gut [3]. The MAIT cell defining surface marker CD161 is a C-type lectin-like membrane receptor that can bind its ligand, the lectin-like transcript 1 (LLT1), with yet unclear function [4,5]. MAIT cells exhibit a tissue-targeting memory phenotype and express high levels of cytokine receptors for IL-18, IL-12 and IL-23 [4,6–8]. Moreover, MAIT cells exhibit specific effector activities such as TNF-α, IFN-γ, IL-17 production as well as granzyme B secretion [4,6,7].

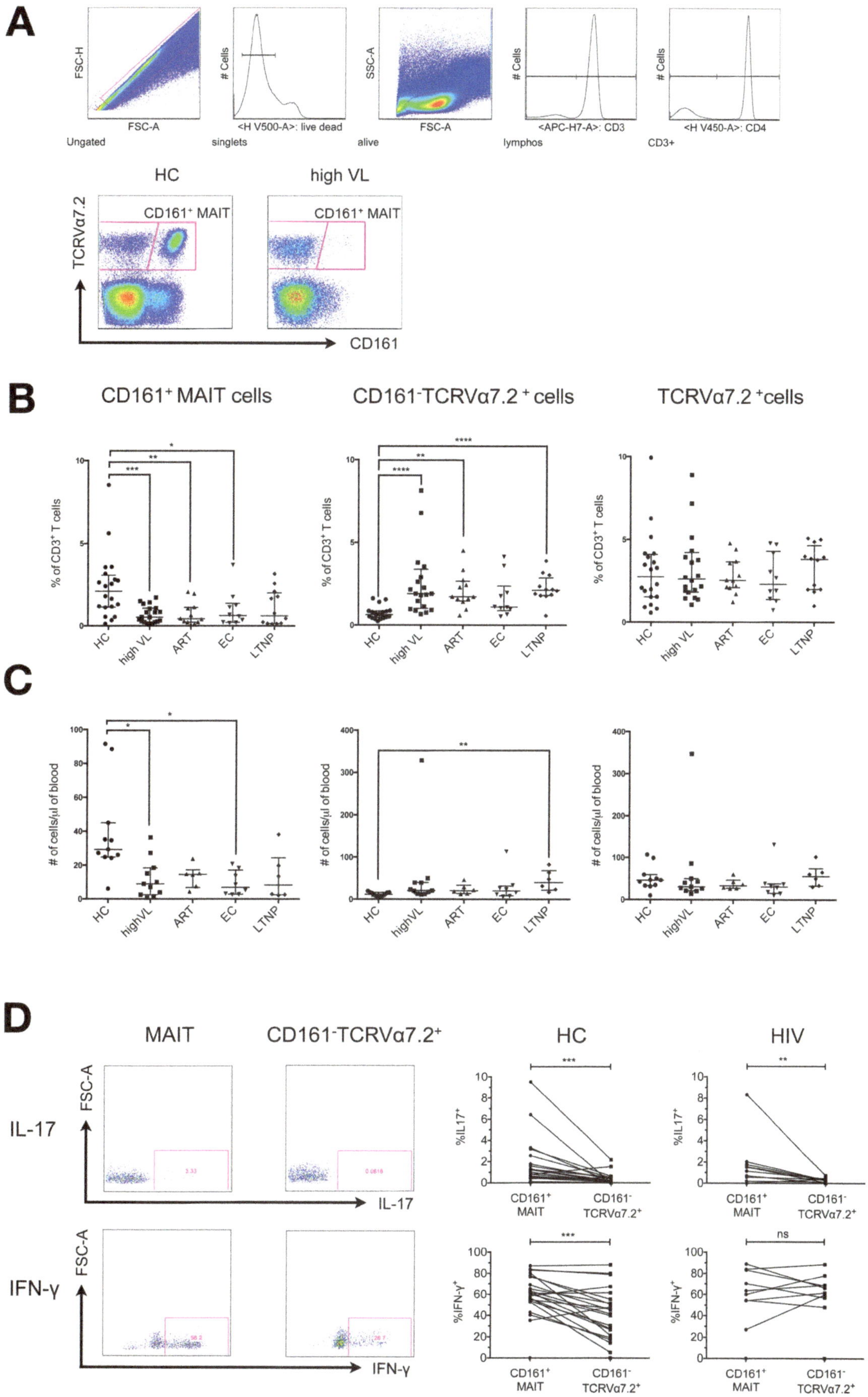
A
FSC-H
FSC-A
Ungated
Cells
<H V500-A>: live dead
singlets
SSC-A
FSC-A
alive
Cells
<APC-H7-A>: CD3
lymphos
Cells
<H V450-A>: CD4
CD3+
HC
high VL
TCRVα7.2
CD161+ MAIT
CD161+ MAIT
CD161
B
CD161+ MAIT cells
CD161-TCRVα7.2+ cells
TCRVα7.2+cells
% of CD3+ T cells
HC
high VL
ART
EC
LTNP
C
# of cells/μl of blood
HC
highVL
ART
EC
LTNP
D
MAIT
CD161-TCRVα7.2+
HC
HIV
IL-17
FSC-A
IL-17
IFN-γ
FSC-A
IFN-γ
%IL17+
%IFN-γ+
CD161+ MAIT
CD161- TCRVα7.2+
ns

Figure 1. CD161$^+$TCRVα7.2$^+$ MAIT cells are severely reduced in the blood of HIV-infected patients. A) Gating Strategy for CD161 and TCRVα7.2 based MAIT cell characterization in the CD4$^-$CD3$^+$T cell subset. All FACS analyses were performed on frozen PBMC samples. Depicted are representative plots from healthy control PBMCs (upper panel). Gating of the MAIT cell subsets comparing a healthy donor (HC) and an HIV patient (lower panel). **B**) Cumulative display of CD161$^+$TCRVα7.2$^+$ MAIT cell frequencies, CD161$^-$TCRVα7.2$^+$ and total TCRVα7.2$^+$ cells in % of CD3$^+$ T cells comparing PBMC samples derived from healthy controls (HC n = 20), untreated patients with high viral loads (high VL n = 20), patients receiving antiretroviral treatment for a at least one year (ART n = 12), elite controller (EC n = 10) and patients with very low viremia and slow progression (< 5000 copies/ml; LTNP n = 12). **C**) Absolute MAIT cell counts, CD161$^-$TCRVα7.2$^+$ and total TCRVα7.2$^+$ cells per µl peripheral blood, calculated based on absolute CD3$^+$ T cell counts (available for 12 HC, 11 high VL, 6 ART, 8 EC and 6 LTNP). All groups were tested for normal distribution with the Kolmogorov-Smirnov test and were compared by the adequate test, ANOVA followed by Tukey's multiple comparisons test or Kruskal-Wallis followed by multiple comparison test, respectively. P-values smaller than 0.05 were considered significant, where *, ** and *** indicate p-values between 0.01 to 0.05, 0.001 to 0.01 and 0.0001 to 0.001, respectively. Bars and lines indicate median, 25% and 75% quartiles. **D**) Representative FACS plots and the percentages of cells that produce the cytokines IL-17 and INF-γ upon stimulation with PMA/ionomycin among MAIT cells and CD161$^-$TCRVα7.2$^+$ cells are shown. PBMC samples derived from healthy donors (n = 22) and HIV-infected patients (ART treated and untreated with high viral loads, n = 10) were analyzed. Asterisks indicate the results of Wilcoxon matched-pairs signed-rank tests.

Recent reports describe a significant loss of CD161$^+$ MAIT cells from the circulation of HIV- infected patients [9–12]. It is thought that the decrease of these cells not only weakens the defense against bacterial pathogens like *Escherichia coli*, *Candida albicans* and *Mycobacterium tuberculosis* (MTB) [1–4], but could also further enhance the intestinal translocation of microbial products, which is related to the chronic activation and exhaustion of the immune system associated with HIV-infection [2,6,9,11,12]. However, the timing, kinetics and mechanisms behind the reduction of peripheral CD161$^+$ MAIT cells in patients with HIV-infection and different disease course has not been fully elucidated. On the one hand, activation induced cell death and accumulation in tissues could explain the severe reduction of MAIT cells. On the other hand a change of phenotype in terms of down-regulation of marker molecules such as CD161 following activation and exhaustion have been suggested as alternative explanation [5–7]. Limited data on the tissue distribution of MAIT cells are available so far, especially with regard to secondary lymphoid tissues. Furthermore, there are extant questions about the early kinetics of MAIT cells during acute infection, and whether patients who exhibit natural control of HIV have spared MAIT cells [8] [11]. In particular, the loss and exhaustion of MAIT cells could have important implications for the mucosal defense against bacterial pathogens in the gut of HIV-infected patients. Latest studies contradict earlier assumptions [9] and show that HIV elite controllers (EC) show activated innate immune responses in comparison to healthy controls despite controlling plasma HIV viremia [13–15]; therefore, these results are consistent with an impaired mucosal barrier.

In the current study, MAIT cells, defined as CD161$^+$ TCR Vα7.2$^+$ CD4$^-$ T cells as well as CD161$^-$TCR Vα7.2$^+$ CD4$^-$ T cells are characterized *ex vivo* and after *in vitro* stimulation in a large cohort of HIV patients with emphasis on patients with slow disease progression and elite controllers (EC). This study aimed to gain further insight into the kinetics as well as possible mechanisms of MAIT cell decline during HIV-infection including the important compartment of lymphoid tissue.

Results

CD161$^+$ MAIT cells are severely reduced in the blood and lymph nodes of HIV-infected patients independently of their disease status

The aim of this study was to comprehensively analyze MAIT cell subsets in the peripheral blood as well as in the lymph node compartment of a large cohort of patients with different HIV disease status.

We first determined the frequency of CD161$^+$ MAIT cells in the peripheral blood in a cohort of healthy, HIV-negative donors (Fig. 1). The vast majority of the CD3$^+$CD161$^+$TCRVα7.2$^+$ MAIT cell population (>90%) either expresses CD8$\alpha\alpha$ or CD8$\alpha\beta$, whereas a smaller subset (<10%) is CD8$^-$CD4$^-$ and only a negligible fraction of these cells expresses the CD4 molecule [10]. For simplicity and for better comparability with previous studies we defined MAIT cells as CD161$^+$TCRVα7.2$^+$CD4$^-$CD3$^+$ T cell population. This gating strategy allowed us to exclude the effect of general CD4$^+$ T cell depletion from the analysis. Our gating strategy is depicted in Fig. 1A. Healthy controls displayed a broad range of MAIT cell frequencies, quantified in two ways: i) as percentage of CD3$^+$ T cells (median = 2.1%, IQR = 1.12–3.06%) and ii) as percentage of CD4$^-$ T cells (mean = 8.12%, IQR = 5.6–12.25%; data not shown) (Fig. 1B). This was reflected in a pattern of similar variation of the absolute number of CD161$^+$ MAIT cells per µl of blood (Fig. 1C) and thus is not merely a consequence of varying parent population sizes. Our results are consistent with previous results from studies that determined MAIT cell frequencies in healthy subjects [5,11,12].

In accordance with previous studies [5–7,13] we observed a severe reduction of the peripheral CD161$^+$ MAIT cell subset of untreated and treated HIV-infected patients (median HC = 2.1%, IQR = 1.12–3.06% vs. median high VL = 0.52%, IQR = 0.22–1.06% and median ART = 0.42%, IQR = 0.22–1.1%, ANOVA followed by Tukey's multiple comparison test: $p<0.001$ and $p<0.01$, respectively) (Fig. 1B, C).

Importantly, we extended the results of the aforementioned studies by characterizing the frequency and function of MAIT cells in a group of elite controllers (n = 10) and long-term nonprogressors (n = 12) (Table 1) to answer the question whether spontaneous viral control or slower disease progression are associated with the preservation of peripheral MAIT cells. Throughout this study LTNPs were defined as: HIV Patients with low viremia (<5000 copies/ml) that maintain a favourable course of infection (CD4 counts>350 cells/µl) over 5 years in the absence of therapy.

Interestingly, we observed a reduction of the CD161$^+$ MAIT cell subset in both groups of patients (LTNP as well as EC) compared to healthy controls (median HC = 2.1%, IQR = 1.12–3.06% vs. median EC = 0.62%, IQR = 0.21–1.37% and median LTNP = 0.61, IQR = 0.14–2.0%) (Fig. 1B). This reduction was slightly less pronounced in EC and not statistically significant for LTNP (ANOVA followed by Tukey's multiple comparison test: $p<0.05$ for EC).

In previously published studies, it has been hypothesized that the disappearance of MAIT cells from the peripheral blood in chronic HIV infection might be best explained by a combination of activation induced cell death and/or homing of MAIT cells to different tissues and the gut [7]. Thus, in order to advance the understanding of possible tissue redistributions of MAIT cells in the course of the HIV infection, we extended our analysis by

Table 1. Cohort (PBMC samples).

	Healthy	high VL	ART	EC	LTNP
number of donors	20	21	12	10	12
% female	53.3	29.4	36.4	57.1	40
age [years]	39.2(±11.2)	39.9(±11.7)	48.9(±16)	46(±11.6)	43.92(±15.3)
time since first diagnosis [month]	–	51.2(±71.6)	101.2(±58.5)	150.5(±69.9)	106.8(±67.1)
viral load [copies/ml]	–	1580000(±3080000)	10 of 12: below detection limit; 2 of 12: <200	below detection limit	986.1 (±1655)
CD4 [c/µl]	798.2(±308.8)	243.6(±289.1)	627.5(±363.1)	780.7(±284.7)	591.8(±176.8)
CD8 [c/µl]	439(±154.1)	951.4(±980.8)	844.3(±266.7)	686.4(±305.9)	1217(±480.9)
CD3 [c/µl]	1323(±418.8)	1594(±1471)	1475(±536.2)	1487(±588.1)	2140(±722.5)
lymphocytes [c/µl]	1785(±527.7)	1613(±1325)	1997(±627.5)	2014(±712.5)	2386(±770)

Shown are means and standard deviation.

inclusion of lymph nodal MAIT cells. As natural killer T cells MAIT cells might have an important role in B cell help [14–16]. Previously, high expression of CCR6 and low expression of CCR7 have been observed on MAIT cells, indicating that these cells are mainly tissue circulating T cells [17].

We also found that lymph node samples of healthy controls and HIV patients (Table 2) generally showed a significantly lower frequency of MAIT cells compared to PBMC of unpaired samples of the same groups ($p<0.01$ in HC and $p<0.0001$ in HIV patients, Mann-Whitney tests), while the frequencies of $CD161^-TCRV\alpha7.2^+$ T cells were not significantly different between the two compartments (Fig. 2A, B). However, analogous to the results obtained for the peripheral blood we observed a further reduction of the lymph nodal $CD161^+$ MAIT cell frequency in HIV-infected patients to a significantly lower median of 0.06% (IQR = 0.04–0.2%, $p = 0.03$) in comparison to healthy controls (Fig. 2). A similar reduction of the $CD161^+$ MAIT frequency was detectable in all LNMC samples of HIV-infected patients regardless of their treatment status (LNMC from 5 untreated and 6 ART-treated patients were included in our analysis). However, it has to be noted that our analysis was limited by the fact that no paired blood - lymph node samples from the same donors were available.

The frequency of the $CD161^-CD4^-$ T cell subset that expressed $TCRV\alpha7.2^+$ but no other MAIT cell-defining markers (e.g. CD161, hence termed: $CD161^-TCRV\alpha7.2^+$ subset), was increased in viremic HIV patients, patients receiving ART and in LTNP (median HC = 0.62%, IQR = 0.44–0.83% vs. median high VL = 1.9%, IQR = 1.0–3.4%, median ART = 1.72%, IQR = 1.46–2.65% and median LTNP = 1.14% IQR = 0.31–4.6%; Kruskal-Wallis test followed by Dunn's multiple comparisons test: $p<0.0001$, $p<0.01$ and $p<0.0001$, respectively) (Fig. 1B middle panel). In the resting state this cell population consists most likely of regular T cells using this Vα chain but their increase in HIV-infected patients might reflect an activation-induced down-regulation of CD161 on the MAIT cell population [13], which was supported by the stable frequency of $TCRV\alpha7.2^+$ T cells within the $CD3^+$ T cell pool (Fig. 1B, right panel). However, only few untreated highly viremic patients showed very high levels of $CD161^-TCRV\alpha7.2^+CD4^-$ T cells. A closer analysis revealed that five of these patients were recently diagnosed as HIV positive and at least three of these patients had a documented primary infection with definite seroconversion (<1 month) (Fig. S1A). For these patients, we used the time since HIV diagnosis as a crude measure for the time of infection (Fig. S1B) as previously described [6]. Therefore, it is intriguing to speculate whether this expansion of the $CD161^-TCRV\alpha7.2^+CD4^-$ T cell subset might be an effect of CD161 down-regulation on former $CD161^+$ MAIT cells, taking place during early stages of infection. While in general, there was a great variation between individual subjects in the frequency of MAIT cells and $CD161^-$ cells in healthy donors as well as in HIV patients, in HIV patients the MAIT/$CD161^-TCRV\alpha7.2^+$ cell ratio was shifted towards the (expanded) $CD161^-TCRV\alpha7.2^+$ portion (Fig. S1). Of note, in lymph nodes we detected a similar shift of this $CD161^+$ MAIT/$CD161^-TCRV\alpha7.2^+$ cell ratio in HIV-infected patients (Fig. 2).

Functional characterization of $CD161^+$ MAIT cells versus $CD161^-TCRV\alpha7.2^+$ cells

MAIT cells are believed to operate by secreting effector cytokines such as TNF-α, IFN-γ as well as IL-17 and IL-22 [1]. In order to assess possible functional impairments of MAIT cells in HIV-infection, we next wanted to explore, whether $CD161^+$ MAIT cells and $CD161^-TCRV\alpha7.2^+CD4^-$ T cells of HIV-infected patients differ in their cytokine secretion profile after unspecific stimulation. Thus, we carried out intracellular cytokine staining assays with PMA/ionomycin-stimulated PBMCs of both groups. Upon PMA/ionomycin-stimulation $CD161^+$ MAIT cells produced slightly more IL-17 ($p<0.001$ and <0.01, for HC and HIV patients respectively) and IFN-γ ($p<0.001$ for HC, no significant difference in HIV patients) as compared to their $CD161^-TCRV\alpha7.2^+$ counterparts (Fig. 1D). This finding is in line with previous results [8] and suggests that both T cell subsets are functionally different, and that $CD161^-TCRV\alpha7.2^+$ cells are less capable to fulfill Tc17 functionality than $CD161^+$ MAIT cells in HIV-infected patients.

Frequencies of activated $CD161^+$ MAIT cells and $CD161^-TCRV\alpha7.2^+$ cells are elevated in the blood of highly viremic HIV patients

In accordance with previous reports [18,19] we observed elevated levels of the soluble activation marker sCD163, a monocyte- and macrophage-specific scavenger receptor, shed during activation, in the plasma of untreated patients (Fig. 3A). A similar trend was observed for levels of sCD14, a marker of monocyte response to LPS [20]. However, this trend did not reach

Table 2. Cohort (LNMC samples).

	Healthy	HIV+(high VL and ART)
number of donors	6	11
age [years]	55 (±16)	44 (±15)
viral load [copies/ml]	–	42516 (±58152)

Shown are means and standard deviation.

statistical significance and was not directly correlated to MAIT cell frequencies (Fig. 3A and data not shown).

In addition to the expression of CD161, MAIT cells are defined by the expression of IL-18R [1]. Therefore, we hypothesized that circulating IL-18 in HIV-infected patients might lead to down-regulation of this receptor as well as to a strong stimulation of these cells. Indeed, IL-18, which is produced by macrophages, dendritic cells and enterocytes, was slightly elevated - though not statistically significant - in the plasma of untreated HIV patients of our cohort when measured in a standard ELISA assay (median high VL = 683.4 pg/ml, IQR = 445.4–1087 pg/ml vs. median HC = 523.4 pg/ml, IQR = 134.2–631 pg/ml) (Fig. 3A). Our results are in line with previous studies that showed that IL-18 is elevated during primary and chronic HIV-infection [21,22].

We next tested the hypothesis whether potent activation of the $CD161^+$ MAIT cell subset could indeed be a possible driving force

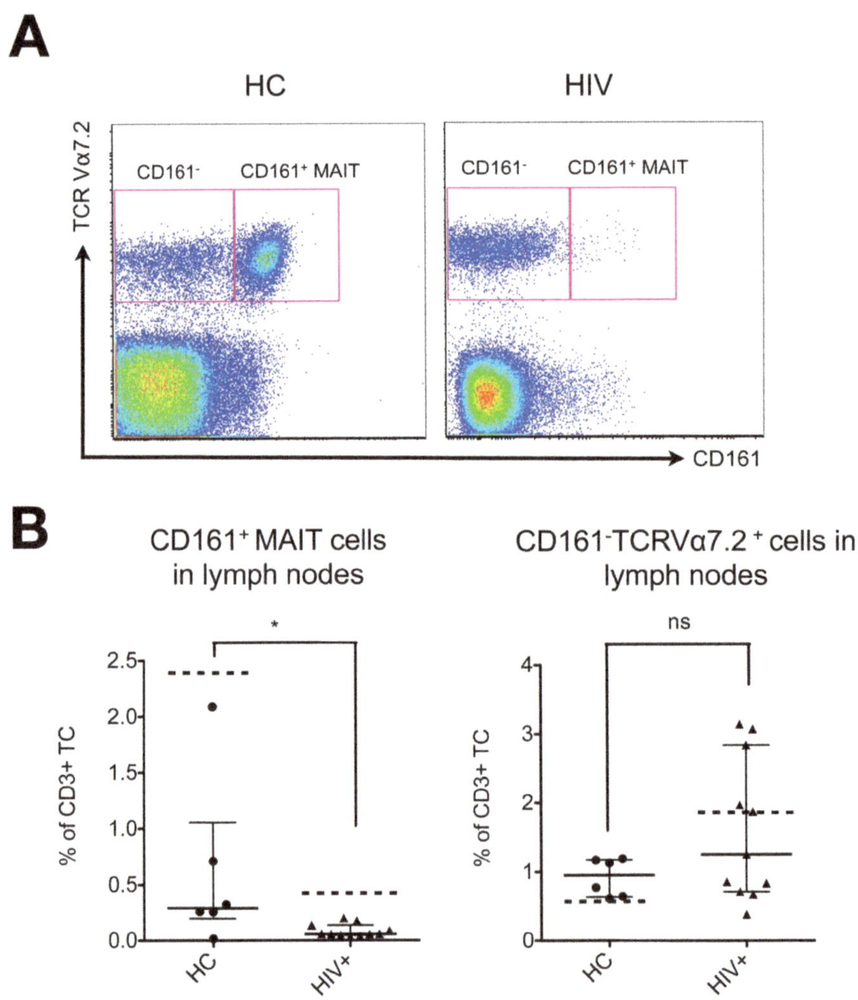

Figure 2. The frequency of $CD161^+$ MAIT cells is severely reduced in lymph nodes of HIV-infected patients. A) Gating strategy for the characterization of MAIT cells and $CD161^-TCRV\alpha7.2^+$ cells within the $CD4^-$ T cell subset of lymph node mononuclear cells (LNMC). Representative FACS plots for LNMC from a healthy control and an HIV-infected patient are shown. **B**) Frequencies of $CD161^+$ MAIT cells and $CD161^-TCRV\alpha7.2^+$ cells as percentages among $CD3^+$ lymphocytes for LNMC samples derived from healthy controls (healthy, n = 6) and HIV-infected patients (HIV, n = 11). Bars and lines indicate median and interquartile range. Dotted lines indicate the frequencies in the PBMC compartment of unmatched but similar groups for comparison. P-values are results of unpaired Mann-Whitney tests.

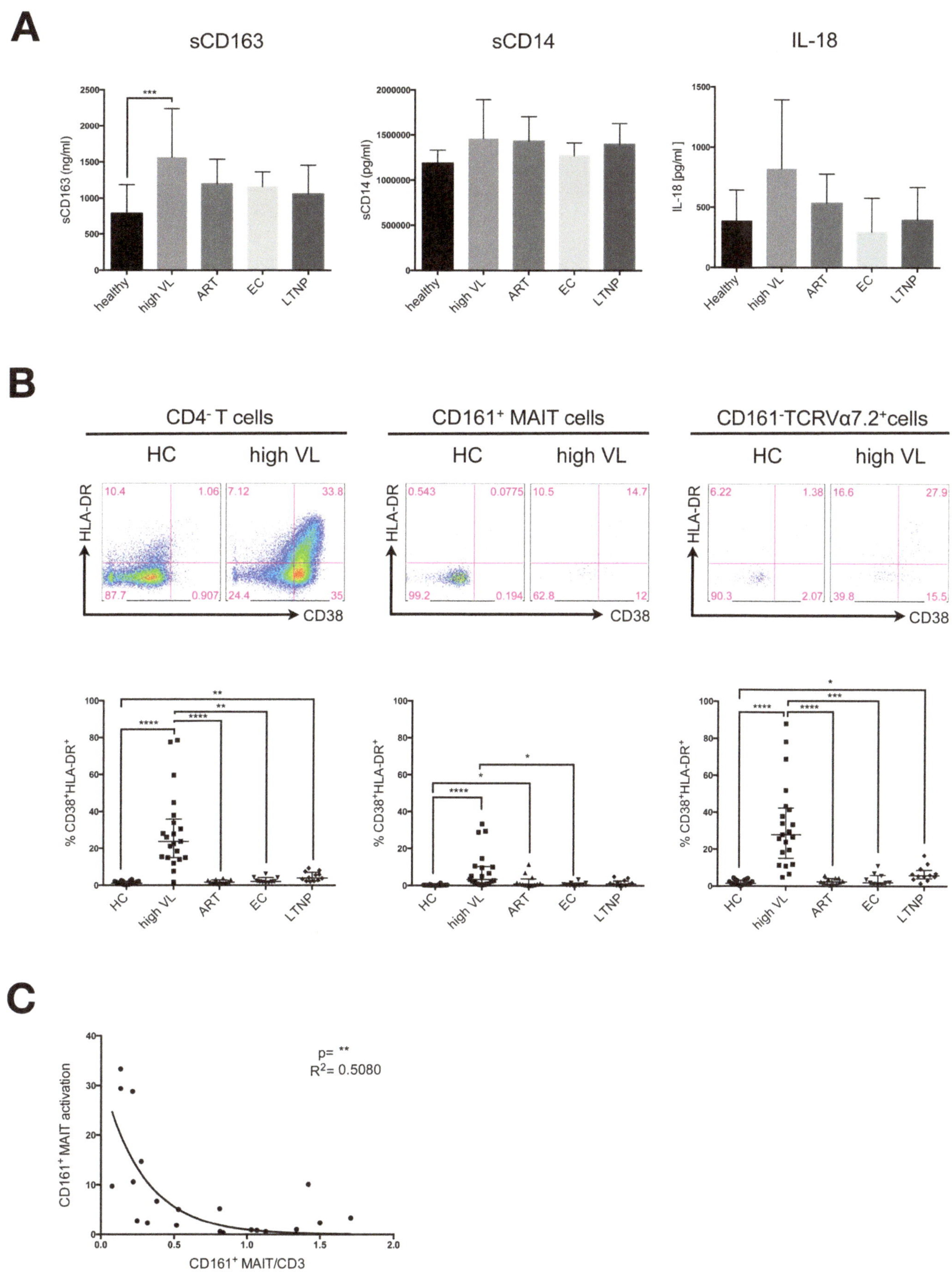
A
sCD163
sCD163 (ng/ml)
***
healthy
high VL
ART
EC
LTNP
sCD14
sCD14 (pg/ml)
IL-18
IL-18 [pg/ml]
Healthy
B
CD4- T cells
CD161+ MAIT cells
CD161-TCRVα7.2+cells
HC
high VL
HLA-DR
CD38
10.4
1.06
7.12
33.8
87.7
0.907
24.4
35
0.543
0.0775
10.5
14.7
99.2
0.194
62.8
12
6.22
1.38
16.6
27.9
90.3
2.07
39.8
15.5
% CD38+HLA-DR+
****
**
*
***
C
p= **
R2= 0.5080
CD161+ MAIT activation
CD161+ MAIT/CD3

Figure 3. Frequencies of activated $CD161^+$ and $CD161^-$ TCR Vα7.2$^+$ cells are elevated in the blood of highly viremic HIV patients. A) Plasma levels of sCD163, sCD14 and IL-18 were measured by ELISA in mostly corresponding samples of healthy controls (HC n = 13), highly viremic HIV-infected patients (high VL n = 18), patients receiving ART (ART n = 17), elite controllers (EC n = 6) and long-term nonprogressors (LTNP n = 6). B) Activated cells were defined as $CD38^+$ and HLA-DR^+ double positive cells and their frequency was assessed within the $CD4^-$, MAIT and $CD161^-$TCRVα7.2$^+$ populations. PBMC samples were derived from healthy controls (HC), highly viremic HIV-infected patients (high VL), patients receiving ART (ART), elite controllers (EC) and long-term nonprogressors (LTNP). Groups were compared by Kruskal-Wallis test followed by Dunn's multiple comparison test. P-values smaller than 0.05 were considered significant, where *, ** and *** indicate p-values between 0.01 to 0.05, 0.001 to 0.01 and 0.0001 to 0.001 respectively. Bars and lines indicate mean and standard deviation. C) Pearson correlation analysis of $CD161^+$ MAIT cell activation and $CD161^+$ MAIT cell frequency of $CD3^+$ T cells from the untreated high VL patient group. R^2 quantifies goodness of fit to the non-linear regression (exponential grow equation). R^2 is a fraction between 0.0 and 1.0, with 1.0 indicating the best fit.

for MAIT cell depletion. We therefore determined expression of the activation markers HLA-DR and CD38 on the $CD161^+$ MAIT cell subset and their parent population ($CD4^-CD3^+$T cells) as well as on the $CD161^-$TCRVα7.2$^+$ cells (Fig. 3B). The frequency of activated cells within the $CD161^+$ MAIT cell subset was significantly elevated in patients with untreated HIV infection and high viral load and slightly in patients receiving ART (median HC = 0.15%, IQR = 0.06–0.28% vs. median high VL = 3.31%, IQR = 0.94–10.35% and median ART = 0.83%, IQR = 0.33–3.63%, Kruskal-Wallis test followed by Dunn's multiple comparisons test: $p<0.0001$ and $p<0.05$, respectively). In fact, the activation level of MAIT cells from elite controllers was also significantly lower compared to highly viremic patients (median EC = 0.39%, IQR = 0.12–1.45%; $p<0.05$).

The $CD4^-$ parent population also showed a very high level of activation in viremic patients in comparison to all other patient groups, which indicates that this activation is part of the general immune activation observed in HIV infection and is not specific for the $CD161^+$ MAIT cell population (Fig. 3B). However, co-expression of CD38 and HLA-DR on the $CD161^+$ MAIT cell subset itself was inversely correlated to the $CD161^+$ MAIT cell frequency (Fig. 3C), indicating that at least an indirect effect of activation (for example at early stages of infection) is likely to be associated with the reduction of the $CD161^+$ MAIT cell subset.

In vitro stimulation of MAIT cells leads to activation and a reduced $CD161^+$ MAIT cell frequency

To determine possible factors that might contribute to the reduction of the $CD161^+$ MAIT cell population in HIV-infection on the one hand or possibly could lead to proliferation on the other hand, we tested the effect of cytokines (i.e. cytokines for which MAIT cells highly express the respective receptor) on $CD161^+$ MAIT cells. Moreover, the hypothesis of microbial translocation as a driving force for MAIT cell reduction in HIV was tested by adding fixed *E.coli* in a bacteria per cell ratio of 100:1 to the *in vitro* culture. In an *in vitro* experiment, PBMCs from healthy donors were stimulated with IL-12, IL-18, IL-7, fixed *E.coli* alone or in combination to elucidate the effect on MAIT cell activation (Fig. 4A, B). No significant alteration in the level of activation or frequency of the $CD161^+$ MAIT cell population was observed with addition of IL-12 or IL-18 alone (Fig. 4A, B). Combined stimulation with IL-12 and IL-18 in contrast led to potent activation of the MAIT cell subset as measured by CD69 expression (unstimulated cells mean = 2.98±1.16% vs. IL-12+IL-18 mean = 53.88±27.04%) accompanied by a slight reduction of the MAIT cell frequency among $CD3^+$ T cells, reflecting synergistic effects of IL-18 and IL-12 (Fig. 4A, B). The reduction of the MAIT cell frequency was confirmed using IL18R or CCR6 expression in addition to CD161 expression as alternative MAIT cell characterization (Fig. S4).

Since IL-7 has been described to be significantly elevated in untreated HIV-Infection [22] and a previous report described IL-7 to be an important cytokine to license MAIT cell effector function [23], the effect of exogenous IL-7 for MAIT cell activation was also tested. In our hands, *in vitro* addition of this cytokine indeed led to the activation of almost the entire $CD161^+$ MAIT cell subset. However, this activation was accompanied by a sharp drop of the $CD161^+$ MAIT cell frequency (Fig. 4A, B).

Addition of fixed *E. coli* also resulted in pronounced $CD161^+$ MAIT cell activation (blank mean = 2.98±1.16% vs. *E. coli* mean = 75.95±14.50%), TCRVα7.2 down-regulation and significant reduction of this cell subset (blank normalized to 1 vs. *E.coli* mean = 0.17±0.15) (Fig. 4A, B).

These results support the hypothesis that the translocation of bacteria and their products as well as consecutively produced pro-inflammatory cytokines (e.g. IL-12, IL-18) contribute to $CD161^+$ MAIT cell over-activation and, in turn to their quantitative reduction in HIV-infected patients [7]. Our results are also in line with a recent report that demonstrated that $CD161^+$ MAIT cells can be stimulated in an TCR independent manner by the cytokines IL-12 and IL-18 [24].

Material and Methods

Study subjects and samples

PBMC as well as lymph node mononuclear cells (derived from hilar and axillary lymph nodes) of in total 63 HIV patients were collected at the University Medical Center Hamburg-Eppendorf and Hannover Medical School, Germany. Healthy individuals (PBMC n = 20, LNMC n = 6) served as controls and for validation of the immunological tests. Written informed consent was obtained from all patients enrolled in this study, which was approved by the Ethics Committee of the Medical Association of Hamburg. The HIV long-term nonprogressor and elite controller cohorts consisted of HIV-infected subjects selected according to viral load, CD4 count, time and duration of HIV infection. The definition of the different stages of the disease were extracted from the electronic databases of the participating centers and confirmed by the treating physicians according to standard classifications and by criteria commonly used in the literature [25,26]. HIV-1 viral load was determined using COBAS amplicor assays with a detection limit of 50 RNA copies/ml. HIV CDC status, antiretroviral treatment, and $CD4^+$ T cell counts were determined via chart review.

Immunophenotypic analysis

For immunophenotypic staining, cryopreserved PBMC or LNMC were thawed using standardized techniques. For exclusion of dead cells PBMCs were stained with the LIVE/DEAD Fixable Aqua Dead Cell Stain Kit (life technologies, Darmstadt, Germany) according to the manufacturer's protocol. To characterize T cell populations, at least 5×10^5 cells were stained with appropriate fluorochrome-conjugated surface antibodies, including anti-CD3 (SK7), anti-CD4 (RPAT4), anti-CD8α (HIT8a), anti-TCRVα7.2 (3C10), anti-CD161 (HP-3G10), anti-HLA-DR (G46-6), anti-CD38 (HIT2, Biolegend), anti-IL-18R (H44), anti-CD69 (FN50),

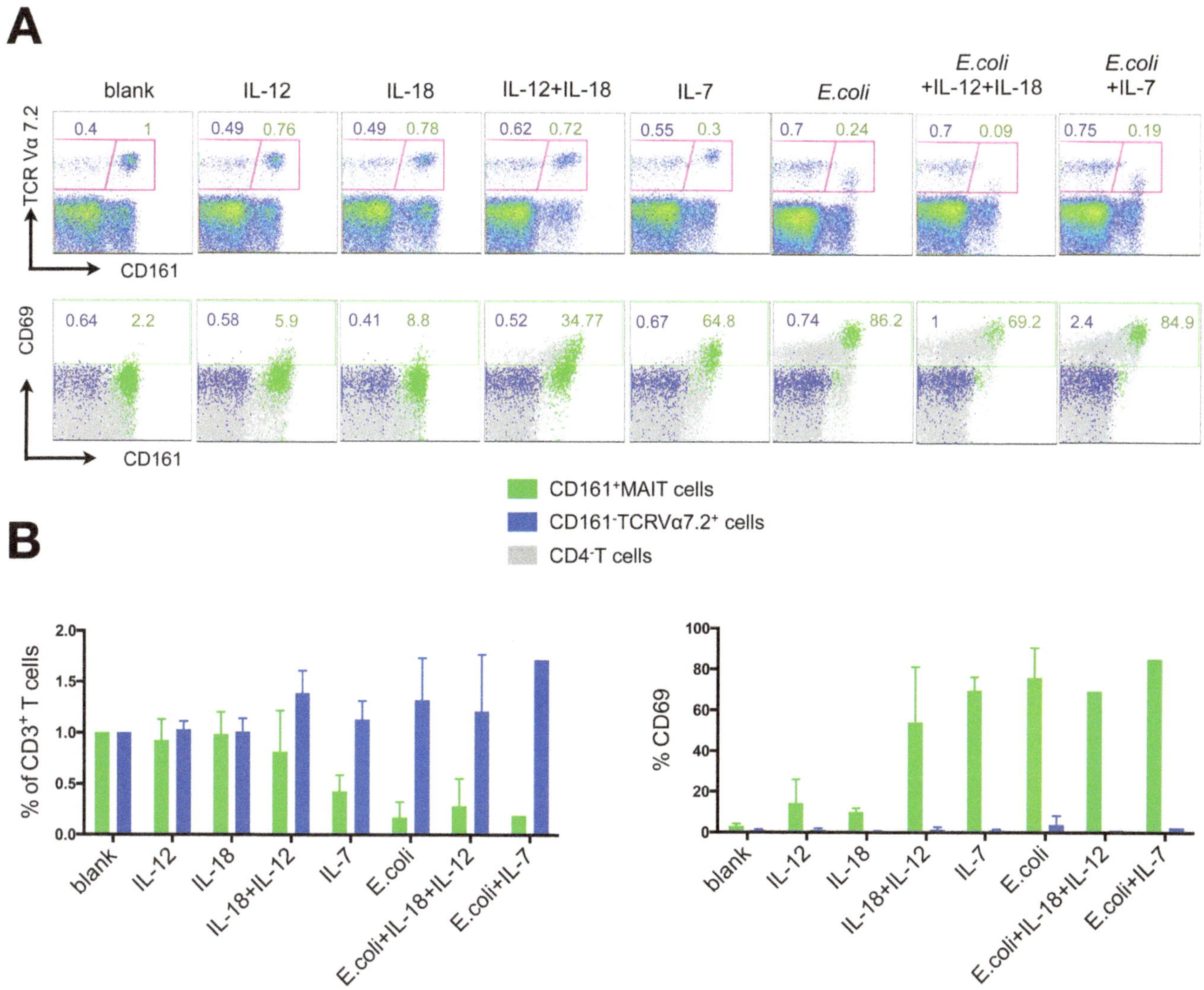

Figure 4. Frequencies of CD161$^+$ MAIT cells are reduced upon *in vitro* stimulation with PFA fixed *E.coli*, IL-7 and combined IL-12 and IL-18. A) Representative FACS plots depicting frequencies of CD161$^-$TCRVα7.2$^+$ cells, CD161$^+$ MAIT cells and all TCRVα7.2$^+$ cells as frequencies of CD3$^+$ T cells after 28 hours of stimulation with IL-12 (100 μg/ml), IL-18 (100 μg/ml) and their combination, IL-7 (100 μg/ml) and PFA fixed *E. coli* (bacteria per cell ratio of 100:1 PBMC). PBMCs were healthy donor-derived and seeded in 1×10^6 cells/well. **B**) Cumulative display of normalized frequencies of CD161$^+$ MAIT cells and CD161$^-$TCRVα7.2$^+$ cells from 3 healthy donors in duplicate measurements for each stimulation setting (apart from *E.coli* in combination with cytokines, which was tested once) measured after 28 hours of stimulation (left panel). Activation levels were assessed by determining the percentage of CD69$^+$ cells within the CD161$^+$ MAIT cell and the CD161$^-$TCRVα7.2$^+$ population.

anti-CCR6 (G034E3) (from Biolegend or BD Biosciences, Heidelberg, Germany) for 20 min at RT in the dark. After surface staining, cells were washed once with PBS and were then resuspended in 0.5% paraformaldehyde. For intracellular cytokine staining, the cells were stimulated with PMA (50 ng/ml) and ionomycin (0.67 μM) for 5 h at 37°C and 5% CO_2 prior to immunophenotypic staining. Brefeldin A (10 g/ml) was added for the last 4 h of the stimulation. Data were collected on a BD LSRII machine using FACS Diva version 5 (BD Biosciences, Heidelberg, Germany).

ELISA of plasma sCD163, sCD14 and IL-18

sCD163 levels in plasma were measured using the Macro163 ELISA kit (Trillium Diagnostics, Bangos, ME). sCD14 levels in plasma were measured using the Human sCD14 Quantikine ELISA kit (R&D Systems, Minneapolis, MN). Plasma levels of IL-18 were measured using the Human IL-18 Platinum ELISA kit (eBioscience, Germany).

Stimulation of PBMCs with cytokines and fixed *E. coli*

PBMCs from healthy donors were freshly isolated and seeded into a 48 well plate (1×10^6 cells/well). IL-12, IL-18 and IL-7 were added with an end concentration of 100 ng/ml. Prior to an experiment, aliquots of 1×10^9 *E.coli* (DH5α)/ml were fixed for 5 min in 1% paraformaldehyde and stored at −80°C. After thawing and washing, *E. coli* was added in a bacteria/cell ratio of 100:1. The PBMCs were stimulated for either 14 or 28 h before surface staining and FACS analysis.

Statistical analysis

All flow cytometric data were analyzed using FlowJo version 9.2 software (Treestar). Statistical analysis was carried out using Prism

5.0 software (GraphPad Software, San Diego, CA). All groups were tested for normal distribution with the Kolmogorov-Smirnov test and were compared by the adequate test. For normally distributed data, parametric tests were applied: for two groups t-tests, for more than two groups ANOVA followed by Tukey's multiple comparisons test. Data that was not normally distributed was tested by the Mann-Whitney test for two unpaired groups, by the Wilcoxon test for paired groups, or Kruskal-Wallis test followed by Dunn's multiple comparisons test for more then two groups, respectively. P-values smaller than 0.05 were considered significant, where *, ** and *** indicate p-values between 0.01 to 0.05, 0.001 to 0.01 and 0.0001 to 0.001, respectively. Pearson's correlation was applied for bivariate correlation analyses. Data are expressed as median, 25% and 75% quartiles or means with standard deviation, respectively (as indicated in the figure legend). $CD161^+$ MAIT cell frequencies were normalized for the *in vitro* stimulation data.

Discussion

Only in the last couple of years the important role of $CD161^+TCRV\alpha7.2^+CD4^-CD3^+$ MAIT cells in the defense of different bacterial (and indirectly in viral) infections has become clear [1,2,6,12,24,27–29]. While great progress has been made in characterizing the phenotypic and functional properties of MAIT cells [1,4,23,24,30–33], many details of MAIT cell function still have to be elucidated.

The current study adds further detail to the recent body of data suggesting diminishing function and decreasing numbers of MAIT cells in HIV infection [5–7]. In particular, frequency and phenotype of MAIT cells during HIV infection with regards to disease status, including HIV LTNP and elite controllers, were analyzed in detail. In accordance with data from a recent study [6] we confirm an irreversible reduction of the $CD161^+$ MAIT cell population in peripheral and lymph nodal tissue of patients with treated and untreated chronic HIV infection. However, while the preliminary results of the study by Leeansyah and coworkers [6] suggests that elite controllers maintain a similar size of their MAIT cell population as healthy controls, we found a significantly reduced MAIT cell frequency, as well as reduced MAIT cell numbers in the ten elite controller patients and a similar trend in twelve long-term nonprogressors included in the present study. These data are potentially of clinical importance and further studies have to elucidate whether the higher general immune activation detected in elite controllers in comparison to healthy controls is in parts due to a lower level of MAIT cells in these patients [34–36].

In functional *in vitro* experiments (Fig. 4) we were able to replicate the proposed model of a constitutive down-regulation of functional MAIT cell markers (i.e. CD161, IL-18R, CCR6) and eventual loss of $TCRV\alpha7.2^+CD4^-CD3^+$ T cells by stimulation with bacterial antigens and pro-inflammatory cytokines in HIV infection [7]. Importantly, we and others found that inflammatory cytokines like IL-12 or IL-18 can activate MAIT cells in a TCR independent manner [24,37]. It is not quite clear in how far the *in vitro* conditions replicate the *in vivo* milieu, but significant shifts towards inflammatory cytokines have been described and it has been proposed that these cytokines add to the pathogenesis of HIV infection [21,22].

Clearly, the current study is limited by the fact that no mucosal tissue was available for any of the patients studied and homing of the MAIT cell population to the gut might be in part responsible for the decrease of the peripheral MAIT cell frequencies. However, two independent studies previously showed a loss of mucosal gut resident MAIT cells in HIV-infected patients [5,6]. In preliminary experiments, we also see high expression of the gut-homing markers CCR9 and beta7 integrin [38] on MAIT cells in the jejunum of healthy controls (data not shown) and up-regulation of CCR9 and beta7 integrin was detected in peripheral MAIT cells in HIV patients (Fig. S3). The frequency of $CCR9^+\beta7^+$ integrin on MAIT cells was inversely correlated with the frequency of MAIT cells supporting the model of partial homing of MAIT cells to the gut in HIV infection [5]. In future prospective efforts it is planned to analyze the gut resident MAIT cell frequencies in HIV patients with different disease course, including HIV elite controllers obtained during routine screening colonoscopies.

In the present study, we also looked at a small number of patients with a recent history of acute retroviral syndrome, early primary HIV infection and/or confirmed recent seroconversion. In line with the results of the recently published studies [5–7], our data indicate that the decrease of peripheral $CD161^+$ MAIT cell numbers seems to be an early event in HIV infection. However, very early in the course of the primary infection we find a relative increase of the $CD161^-$ $TCRV\alpha7.2^+CD4^-CD3^+$ T cell subset suggestive of a down-regulation of CD161 on these cells. This elevation can still be detected at later stages and in different patient groups (Fig. 1B, middle panel). These $CD161^-TCRV\alpha7.2^+CD4^-CD3^+$ T cells were also recently described [5] and appear to have a larger proportion of cells with a similar TCRVβ usage as seen in MAIT cells in HIV-infected patients. In our hands, these highly activated $CD161^-TCRV\alpha7.2^+CD4^-CD3^+$ T cells rapidly develop after *in vitro* stimulation of $CD161^+$ MAIT cells and seem to be less functional *ex vivo* than their $CD161^+$ MAIT cell counterparts (Fig. 1D). In one patient who is included in our study and was treated during early primary infection, the MAIT cell frequency indeed recovered (Fig. S2). In a next step, further prospective clinical studies of patients with primary HIV infection have to establish whether very early initiation of ART can indeed "rescue" the MAIT cell population [39,40].

In ongoing experiments we are now characterizing the transcription factor expression profile (RORγt, Tbet, Gata3, PLZF) of $CD161^+$ MAIT cells versus $CD161^-$ $TCRV\alpha7.2^+CD4^-CD3^+$ T cells in uninfected donors as well as HIV-infected patients in order to explain some of the detected results of this study and to further discriminate relevant MAIT cell subpopulations [14,32,41–43]. For example the ability to secrete IL-17 could well be correlated with expression of the transcription factor RORγt [41]. Of importance, recent studies suggest that iNKT cells and MAIT cells exhibit a proapoptotic propensity with elevated expression of activated caspases, which is correlated with expression of transcription factor PLZF/ZBTB-16 [32]. This would make the loss of MAIT cells due to activation-induced cell death in HIV even more plausible. Also, the manipulation of these transcription factors represents an intriguing target for future therapeutic approaches [44]. The proof of "successful genetic manipulation and reprogramming to pluripotency and re-differentiation of functional MAIT cells" opens at least theoretically further therapeutic options [44,45]. In our hands, it was difficult to culture and expand primary MAIT cells *in vitro* and novel *in vitro* MAIT cell expansion protocols should be developed.

For the time being, it will be important to prospectively examine patients at the first stages of acute HIV infection to understand the exact kinetics of the MAIT cell loss and whether very early initiation of ART during primary HIV infection can indeed rescue the MAIT cell population and thereby possibly minimize subsequent microbial translocation [40]. Other theoretical therapeutic options include the immunomodulatory blockade of circulating cytokines (eg. IL-18) or the use of probiotics to stimulate MAIT cell regeneration and proliferation by activation of the commensal bacterial flora [2,46]. In a next step, the MAIT cell frequency and function have to be comprehensively examined in different tissues, e.g. lung tissue (via BAL) [28,47] or the liver [23] of HIV-infected patients (including elite controllers) in comparison to uninfected controls and, importantly, in HIV/TB or HIV/HCV coinfection [47]. Further studies should also comprehensively look at the different immune cell populations with antibacterial activity (e.g. $\gamma\delta$ T cells, NKT cells or innate lymphoid cells [48,49]) as other cells might compensate the loss of the MAIT cell population. For example, we find a relative expansion of $\gamma\delta$ T cell subsets in HIV infection ([49] and data not shown). Further analysis of MAIT cells might be assisted by the use of MAIT cell tetramer technology [31]. It will also be interesting to see whether the riboflavin metabolites are in itself more reliable and stable markers for bacterial translocation than LPS [30].

In summary, the current study confirms and extends previous studies and suggests that an irreversible reduction of the peripheral $CD161^+$ MAIT as well as an expansion of the $CD161^-$TCR $V\alpha7.2^+$ subset are early events in HIV infection [5–7,24,47]. The loss is most likely caused by a combination of increased homing to the gut as well as a lacking resistance towards stimulation by microbial products and cytokines leading to a) a change of phenotype, b) loss of function and c) possibly cell death, which takes place in all patients including HIV long-term nonprogressors and elite controllers independently of disease progression.

Supporting Information

Figure S1 The $CD161^+$ MAIT/$CD161^-$TCR$V\alpha^+$ ratio is shifted in HIV infection. **A**) Bars indicate each individual's frequency of $CD161^+$ MAIT cells (light grey) and $CD161^-$TCR$V\alpha^+$ cells (dark grey). Patients with confirmed or suspected acute HIV-infection (n = 5) below 1 month post first diagnosis are marked in red. **B**) Comparison of $CD4^-$T cell frequencies (grey), $CD161^-$TCR$V\alpha7.2^+$ cell frequencies (blue), $CD161^+$ MAIT cell frequencies (green) of high VL patients below 1 month vs. above 1 month of known HIV-infection. The indicated p-value results from a Mann Whitney test. P-values smaller than 0.05 were considered significant.

Figure S2 Longitudinal $CD161^+$ MAIT cell increase in a patient after early treatment initiation. FACS plots depicting frequencies of $CD161^+$ MAIT (upper right number in green) and $CD161^-$TCR$V\alpha^+$ cells of the $CD4^-$ T cell population (upper left number in blue) of a patient during acute HIV-infection (Fiebig stage III: ELISA +, Immunoblot -) and 28 month later after immediate initiation of ART.

Figure S3 Migration to the gut is specifically elevated in the $CD161^+$ MAIT cell population. Migrating cells are measured by frequencies of $CCR9^+\beta7integrin^+$ double positive cells of $CD161^+$ MAIT cells and $CD161^-$TCR$V\alpha7.2^+$ cells, respectively. PBMC samples were derived from healthy controls, highly viremic HIV-infected patients and patients under ART. **A**) Groups were tested for normal distribution by Kolmogorov-Smirnov test and compared by Kruskal-Wallis test followed by Dunn's multiple comparisons test. P-values smaller than 0.05 were considered significant, where *, ** and *** indicate p-values between 0.01 to 0.05, 0.001 to 0.01 and 0.0001 to 0.001 respectively. Bars and lines indicate median and interquartile ranges. **B**) Correlation analysis of $CD161^+$ MAIT cell frequency or $CD161^-$TCR$V\alpha7.2^+$ cell frequency with the corresponding frequency of $CCR9^+/\beta7^+$ $CD161^+$MAIT cells. R^2 is a fraction between 0.0 and 1.0, with 1.0 indicating the best fit to the linear regression.

Figure S4 The MAIT cell defining markers CD161, IL18R and CCR6 are reduced within the TCR$V\alpha7.2^+$ subset upon stimulation with IL-12 and IL-18, IL-7 and *E.coli*. **A**) Representative FACS plots depicting frequencies of $CD161^-$TCR$V\alpha7.2^+$ cells, $CD161^+$ MAIT cells and all TCR$V\alpha7.2^+$ cells as frequencies of $CD3^+$ T cells after 28 hours of stimulation with IL-12 (100 µg/ml), IL-18 (100 µg/ml) and their combination, IL-7 (100 µg/ml) and PFA fixed *E. coli* (bacteria per cell ratio of 100:1 PBMC). PBMCs were healthy donor-derived and seeded in 1×10^6 cells/well.

Acknowledgments

We thank the patients who participated in this study. Furthermore we want to thank Benjamin Otto, from the Department of Clinical Chemistry/ Central Laboratories, UKE for providing statistical advice.

Author Contributions

Conceived and designed the experiments: JSzW PH JME JvL. Performed the experiments: JME PH SK. Analyzed the data: JME PH JSzW. Contributed reagents/materials/analysis tools: JvL RES MB CL. Wrote the paper: JME PH JSzW JH JvL. Provided clinical samples: JvL RES MB CL. Carried out the soluble activation marker assays: AB.

References

1. Le Bourhis L, Mburu YK, Lantz O (2013) MAIT cells, surveyors of a new class of antigen: development and functions. Curr Opin Immunol 25: 174–180.
2. Le Bourhis L, Dusseaux M, Bohineust A, Bessoles S, Martin E, et al. (2013) MAIT cells detect and efficiently lyse bacterially-infected epithelial cells. PLoS pathogens 9: e1003681.
3. Le Bourhis L, Martin E, Peguillet I, Guihot A, Froux N, et al. (2010) Antimicrobial activity of mucosal-associated invariant T cells. Nat Immunol 11: 701–708.
4. Patel O, Kjer-Nielsen L, Le Nours J, Eckle SB, Birkinshaw R, et al. (2013) Recognition of vitamin B metabolites by mucosal-associated invariant T cells. Nature communications 4.
5. Cosgrove C, Ussher JE, Rauch A, Gartner K, Kurioka A, et al. (2013) Early and nonreversible decrease of CD161++/MAIT cells in HIV infection. Blood 121: 951–961.
6. Leeansyah E, Ganesh A, Quigley MF, Sonnerborg A, Andersson J, et al. (2013) Activation, exhaustion, and persistent decline of the antimicrobial MR1-restricted MAIT-cell population in chronic HIV-1 infection. Blood 121: 1124–1135.
7. Sandberg JK, Dias J, Shacklett BL, Leeansyah E (2013) Will loss of your MAITs weaken your HAART [corrected]? AIDS 27: 2501–2504.
8. Walker BD (2007) Elite control of HIV Infection: implications for vaccines and treatment. Top HIV Med 15: 134–136.
9. Bello G, Velasco-de-Castro CA, Bongertz V, Rodrigues CA, Giacoia-Gripp CB, et al. (2009) Immune activation and antibody responses in non-progressing elite controller individuals infected with HIV-1. J Med Virol 81: 1681–1690.
10. Walker LJ, Kang Y-H, Smith MO, Tharmalingham H, Ramamurthy N, et al. (2012) Human MAIT and CD8αα cells develop from a pool of type-17 precommitted CD8+ T cells. Blood 119: 422–433.
11. Dusseaux M, Martin E, Serriari N, Peguillet I, Premel V, et al. (2011) Human MAIT cells are xenobiotic-resistant, tissue-targeted, CD161hi IL-17-secreting T cells. Blood 117: 1250–1259.
12. Billerbeck E, Kang YH, Walker L, Lockstone H, Grafmueller S, et al. (2010) Analysis of CD161 expression on human CD8+ T cells defines a distinct functional subset with tissue-homing properties. Proc Natl Acad Sci U S A 107: 3006–3011.

13. Wong EB, Akilimali NA, Govender P, Sullivan ZA, Cosgrove C, et al. (2013) Low levels of peripheral CD161++CD8+ mucosal associated invariant T (MAIT) cells are found in HIV and HIV/TB co-infection. PLoS One 8: e83474.
14. Chang PP, Barral P, Fitch J, Pratama A, Ma CS, et al. (2012) Identification of Bcl-6-dependent follicular helper NKT cells that provide cognate help for B cell responses. Nat Immunol 13: 35–43.
15. King IL, Fortier A, Tighe M, Dibble J, Watts GF, et al. (2012) Invariant natural killer T cells direct B cell responses to cognate lipid antigen in an IL-21-dependent manner. Nat Immunol 13: 44–50.
16. Martin E, Treiner E, Duban L, Guerri L, Laude H, et al. (2009) Stepwise development of MAIT cells in mouse and human. PLoS Biol 7: e54.
17. Le Bourhis L, Guerri L, Dusseaux M, Martin E, Soudais C, et al. (2011) Mucosal-associated invariant T cells: unconventional development and function. Trends Immunol 32: 212–218.
18. Burdo TH, Lo J, Abbara S, Wei J, DeLelys ME, et al. (2011) Soluble CD163, a novel marker of activated macrophages, is elevated and associated with noncalcified coronary plaque in HIV-infected patients. J Infect Dis 204: 1227–1236.
19. Burdo TH, Lentz MR, Autissier P, Krishnan A, Halpern E, et al. (2011) Soluble CD163 made by monocyte/macrophages is a novel marker of HIV activity in early and chronic infection prior to and after anti-retroviral therapy. J Infect Dis 204: 154–163.
20. Sandler NG, Wand H, Roque A, Law M, Nason MC, et al. (2011) Plasma levels of soluble CD14 independently predict mortality in HIV infection. J Infect Dis 203: 780–790.
21. Ahmad R, Sindhu ST, Toma E, Morisset R, Ahmad A (2002) Elevated levels of circulating interleukin-18 in human immunodeficiency virus-infected individuals: role of peripheral blood mononuclear cells and implications for AIDS pathogenesis. J Virol 76: 12448–12456.
22. Napolitano LA, Grant RM, Deeks SG, Schmidt D, De Rosa SC, et al. (2001) Increased production of IL-7 accompanies HIV-1-mediated T-cell depletion: implications for T-cell homeostasis. Nat Med 7: 73–79.
23. Tang XZ, Jo J, Tan AT, Sandalova E, Chia A, et al. (2013) IL-7 licenses activation of human liver intrasinusoidal mucosal-associated invariant T cells. J Immunol 190: 3142–3152.
24. Ussher JE, Bilton M, Attwod E, Shadwell J, Richardson R, et al. (2014) CD161++ CD8+ T cells, including the MAIT cell subset, are specifically activated by IL-12+ IL-18 in a TCR-independent manner. European journal of immunology 44: 195–203.
25. Deeks SG, Walker BD (2007) Human immunodeficiency virus controllers: mechanisms of durable virus control in the absence of antiretroviral therapy. Immunity 27: 406–416.
26. Pereyra F, Addo MM, Kaufmann DE, Liu Y, Miura T, et al. (2008) Genetic and immunologic heterogeneity among persons who control HIV infection in the absence of therapy. J Infect Dis 197: 563–571.
27. Northfield JW, Kasprowicz V, Lucas M, Kersting N, Bengsch B, et al. (2008) CD161 expression on hepatitis C virus-specific CD8+ T cells suggests a distinct pathway of T cell differentiation. Hepatology 47: 396–406.
28. Meierovics A, Yankelevich WJ, Cowley SC (2013) MAIT cells are critical for optimal mucosal immune responses during in vivo pulmonary bacterial infection. Proc Natl Acad Sci U S A 110: E3119–3128.
29. Grimaldi D, Le Bourhis L, Sauneuf B, Dechartres A, Rousseau C, et al. (2014) Specific MAIT cell behaviour among innate-like T lymphocytes in critically ill patients with severe infections. Intensive Care Med 40: 192–201.
30. Birkinshaw RW, Kjer-Nielsen L, Eckle SB, McCluskey J, Rossjohn J (2014) MAITs, MR1 and vitamin B metabolites. Curr Opin Immunol 26: 7–13.
31. Reantragoon R, Corbett AJ, Sakala IG, Gherardin NA, Furness JB, et al. (2013) Antigen-loaded MR1 tetramers define T cell receptor heterogeneity in mucosal-associated invariant T cells. J Exp Med 210: 2305–2320.
32. Gérart S, Sibéril S, Martin E, Lenoir C, Aguilar C, et al. (2013) Human iNKT and MAIT cells exhibit a PLZF-dependent proapoptotic propensity that is counterbalanced by XIAP. Blood 121: 614–623.
33. Lee OJ, Cho YN, Kee SJ, Kim MJ, Jin HM, et al. (2014) Circulating mucosal-associated invariant T cell levels and their cytokine levels in healthy adults. Exp Gerontol 49: 47–54.
34. Krishnan S, Wilson EM, Sheikh V, Rupert A, Mendoza D, et al. (2014) Evidence for Innate Immune System Activation in HIV Type 1-Infected Elite Controllers. J Infect Dis 209: 931–939.
35. Chun T-W, Shawn Justement J, Murray D, Kim CJ, Blazkova J, et al. (2013) Effect of Antiretroviral Therapy on HIV Reservoirs in Elite Controllers. Journal of Infectious Diseases 208: 1443–1447.
36. Pereyra F, Lo J, Triant VA, Wei J, Buzon MJ, et al. (2012) Increased coronary atherosclerosis and immune activation in HIV-1 elite controllers. AIDS 26: 2409–2412.
37. Turtle CJ, Delrow J, Joslyn RC, Swanson HM, Basom R, et al. (2011) Innate signals overcome acquired TCR signaling pathway regulation and govern the fate of human CD161hi CD8α+ semi-invariant T cells. Blood 118: 2752–2762.
38. Mavigner M, Cazabat M, Dubois M, L'Faqihi FE, Requena M, et al. (2012) Altered CD4+ T cell homing to the gut impairs mucosal immune reconstitution in treated HIV-infected individuals. J Clin Invest 122: 62–69.
39. Chen J, Han X, An M, Liu J, Xu J, et al. (2013) Immunological and virological benefits resulted from short-course treatment during primary HIV infection: a meta-analysis. PLoS One 8: e82461.
40. Investigators ST, Fidler S, Porter K, Ewings F, Frater J, et al. (2013) Short-course antiretroviral therapy in primary HIV infection. N Engl J Med 368: 207–217.
41. Constantinides MG, Bendelac A (2013) Transcriptional regulation of the NKT cell lineage. Curr Opin Immunol 25: 161–167.
42. Gordon SM, Carty SA, Kim JS, Zou T, Smith-Garvin J, et al. (2011) Requirements for eomesodermin and promyelocytic leukemia zinc finger in the development of innate-like CD8+ T cells. J Immunol 186: 4573–4578.
43. Alonzo ES, Sant'Angelo DB (2011) Development of PLZF-expressing innate T cells. Curr Opin Immunol 23: 220–227.
44. Wakao H, Fujita H (2013) Toward the realization of cell therapy: the advent of MAIT cells from iPSCs. Cell Cycle 12: 2341–2342.
45. Wakao H, Yoshikiyo K, Koshimizu U, Furukawa T, Enomoto K, et al. (2013) Expansion of functional human mucosal-associated invariant T cells via reprogramming to pluripotency and redifferentiation. Cell Stem Cell 12: 546–558.
46. Wilson NL, Moneyham LD, Alexandrov AW (2013) A systematic review of probiotics as a potential intervention to restore gut health in HIV infection. J Assoc Nurses AIDS Care 24: 98–111.
47. Wong EB, Akilimali NA, Govender P, Sullivan ZA, Cosgrove C, et al. (2013) Low Levels of Peripheral CD161++ CD8+ Mucosal Associated Invariant T (MAIT) Cells Are Found in HIV and HIV/TB Co-Infection. PloS one 8: e83474.
48. Sutton CE, Mielke LA, Mills KHG (2012) IL-17-producing γδ T cells and innate lymphoid cells. European Journal of Immunology 42: 2221–2231.
49. Hartjen P, Meyer-Olson D, Lehmann C, Stellbrink HJ, van Lunzen J, et al. (2013) Vgamma2Vdelta2 T cells are skewed toward a terminal differentiation phenotype in untreated HIV infection. J Infect Dis 208: 180–182.

12

Whole Blood Transcriptional Profiling Reveals Deregulation of Oxidative and Antioxidative Defence Genes in Myelofibrosis and Related Neoplasms. Potential Implications of Downregulation of Nrf2 for Genomic Instability and Disease Progression

Hans Carl Hasselbalch[1]*, Mads Thomassen[2], Caroline Hasselbalch Riley[3], Lasse Kjær[1], Thomas Stauffer Larsen[4], Morten K. Jensen[1], Ole Weis Bjerrum[5], Torben A. Kruse[2], Vibe Skov[1]

1 Department of Hematology, Roskilde Hospital, University of Copenhagen, Roskilde, Denmark, **2** Department of Clinical Genetics, Odense University Hospital, Odense, Denmark, **3** Department of Hematology L, Herlev Hospital, University of Copenhagen, Herlev, Denmark, **4** Department of Hematology X, Odense University Hospital, Odense, Denmark, **5** Department of Hematology L, Rigshospitalet, University of Copenhagen, Copenhagen, Denmark

Abstract

The Philadelphia-negative chronic myeloproliferative neoplasms - essential thrombocythemia (ET), polycythemia vera (PV), and myelofibrosis (MF) (MPNs) - have recently been shown to be associated with chronic inflammation, oxidative stress and accumulation of reactive oxygen species (ROS). Using whole blood transcriptional profiling, we report that several oxidative stress and anti-oxidative stress genes are significantly deregulated in MPNs. Among the twenty most up- and downregulated genes, ATOX1, DEFB122, GPX8, PRDX2, PRDX6, PTGS1, and SEPP1 were progressively upregulated from ET over PV to PMF, whereas AKR1B1, CYBA, SIRT2, TTN, and UCP2 were progressively downregulated in ET, PV and PMF (all FDR <0.05). The gene Nrf2, encoding the transcription factor nuclear factor erythroid 2-related factor 2 (NFE2L2 or Nrf2) was significantly downregulated in all MPNs. Nrf2 has a key role in the regulation of the oxidative stress response and modulates both migration and retention of hematopoietic stem cells (HSCs) in their niche. The patogenetic importance of Nrf2 depletion in the context of expansion of the hematopoietic progenitor pool in MPNs is discussed with particular focus upon the implications of concomitant downregulation of Nrf2 and CXCR4 for stem cell mobilization.

Editor: Ken Mills, Queen's University Belfast, United Kingdom

Funding: The study has received grants from the The Danish Council for Independent Research Medical Sciences (http://fivu.dk/forskning-og-innovation/rad-og-udvalg/det-frieforskningsrad/radet/dff-sundhed-og-sygdom). The funders had no role in study design, data Collection and analysis, decision to publish, or preparation of the manuscript.

Competing Interests: The authors have declared that no competing interests exist.

* Email: hans.hasselbalch@dadlnet.dk

Introduction

The Philadelphia-negative chronic myeloproliferative neoplasms (MPNs) – essential thrombocythemia (ET), polycythemia vera (PV) and primary myelofibrosis (PMF) – are clonal stem cell diseases, arising due to an acquired genetic defect in the pluripotent stem cell. The nature of the initiating genetic defect remains to be established but several "second hit" genetic aberrations have been identified giving rise to dysregulation of various signaling pathways of importance in controlling blood cell production. One of these is the JAK2V617F mutation, which is present in virtually all patients with PV and in half of those with ET and PMF [1]. According to "The Biological Continuum" concept, these neoplasms evolve from an early disease stage (ET) to the advanced myelofibrosis stage, implying in the JAK2V617F-positive patients a steady increase in the JAK2V617F mutational load from "low burden" JAK2V617F-positive ET over PV to the advanced burnt-out myelofibrosis stage [1–3].

The MPNs are associated with a chronic inflammatory state due to the continuous release of inflammation products from in vivo activated leukocytes and platelets [4]. Indeed, the MPNs may be described as a "Human Inflammation Model", illustrating the devastating consequences of chronic inflammation in MPNs – premature atherosclerosis, immune deregulation with loss of tumor immune surveillance, clonal evolution with myelofibrotic and leukemic transformation and an increased risk of second cancer as well [5–8]. Most recently the potential link between chronic inflammation and the development of myeloproliferative cancer has been described [6].

Inflammation generates reactive oxygen species (ROS), and most recently the JAK2V617F mutation per se has been shown to induce the accumulation of ROS in the hematopoietic stem cell compartment, overproduction of ROS being a mediator of JAK2V617F-induced oxidative stress, genomic instability and DNA-damage [9]. In the context of oxidative stress, the transcription factor nuclear factor erythroid 2-related factor 2 (NFE2L2 or Nrf2) has a key role in the regulation of the oxidative stress response [10]. Furthermore, most recently Nrf2 has been shown to modulate both migration and retention of hematopoietic stem cells (HSCs) in their niche, Nrf2 depletion giving rise to an expansion of the hematopoietic stem and progenitor cell (HSPC) compartment [11]. Myelofibrosis is characterized by an expansion of the HSPC pool and by egress of CD34+ positive cells from stem cell niches into the circulation to seed extramedullarily in the spleen and liver [12]. Accordingly, taken into account that chronic inflammation with ROS accumulation might induce an altered redox balance of pivotal significance for stem cell mobilization in myelofibrosis, we speculated if oxidative and anti-oxidative stress genes might be deregulated in MPNs with particular attention to the Nrf2 gene which plays such a central role in the regulation of hematopoietic stem cell (HSC) function. Using whole blood transcriptional profiling, we have identified a massive deregulation of several genes involved in oxidative stress and anti-oxidative stress mechanisms.

Patients and Methods

Whole blood was collected from control subjects (n = 21) and patients with ET (n = 19), PV (n = 41), and PMF (n = 9) (data set 1). Patient characteristics and hematological data are shown in Table 1 and Table 2, which have been previously published [3]. Patients were diagnosed and followed in two institutions in Denmark. Most patients were studied on cytoreductive therapy, which for the large majority included hydroxyurea, being administered to 10 patients with ET, 26 patients with PV and in 1 patient with PMF (8 PMF patients received no therapy). In ET, PV and PMF patients, 9, 40 and 2 patients were JAK2V617F-positive, respectively. Whole blood from a cohort of patients with ET (n = 8), PV (n = 21) and PMF (n = 4) was collected (data set 2), compared to the control subjects (n = 21), and used to evaluate results from data set 1. Patient characteristics are shown in Table 3. Samples were collected in Paxgene tubes (Preanalytix, Hombrechtikon, Switzerland) and stored at room temperature for 24 hours, then at −20°C for minimum one day, and finally transferred to a −80°C freezer. Total RNA was extracted from each sample using the Paxgene Blood RNA kit (Qiagen, Franklin Lakes, NJ, USA). The quantity and quality of RNA were tested with NanoDrop spectrophotometer ND-8000 (NanoDrop Technologies) and Agilent 2100 Bioanalyzer (Agilent Technologies, Palo Alto, CA), respectively. The Message-AmpTM III RNA amplification kit (Ambion, Austin, TX) was applied to convert 300 ng of purified total RNA to biotin-labeled aRNA. Labeled aRNA was fragmented and hybridized to Affymetrix HGU133 Plus 2.0 chips.

Background correction, normalization, and gene expression index calculation of probe intensities were done in R [13] using the robust multi-array average (rma) method [14]. Only perfect match probes were used for data analysis. The regularized t-test limma [15] was applied to calculate differences in gene expression between patients and controls, and the Benjamini Hochberg method using the false discovery rate (FDR) was used to correct for multiple hypothesis testing [16]. An FDR <0.05 was considered significant. Data from both data set 1 and 2 have been deposited into Gene Expression Omnibus (http://www.ncbi.nlm.nih.gov/geo; accession no. GSE26049/GSE61629, respectively).

Table 1. Patient characteristics–Data set 1.

	No	Gender (m/f)	Age (years)	Disease duration (months)	JAK2V617F (+/−)	V617F allele burden %	Therapy	Thrombosis (+/−)
ET	19	9/10	60 (35–87)	40 (15–278)	9/10	23 (1–55)	HU = 10 IFN = 3 ANA = 5 BU = 1	9/10
PV	41	21/20	69 (35–85)	39 (2–171)	40/1	37 (28–48)	None = 3 HU = 26 IFN = 5 ANA = 1 BU = 6	19/22
PMF	9	3/6	68 (53–74)	31 (11–204)	2/7	59	None = 8 HU = 1	1/8

Age: Median and range; Disease duration: Median and range; V617F allele burden %: median and 95% confidence interval. Therapy: HU = hydroxyurea, IFN = recombinant interferon-alfa, ANA = anagrelide; BU = busulfan.

Table 2. Hematological data–Data set 1.

	ET	PV	PMF	P-value
Hemoglobin g/dl	13.4 (11.6–14.4)	13.5 (12.9–13.7)	11.1 (9.7–11.8)	<.00001
Leucocytes $\times 10^9$/l	5.3 (4.2–8.1)	7.6 (6.6–8.8)	7.3 (2.3–18.7)	NS
Neutrophils $\times 10^9$/l	3.65 (2.31–5.63)	5.32 (4.22–6.21)	4.31 (1.10–9.82)	NS
Lymphocytes $\times 10^9$/l	1.60 (0.35–0.56)	1.44 (0.33–0.55)	1.06 (0.60–3.08)	NS
Monocytes $\times 10^9$/l	0.45 (0.35)	0.44 (0.33–0.55)	0.80 (0.17–2.31)	NS
Immatures $\times 10^9$/l	NA	NA	0.36 (0.0–4.81)	NA
Platelets $\times 10^9$/l	400 (310–519)	386 (319–450)	80 (32–232)	0.0001

Hemoglobin concentration and cell counts are presented as medians with 95% confidence intervals in parenthesis. NA: Not applicable. NS: Not significant.

Ethics statement

The study was approved by The Regional Scientific Ethical Committees for Southern Denmark and was performed in accordance with the Helsinki Declaration. All patients provided written informed consent to participate in the study.

Results

In data set 1, 20,439, 25,307, and 17,417 probe sets were identified to be differentially expressed between controls and patients with ET, PV, and PMF, respectively (FDR <0.05). 148 of these genes were found to be included in previous studies focusing on deregulation of oxidative stress genes in various diseases and were chosen for further analysis (Table S1). 35, 40, and 46 oxidative stress genes were significantly upregulated and 33, 37, and 23 were significantly downregulated in patients with ET, PV, and PMF, respectively. The twenty most up- and downregulated genes are shown in Table 4 and Table 5, respectively. ATOX1, DEFB122, GPX8, PRDX2, PRDX6, PTGS1, and SEPP1 were progressively upregulated from ET over PV to PMF (Figure 1), whereas AKR1B1, CYBA, SIRT2, TTN, and UCP2 were progressively downregulated in ET, PV and PMF (Figure 2) (all FDR <0.05). Since inactivation of certain genes - e.g. FoxO3, TP53 and ATM - are associated with increased ROS levels and impairment of hematopoietic stem cell function, the expression of these genes was included as well. The FoxO1 gene was significantly downregulated in PV: (Fold Change (FC) = −1.22; FDR = 0.01) and PMF: (FC = −2.0; FDR = 4.4E-06). The FoxO3 gene was significantly upregulated in PV: FC = 1.6, FDR = 6.3E-05 and PMF: FC = 1.7, FDR = 0.008). The TP53 gene was highly significantly downregulated in ET, PV and PMF: (FC −1.5, −1.5 and −1.5, respectively; FDR = 2.6E-07, 2.6E-14, and 3.4E-05, respectively. The ATM gene was significantly and progressively downregulated in ET, PV and PMF: (ET: FC = −1.3; FDR = 0.0006; PV: FC = −1.3, FDR = 2.3E-06; PMF: FC = −1.5, FDR = 0.0002). CCND1 was highly significantly upregulated in ET, PV and PMF: FC = 1.3, 1.3, 1.9, respectively; FDR = 8.9E-06, 2.9E-06, 0.009, respectively; and CXCR4 was highly significantly downregulated in ET, PV and PMF: FC = −2.1, −2.0, −2.8, respectively; FDR = 3.7E-09, 1.1E-11, 1.5E-09, respectively. No significant differences in white blood cell counts and differential counts were recorded between the three subgroups of patients (Table 2). The 20 most up- and downregulated genes from data set 1 are evaluated in data set 2 and shown in Table 4 and 5, respectively.

Discussion

Myelofibrosis and related neoplasms are associated with a marked increase in several inflammatory cytokines [7]. Likewise, whole blood transcriptional profiling studies have unraveled a massive deregulation of inflammation and immune genes, which may be of crucial importance for disease progression [3,17,18]. Thus, chronic inflammation has been proposed to be both a trigger and a driver of clonal evolution, premature atherosclerosis and second cancer in MPNs [5]. Furthermore, it has been suggested that MPNs depict "A Human Inflammation Model for Cancer Development", chronic inflammation being the driving force from early cancer stage (ET) over PV (in the JAK2V617F-positive patients) to the advanced myelofibrotic cancer stage [6].

Several biological processes are deeply dependent upon appropriate intracellular levels of ROS, including e.g. those processes being involved in the activation of signaling pathways in response to cytokines and the gene expression elicited by this signaling. However, oxidative stress may occur if ROS is produced in excessive amounts and/or if the cell's normal antioxidant defence system is defective. Chronic inflammation is associated with the generation of ROS which may ultimately give rise to oxidative stress, genomic instability, DNA-damage, and risk of mutations with the development or progression of cancer [19,20]. A prerequisite in the defence against clonal evolution and cancer development during chronic inflammation is an effective DNA

Table 3. Patient characteristics–Data set 2.

	No	Gender (m/f)	Age (years)	JAK2V617F(+/)	V617Fallele burden (%)	Therapy
ET	8	4/4	57(45–66)	6/2	14(1–48)	HU = 5 None = 3
PV	21	10/11	62(26–69)	21/0	20(10–79)	HU = 14 None = 5 ANA = 2
PMF	4	2/2	68(55–73)	4/0	30(6–92)	None = 4

Age: Median and range; Disease duration: Median and range; V617F allele burden %: median and 95% confidence interval. HU = hydroxyurea, ANA = anagrelide.

Table 4. The top 20 most upregulated oxidative stress and antioxidative defense genes in patients with ET, PV, and PMF (FDR <0.05).

ET					PV					PMF				
	Data set 1		Data set 2			Data set 1		Data set 2			Data set 1		Data set 2	
Gene Symbol	FC	FDR	FC	Pvalue	Gene Symbol	FC	FDR	FC	Pvalue	Gene Symbol	FC	FDR	FC	Pvalue
MT2A	1.6	8.7E-05	1.4	0.001	MT2A	1.8	6.7E-07	1.5	0.0002	DEFA4	11.9	9.4E-07	5.0	4.6E-04
PRDX2	1.6	0.01	1.6	0.01	PRDX2	1.7	0.0004	1.4	0.006	MPO	5.5	5.8E-05	3.3	1.7E-05
PTGS1	1.5	0.003	1.9	5.5E-05	PTGS1	1.5	0.0001	1.6	6.6E-05	PRDX2	4.4	9.1E-06	3.2	2.4E-06
GPX1	1.4	0.002	1.5	4.2E-05	PRDX6	1.5	5.2E-05	1.5	3.5E-05	DEFA1	3.5	0.0002	1.9	0.1
PRDX6	1.3	0.03	1.6	6.3E-04	GCLM	1.5	9.2E-05	1.4	0.008	SEPP1	3.5	0.0002	2.1	0.0001
MPO	1.3	0.005	1.2	0.03	GCLC	1.4	0.008	1.5	0.002	GCLM	3.3	7.5E-07	2.0	5.6E-04
GPR156	1.3	0.0001	1.06	0.3	TXN	1.4	0.007	1.3	0.08	GCLC	2.4	0.0002	2.5	5.2E-06
SOD3	1.3	0.0003	1.1	0.1	FTH1	1.4	0.0002	1.4	3.1E-05	TXN	2.2	0.0003	1.6	0.04
LPO	1.3	0.001	−1.0	1.0	ALOX12	1.3	0.03	1.5	0.01	MGST3	1.8	1.7E-05	1.2	0.1
DUOX1	1.3	1.3E-05	1.02	0.8	GPX1	1.3	0.001	1.3	0.004	DEFT1P	1.8	0.0002	1.5	7.9E-05
SQSTM1	1.3	5.1E-05	1.08	0.1	SEPP1	1.3	0.0001	1.2	3.6E-04	GLRX	1.8	0.002	1.3	0.2
DEFB103A	1.3	0.0007	1.08	0.2	GPR156	1.3	7.0E-06	1.1	0.009	PRDX6	1.8	0.0008	2.4	3.4E-07
ATOX1	1.3	0.001	1.1	0.04	ATOX1	1.3	5.2E-06	1.2	7.0E-05	PRDX4	1.8	0.007	1.05	0.8
ADH7	1.2	0.005	1.01	0.9	LPO	1.3	1.7E-05	1.06	0.3	PRG3	1.8	0.004	1.1	0.2
SEPP1	1.2	0.0005	1.1	0.03	SQSTM1	1.2	4.6E-06	1.1	0.0002	GPX1	1.7	6.7E-05	1.7	8.0E-06
GSTZ1	1.2	0.0004	1.05	0.4	MPO	1.2	0.006	1.3	0.02	MT2A	1.7	0.0009	1.4	0.006
GPX2	1.2	0.002	1.1	0.1	ADH7	1.2	0.0004	1.04	0.3	NUDT1	1.7	3.8E-05	1.1	0.1
DEFB129	1.2	0.0009	1.2	0.001	DEFB103A	1.2	5.0E-06	1.08	0.06	PTGS1	1.6	0.02	1.8	0.009
TXNDC2	1.2	0.006	−1.0	1.0	DUOX1	1.2	3.3E-06	1.01	0.7	GSR	1.5	7.0E-06	−1.0	0.9
DEFB121	1.2	0.02	1.02	0.6	GSTZ1	1.2	4.8E-05	1.03	0.4	ATOX1	1.5	0.001	1.2	0.01

FC: fold change. FDR: false discovery rate.
The results from data set 1 are compared with results from data set 2.

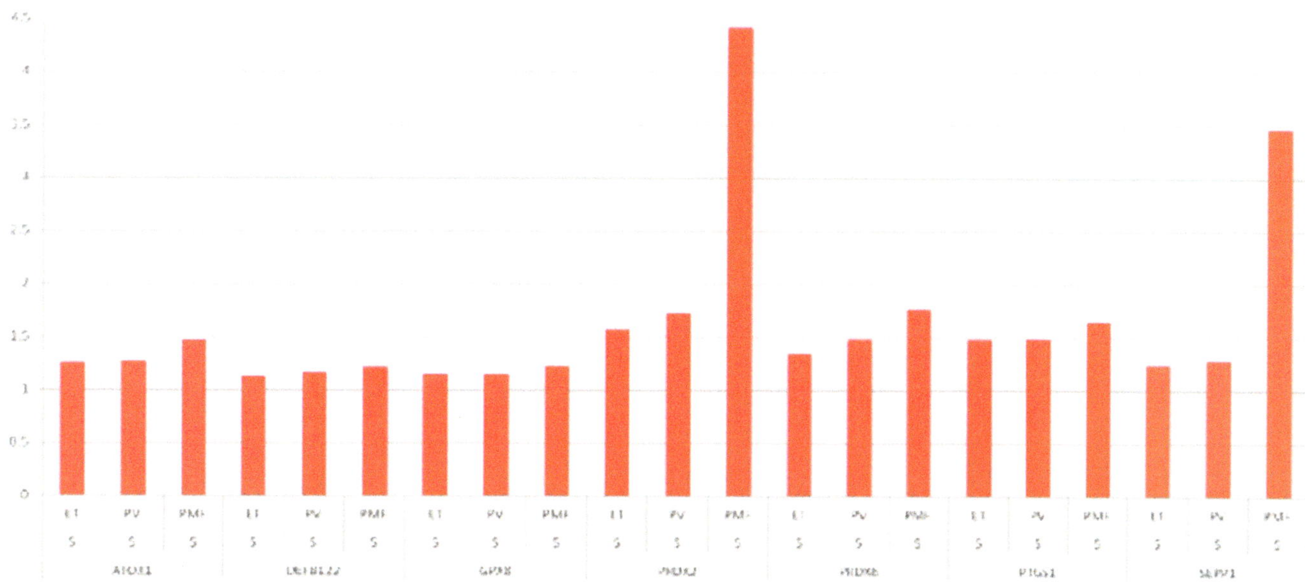

Figure 1. ATOX1, DEFB122, GPX8, PRDX2, PRDX6, PTGS1, and SEPP1 were progressively and significantly upregulated in patients with ET, PV, and PMF (FDR <0.05). Fold changes for each gene are shown on the y-axis.

repair mechanism of the sustained oxidative stress induced by the chronic inflammatory drive. Accordingly, mutations in DNA repair mechanisms may likely increase the risk of clonal evolution in MPNs as well.

The importance of ROS for HSC function and integrity of the stem cell niche is being increasingly recognized [21,22], and recently the link between oxidative DNA damage, genomic instability and leukemogenesis has been reviewed [23,24]. Most recently, it has been hypothesized that the acquired stem cell lesion in MPNs might arise due to a chronic sustained inflammation stimulus being further enhanced in a selfperpetuating vicious circle by the malignant clone, which per se continuously generates inflammatory products in the bone marrow [5–7]. These products – e.g. tumor necrosis factor alpha (TNF-alpha) – further stimulate clonal expansion [25,26] thus creating a positive feedback loop and a vicious circle [5–7]. The sustained release of inflammatory

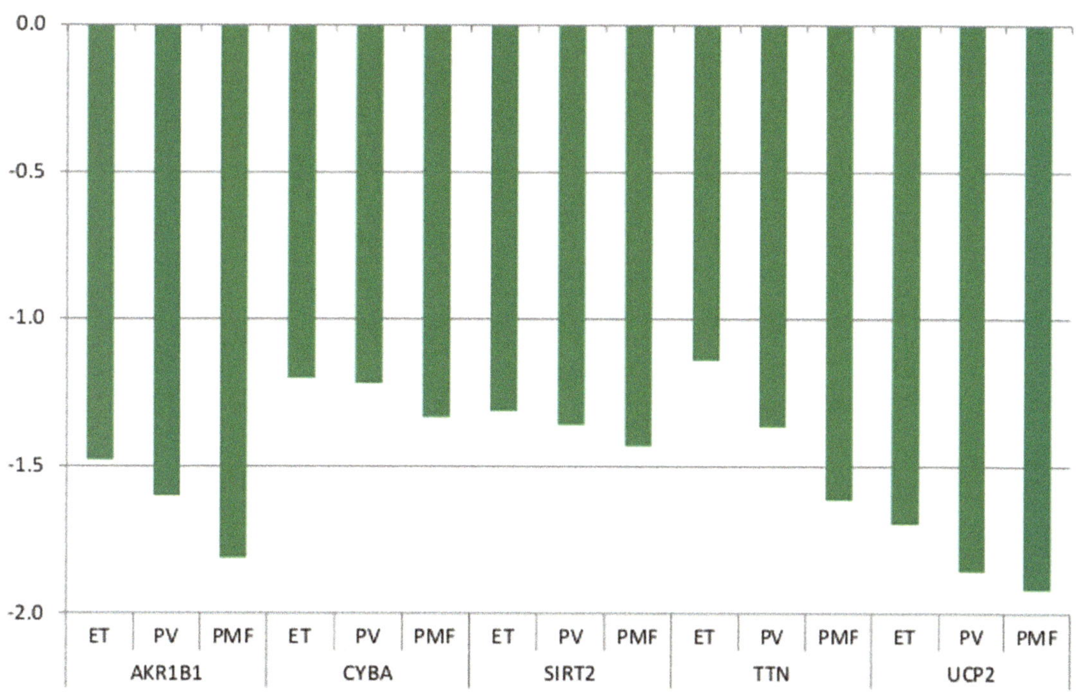

Figure 2. AKR1B1, CYBA, SIRT2, TTN, and UCP2 were progressively and significantly downregulated in patients with ET, PV, and PMF (FDR <0.05). Fold changes for each gene are shown on the y-axis.

Table 5. The top 20 most downregulated oxidative stress and antioxidative defense genes in patients with ET, PV, and PMF (FDR <0.05).

ET					PV					PMF				
	Data set 1		Data set 2			Data set 1		Data set 2			Data set 1		Data set 2	
Gene Symbol	FC	FDR	FC	Pvalue	Gene Symbol	FC	FDR	FC	Pvalue	Gene Symbol	FC	FDR	FC	Pvalue
CAT	−2.4	1.3E-08	−1.3	0.04	UCP2	−1.9	9.0E-09	−1.6	4.7E-07	PREX1	−2.6	2.3E-07	−1.6	9.2E-04
GTF2I	−1.9	4.8E-08	−1.2	0.01	CAT	−1.9	6.4E-06	−1.07	0.5	DUSP1	−2.2	0.0008	−1.6	0.01
SOD2	−1.8	0.0003	−1.4	0.1	GTF2I	−1.6	1.2E-07	−1.1	0.006	SOD2	−2.1	0.006	−1.6	0.1
HSPA1A	−1.8	0.0002	−1.04	0.7	AKR1B1	−1.6	4.4E-07	−1.4	7.5E-05	UCP2	−1.9	3.9E-06	−1.7	3.6E-05
TKT	−1.8	7.3E-06	−1.2	0.1	CYBB	−1.6	7.3E-06	−1.4	0.0001	AKR1B1	−1.8	0.0002	−1.6	9.4E-05
PREX1	−1.8	0.0002	−1.3	0.02	TKT	−1.6	2.0E-07	−1.06	0.4	PRNP	−1.7	0.002	−1.6	0.01
CYBB	−1.7	0.0003	−1.3	0.02	SOD2	−1.6	0.004	−1.5	0.008	NCF2	−1.7	4.7E-05	−1.1	0.4
UCP2	−1.7	1.8E-07	−1.3	0.02	PRPS1	−1.5	5.1E-13	−1.2	3.0E-05	GTF2I	−1.7	2.0E-05	−1.2	0.02
PGD	−1.7	0.0006	−1.02	0.9	NFE2L2	−1.5	1.5E-11	−1.2	0.0008	CCL5	−1.7	0.03	−1.3	0.2
PRNP	−1.6	0.008	−1.5	0.004	OXR1	−1.5	9.6E-09	−1.1	0.09	NCF1	−1.6	0.002	−1.1	0.5
OXR1	−1.5	4.1E-07	−1.1	0.1	GPI	−1.5	3.4E-05	−1.1	0.09	TTN	−1.6	7.8E-06	−1.3	0.008
AKR1B1	−1.5	1.5E-05	−1.2	0.02	SELS	−1.4	5.2E-06	−1.2	0.006	HSPA1A	−1.6	0.009	−1.1	0.5
CSDE1	−1.5	1.3E-05	−1.06	0.2	PREX1	−1.4	0.001	−1.1	0.1	TKT	−1.6	0.001	−1.1	0.3
PRPS1	−1.4	1.3E-09	−1.2	2.7E-04	TTN	−1.4	4.4E-06	−1.2	0.04	SIRT2	−1.4	2.6E-04	−1.2	0.05
PRDX3	−1.4	0.0004	−1.3	0.003	SIRT2	−1.4	3.2E-06	−1.02	0.7	NFE2L2	−1.4	0.001	−1.1	0.3
NFE2L2	−1.4	1.1E-05	−1.1	0.06	CSDE1	−1.3	4.8E-05	−1.09	0.1	EPHX2	−1.4	1.9E-05	−1.2	0.02
SELS	−1.4	0.0006	−1.2	0.04	CCL5	−1.3	0.03	−1.2	0.2	GSTM4	−1.4	0.02	1.1	0.4
TALDO1	−1.3	0.009	1.03	0.7	PRNP	−1.3	0.04	−1.4	0.01	ALDOA	−1.4	0.01	−1.2	0.07
GPI	−1.3	0.004	1.03	0.7	EPHX2	−1.3	8.3E-07	−1.1	0.06	CYBA	−1.3	2.6E-06	−1.0	1.0
EPHX2	−1.3	6.0E-06	−1.07	0.3	GSTP1	−1.3	0.003	−1.3	0.003	OXR1	−1.3	0.03	−1.1	0.4

FC: fold change. FDR: false discovery rate.
The results from data set 1 are compared with results from data set 2.

products with ensuing chronic oxidative stress due to elevated levels of ROS in the bone marrow might likely create a high-risk microenvironment for induction of oxidative damage to DNA in hematopoietic cells and mutations [6].

By whole blood transcriptional profiling we herein for the first time demonstrate that MPNs are associated with a significant upregulation of several oxidative stress genes in concert with downregulation of important antioxidative defence genes, among others a significant downregulation of the Nrf2 gene – the master regulator of the antioxidant response ensuring that chronic inflammation in normal cells slowly ceases [10]. The Nrf2 gene was significantly downregulated across all three disease categories – ET, PV and PMF. Under normal conditions, chronic inflammation is dampened due to IL-1beta induced activation of Nrf2, which subsequently activates several antioxidant genes of crucial importance for protection of cells against oxidative stress. Thus, increased Nrf2 expression up-regulates antioxidant response element (ARE)-dependent genes causing increased ARE-transcriptional activity, thereby augmenting expression of several ARE-dependent antioxidant and cytoprotective enzymes [10].

In addition to being the master regulator of the antioxidant response, Nrf2 also has a major role for normal stem cell function and is required for HSPC survival and myeloid development [11]. The role of Nrf2 in this context has been found to be independent of ROS [27]. In regard to oxidative stress and stem cell function, levels of ROS have been shown to regulate normal hematopoietic stem cells [28], implying high levels to be associated with stem cell dysfunction [29]. Lower levels in hematopoietic stem cells may explain their sustained self-renewal potential by inhibiting differentiation [30]. Thus, the marked downregulation of Nrf2 in MPNs may have a major impact upon stem cell function and behavior for several reasons. First, Nrf2 deficiency may likely compromise the antioxidant defence mechanisms against increased oxidative stress and accumulation of ROS, being induced by the inflammatory products generated by the myeloproliferation per se [5–7] and in the JAK2V617F positive patients also being generated by the JAK2V617F-mutation per se [9]. By an impaired defence against the increased oxidative stress in the bone marrow, accumulation of ROS may favour genotoxic damage to hematopoietic cells and stromal cells as well thereby enhancing the risk of triggering mutations [6,7]. In this setting, increased intracellular ROS levels may also induce activation of redox-sensitive transcription factors and thereby enhancing clonal evolution and progression [31]. Second, most recently, it has been demonstrated that Nrf2 deficiency also results in an expansion of the hematopoietic stem and progenitor cell pool and a disturbed differentiation [11] which may likely contribute to enhanced clonal myeloproliferation and defective differentiation in myelofibrosis (immature red and white blood cells in the peripheral blood, respectively). Third, taking into account that Nrf2 functions as a negative regulator of cell-cycle entry in HSCs, maintaining the delicate balance between HSC quiescence and self-renewal [11] and Nrf2 also has a key role in governing the retention of HSCs and their homing to the bone marrow niche [11], Nrf2 deficiency in MPNs may likely contribute to the egress of CD34+ cells from bone marrow niches to seed preferentially in the spleen and liver (myelofibrosis with myeloid metaplasia). Of note, in regard to Nrf2 being a negative regulator of cell-cycle entry in HSCs, Nrf2 deficiency might be anticipated to be associated with higher levels of cyclin D (being synthesized during G1 phase and required for the transition to S-phase) which was also recorded in the study by Tsai et al. [11]. Importantly, we found that the cyclin D gene (CCND1) was significantly upregulated in MPNs, being most deregulated in myelofibrosis similar to Nrf2. In regard to the role of Nrf2 for efficient homing of bone marrow cells and in maintaining HSC quiescence, it has most recently been shown that Nrf2 exerts its influence, at least in part, through direct regulation of the expression of the chemokine CXCR4 which was found to be significantly reduced in HSCPs in Nrf2 deficient mice [11]. In addition, it was shown that Nrf2 directly binds to the CXCR4 promoter and activates its expression [11] explaining the dysregulation of CXCR4 in Nrf2 deficient mice. The CXCR4 chemokine has a well-established major role for HSCP homing and retention [32] but recently there has been considerable interest in CXCR4 signalling for its role in maintaining HSC quiescence as well [33,34]. Highly interesting, CXCR4 was significantly downregulated across all three MPN categories being most pronounced in patients with myelofibrosis. This observation is consistent with previous studies displaying an altered SDF-1/CXCR4 axis with downregulation of CXCR4 in the CD34+ cells in myelofibrosis [35,36]. Accordingly, it is intriguing to consider if the significant downregulation of Nrf2 in MPNs may not only have a profound impact upon the balance between stem cell quiescence and proliferation, between self-renewal and differentiation, but also significantly influencing homing and retention of HSCs in the bone marrow niche. Fourth, defective antioxidative defence mechanisms with excessive ROS accumulation and oxidative stress – consequent to among others Nrf2 deficiency – may likely also contribute to aberrant DNA methylation [37], which has been reported in patients with MPNs [38], including hypermethylation of the CXCR4 promoter in CD34+ cells from patients with primary myelofibrosis.

As noted above, chronic inflammation has been suggested to have a major role for disease progression in MPNs – likely being a mediator of premature atherosclerosis (and premature ageing?), clonal evolution and myelofibrotic and leukemic transformation [5–7]. In this context, the impact of TNF-alpha as a tumor promoter [39] and its ability to facilitate clonal expansion of JAK2V617-positive cells is of crucial importance [25], since the JAK2V617F mutation per se has most recently been shown to induce excessive ROS accumulation and accordingly oxidative stress, DNA strand breaks and mutations [9]. Furthermore, oxidative stress is associated with overproduction of several proinflammatory cytokines (e.g. TNF-alpha, IL-1beta, IL-2, IL-6, IL-8, IL-12), when the redox-sensitive NF-kappabeta is activated by oxidative stress. These cytokines, in turn, can cause oxidative stress in HSC and circulating hematopoietic cells. Considering the MPNs as "A Human Inflammation Model" with a selfperpetuating vicious circle [6] being fueled by inflammation products and excessive ROS accumulation, implying an imbalance between NF-E2 and Nrf2 [40], it is evident that this vicious circle (chronic inflammation – NF-kappa-beta-activation – production of inflammatory cytokines – ROS-generation – oxidative stress – genomic instability – clonal evolution – chronic inflammation) is only disrupted by dampening one of its very important driving forces - chronic inflammation [5–7]. This novel concept on pathogenesis of MPNs also dictates early upfront intervention with agents having the potential of blocking the vicious circle – interferon-alpha2 (IFN-alpha2), statins and JAK2-inhibitor treatment being potential candidates [5–7,41] – both by inhibiting clonal myeloproliferation but also by impairment of ROS generation due to their very potent anti-inflammatory capacities [5–7]. To this end, oxidative stress and inflammation impairs IFN-alpha signaling [42] which may likely cause resistance to the effects of IFN-alpha in MPNs, including the effects of IFN-alpha2 on immune cells [43].

Inactivation of several genes – e.g. transcription factor p53 and FoxO3 – has been shown to increase ROS levels and to be associated with the loss of hematopoietic stem cell function [44,45]. Of note, we found that the tumor suppressor p53 gene – TP53 – was significantly and progressively downregulated across all three disease categories (ET, PV and PMF). The TP53 gene has a key role in protecting the genome from oxidation by ROS with ensuing DNA damage and genetic instability. Thus, the highly significant downregulation of TP53 in our patients may result in excessive oxidation of DNA, increased mutation rate and karyotype instability [44]. The FoxO3 gene decreases ROS levels by influencing the regulation of the ataxia telangiectasia mutated (ATM) gene [34,46], which also has a crucial role in mediating the cellular response to DNA and oxidative damage. Accordingly, downregulation of the ATM gene might profoundly enhance genomic instability consequent to increased ROS levels. In our MPN patients, the ATM gene was significantly and progressively downregulated from ET over PV to PMF, which – together with downregulation of TP53 - may have a profound negative impact upon DNA-stability. The downregulation of ATM was not associated with a downregulation of FoxO3 – actually significantly increased in our patients with PV and PMF – which accordingly may not be the main regulator of the ATM gene in our patients.

The genes UCP2 and SIRT2 were significantly and progressively downregulated in ET, PV and PMF. Both genes are involved in the regulation of NF-kappabeta, implying constitutively increased NF-kappabeta activity and production of inflammatory cytokines when these genes are deactivated or downregulated [47]. In addition, sirtuins have been described as major players in sensing and coordinating oxidative stress response and having an essential role in promoting DNA repair, telomere stability and in stem cell differentiation as well [47]. Thus, some sirtuins, such as SirT2 and SirT6, seem to work as tumor suppressors. We have previously reported significant downregulation of several sirtuins in MPNs, including – in addition to SirT2 and SirT6 – SirT3 and SirT7 [48]. Accordingly, downregulation of these genes may further prime for enhancement of inflammation, oxidative stress and genomic instability in MPNs.

As underscored above, oxidative stress induces activation of several signaling pathways including PI3K/AKT which may likely participate in the development of MPNs [49]. AKT negatively regulates the Forkhead O transcription factor family (FoxO) which targets expression of several anti-oxidant enzymes, including the GPx, catalase (CAT) and SODs. The FoxO3 gene was significantly upregulated in all three MPNs and several GPx as well. Regarding SODs, SOD2 was significantly downregulated across all three MPNs. Interestingly, the CAT gene was highly significantly downregulated in our patients with ET and PV but not in myelofibrosis. The absence of a significant downregulation of CAT in PMF was surprising, but might be related to the fact that only 2 out 9 patients were JAK2V617F-positive. Thus, most recently ROS accumulation in JAK2V617F-positive cells has been shown to be associated with a significant decrease in gene expression of CAT - both in a mouse model and in CD34+ cells from PV and myelofibrosis patients [9].

Our study has limitations and strengths. First, in the interpretation of the different genes being deregulated, it should be taken into account that our patients were not newly diagnosed but investigated at different time points after diagnosis. Second, many patients were treated with hydroxyurea (HU) at the time of investigation, which potentially might have impacted the "global signature" of increasing genomic instability (e.g. evidenced by significant downregulation of Nrf2, TP53 and ATM genes). Third, in data set 2, Nrf2 was significantly downregulated in patients with PV, showed a tendency towards downregulation in ET ($P = 0.06$), and was not significantly downregulated in PMF. The lack of significance in the PMF group may be due to the limited number of patients ($n = 4$). Fourth, we used whole blood instead of e.g. isolated granulocytes, CD34+ cells and mononuclear cells, which have been used in many previous transcriptional profiling studies in MPNs. In the context of describing "the signature of oxidative stress in haematopoietic cells", we believe that a signature of oxidative stress and antioxidative defence genes may be more reliably obtained from transcriptional profiling of whole blood than if isolated cell types were analysed. Indeed, our previous studies of whole blood transcriptional profiling are strongly supportive, since these studies – in addition to confirming gene signatures obtained by analyzing single cells by others but generally with much stronger signals [3,17,18,48,50,51] – also have unravelled deregulation of several genes which may be involved in disease pathogenesis and progression [3,17,18,50,51]. Our approach certainly also makes sense when considering that the "tumor tissue" being studied – whole blood – is composed of clonal "tumor" cells (being both myeloid cells, platelets, B-cells and T-cells) and non-clonal cells, including immune cells, which may also be activated due to oxidative stress fueled by clonal myeloproliferation. In this setting, whole blood transcriptional profiling is actually very similar to all other studies of gene signatures in tumor tissue. Accordingly, in the context of studying gene signatures of inflammation and oxidative stress/antioxidative defence genes in MPNs, our approach with whole blood transcriptional profiling is more a strength than a limitation. To this end, whole blood has also been used successfully in a most recent study of DNA-methylation profiles in MPNs, arguing unfractionated whole blood to be suitable for analysis [38]. Fifth, although several ROS-related genes displayed a gradual deregulation from ET, PV to PMF, we cannot definitely conclude that these changes are linked to disease progression, since the cohort did not include matched samples with identical timepoints during the course of the disease. Prospective studies of larger cohorts with serial gene expression profiling studies are needed to confirm our observations.

In conclusion, our results highlight the MPNs as novel disease categories to be listed as "Oxyradical Overload Disorders" and thereby potentially being at a risk of premature atherosclerosis and ageing in addition to the inherent risk of clonal evolution, genomic instability, leukemic transformation, and development of second cancer as well. Since chronic inflammation is likely an important trigger and driver of oxidative stress contributing to "oxyradical overload" in MPNs, this study substantiates the urgent need for early upfront interruption with agents having the potential to stop the delivery of "fuel to the fire", implying potent anti-inflammatory and antiproliferative capacities. These agents include among others IFN-alpha2 and JAK2-inhibitors, which as monotherapies have been very promising with induction of deep and sustained molecular remissions in ET and PV patients, even after discontinuation of therapy (IFN-alpha2), rapid resolution of huge splenomegaly and constitutional symptoms (JAK2-inhibitor) and also resolution of bone marrow fibrosis after long term treatment (IFN-alpha2 and JAK2-inhibitor). In the context of dampening inflammation and oxidative stress, statins may also be highly efficacious - likely in a combinatorial approach -, since statins have been demonstrated to impair MPN cell growth and enhancing the effect of JAK2-inhibition as well [5–7].

Supporting Information

Table S1 Fold change (FC) and false discovery rate (FDR) of 148 oxidative stress genes.

Author Contributions

Conceived and designed the experiments: HCH TSL MT OWB VS TAK MKJ CHR. Performed the experiments: HCH VS TSL MT. Analyzed the data: VS HCH LK. Contributed reagents/materials/analysis tools: HCH TAK MKJ OWB CHR. Wrote the paper: HCH VS.

References

1. Campbell PJ, Green AR (2006) Mechanisms of disease: the myeloproliferative disorders. N Engl J Med 355(23): 2452–66.
2. Larsen TS, Pallisgaard N, Moller MB, Hasselbalch HC (2007) The JAK2 V617F allele burden in essential thrombocythemia, polycythemia vera and primary myelofibrosis–impact on disease phenotype. Eur J Haematol 79(6): 508–15.
3. Skov V, Thomassen M, Riley CH, Jensen MK, Bjerrum OW, et al. (2012) Gene expression profiling with principal component analysis depicts the biological continuum from essential thrombocythemia over polycythemia vera to myelofibrosis. Exp Hematol 40(9): 771–80.
4. Barbui T, Carobbio A, Finazzi G, Vannucchi AM, Barosi G, et al. (2011) Inflammation and thrombosis in essential thrombocythemia and polycythemia vera: different role of C-reactive protein and pentraxin3. Haematologica 96(2): 315–8.
5. Hasselbalch HC (2012) Perspectives on chronic inflammation in essential thrombocythemia, polycythemia vera, and myelofibrosis: is chronic inflammation a trigger and driver of clonal evolution and development of accelerated atherosclerosis and second cancer? Blood 119(14): 3219–25.
6. Hasselbalch HC (2013) Chronic Inflammation as a Promoter of Mutagenesis in Essential Thrombocythemia, Polycythemia Vera and Myelofibrosis. A Human Inflammation Model for Cancer Development? Leuk Res 37(2): 214–20.
7. Hasselbalch HC (2013) The role of cytokines in the initiation and progression of myelofibrosis. Cytokine Growth Factor Rev 24(2): 133–45.
8. Frederiksen H, Farkas DK, Christiansen CF, Hasselbalch HC, Sørensen HT (2011) Chronic myeloproliferative neoplasms and subsequent cancer risk: a Danish population-based cohort study. Blood 118(25): 6515–20.
9. Marty C, Lacout C, Droin N, Le Couédic JP, Ribrag V, et al. (2013) A role for reactive oxygen species in JAK2(V617F) myeloproliferative neoplasm progression. Leukemia 27(11): 2187–95.
10. Kim J, Cha YN, Surh Y-JYJ (2010) A protective role of nuclear factor-erythroid 2- related factor-2 (Nrf2) in inflammatory disorders. Mutat Res 690: 12–23.
11. Tsai JJ, Dudakov JA, Takahashi K, Shieh JH, Velardi E, et al. (2013) Nrf2 regulates haematopoietic stem cell function. Nature Cell Biology 15(3): 309–316.
12. Barosi G, Viarengo G, Pecci A, Rosti V, Piaggio G, et al. (2001) Diagnostic and clinical relevance of the number of circulating CD34(+) cells in myelofibrosis with myeloid metaplasia. Blood 98(12): 3249–55.
13. Ihaka R, Gentleman R (1996) R: A language for data analysis and graphics. J Comp Graph Stat 5: 299–314.
14. Irizarry RA, Hobbs B, Collin F, Beazer-Barclay YD, Antonellis KJ, et al. (2003) Exploration, normalization, and summaries of high density oligonucleotide array probe level data. Biostatistics 4: 249–264.
15. Smyth GK (2004) Linear models and empirical bayes methods for assessing differential expression in microarray experiments. Stat Appl Genet Mol Biol 3: Article3.
16. Benjamini Y, Hochberg Y (1995) Controlling the false discovery rate: a practical and powerful approach to multiple testing. J R Statist Soc B 57: 289–300.
17. Skov V, Larsen TS, Thomassen M, Riley CH, Jensen MK, et al. (2011) Whole-blood transcriptional profiling of interferon-inducible genes identifies highly upregulated IFI27 in primary myelofibrosis. Eur J Haematol. 87(1): 54–60.
18. Skov V, Larsen TS, Thomassen M, Riley CH, Jensen MK, et al. (2012) Molecular profiling of peripheral blood cells from patients with polycythemia vera and related neoplasms: identification of deregulated genes of significance for inflammation and immune surveillance. Leuk Res 36(11): 1387–92.
19. Grivennikov SI, Greten FR, Karin M (2010). Immunity, inflammation, and cancer. Cell 140: 883–99.
20. Ferguson LR (2010) Chronic inflammation and mutagenesis. Mutat Res 690: 3–11.
21. Yahata T, Takanashi T, Muguruma Y, Ibrahim AA, Matsuzawa H, et al (2011) Accumulation of oxidative DNA damage restricts the self-renewal capacity of human hematopoietic stem cells. Blood 118(11): 2941–50.
22. Shao L, Li H, Senthil K. Pazhanisamy SK, Meng A, et al. (2011) Reactive oxygen species and hematopoietic stem cell senescence. Int J Hematol 94: 24–32.
23. Austin C (2009) Does oxidative damage contribute to the generation of leukemia? Leuk Res 33: 1297.
24. Hole PS, Darley RL, Tonks A (2011) Do reactive oxygen species play a role in myeloid leukemias? Blood 2;117(22): 5816–5826.
25. Fleischman AG, Aichberger KJ, Luty SB, Bumm TG, Petersen CL, et al. (2011) Tumor necrosis factor-alpha facilitates clonal expansion of JAK2V617F positive cells in myeloproliferative neoplasms. Blood 118(24): 6392–8.
26. Hermouet S, Vilaine M (2011) The JAK2 46/1 haplotype: a marker of inappropriate myelomonocytic response to cytokine stimulation, leading to increased risk of inflammation, myeloid neoplasm, and impaired defense against infection? Haematologica 96(11): 1575–9.
27. Merchant AA, Singh A, Matsui W, Biswal S (2011) The redox-sensitive transcription factor Nrf2 regulates murine hematopoietic stem cell survival independently of ROS levels. Blood 118(25): 6572–9.
28. Ghaffari S (2008) Oxidative stress in the regulation of normal and neoplastic hematopoiesis. Antioxidants & Redox Signaling 10(11): 1923–1940.
29. Naka K, Muraguchi T, Hoshii T, Hirao A (2008) Regulation of reactive oxygen species and genomic stability in hematopoietic stem cells. Antioxidants & Redox Signaling 10(11): 1883–1894.
30. Jang YY, Sharkis SJ (2007) A low level of reactive oxygen species selects for primitive hematopoietic stem cells that may reside in the low-oxygenic niche. Blood 110: 3056–63.
31. Trachootham D, Lu W, Ogasawara MA, Nilsa RD, Huang P (2008) Redox regulation of cell survival. Antioxid Redox Signal 10(8): 1343–74.
32. Moll NM, Ransohoff RM (2010) CXCL12 and CXCR4 in bone marrow physiology. Expert Rev Hematol 3(3): 315–22.
33. Nie Y, Han YC, Zou YR (2008) CXCR4 is required for the quiescence of primitive hematopoietic cells. J Exp Med 205: 777–83.
34. Tzeng YS, Li H, Kang YL, Chen WC, Cheng WC, et al. (2011) Loss of Cxcl12/Sdf-1 in adult mice decreases the quiescent state of hematopoietic stem/progenitor cells and alters the pattern of hematopoietic regeneration after myelosuppression. Blood 117: 429–39.
35. Rosti V, Massa M, Vannucchi AM, Bergamaschi G, Campanelli R, et al. (2007) The expression of CXCR4 is down-regulated on the CD34+ cells of patients with myelofibrosis with myeloid metaplasia. Blood Cells Mol Dis 38(3): 280–6.
36. Migliaccio AR, Martelli F, Verrucci M, Migliaccio G, Vannucchi AM, et al. (2008) Altered SDF-1/CXCR4 axis in patients with primary myelofibrosis and in the Gata1 low mouse model of the disease. Exp Hematol 36(2): 158–71.
37. Cencioni C, Spallotta F, Martelli F, Valente S, Mai A, et al. (2013) Oxidative stress and epigenetic regulation in ageing and age-related diseases. Int J Mol Sci 14(9): 17643–63.
38. Pérez C, Pascual M, Martin-Subero JI, Bellosillo B, Segura V, et al. (2013) Aberrant DNA methylation profile of chronic and transformed classic Philadelphia-negative myeloproliferative neoplasms. Haematologica 98(9): 1414–20.
39. Balkwill F (2002). Tumor necrosis factor or tumor promoting factor? Cytokine Growth Factor Rev 13(2): 135–141.
40. Hasselbalch HC (2013) A Role of NF-E2 in Chronic Inflammation and Clonal Evolution in Essential Thrombocythemia, Polycythemia Vera and Myelofibrosis? Leuk Res 38(2): 263–6.
41. Silver RT, Kiladjian JJ, Hasselbalch HC (2013) Interferon and the treatment of polycythemia vera, essential thrombocythemia and myelofibrosis. Expert Rev Hematol 6(1): 49–58.
42. Di Bona D, Cippitelli M, Fionda C, Cammà C, Licata A, et al. (2006) Oxidative stress inhibits IFN-alpha-induced antiviral gene expression by blocking the JAK-STAT pathway. J Hepatol 45(2): 271–9.
43. Riley CH, Jensen MK, Brimnes MK, Hasselbalch HC, Bjerrum OW, et al. (2011) Increase in circulating CD+CD25+Foxp3+ T cells in patients with Philadelphia-negative chronic myelopoliferative neoplasms during treatment with IFN-alpha2. Blood 118(8): 2170–3.
44. Sablina AA, Budanov AV, Ilyinskaya GV, Agapova LS, Kravchenko JE at al. (2005) The antioxidant function of the p53 tumor suppressor. Nat Med 11(12): 1306–13.
45. Tothova Z, Gilliland DG (2007) FoxO transcription factors and stem cell homeostasis: insights from the hematopoietic system. Cell Stem Cell 1(2): 140–52.
46. Barzilai A, Rotman G, Shiloh Y (2002) ATM deficiency and oxidative stress: a new dimension of defective response to DNA damage. DNA Repair (Amst) 1(1): 3–25.
47. Rodrigues RM, Fernandez AF, Fraga MF (2013) Role of sirtuins in stem cell differentiation. Genes Cancer 4(3–4): 105–11.
48. Skov V, Larsen TS, Thomassen M, Riley CH, Jensen MK, et al. (2012) Increased gene expression of histone deacetylases in patients with Philadelphia-negative chronic myeloproliferative neoplasms. Leuk Lymphoma 53(1): 123–9.
49. Yalcin S, Marinkovic D, Mungamuri SK, Zhang X, Tong W, et al. (2010) ROS-mediated amplification of AKT/mTOR signalling pathway leads to myeloproliferative syndrome in Foxo3(_/_) mice. EMBO J 29: 4118–4131.
50. Hasselbalch HC, Skov V, Larsen TS, Thomassen M, Riley CH, et al. (2011) High expression of carcinoembryonic antigen-related cell adhesion molecule (CEACAM) 6 and 8 in primary myelofibrosis. Leuk Res 35(10): 1330–4.
51. Skov V, Riley CH, Thomassen M, Larsen TS, Jensen MK, et al. (2013) Whole blood transcriptional profiling reveals significant down-regulation of human leukocyte antigen class I and II genes in essential thrombocythemia,polycythemia vera and myelofibrosis. Leuk Lymphoma 54(10): 2269–73.

13

Filament-Producing Mutants of Influenza A/Puerto Rico/8/1934 (H1N1) Virus Have Higher Neuraminidase Activities than the Spherical Wild-Type

Jill Seladi-Schulman, Patricia J. Campbell, Suganthi Suppiah, John Steel, Anice C. Lowen*

Department of Microbiology and Immunology, Emory University School of Medicine, Atlanta, Georgia, United States of America

Abstract

Influenza virus exhibits two morphologies – spherical and filamentous. Strains that have been grown extensively in laboratory substrates are comprised predominantly of spherical virions while clinical or low passage isolates produce a mixture of spheres and filamentous virions of varying lengths. The filamentous morphology can be lost upon continued passage in embryonated chicken eggs, a common laboratory substrate for influenza viruses. The fact that the filamentous morphology is maintained in nature but lost in favor of a spherical morphology *in ovo* suggests that filaments confer a selective advantage within the infected host that is not necessary for growth in laboratory substrates. Indeed, we have recently shown that filament-producing variant viruses are selected upon passage of the spherical laboratory strain A/Puerto Rico/8/1934 (H1N1) [PR8] in guinea pigs. Toward determining the nature of the selective advantage conferred by filaments, we sought to identify functional differences between spherical and filamentous particles. We compared the wild-type PR8 virus to two previously characterized recombinant PR8 viruses in which single point mutations within M1 confer a filamentous morphology. Our results indicate that these filamentous PR8 mutants have higher neuraminidase activities than the spherical PR8 virus. Conversely, no differences were observed in HAU:PFU or HAU:RNA ratios, binding avidity, sensitivity to immune serum in hemagglutination inhibition assays, or virion stability at elevated temperatures. Based on these results, we propose that the pleomorphic nature of influenza virus particles is important for the optimization of neuraminidase functions *in vivo*.

Editor: Ralph Tripp, University of Georgia, United States of America

Funding: This work was funded by the National Institutes of Health/National Institute of Allergy and Infectious Disease under Centers for Excellence in Influenza Research and Surveillance (CEIRS) contract number HHSN266200700006C (http://www.niaid.nih.gov/labsandresources/resources/ceirs). The funders had no role in study design, data collection and analysis, decision to publish, or preparation of the manuscript.

Competing Interests: The authors have declared that no competing interests exist.

* Email: anice.lowen@emory.edu

Introduction

Influenza A virus (IAV) is an enveloped virus containing eight negative-sense RNA gene segments [1]. It is the causative agent of seasonal epidemics of respiratory illness as well as occasional pandemics, the most recent of which occurred in 2009 [2]. IAV is pleomorphic, producing virions of spherical and filamentous morphology [3]. Strains that produce predominantly spherical or ovoid virions have typically been passaged many times within laboratory substrates, while filament-producing strains occur in primary or low passage isolates [4,5]. Filaments are of variable length and can be up to 30 µm long [6]. Herein, we define filaments as any virion 300 nm in length or longer (≥3x the diameter of a typical spherical virion). Studies performed using reverse genetics systems have identified the M1 matrix protein as the major genetic determinant of virion morphology, however portions of the viral nucleoprotein (NP) as well as the cytoplasmic tails of the M2 ion channel, hemagglutinin (HA) and neuraminidase (NA) proteins have been shown to affect virion morphology as well [7–13].

Early observations showed that the filamentous morphology is gradually lost upon continued passage in embryonated chicken eggs in favor of a more spherical morphology [14,15]. We also observed that filaments could be lost following ten passages in eggs or MDCK cells, but that this phenotypic change was not required for robust adaptation to either substrate [5]. The fact that filaments are maintained in nature while dispensable for growth in laboratory substrates suggests that the filamentous morphology provides a selective advantage within the infected host that is not necessary for growth in the laboratory. Previously, we showed that passaging of the spherical laboratory strain A/Puerto Rico/8/1934 (H1N1) [PR8] twelve times in guinea pigs led to the emergence of virions that are filamentous in morphology [5]. Through sequencing of the M1 matrix gene of the passage 12 (P12) virus pool, we identified several coding mutations within M1. Individual introduction of four of these amino acid changes using reverse genetics yielded mutant viruses that produced significantly more filaments than the wild-type [$p<0.05$; difference in proportions test] [5].

While selection for a filamentous morphology through passaging in an animal host confirms an advantage of filamentous virions *in vivo*, the nature of the selective advantage remains unclear. To determine the advantage filament-producing viruses have over their spherical counterparts, we used recombinant wild-type PR8 (rPR8wt) and two previously characterized filamentous M1 mutants – rPR8 M1 N87S (N87S) and rPR8 M1 R101G (R101G) [5]. Our published particle counts showed that 16% and 41% of virions were filamentous for N87S and R101G viruses, respectively, compared to 4% for PR8wt [5]. These three viruses present an ideal system in which to address the differences between exclusively spherical and filament-producing IAV, for the following reasons: i) the mutant strains are highly similar genetically to the rPR8wt, simplifying the interpretation of results; ii) the mutations used arose naturally, minimizing the likelihood of disrupting viral functions through their introduction; and iii) the mutant viruses differ significantly from rPR8wt in terms of filament production. Thus, rPR8wt, N87S, and R101G viruses were analyzed in a series of *in vitro* assays. We hypothesized that functional differences between spherical and filamentous virions might arise due to their differing surface areas, and therefore focused our efforts on the two surface glycoproteins of IAV, HA and NA. We tested whether the HA avidity or NA activity per virion differed between the spherical rPR8wt virus and filament producing strains. In addition, the ratio of hemagglutination units (HAU) to plaque forming units (PFU), the ratio of HAU to RNA copies, and virion stability at elevated temperatures were investigated. Our findings suggest a role of the viral NA protein in the fitness advantage conferred by filamentous virion morphology: by two independent measures, the two filamentous rPR8 mutants displayed higher neuraminidase activities compared to rPR8wt, but did not differ significantly in binding avidity, inhibition of binding by antiserum, infectivity or thermostability.

Material and Methods

Ethics statement

This study was performed in accordance with the recommendations in the Guide for the Care and Use of Laboratory Animals of the National Institutes of Health. Animal husbandry and experimental procedures were approved by the Emory University Institutional Animal Care and Use Committee (IACUC protocol #2000719).

Viruses and cells

The rPR8wt, rPR8 M1 N87S, and rPR8 M1 R101G viruses were generated using reverse genetics as previously described [16–18]. Briefly, rPR8-based viruses were recovered following eight (pDZ) plasmid transfection of 293T cells and subsequent inoculation of transfected cells and culture medium into 9–11 day old embryonated chicken's eggs. Stocks of the rPR8 wild-type virus and mutants were generated in 9–11 day old embryonated chicken's eggs. Influenza A/Udorn/301/1972 (H3N2) virus was grown in MDCK cells. Influenza A/Anhui/1/2013 (H7N9) virus was grown in eggs under enhanced BSL3 containment and inactivated by addition of beta-propiolactone (BPL) prior to removal from the BSL3 facility.

Washed chicken red blood cells from Lampire Biological were used for all hemagglutination-based assays. MDCK cells, a kind gift of Peter Palese, were maintained in minimal essential medium supplemented with 10% fetal bovine serum and penicillin/streptomycin. 293T cells (ATCC), used for virus rescue by reverse genetics, were maintained in Dulbecco's minimal essential medium supplemented with 10% fetal bovine serum. Embryonated chickens' eggs were obtained from Hy-Line International and incubated at 37°C, with rocking, for 9–11 days prior to inoculation with IAV.

Infectious titer comparison

Viruses were diluted to concentration of 128 HAU. Hemagglutination units, or HAU, are defined as the reciprocal of the highest dilution of virus still allowing agglutination of red blood cells. After confirming the HA titer, viruses were titrated in triplicate by plaque assay of 10-fold serial dilutions on MDCK cells. A Student *t*-test was used to compare the infectious titers of each mutant virus to rPR8wt virus.

C_q value comparison

Viruses were diluted to concentration of 128 HAU. After confirming the HA titer, RNA was extracted from 160 µl of each diluted virus sample using the QIAamp Viral RNA Mini Kit (QIAGEN), according to the manufacturer's instructions. cDNA was generated using Maxima reverse transcriptase (Thermo Scientific) and a universal forward primer (GGCCAGCAAAAGCAGG). Quantitative PCR was then performed on a Bio-Rad CFX384 thermocycler using the cDNA as template, SsoFast EvaGreen Supermix (Bio-Rad), and primers specific for the NP segment (F: TATTCGTCTCAGGGAGCAAAAGCAGG [19] and R: CTGATTTCAGTGGCATTCTGGC). Each cDNA was analyzed in triplicate and the resulting cycle threshold (C_q) values were recorded. Average C_q values shown in Table 1 were calculated by first converting each C_q value to $2^{(-Cq)}$, calculating the arithmetic mean, and then taking the $-\log_2$ of the arithmetic mean.

Red blood cell elution assay

Each virus was standardized to a concentration of 128 HAU. Duplicate HA assays were then set up in parallel using 1:2 serially diluted viruses and allowed to develop at 4°C. One set of plates was then transferred to 37°C (t = 0 hours) to trigger neuraminidase activity, while the second set of plates was left at 4°C to act as a negative control. Red blood cells were monitored for elution (visible as the formation of a red blood cell pellet at the bottom of the well) at the following time points: 1, 2, 3, 4, 6, and 8 hours.

MUNANA neuraminidase activity assay

Neuraminidase activity assays using the soluble substrate methylumbelliferyl N-acetylneuraminic acid (MUNANA) were performed as previously described by Campbell et al. [20]. Virus was diluted to 5×10^5 PFU/ml and 80 µl was added to each well of a black 96-well plate (CoStar). A sample of each diluted virus preparation was retained for quantification of viral RNA therein by RT-qPCR. Concentrations of MUNANA substrate ranging from 1.17 µM to 150 µM were used. When cleaved by the viral NA, MUNANA produces a fluorescent product. Fluorescence was quantified using a Biotek Synergy H1 plate reader every minute over the course of an hour. Fluorescence curves were then fitted to the Michaelis-Menton equation to determine values of V_{max} (maximal enzyme velocity) and K_m (the Michaelis constant, the substrate concentration at which the reaction rate is half of V_{max}). Each experiment included triplicate samples of each virus.

Virus concentration for Western blot analysis

Each virus was purified from allantoic fluid collected from 9–11 day embryonated chicken eggs infected with 250 PFU of virus. Allantoic fluid was spun at 3,000 rpm for 10 minutes at 4°C in a Sorvall tabletop centrifuge after which the supernatant was transferred to ultracentrifuge tubes (Beckman Coulter). Samples

Table 1. 128 HAU of rPR8wt, rPR8 M1 N87S and rPR8 M1 R101G viruses comprise comparable infectious titers and genome copies.

Virus	Infectious titer (PFU/ml)[a]	Average infectious titer (PFU/ml)	C_q value[b]	Average C_q value
rPR8wt	6.00×10^7	1.15×10^8	19.06	19.16
	1.55×10^8		19.37	
	1.30×10^8		19.08	
rPR8 M1 N87S	5.00×10^7	7.60×10^7	19.23	19.32
	5.00×10^7		19.42	
	1.30×10^8		19.32	
rPR8 M1 R101G	4.00×10^7	7.80×10^7	18.86	18.94
	6.50×10^7		18.92	
	1.30×10^8		19.04	

[a]rPR8wt to rPR8 M1 N87S comparison (p = 0.38), rPR8wt to rPR8 M1 R101G comparison (p = 0.40). A two-tailed Student *t*-test was used to assess significance.
[b]rPR8wt to rPR8 M1 N87S comparison (p = 0.23), rPR8wt to rPR8 M1 R101G comparison (p = 0.10). To assess significance, a two-tailed Student *t*-test was applied to values of $2^{(-Cq)}$.

were spun in an SW32 rotor at 10,000 rpm for 30 minutes at 4°C and supernatant was then transferred to a fresh tube where a 5-ml 30% sucrose cushion was added. Samples were spun in an SW32 rotor at 25,000 rpm for 1.5 hours at 4°C. All supernatant was removed and 100 µl of PBS was added to the virus pellet and allowed to resuspend at 4°C overnight.

NP normalization and Western blot

Concentrated virus samples were denatured by boiling for 10 minutes and treated with PNGaseF (New England Biolabs) for 1 hour at 37°C to allow for deglycosylation. The amount of NP in each virus sample was quantified by polyacrylamide gel electrophoresis followed by Coomassie staining (GelCode Blue – Thermo Scientific) and analysis with Image Lab software (Bio-Rad). The volume of each sample used for western blotting was then normalized based on NP content. Samples were loaded on a 4–15% SDS gradient gel (Bio-Rad Mini Protean) and electrophoresed at 130 V for 1 hour and 5 minutes. Protein was transferred (semi-dry) onto nitrocellulose membrane for 1 hour at 100 mA and blocking was performed overnight. NA was detected using a goat anti-NA primary antibody (BEI NR-9598) and a donkey anti-goat alexa 647-conjugated secondary antibody. NP was detected using a rabbit anti-NP primary antibody (a kind gift of Peter Palese) and a donkey anti-rabbit alexa 488-conjugated secondary antibody. Band intensity was quantified using Image Lab software (Bio-Rad).

Red blood cell-based avidity assay

The red blood cell-based avidity assay was performed similarly to those described in [21]. Briefly, a 1.3% solution of red blood cells in PBS was treated with a series of dilutions of *C. perfringens* neuraminidase (Sigma) for 30 minutes at 37°C. Neuraminidase concentrations incremented by 5 mU/ml for the PR8-based viruses and 10 mU/ml for the H3 and H7 subtype viruses. Treated red blood cells were then added to virus at a standardized concentration of 8 HAU in a v-bottom, 96-well plate. Hemagglutination was assessed after 2 hours at 4°C. To rule out the activity of the viral NA in interpreting results, virus was diluted in PBS containing oseltamivir carboxylate (GS4071) and the assay was allowed to develop at 4°C.

Trypsin-heat-periodate treatment

In order to remove nonspecific inhibitors of hemagglutination, serum treatment was performed as outlined in [22]. Briefly, serum was treated with L -1-Tosylamide-2-phenylethyl chloromethyl ketone (TPCK) trypsin for 30 minutes at 56°C. After cooling to room temperature, serum was then treated with 0.011 M metapotassium periodate (KIO_4) for 15 minutes at room temperature. After KIO_4 treatment, serum was treated with 1% glycerol in PBS for 15 minutes at room temperature after which an 85% PBS solution was added to reach a final serum dilution of 1:10.

Hemagglutination inhibition (HI) assay

Trypsin-heat-periodate-treated anti-PR8 guinea pig serum was diluted in PBS either 1:2 or 1:1.5 across a v-bottom, 96-well plate. Each virus was standardized to a concentration of 8 HAU and was then added to the diluted serum. Serum and virus were incubated together at 4°C for 30 minutes after which 0.5% red blood cells in PBS were added to each well. The assay was allowed to develop at 4°C. Naïve guinea pig serum was used as a negative control. The HI titers reported reflect HI activity above background levels.

Plaque reduction assay

Each virus was diluted to approximately 250 PFU. Trypsin-heat-periodate treated anti-PR8 guinea pig serum was serially diluted 1:80, 1:160, 1:320, and 1:640 in PBS. Control serum obtained from a naïve guinea pig was also used. Virus was added to the diluted serum and incubated for 30 minutes at 37°C. The infectious titer of each serum/virus sample then quantified by plaque assay in MDCK cells. This assay was performed in triplicate.

Thermostability assay

Each virus was diluted to approximately 1×10^6 PFU. Fifteen 120 µl aliquots of each virus were incubated at 50°C and three aliquots of each virus were removed at 0, 15, 30, 60, and 120 minutes. Titers for each sample were quantified via plaque assay on MDCK cells.

Results

Equivalent HAU of the rPR8wt, rPR8 M1 N87S, and rPR8 M1 R101G viruses do not differ in infectivity or RNA copy number

Each of the functional assays that we applied to our spherical and filamentous PR8 viruses required normalization of the input of each virus. Ideally, this normalization would be achieved by counting virus particles in transmission electron micrographs, but this approach was not practical given that the preparations used were relatively dilute and concentration by centrifugation can alter virus morphology. We therefore performed the following experiment to determine the relationships between the hemagglutination-based titer, infectious (PFU) titer and RNA copy number for each virus. rPR8wt, N87S, and R101G viruses were diluted to 128 HAU and HA titers were confirmed. Diluted virus samples were then titrated in triplicate by plaque assay. The mutant viruses showed lower PFU titers compared to rPR8wt, but the differences were not statistically significant (Table 1). RNA was extracted from 160 µl of each diluted virus and quantified by reverse transcription followed by quantitative PCR. C_q values obtained were consistent across all three viruses (Table 1). Thus, for all three viruses, the HAU to PFU and HAU to RNA copy number ratios were comparable. To assess the precision and consistency of the hemagglutination assay, we furthermore evaluated the PFU titers and relative RNA copy numbers of three 128 HAU samples of rPR8wt virus that had been obtained through independent dilution series. The average PFU titers obtained ranged from 1.66 to 1.78×10^8 PFU/ml (n = 3 per 128 HAU sample). The average C_q values were also very similar, ranging from 18.64 to 18.85. Taken together, these results indicate that similar results would be expected following normalization of rPR8wt, N87S, and R101G viruses by PFU, HAU or RNA copy number.

The rPR8 M1 N87S and rPR8 M1 R101G filamentous mutants have higher neuraminidase activity than rPR8wt virus

The NA activities of the spherical and filament-producing viruses were assessed by comparing rPR8wt, N87S, and R101G viruses in a red blood cell elution assay. To test our hypothesis that filamentous and spherical virions differ at the level of the whole virus particle, due to differing surface areas, we aimed to evaluate NA activity per virion rather than per NA protein. We therefore normalized virus input by hemagglutination titer rather than protein levels. Briefly, HA assays were set up in parallel using a standardized amount of virus (128 HAU) and allowed to develop at 4°C. At that point, one set of plates was transferred to 37°C. At this temperature, the viral NA is active and begins cleaving the sialic acids on the surface of the red blood cells, causing them to drop to the bottom of the well (elution). We monitored the plates for elution over the course of 8 hours. Progressive elution was observed at 37°C, while no elution was seen over the same time period at 4°C. We found that, when incubated with the R101G mutant virus, red blood cells eluted at a faster rate compared to those incubated with rPR8wt (Figure 1A). The N87S mutant had a less marked phenotype than the R101G mutant, but also eluted red blood cells at a faster rate than the rPR8wt – particularly at the later time points (Figure 1B).

The rPR8 M1 N87S and rPR8 M1 R101G filamentous mutants have higher neuraminidase activity in the MUNANA assay than rPR8wt virus

To confirm that the differing elution phenotypes observed were due to differing NA activities, we compared the spherical and filamentous rPR8 viruses using a MUNANA-based assay. MUNANA (methylumbelliferyl N-acetylneuraminic acid) is a soluble substrate that produces a fluorescent product when cleaved by the viral NA. For this assay, viruses were standardized to equivalent PFU and RNA titers and concentrations of MUNANA substrate ranging from 1.17 µM to 150 µM were used. Levels of fluorescence were measured every minute over a sixty-minute period. The resulting fluorescence curves were then fitted to the Michaelis-Menton equation for calculation of K_m and V_{max} values associated with each virus. It is important to note that, in line with our aim of evaluating NA enzyme kinetics per virion, NA protein levels contained within each virus sample were not normalized for this assay.

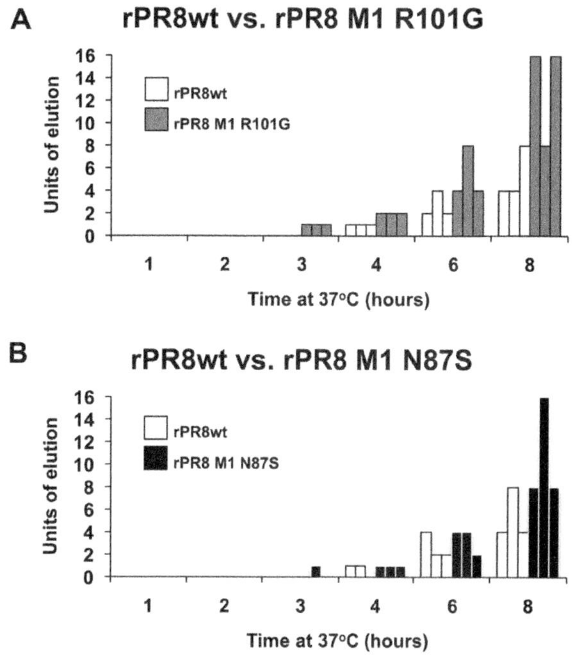

Figure 1. rPR8 M1 R101G and rPR8 M1 N87S viruses elute red blood cells at a faster rate than rPR8wt virus. HA assays were set up using virus diluted to a concentration of 128 HAU. After the assays had developed, plates were transferred to 37°C to allow for red blood cell elution by the viral neuraminidase. A second set of plates remained at 4°C where no elution occurred (not shown). The results of three independent experiments are shown, with each experiment represented by a separate bar. Within each experiment, viruses were analyzed in triplicate (standard deviation for each virus = 0). "Units of elution" is defined as the reciprocal of the highest virus dilution showing elution. A) Elution of rPR8 M1 R101G virus is compared to that of rPR8wt virus. B) Elution of rPR8 M1 N87S virus is compared to that of rPR8wt virus.

The results obtained correlated well with those observed from the red blood cell elution assay (Figure 2). We confirmed that equivalent amounts of each virus were assayed by performing RT-qPCR on viral RNA extracted from the same diluted virus preparations employed in the MUNANA assay (Figure 2B). The R101G mutant virus displayed the highest V_{max}, followed by the N87S mutant. rPR8wt had the lowest V_{max} (Table 2). The K_m for all three viruses was found to be consistent, as expected considering the NA protein is the same for all three viruses (Table 2). Based on the results of both the elution assay and the MUNANA assay, we concluded that the filament-producing M1 mutant viruses had a higher neuraminidase activity per virion than the spherical wild-type virus.

When standardized to NP protein levels, NA and M1 protein incorporation among rPR8wt, rPR8 M1 N87S, and rPR8 M1 R101G is similar

Because filamentous virions can be much greater in size than spherical virions, a logical explanation for our NA activity results is that filamentous virions have more NA adorning their surface. Indeed, the consistent K_m values across all three viruses obtained

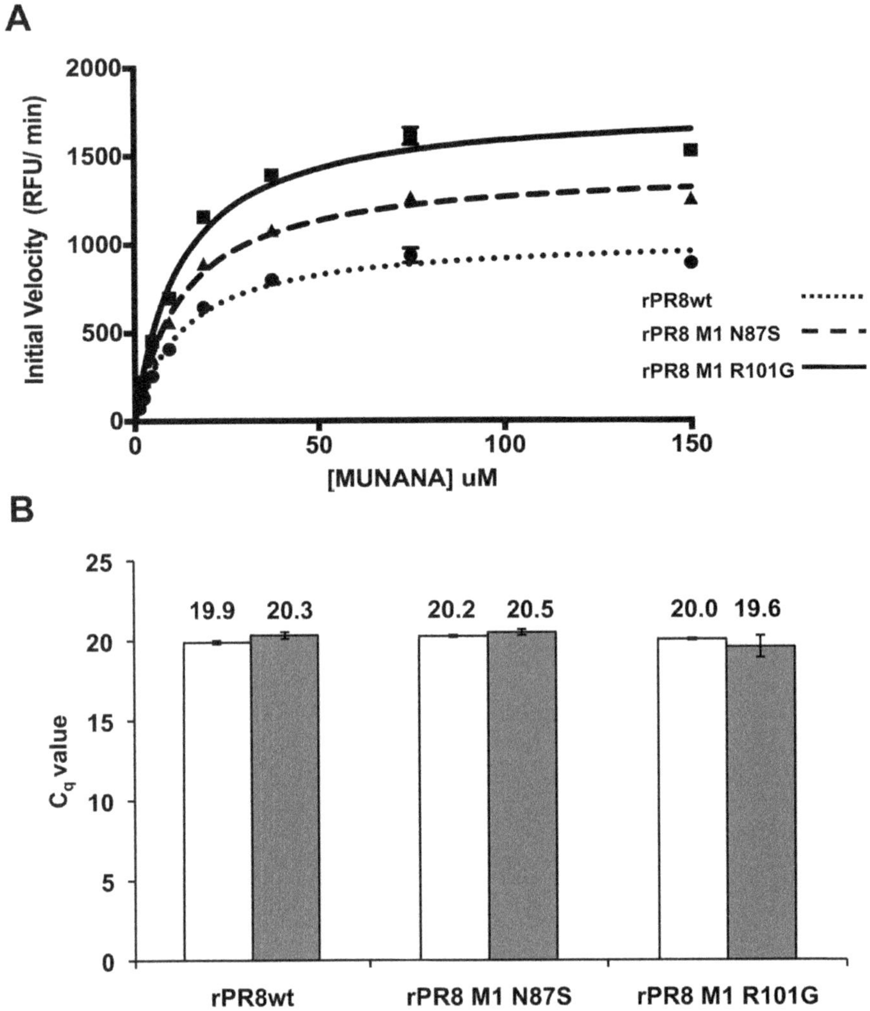

Figure 2. rPR8 M1 R101G and rPR8 M1 N87S viruses have higher neuraminidase activity than rPR8wt virus. A) Neuraminidase enzyme kinetics. Virus input was standardized to 5×10^5 PFU and concentrations of MUNANA substrate ranging from 1.17 μM to 150 μM were used. Fluorescence generated at each time point (every minute over the course of 1 hour) was detected using a Biotek Synergy H1 plate reader. The resulting fluorescence curves were then fitted to the Michaelis-Menton equation. B) That equivalent amounts of each virus were used in the MUNANA assay was confirmed by RT-qPCR for the viral NP segment. The arithmetic mean (n = 3) and standard deviation of $2^{(-C_q)}$ values were calculated and then converted back to a C_q scale by taking the $\log_2$. Two biological replicates of each virus are included in white and grey bars; each biological replicate comprised three technical replicates.

from the MUNANA assay suggest that the intrinsic NA activity is unaffected. To test this hypothesis, we performed Western blots on concentrated virus preparations of rPR8wt, N87S, and R101G, and probed for NP, NA, and M1 proteins. The fluorescence intensity of bands was quantified using a Bio-Rad Chemidoc imager. NP and M1 were included as controls: due to its association with the viral genome, NP levels would be expected to be constant among viruses of differing morphology, while M1 levels would be expected to increase with surface area. For a given amount of NP, the filamentous mutant viruses did not show increased quantities of NA or M1 proteins in virions (Figure 3A and 3B). Similar results were obtained when egg-grown virus

Table 2. rPR8 M1 N87S and rPR8 M1 R101G viruses have a higher neuraminidase activity than rPR8 wt virus in a MUNANA-based assay.

Virus	V_{max}	V_{max} 95% confidence interval	K_m	K_m 95% confidence interval
rPR8wt	1040	978–1101	13.02	10.41–15.63
rPR8 M1 N87S	1434	1370–1497	13.15	11.17–15.14
rPR8 M1 R101G	1785	1669–1901	15.52	10.60–20.44

stocks were analyzed directly (rather than concentrating them first), and when inputs were normalized by viral RNA content, rather than normalization to NP (data not shown). Based on our inability to detect increases in M1:NP ratios for the filament-producing viruses relative to rPR8wt, we concluded that the Western blot assay used was not sufficiently sensitive to detect differences (or lack thereof) in NA or M1 incorporation. The preponderance of spherical viruses present in the N87S and R101G virus stocks most likely obscures any differences in protein content between spherical and filamentous particles.

No difference in binding avidity is observed between rPR8wt, rPR8 M1 N87S, and rPR8 M1 R101G

After assessing the NA activity between spherical and filamentous viruses, we compared the function of the viral HA in a red blood cell-based avidity assay. We treated chicken red blood cells with a series of dilutions of *C. perfringens* neuraminidase. This treatment removes alpha 2,3-, alpha 2,6- and alpha 2,8-linked sialic acids. Thus, red blood cells treated with higher concentrations of neuraminidase had fewer sialic acids on their surface than those treated with lower concentrations of neuraminidase. We then added a standardized amount of virus (8 HAU) to the treated red blood cells and allowed agglutination to occur. We found that the neuraminidase concentration that prevented agglutination was the same for the rPR8wt, N87S, and R101G viruses, indicating that red blood cell binding avidity is not affected by the changes in morphology seen with these viruses (Figure 4). Additionally, to validate that the assay was sufficiently sensitive to detect differences in red blood cell binding avidity, we compared avidity of the rPR8-based viruses to those of viruses with differing HA types (specifically, H3 and H7). We found that A/Udorn/301/1972 (H3N2) and BPL-inactivated A/Anhui/1/2013 (H7N9) virus had higher red blood cell binding avidities than the PR8-based viruses. From these results, we concluded that the changes in virion morphology mediated by the N87S and R101G mutations do not affect the binding avidity of rPR8 virus.

No difference in hemagglutination inhibition and little difference in plaque reduction was observed among rPR8wt, rPR8 M1 N87S, and rPR8 M1 R101G

Next, we compared hemagglutination inhibition (HI) between rPR8wt, N87S, and R101G viruses, reasoning that, due to their increased size, filaments may be more difficult to neutralize than spheres. Using 1:2 dilutions of trypsin-heat-periodate treated anti-PR8 guinea pig immune serum and virus standardized to 8 HAU, we found no difference in HI among rPR8wt, N87S, and R101G (Table 3). Since we were working with populations of mixed morphology, which may make differences between filaments and spheres difficult to detect, we sought to improve the sensitivity of the assay by using a series of 1:1.5 serum dilutions. Similar to the assays utilizing 1:2 dilutions, we observed little difference in HI between the spherical wild-type and filamentous mutants (Table 3).

To substantiate the relationship between particle morphology and sensitivity of virus to immune serum, we also performed a plaque reduction assay. Briefly, trypsin-heat-periodate treated anti-PR8 guinea pig serum was diluted to 1:80, 1:160, 1:320, or 1:640 in PBS. The same dilutions of a naïve guinea pig serum were used as controls. Virus was diluted to approximately 250 PFU and incubated with the diluted serum for 30 minutes at 37°C.

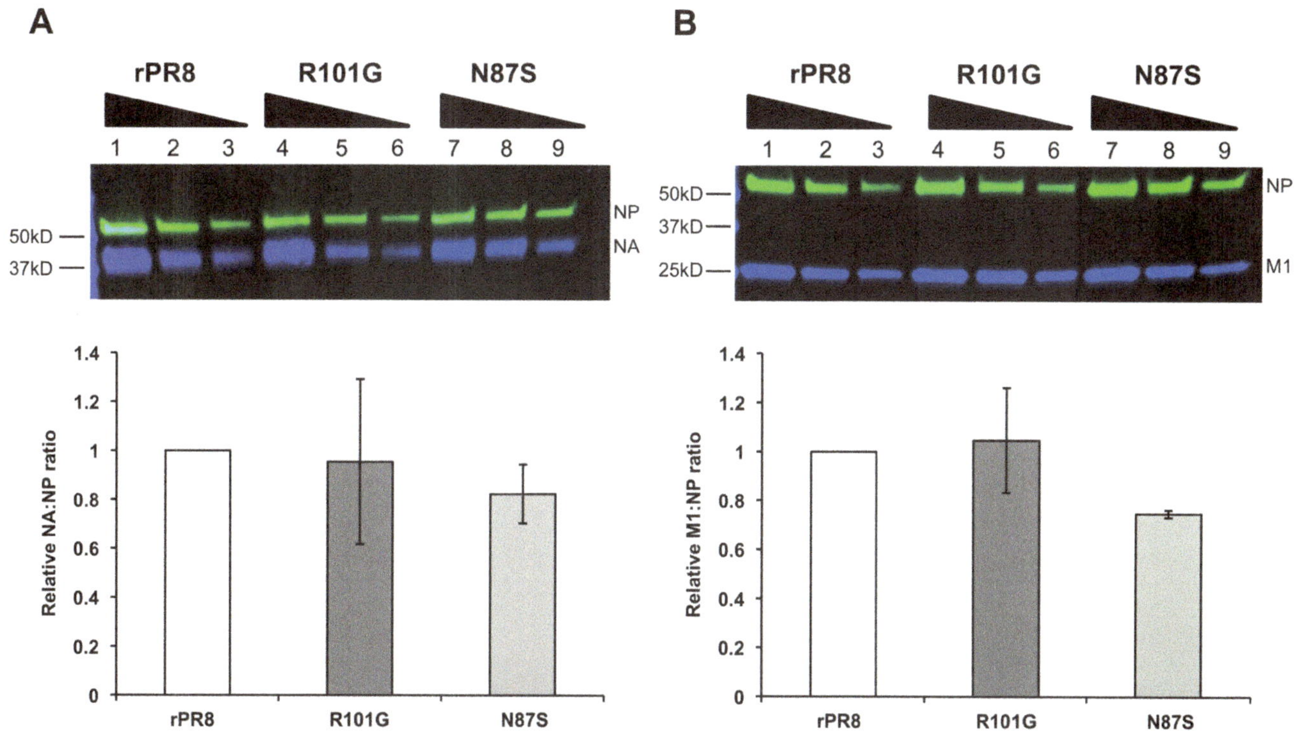

Figure 3. NA and M1 protein levels between rPR8wt, rPR8 M1 N87S, and rPR8 M1 R101G are similar when normalized to NP protein levels. Virus samples were concentrated via ultracentrifugation through a 30% sucrose cushion and resuspended in PBS. Samples were then deglycosylated and denatured, after which NP protein levels were standardized via Coomassie. For the Western blot, protein was detected using primary antibodies specific for NA, M1, and NP and fluorophore-conjugated secondary antibodies. All bands were quantified using Image Lab software (Bio-Rad). Error bars represent standard deviation.

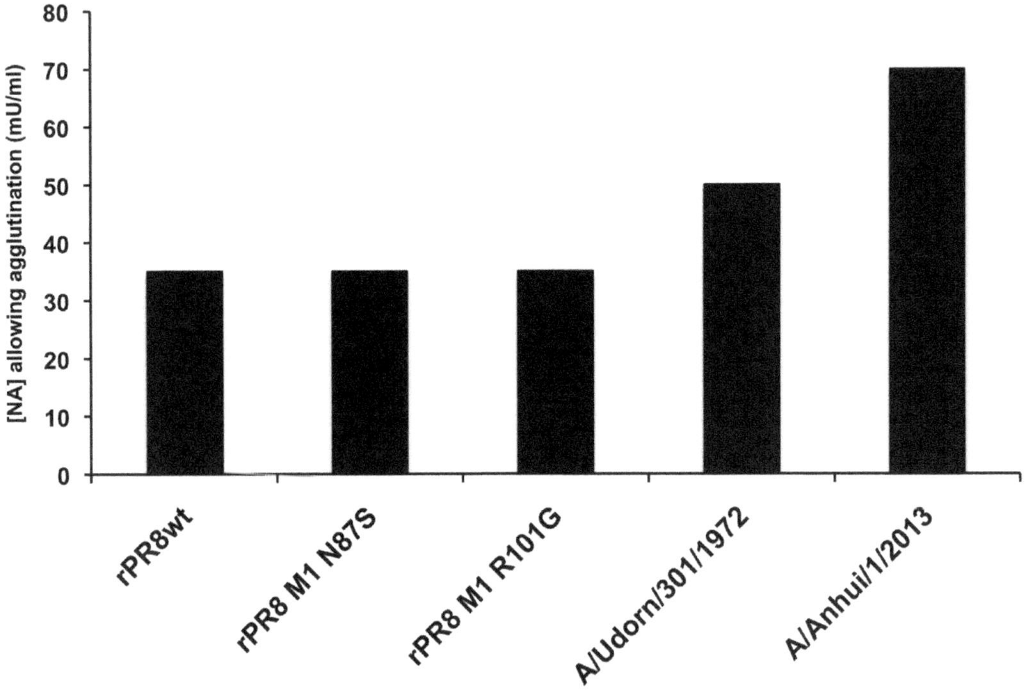

Figure 4. rPR8wt, rPR8 M1 N87S, and rPR8 M1 R101G viruses have the same red blood cell binding avidity. Chicken red blood cells were treated with a series of dilutions of *C. perfringens* neuraminidase. Treated red blood cells were then added to a standardized amount of each virus (8 HAU) and allowed to develop at 4°C. The assay was run in triplicate (standard deviation for each virus = 0). The highest concentration of neuraminidase that still allowed agglutination by each virus is plotted.

Following the incubation period, virus titer was determined in triplicate for each serum/virus sample by plaque assay on MDCK cells. Plaque numbers were compared to those obtained when virus was incubated with the control serum. All three viruses showed reductions in titer with immune serum diluted 1:80 and 1:160, but not with immune serum diluted 1:320 or 1:640 (Figure 5). The extent of reduction seen with the wt vs. mutant viruses at the 1:160 dilution was found to be significantly different for both mutants ($p<0.05$, t-test) and suggested that the two filamentous viruses are slightly more sensitive to antibody neutralization than is the spherical PR8wt strain (Figure 5). We interpret these results with caution, however, since the number of plaques remaining after incubation with 1:160 diluted immune serum was near the limit of detection. Overall, the results from the HI assays and the plaque reduction assay indicate that the greater surface area of filamentous compared to a spherical viruses does not confer resistance to antibody neutralization.

No difference in virion stability is observed between rPR8wt, rPR8 M1 N87S, and rPR8 M1 R101G

Due to potential differences in the structure of the matrix layer [23], we hypothesized that filamentous and spherical viruses might differ in their sensitivity to environmental stresses, such as fluctuations in temperature. To test this hypothesis, we evaluated virion stability at high temperatures. Each virus was diluted to a concentration of 1×10^6 PFU and incubated at 50°C for one of the following lengths of time: 0, 15, 30, 60, or 120 minutes. Following heat exposure, the titer of each sample was quantified in triplicate via plaque assay in MDCK cells. All three viruses had similar infectious titers remaining at each time point, indicating that the observed changes in virion morphology do not affect virion stability at elevated temperatures (Figure 6).

Table 3. There are no differences in hemagglutination inhibition among rPR8wt, rPR8 M1 N87S, rPR8 M1 R101G viruses.

	1:2 serum dilutions			**1:1.5 serum dilutions**		
	HI titer[a]			**HI titer[a]**		
Virus	**A**	**B**	**C**	**A**	**B**	**C**
rPR8wt	160	160	320	256	256	384
rPR8 M1 N87S	160	160	160	256	256	384
rPR8 M1 R101G	160	160	320	171	256	384

[a]The reciprocal of the highest dilution of serum that prevented hemagglutination is shown for three replicates (A, B and C).

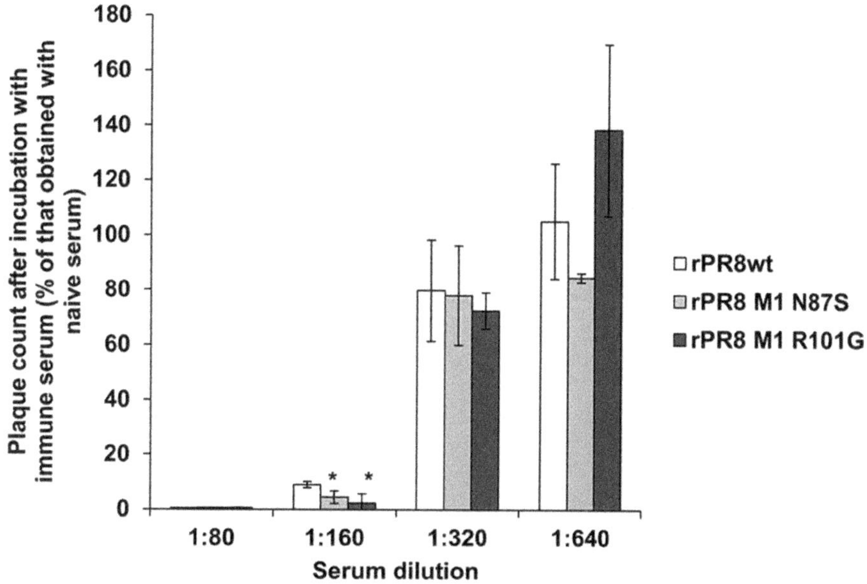

Figure 5. There is little difference in plaque reduction among rPR8wt, rPR8 M1 N87S, and rPR8 M1 R101G viruses. Each virus was diluted to approximately 250 PFU. Trypsin-heat-periodate treated serum was diluted 1:80, 1:160, 1:320, and 1:640 in PBS. Virus was added to serum dilutions and incubated for 30 minutes at 37°C. Virus titer for each serum/virus sample was then quantified by plaque assay on MDCK cells. The number of plaques obtained following incubation with immune serum is plotted as a percentage of the plaques obtained following incubation with naïve serum. The mean of three replicates is plotted, and error bars indicate standard deviation. $^{*}p<0.05$ compared to rPR8wt virus. The limit of detection for the plaque assays was 5 PFU/ml.

Discussion

The fact that the filamentous morphology of IAV is maintained in nature but not in the laboratory suggests that filaments have a functional significance within the infected host. Due to the greater surface area of filaments relative to spheres, we hypothesized that functional differences between the two morphologies may lie with the HA and NA surface glycoproteins. We therefore focused our study on the HA and NA functions of strains with differing morphological phenotypes. We took advantage of two M1 point mutants selected during serial adaptation of rPR8 virus to an animal host [5]. By measuring particles in electron micrographs, the R101G mutant was previously shown to comprise 41% filamentous particles, while the N87S had 16% filaments and the rPR8wt virus had 4% filaments [5].

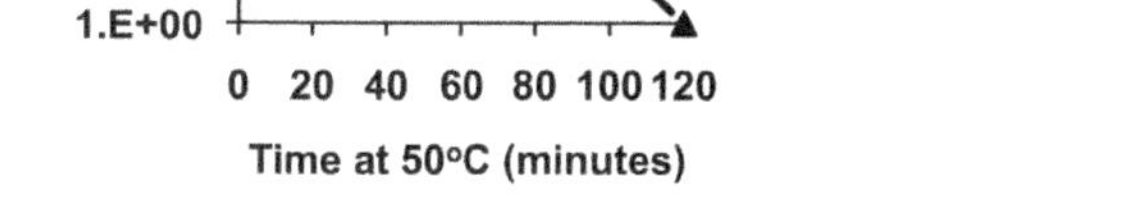

Figure 6. No difference in virion stability at an elevated temperature was observed between rPR8wt, rPR8 M1 N87S, and rPR8 M1 R101G viruses. Each virus was diluted to 1×10^{6} PFU and incubated in triplicate at 50°C for one of the following lengths of time: 0, 15, 30, 60, and 120 min. Results shown are the average of four separate assays performed in triplicate (thus $n=12$). The titers of each mutant virus were compared to that of the wt virus at each time point using Student's *t* test. All p values were >0.05 except that obtained for wt vs. N87S viruses at the 0 h time point ($p=0.0094$). The dotted line indicates the limit of detection.

Our approach, focused on the surface of the virion, assumes that the internal components of spherical and filamentous particles are similar. Our results indicating comparable infectivity and RNA content per HAU for spherical and filament-producing strains supports this assumption. Similar results were also reported by Roberts et al. for the A/Udorn/301/1972 (H3N2) strain [10]. Nevertheless, the literature contains conflicting reports on the genomic content of filaments versus spheres. Early studies suggested that filamentous virions could be polyploid (containing more than one copy of the genome) or contain more RNA than their spherical counterparts [24,25]. In contrast, a recent cryo-electron tomography study has shown that many longer filaments produced by A/Udorn/301/1972 (H3N2) virus lack RNPs [26]. Lastly, sectioning TEM and cryo-electron tomography studies have shown that filamentous virions contain a single copy of the viral genome located at the apical tip of the budding virion [23,27]. These apparently contradictory results can be partially reconciled by noting that the absence of genomes from filamentous particles appears to apply mainly to very long filaments [26]. In some cases, IAV strain specific differences in the properties of filaments may also play a role.

Our observations through two independent functional assays show that the two filament-producing rPR8 mutants have higher NA activities than the spherical rPR8wt virus. Replacement of the PR8 M segment with that of the filamentous 2009 pandemic strain A/Netherlands/602/2009 (H1N1) was also shown to increase both filament production and NA activity compared to the rPR8wt virus [20]. Now we show that significant increases in NA activity can be conferred through a single point mutation that changes virion morphology, thereby strengthening the causal link between morphology and NA activity. We predict that the increased NA activities associated with filament-containing virus preparations are due to greater numbers of NA proteins adorning the surface of filaments compared to spheres. We were not able to test this prediction robustly, however, due to limitations in the sensitivity of our Western blot assay. An alternative mechanism by which morphology could impact NA activity relates to the distribution of NA molecules on the virion surface. If filaments and spheres differ in terms of the positioning of NA on the particle, increased neuraminidase activity could be due to a cooperative effect mediated by greater NA protein clustering on filamentous virions. Consistent with this idea, clustering of NA at the tip of the virus particle proximal to the cell membrane has been reported [23,28,29]. Such an arrangement was suggested to promote destruction of host cell receptors as the virus is budding.

Contrary to what was observed for NA activity, we found no difference in binding avidity to red blood cells between the spherical and filamentous rPR8 viruses. Similarly, we did not observe marked differences in HI titer or in plaque reduction between spherical and filamentous viruses. These results suggest that the mechanism by which NA activity is increased for filament-producing viruses does not apply to HA. For example, if incorporation of both glycoproteins increases with filament size, then our data would suggest that avidity does not increase linearly with the valency of the virus particle. Lastly, we did not observe a difference in thermostability between spherical and filamentous viruses. Thus our data suggest that, at least in the PR8 background and in a guinea pig host, the selective advantage of a filamentous morphology lies with increased NA activity.

Enhanced NA activity could be advantageous to the virus by promoting release from infected cells and/or spread within the respiratory tract to new target cells [30]. Indeed, Roberts et al. suggested that increased amounts of NA protein per virion could aid movement through the mucus lining the airway [31]. Additionally, increased NA activity was shown to improve transmission in guinea pigs [20,32]. Importantly, the M segment has been shown to affect virus transmission as well [20,33]. Whether this effect on transmission is directly mediated by viral morphology has not yet been established. However, the fact that a single point mutation in the M1 matrix protein can both significantly alter virion morphology and confer increased NA activity suggests a mechanism by which the M segment may affect transmission. We know from previous work that the rPR8 M1 N87S mutant virus, which has both a significantly more filamentous morphology as well as a higher NA activity than rPR8wt, is not transmissible by a contact route in the guinea pig transmission model [5]. It is likely that N87S and the other point mutations identified in M1 following serial passage need to be coupled with additional permissive mutations on the M segment and/or elsewhere in the genome to promote transmission [34].

In summary, we have shown that filament-producing viruses have a higher neuraminidase activity than their spherical counterparts. Other properties such as HA binding avidity, HI titer, and thermostability were unaffected by changes in virion morphology. The viruses used herein were single M1 point mutants generated on a PR8 background and produced significantly more filaments than rPR8wt. The fact that these point mutations, when introduced individually, confer both a filamentous morphology and increased NA activity further strengthens the idea that the selective advantage conferred by filamentous virions lies in their increased NA activity over spherical virions.

Author Contributions

Conceived and designed the experiments: AL JSS JS. Performed the experiments: JSS PJC SS. Analyzed the data: AL JSS JS. Contributed to the writing of the manuscript: JSS AL JS.

References

1. Palese P, Shaw ML (2007) Orthomyxoviridae: the viruses and their replication. In: Knipe DM, Howley PM, editors. Fields Virology 5th edition Philadelphia: Lippincott Williams & Wilkins. pp 1647–1689.
2. Novel Swine-Origin Influenza A (H1N1) Virus Investigation Team, Dawood FS, Jain S, Finelli L, Shaw MW, Lindstrom S, et al. (2009) Emergence of a novel swine-origin influenza A (H1N1) virus in humans. N Engl J Med. 360: 2605–2615.
3. Chu CM, Dawson IM, Elford WJ (1949) Filamentous forms associated with newly isolated influenza virus. Lancet. 1: 602.
4. Itoh Y, Shinya K, Kiso M, Watanabe T, Sakoda Y, et al. (2009) In vitro and in vivo characterization of new swine-origin H1N1 influenza viruses. Nature. 460: 1021–1025.
5. Seladi-Schulman J, Steel J, Lowen AC (2013) Spherical influenza viruses have a fitness advantage in embryonated eggs, while filament-producing strains are selected in vivo. Journal of Virol. 87: 13343–13353.
6. Mosley VM, Wyckoff RW (1946) Electron micrography of the virus of influenza. Nature. 157: 263.
7. Burleigh LM, Calder LJ, Skehel JJ, Steinhauer DA (2005) Influenza A viruses with mutations in the M1 helix six domain display a wide variety of morphological phenotypes. J Virol. 79: 1262–1270.
8. Bourmakina SV, Garcia-Sastre A (2003) Reverse genetics studies on the filamentous morphology of influenza A virus. J Gen Virol. 84: 517–527.
9. Elleman CJ, Barclay WS (2004) The M1 matrix protein controls the filamentous phenotype of influenza A virus. Virology. 321: 144–153.
10. Roberts PC, Lamb RA, Compans RW (1998) The M1 and M2 proteins of influenza A virus are important determinants in filamentous particle formation. Virology. 240: 127–137.
11. Jin H, Leser GP, Zhang J, Lamb RA (1997) Influenza virus hemagglutinin and neuraminidase cytoplasmic tails control particle shape. EMBO J. 16: 1236–1247.
12. Bialas KM, Bussey KA, Stone RL, Takimoto T (2014) Specific nucleoprotein residues affect influenza virus morphology. J Virol. 88: 2227–2234.
13. Mitnaul LJ, Castrucci MR, Murti KG, Kawaoka Y (1996) The cytoplasmic tail of influenza A virus neuraminidase (NA) affects NA incorporation into virions, virion morphology, and virulence in mice but is not essential for virus replication. J Virol. 70: 873–879.
14. Kilbourne ED, Murphy JS (1960) Genetic studies of influenza viruses. I Viral morphology and growth capacity as exchangeable genetic traits Rapid in ovo adapation of early passsage Asian strain isolates by combination with PR8. J Exp Med. 111: 387–406.
15. Choppin PW, Murphy JS, Tamm I (1960) Studies of two kinds of virus particles which comprise influenza A2 virus strains. III. Morphological characteristics: independence to morphological and functional traits. J Exp Med. 112: 945–952.
16. Fodor E, Devenish L, Engelhardt OG, Palese P, Brownlee GG, et al (1999) Rescue of influenza A virus from recombinant DNA. J Virol 73: 9679–9682.
17. Steel J, Lowen AC, Mubareka S, Palese P (2009) Transmission of influenza virus in a mammalian host is increased by PB2 amino acids 627K or 627E/701N. PLoS Pathog. 5: e100052.
18. Quinlivan M, Zamarin D, Garcia-Sastre A, Cullinane A, Chambers T, et al. (2005) Attentuation of equine influenza viruses through truncations of the NS1 protein. J Virol. 79: 8431–8439.
19. Hoffmann E, Stech J, Guan Y, Webster RG, Perez DR (2001) Universal primer set for the full-length amplification of all influenza A viruses. Arch Virol. 146: 2275–2289.
20. Campbell PJ, Danzy S, Kyriakis CS, Deymier MJ, Lowen AC, et al (2014) The M segment of the 2009 pandemic influenza virus confersincreased NA activity, filamentous morphology, and efficient contact transmissibility to A/Puerto Rico/8/1934-based reassortant viruses Journal of Virol. 88: 3802–3814.
21. Hensley SE, Das SR, Bailey AL, Schmidt LM, Hickman HD, et al (2009) Hemagglutinin receptor binding avidity drives influenza A virus antigenic drift. Science. 326: 734–736.
22. Webster RG, Cox NJ, Sthor K (2002) WHO manual on animal influenza diagnosis and surveillance. World Health Organization, Geneva, Switzerland. Available: http://www.who.int/csr/resources/publications/influenza/en/whocdscsrncs20025rev.pdf.
23. Calder LJ, Wasilewski S, Berriman JA, Rosenthal PB (2010) Structural organization of a filamentous influenza A virus. Proc Natl Acad Sci USA 107: 10685–10690.
24. Ada GL, Perry BT (1958) Properties of the nucleic acid of the Ryan strain of filamentous influenza virus. J Gen Virol. 19: 40–54.
25. Smirnov YA, Kuznetsova MA, Kaverin NV (1991) The genetics aspects of influenza virus filamentous particle formation. Arch Virol. 118: 279–284.

26. Vijayakrishnan S, Loney C, Jackson D, Suphamungmee W, Rixon FJ, et al. (2013) Cryotomography of budding influenza A virus reveals filaments with diverse morphologies that mostly do not bear a genome at their distal end. PLoS Pathog. 9: e1003413.
27. Noda T, Sagara H, Yen A, Takada A, Kida H, et al. (2006) Architecture of ribonucleoprotein complexes in influenza A virus particles. Nature. 439: 490–492.
28. Murti KG, Webster RG (1986) Distribution of hemagglutinin and neuraminidase on influenza virions as revealed by immunoelectron microscopy. Virology. 149: 36–43.
29. Harris A, Cardone G, Winkler DC, Heymann JB, Brecher M, et al. (2006) Influenza virus pleiomorphy characterized by cryoelectron tomography. Proc Natl Acad Sci USA. 103: 19123–19127.
30. Matrosovich MN, Matrosovich TY, Gray T, Roberts NA, Klenk HD. (2004) Neuraminidase is important for the initiation of influenza virus infection in human airway epithelium. J Virol. 78: 1265–1267.
31. Roberts PC, Compans RW (1998) Host cell dependence of viral morphology. Proc Natl Acad Sci USA. 95: 5746–5751.
32. Bouvier NM, Lowen AC, Palese P (2008) Oseltamivir-resistant influenza A viruses are transmitted efficiently among guinea pigs by direct contact but not by aerosol. J Virol. 82: 10052–10058.
33. Chou YY, Albrecht RA, Pica N, Lowen AC, Richt JA, et al. (2011) The M segment of the 2009 new pandemic H1N1 influenza virus is critical for its high transmission efficiency in the guinea pig model J Virol. 85: 11235–11241.
34. Gong LI, Suchard MA, Bloom JD (2013) Stability-mediated epistatis constrains the evolution of an influenza protein. Elife. 2: e00631.

14

In Vivo Characterization of Neutrophil Extracellular Traps in Various Organs of a Murine Sepsis Model

Koji Tanaka[1]*, Yuhki Koike[1], Tadanobu Shimura[1], Masato Okigami[1], Shozo Ide[1], Yuji Toiyama[1], Yoshinaga Okugawa[1], Yasuhiro Inoue[1], Toshimitsu Araki[1], Keiichi Uchida[1], Yasuhiko Mohri[1], Akira Mizoguchi[2], Masato Kusunoki[1]

1 Departments of Gastrointestinal and Paediatric Surgery, Mie University Graduate School of Medicine, Tsu, Mie, Japan, **2** Departments of Neural Regeneration and Cell Communication, Mie University Graduate School of Medicine, Tsu, Mie, Japan

Abstract

Neutrophil extracellular traps (NETs) represent extracellular microbial trapping and killing. Recently, it has been implicated in thrombogenesis, autoimmune disease, and cancer progression. The aim of this study was to characterize NETs in various organs of a murine sepsis model *in vivo* and to investigate their associations with platelets, leukocytes, or vascular endothelium. NETs were classified as two distinct forms; cell-free NETs that were released away from neutrophils and anchored NETs that were anchored to neutrophils. Circulating cell-free NETs were characterized as fragmented or cotton-like structures, while anchored NETs were characterized as linear, reticular, membranous, or spot-like structures. In septic mice, both anchored and cell-free NETs were significantly increased in postcapillary venules of the cecum and hepatic sinusoids with increased leukocyte-endothelial interactions. NETs were also observed in both alveolar space and pulmonary capillaries of the lung. The interactions of NETs with platelet aggregates, leukocyte-platelet aggregates or vascular endothelium of arterioles and venules were observed in the microcirculation of septic mice. Microvessel occlusions which may be caused by platelet aggregates or leukocyte-platelet aggregates and heterogeneously decreased blood flow were also observed in septic mice. NETs appeared to be associated with the formation of platelet aggregates or leukocyte-platelet aggregates. These observational findings may suggest the adverse effect of intravascular NETs on the host during a sepsis.

Editor: Marc van Zandvoort, Maastricht University, Netherlands

Funding: This work was partly supported by grants from the Ministry of Education, Culture, Sports, Science, and Technology of Japan (KAKENHI 25462052 to KT and 25462771 to YK). No additional external funding was received for this study. The funder had no role in study design, data collection and analysis, decision to publish, or preparation of the manuscript.

Competing Interests: The authors have declared that no competing interests exist.

* Email: qouji@clin.medic.mie-u.ac.jp

Introduction

Neutrophil extracellular traps (NETs) are known to be part of an antimicrobial defense system. They are released from neutrophils activated by phorbol myristate acetate, interleukin-8, lipopolysaccharide (LPS), and various pathogens [1]. They exhibit fibrous mesh-like, web-like, or string-like structures and are composed of DNA, histones, and granule proteins such as neutrophil elastase or myeloperoxidase [2]. At present, NETs research focused on not only exploring its physiological role [3,4], but also its pathophysiological relevance in various diseases including thrombogenesis [5,6], atherosclerosis [7,8], autoimmune disease [9,10], and cancer metastasis [11,12]. In addition to the function of extracellular bacterial trapping and killing, the adverse effect of NETs on the host in inflammation has been studied extensively.

To understand the beneficial and harmful effect of NETs on host cells, dynamic observations of when, where, and how neutrophils release NETs is needed.

Both a spinning disk confocal microscopy [11,13–15] and a multiphoton microscopy (MPM) [7,8] have been used for *in vivo* NETs imaging, which contribute to analyze the dynamics of neutrophils at the cellular level. To explore the physiological or pathophysiological relevance of NETs, intravital imaging is necessary for direct observation of when, where, and how neutrophils release NETs.

We have developed a method of intravital imaging for intra-abdominal organs using a MPM which provides higher resolution, increased tissue penetration, and reduced photo-damage [16,17]. The system allows us to capture high-magnification, high-resolution images of exteriorized living tissue, from the surface to several micrometers depth [18–23]. Previously, we have visualized in vivo real-time bacterial translocation in dextran sodium sulfate-induced colitis [18], thrombus formation in the laser-induced endothelium injury [19], three-dimensional steroid efficacy for DSS-induced colitis [20], colorectal liver metastatic formation [21], and chemotherapy response on the tumor microenvironment of colorectal liver metastases [22,23].

In this study, we characterized NETs *in vivo* in various organs of a LPS-induced sepsis model using green fluorescent protein transgenic mice. We also investigate the associations between intravascular NETs and platelets, leukocytes, or vascular endothelium in a murine sepsis model.

Materials and Methods

Ethics Statement

This study was reviewed and approved by the Institutional Review Board and the Local Ethics Committee of the Mie University Graduate School of Medicine (No. 2225). Written informed consent was obtained from all the patients (adults) enrolled onto the study. The experimental protocols of in vivo studies were reviewed and approved by the Animal Care and Use Committee at the Mie University Graduate School of Medicine.

Antibodies and Reagents

Goat anti-mouse histone H2AX and goat anti-mouse neutrophil elastase (NE) antibodies were purchased from Santa Cruz Biotechnology (Santa Cruz, CA, USA). SYTOX Green and Orange nucleic acid stains and Zenon Alexa Fluor immunoglobulin G (IgG) labeling kits were purchased from Invitrogen (Carlsbad, CA, USA). LPS (Escherichia coli, serotype 0111:B4) was purchased from Sigma-Aldrich (St. Louis, MO, USA). Deoxyribonuclease I (DNase I) was purchased from Roche Applied Science (Mannheim, Germany). Isolectin GS-IB4 conjugated with Alexa Fluor 594 was purchased from Invitrogen (Carlsbad, CA, USA). Rat anti-mouse monoclonal antibodies against Gr-1 and CD31 were purchased from BD Pharmingen (San Diego, CA, USA).

Mice

Wild-type C57/BL6 mice and enhanced GFP (EGFP)-transgenic C57/BL6-Tg (CAG-EGFP) mice [24] were purchased from Japan SLC (Shizuoka, Japan). The 10- to 12-week-old male mice were bred, housed in groups of six mice per cage, and fed with a pelleted basal diet (CE-7; CLEA Japan, Tokyo, Japan) and had free access to drinking water. Mice were kept in the animal house facilities at the Mie University School of Medicine under standard conditions of humidity (50%±10%), temperature (23±2°C) and light (12/12-h light/dark cycle), according to the Institutional Animal Care Guidelines.

Isolation of Human Neutrophils

Venous blood (6ml each) was obtained from healthy human volunteers (n = 5). Neutrophils were isolated by density gradient centrifugation (at 500 g for 30 min) using Polymorphprep solution (Axis Shield PoC AS, Oslo, Norway) according to the manufacturer's instructions. Neutrophils were resuspended in RPMI 1640 without phenol red supplemented with 1% fetal bovine serum. Neutrophil purity was confirmed to be routinely >90%, as assessed by May-Grünwald Giemsa staining on the blood smear. The institutional review board of the Mie University Graduate School of Medicine approved the study (No. 2225). All patients provided written informed consent for collection of samples and subsequent analysis.

Isolation of Murine Leukocytes

Heparinized blood was withdrawn from the inferior vena cava of anesthetized wild-type C57/BL6 mice or GFP mice. Ammonium-chloride-potassium (ACK) lysing buffer (Lonza, Walkersville, MD, USA) was used to lyse the red blood cells. After ACK treatment, the blood cells that remained included white blood cells (leukocytes) and platelets. They were suspended in the above mentioned medium. Final leukocyte concentration was determined by hemacytometer. The Animal Care and Use Committee at the Mie University Graduate School of Medicine reviewed and approved the experimental protocols (No. 24–26).

LPS-Induced Sepsis Model

LPS at a dose of 20 mg/kg was administered intraperitoneally to wild-type C57/BL6 mice or GFP mice.

Quantification of Plasma DNA

Heparinized blood was obtained from control (LPS-untreated) and LPS-treated mice (5–10 mice at each time point). Blood plasma was separated by centrifugation and stored at −80°C until analysis. Plasma DNA was quantified using a Quant-iTTM PicoGreen dsDNA Assay Kit according to the manufacturer's instructions. In brief, plasma was diluted 10-fold with Tris-EDTA buffer and mixed with an equal volume of PicoGreen reagent. The PicoGreen dye that was bound to double-stranded DNA (dsDNA) was measured using a fluorescence microplate reader (2030 ARVO X; Perkin Elmer, Waltham, MA, USA). The DNA concentration was calculated using a standard curve generated from a series of Lambda DNA standard (100 µg/ml) provided by the manufacturer.

Quantification of *Ex Vivo* NETs

Human neutrophils or murine leukocytes obtained from wild-type C57/BL6 mice were suspended in the above-mentioned medium. Human neutrophils or murine leukocytes (1×10^4 per well) were seeded in 96-well plates and stimulated with LPS at indicated concentrations (2, 20, 100, and 200 µg/mL). The plates were placed in a humidified incubator at 37°C with CO2 (5%) for 6 h. To detect NETs in the culture supernatants, the culture supernatant of each well (100 µL) was collected and transferred to another well. dsDNA in the culture supernatants were measured by a PicoGreen dsDNA Assay Kit. After removal of culture supernatants, fresh medium was added to each well. The PicoGreen dsDNA Assay Kit was also used to detect NETs anchored to neutrophils on the culture well.

Visualization of *Ex Vivo* Nets by Fluorescence Microscopy

Human neutrophils or murine leukocytes obtained from wild-type C57/BL6 mice (1×10^4 per well) were stimulated with LPS for 6 h. A cell-impermeable DNA binding dye, SYTOX Green (5 µM), was added to each well. Ex vivo NETs stained by SYTOX Green were visualized and identified as extracellular DNAs with fibrous structures by fluorescence microscopy (IX71; Olympus, Tokyo, Japan).

Visualization of *Ex Vivo* NETs by MPM

Human neutrophils or murine leukocytes obtained from GFP mice (5×10^5 per well) were seeded onto 16-mm polylysine-coated coverslips in 12-well tissue culture plates and allowed to adhere at 37°C and 5% CO2 for 15 min. Then, cells were stimulated with LPS (20 µg/mL) for 6 h. Zenon Alexa Fluor IgG labeling kits were used to make Alexa Fluor 594-labeled anti-histone or anti-NE antibodies with a modified procedure [14].

For visualization of in vivo NETs by MPM, we confirmed whether SYTOX Orange, Alexa Fluor 594-labeled anti-histone, or anti-NE antibodies can interact with ex vivo NETs and whether their interactions can be visualized immediately by MPM without cell fixation (ex vivo live cell imaging).

Ex vivo NETs on coverslips were directly stained with SYTOX Orange (for human neutrophils and murine leukocytes), Alexa Fluor 594 labeled anti-histone, or anti-NE antibodies (for murine leukocytes) without cell fixation. They were visualized immediately using MPM (FV1000-2P laser-scanning microscope system; FLUOVIEW FV1000MPE, Olympus, Tokyo, Japan).

Setup of MPM

Experiments were performed using an upright microscope (BX61WI; Olympus, Tokyo, Japan) and a FV1000-2P laser-scanning microscope system (FLUOVIEW FV1000MPE; Olympus, Tokyo, Japan) as described previously [18,19]. The use of special stage risers enabled the unit to have an exceptionally wide working distance. This permitted the stereotactically immobilized, anesthetized mouse to be placed on the microscope stage. The microscope was fitted with several lenses with high numeric apertures to provide the long working distances required for in vivo work, and with water-immersion optics. The excitation source in MPM mode was Mai Tai Ti:sapphire lasers (Spectra Physics, Mountain View, CA), tuned and mode-locked at 910 nm. The Mai Tai produces light pulses of about 100 fs width (repetition rate 80 MHz). Laser light reached the sample through the microscope objectives, connected to an upright microscope (BX61WI; Olympus, Tokyo, Japan).

A mean laser power at the sample was between 10 and 40 mW, depending on the depth of imaging. Microscope objective lens used in this study were 20× UPlanSApo (numerical aperture 0.75) for ex vivo imaging and 60×LUMPlanFI/IR (water dipping, numerical aperture of 0.9, working distance 2 mm) for in vivo imaging, respectively. Data were analyzed using a FV10-ASW (Olympus, Tokyo, Japan). MPM images were acquired with 512×512 pixels spatial resolution, from 211-μm field of view dimension, using a pixel dwelling time 4 μs.

Surgical Procedures for *In Vivo* MPM Imaging

As previously described [20–23], GFP mice were anesthetized with isofluorane 4 L/min (4%; Forane, Abbott, Japan). Body temperature was kept at 37°C using a heating pad. For imaging postcapillary venules, the cecum was identified and exteriorized through a laparotomy. The exteriorized cecum was optimally inflated by introducing air using a syringe with a small-bore needle. The inflated cecum was placed on an organ-stabilizing system (Japanese Patent No. 5268282) to reduce the effect of heartbeats and respiratory movements. For imaging hepatic sinusoids, the left lateral lobe of the liver was identified and exteriorized through a laparotomy. The liver lobe was put on an organ-stabilizing system using a solder lug terminal with an instant adhesive agent.

Imaging Methods

The surface of the cecum or liver was initially screened at lower magnifications by setting out the X/Y plane and adjusting the Z axis manually to detect the optimal observation area [19–22]. Each area of interest was subsequently scanned at a higher magnification (water-immersion objective 60× with or without 2× zoom) by manually setting the X/Y plane and adjusting the Z axis (either automatically or manually) to obtain high-resolution, clear MPM images. The scanning areas were 211×211 μm (600×) or 106×106 μm (600× with 2×zoom) respectively. The imaging depth was determined as a length from the tissue surface. In our experimental setting, the imaging depth ranged from 100 μm to 400 μm. The optimal high resolution images were obtained from the tissue surface up to 100 to 200 μm depth. The laser power was adjusted according to the imaging depth. When imaging at larger depths, we increase the laser power level (up to 100%) manually using laser power level controller. To image the optimal simultaneous imaging of EGFP and Alexa Fluor 594, detection sensitivity (brightness by HV) was adjusted manually for EGFP (485–510) or Alexa Fluor 594 (to 585–635), respectively.

Visualization of *In Vivo* NETs by MPM

LPS (20 mg/kg i.p.) was administered to GFP mice. After 12–24 h, systemic clinical signs such as reduced motor activity, lethargy, shivering, and piloerection were observed. The mice with these signs were used as LPS treated mice. To administer regents precisely and reliably, a catheter (M-FAC/FVC, Neuroscience, Tokyo, Japan) was placed in the femoral vein of the anaesthetized mice under surgical microscopy. After laparotomy, the cecum or liver was exteriorized and fixed using the organ-stabilizing system.

After identifying optimal areas, SYTOX Orange, Alexa Fluor 594-labeled anti-histone, or anti-NE antibodies were administered intravenously via a catheter. NETs were detected and visualized in the living mice. Color-coded green (EGFP) and red (SYTOX Orange and Alexa Fluor 594) images were recorded at the same time. Subsequently, they were merged to produce single dual-color images.

Alexa Fluor 594-labeled mouse IgG was used as isotype control for either the LPS-treated or normal control mice.

DNase I Treatment for *In Vivo* NETs

DNase I treatment has been used for the confirmation of the presence of NETs either in vitro or in vivo, since NETs (extracellular DNAs) were degraded or subtracted by DNase I [11,13–15].

After the identification of in vivo NETs in postcapillary venules of the cecum of LPS treated mice, DNase I at a dose of 1000 U was administered intravenously via a catheter (DNase I treatment group, n = 5). In control group (n = 5), the equal amount of phosphate buffered saline (PBS) was administered after NETs identification.

To minimize the photobleaching for NETs during the observation, we recorded the time course of change in NETs by a method of 30 sec-imaging followed by 90 sec-pause for at least 30 min (at least 15 cycles) manually.

Quantification of Leukocyte-Endothelial Interaction *In Vivo*

We observed that leukocytes were adhering to the vascular endothelium of the postcapillary venules in LPS-injected mice.

The number of leukocyte-endothelial interactions was counted in 10 randomly selected fields (×600; 211 μm×211 μm square) with intravital MPM imaging.

The average number per field (211 μm×211 μm square) was expressed as the number of leukocyte-endothelial interaction per field of view (FOV).

Quantification of *In Vivo* NETs

Intravascular NETs were identified by SYTOX Orange, Alexa Fluor 594-labeled anti-histone antibody, or Alexa Fluor 594-labeled anti-NE antibody.

The number of NETs present in intravascular spaces, hepatic sinusoids, and pulmonary capillaries was counted in 10 randomly selected fields (×600; 211 μm×211 μm square) with intravital MPM imaging. The sum of them (a total number of 10 fields) was expressed as the number of NETs per field of view (FOV).

Quantification of Endothelial Injury Using Isolectin GS-IB4

To visualize vascular endothelium in vivo real-time, isolectin GS-IB4 conjugated with Alexa Fluor 594 (invitrogen, Carlsbad, CA, USA) were administered to the living mice [19] Isolectin GS-IB4 positive endothelial cells were visualized in hepatic sinusoids (in vivo) or pulmonary capillaries (ex vivo). Endothelial injury was defined as isolectin GS-IB4 negative microvascular area.

Isolectin GS-IB4 positive endothelial cells were evaluated in 10 randomly selected fields (×600; 211 μm×211 μm square) by MPM imaging. The percentage of endothelial integrity (isolectin GS-IB4 positive staining) was calculated by dividing the area of isolectin GS-IB4 positive staining by the total area of microvascular area.

Finally, endothelial integrity was scored as 0 (0%), 1 (1–25%), 2 (26–50%), 3 (51–75%), and 4 (76–100%) according to the percentage of isolectin GS-IB4 positive endothelial cells. The endothelial integrity per FOV (211 μm×211 μm square) was determined by averaging the scores of 10 FOVs.

Measurement of Blood Flow Speed

Blood flow speed was evaluated using the line-shift-diagram method in a 100-μm segment of the vessel [19]. In brief, platelet velocity was calculated by measuring the distance of platelet traveled between two consecutive images divided by the time interval between these two images. The platelet for blood velocity measurement was carefully selected after confirming to be identical between two consecutive images.

Immunohistochemistry for Gr-1 and CD31

Tissue sections (7 μm thick) were washed in phosphate-buffered saline (PBS), and immersed in a 0.3% hydrogen peroxide in methanol for 5 min to block endogenous peroxidase activity. Nonspecific-binding sites were blocked with normal goat serum (Vector Laboratories Inc., Burlingame, CA, USA) for 60 min. Sections were then incubated with primary rat anti-mouse monoclonal antibodies against Gr-1 (1:250; BD Pharmingen, San Diego, CA, USA) and CD31 (1:100; BD Pharmingen, San Diego, CA, USA) for 2 h at 4°C. After washing with PBS, sections were incubated with a horseradish peroxidase (HRP)-conjugated goat anti-mouse IgG (H+L) (KPL, Gaithersburg, MD, USA) at a 1:200 dilution for 30 min at room temperature. The specific staining was visualized via a 3,3′-diaminobenzidine (DAB) substrate. The sections were counterstained with Mayer's hematoxylin. As negative control, tissue sections were prepared by omitting the primary antibody.

Quantification of Neutrophil Recruitment By Gr-1 Immunostaining

Neutrophils were identified as Gr-1 immunoreactive cells. Gr-1 positive neutrophils were counted in a high-power field (HPF; ×200) of 10 randomly selected areas by a light microscopy. The number of neutrophil recruitment per HPF was determined by averaging the counts of 10 HPFs.

Quantification of Endothelial Injury by CD31 Immunostaining

Endothelial cells were quantified by CD31 immunostaining. CD31 positive staining was detected in hepatic sinusoids or pulmonary capillaries. Endothelial injury was defined as CD31 negative microvascular area.

CD31 immunostaining was evaluated in a high-power field (HPF; ×200) of 10 randomly selected areas by a light microscopy. The percentage of endothelial integrity (CD31 positive staining) was calculated by dividing the area of CD31 positive staining by the total area of microvascular area.

Finally, endothelial integrity was scored as 0 (0%), 1 (1–25%), 2 (26–50%), 3 (51–75%), and 4 (76–100%) according to the percentage of CD31 positive endothelial cells.

The endothelial integrity per HPF was determined by averaging the scores of 10 HPFs.

Statistical Analysis

Statistical analyses were performed using JMP version 5 (SAS Institute Inc. Cary, NC, USA). The data were presented as the mean+standard error (SE) and were analyzed by Mann-Whitney U test. P value of less than 0.05 was considered statistically significant.

Results

Cell-Free and Anchored Nets *In Vitro*

NETs have two distinct forms [11,13–15]. One form is NETs that are released away from neutrophils (cell-free NETs), and the other is those that are anchored to neutrophils (anchored NETs). We examined the LPS induced cell-free and anchored NETs in vitro.

SYTOX Green detected NETs was significantly higher in culture supernatants than that of control in an LPS dose-dependent manner (Figure S1-A). Anchored NETs on culture wells after removal of culture supernatants was significantly higher than that of control wells in an LPS dose-dependent manner (Figure S1-B). Fluorescence microscopy showed that SYTOX Green stained both extracellular DNAs that were anchored to neutrophils (anchored NETs) and nuclei of non-viable neutrophils (Figure S1-C).

Morphological Characteristics of Nets *Ex Vivo*

We examined morphological features of NETs ex vivo. NETs were stained by SYTOX Orange (A), Alexa Fluor 594-labeled anti-histone antibody (B), and Alexa Fluor 594-labeled anti-NE antibody (C).

By SYTOX Orange staining, NETs were characterized as linear structures (Figure S2-A-i), reticular structures anchored to leukocytes (Figure S2-A-ii), reticulolinear structures anchored to leukocytes (Figure S1-A-iii), and spot-like structures anchored to leukocytes (Figure S2-A-iv).

Morphological characteristics of NETs stained by Alexa Fluor 594-labeled anti-histone (Figure S2-B) or NE (Figure S2-C) antibody were similar to those stained by SYTOX Orange. NETs were also characterized as membranous structures (Figure S2-C-iii).

Plasma Cell-Free DNA in a Murine Sepsis Model

Plasma cell-free DNA has been used as a surrogate marker of circulating cell-free NETs [5,6]. To determine the optimal timing of the observation of in vivo NETs, we examined the amount of plasma DNA at the indicated time points after LPS administration.

As shown in Figure S3, plasma DNA was significantly increased in LPS-treated mice compared with normal control mice with a peak at 24 h after the intraperitoneal administration of LPS at a dose of 20 mg/kg whose mortality rate was approximately 50%.

In Vivo Nets in Postcapillary Venules of the Cecum

The leukocyte-endothelial interaction was frequently initiated at the postcapillary venules [25]. Since the LPS-induced adhesion of leukocytes or platelet binding leukocytes to the vascular endothelium was observed in postcapillary venules of the cecum, we hypothesized that anchored NETs might be observed there most frequently.

After the intraperitoneal administration of LPS at a dose of 20 mg/kg, NETs were observed as reticular structures anchored to leukocytes (Figure 1-A-i; Movie S1), reticulolinear structures (Figure 1-A-ii), spot-like structures anchored to leukocytes (Figure 1-A-iii, iv), membranous structures on the surface of leukocytes (Figure 1-A-v) and linear structures anchored to leukocytes (Figure 1-A-vi; Movie S2). Neither anchored nor circulating cell-free NETs were observed in normal control mice. In addition, no rolling or circulating leukocytes with NETs were seen.

The number of leukocyte-endothelial interactions per FOV and the number of NETs per FOV were determined as described in materials and methods. The number of leukocyte-endothelial interactions per FOV were significantly greater in LPS treated mice than control mice (Fig. 1-B; 14.6±1.6 vs 0.6±0.2, $p<0.01$). The number of in vivo NETs per FOV was also significantly greater in LPS treated mice than control mice (Fig. 1-C; 4.4±0.4 vs 0.2±0.1, $p<0.01$). The percentage of NETs to leukocyte-endothelial interactions was approximately 3% (4.4/146). NETs seemed to be the rare event in vivo, as compared with leukocyte-endothelial interaction.

Interestingly, we observed leukocytes showing cytoplasmic vacuoles that adhered to vascular endothelium in LPS-treated mice at the subcellular level (Figure S4-i, ii; arrows). They were more frequently observed in postcapillary venules of the cecum than arterioles or hepatic sinusoids. Some of them released NETs (Figure S4-iii, iv; arrows). These findings may indicate a NETosis, which is defined as a distinct cell death related to NETs [26,27].

In Vivo NETs in Hepatic Sinusoids of the Liver

Neutrophils recruit to hepatic sinusoids during inflammation [11,13,14]. After LPS administration, leukocyte accumulation and platelet aggregation were observed in hepatic sinusoids of the liver. NETs were also observed as spot-like structures anchored to leukocytes (Figure 2-A-i, ii; Movie S3), cell-free DNA fragments (Figure 2-A-iii; Movie S4), and cell-free DNA fragments within platelet aggregates (Figure 2-A-iv). The number of in vivo NETs per FOV was significantly greater in LPS treated mice than normal control mice (Figure 2-B; 1.7±0.2 vs 0.2±0.1, $p<0.01$).

NETs have been reported to cause endothelial dysfunction or injury [27,28]. To visualize endothelial injury of hepatic sinusoids, isolectin GS-IB4 conjugated with Alexa Fluor 594 was used as described in materials and methods. Isolectin GS-IB4 stained hepatic sinusoidal endothelial cells were observed in LPS-treated mice (Figure 2-A-v) and normal mice (Figure 2-A-vi). The score of endothelial integrity based on the percentage of isolectin GS-IB4 positive endothelial cells was significantly lower in LPS treated mice than control mice (Figure 2-C; 2.0±0.3 vs 3.6±0.2, $p<0.01$).

Contrary to previous reports [11,13], widespread web-like NETs was not observed in hepatic sinusoids. Therefore, the endothelial injury in hepatic sinusoids might be mainly caused by severe LPS-induced inflammation rather than NETs.

NETs in Pulmonary Capillaries of the Lung

After imaging of the cecum and liver, excised lungs (ex vivo) were observed immediately to examine NETs in the lung.

NETs were observed in alveolar space (Figure 3-A-i; arrows) and pulmonary capillaries (Figure 3-A-i; arrowheads) of LPS-treated mice. The number of NETs per FOV was significantly greater in LPS-treated mice than control mice (Figure 3-B; 6.4±1.1 vs 0.3±0.1, $p<0.01$). Circulating cell-free NETs appeared to be entrapped in pulmonary capillaries rather than hepatic sinusoids.

Isolectin GS-IB4 stained alveolar capillary endothelial cells of excised lungs were observed in LPS-treated mice (Figure 3-A-iii) and normal mice (Figure 3-A-iv). The score of endothelial integrity based on the percentage of isolectin GS-IB4 positive endothelial cells was 2.8±0.2 in LPS treated mice and 3.7±0.2 in normal control mice, respectively. The difference was not statistically significant (Figure 3-C; $p = 0.057$).

Contrary to the previous reports [11,14], widespread web-like NETs was not observed in pulmonary capillaries, indicating that the endothelial injury might be mainly caused by LPS-induced inflammation rather than NETs.

Circulating Cell-Free NETs

Circulating cell-free NETs were observed in the blood flow of postcapillary venules of the cecum (Figure 4-i, ii) as well as hepatic sinusoids of the liver (Figure 2-A-iii, iv). Circulating cell-free NETs were characterized as fragmented or cotton-like structures. Their shape seemed to depend on blood flow speed.

Figure 4-iii (Movie S5) shows that NETs were anchored to the leukocyte adhering to the vascular endothelium. Thereafter, NETs were leaving away from leukocyte, changing shape from solid to cotton-like, and flowing down the vessel. These cotton-like NETs were arrested far away from the leukocyte (Figure 4-iv).

Association between *In Vivo* Nets and Platelets, Endothelial Cells, or Leukocyte-Platelet Aggregates

NETs have been reported to induce platelet aggregation followed by thrombus formation [5], and also induce endothelial damage or dysfunction [28,29]. We observed the association between in vivo NETs and platelets, leukocytes, or vascular endothelium.

Circulating cell-free NETs were binding to platelet aggregates (Figure 5-i; Movie S6). Platelets were aggregating to cell-free NETs (Figure 5-ii; arrow). Furthermore, cell-free NETs appeared to be a template for platelet thrombus formation (Figure 5-ii; arrowhead). Circulating cell-free NETs were also adhering to vascular endothelium in both venule (Figure 5-iii) and arteriole (Figure 5-iv; Movie S7). NETs-leukocyte-platelet aggregates were observed in venules (Figure 5-v, vi). NETs seemed to be released from the leukocyte with cytoplasmic vacuoles (Figure 5-vi; arrowhead, arrow, Movie S8) [25,26].

These observations may suggest that cell-free NETs seem to interact with platelets, leukocytes, or vascular endothelium.

Although the direct effect of NETs on these phenomena could not yet be clarified in this study, our observational findings may support the previous reports about the association between NETs and thrombus formation or endothelial cell damage [5,28,29].

Association between *In Vivo* Nets and Microcirculation

Microvascular thrombosis may cause microvascular occlusions, resulting in tissue ischemia and organ failure [30,31].

Since the mortality rate at 24 h after the intraperitoneal administration of LPS at a dose of 20 mg/kg was approximately 50%, the survived mice (the other 50% of LPS administered mice) were used as LPS treated mice in this study. We observed that the microvessel appeared to be occluded by platelet aggregates or leukocyte-platelet aggregates in the almost dying mice. (Figure 6-A-i, ii; arrows, Movie S9). In some of them, cell-free NETs appeared to be a template for leukocyte-platelet aggregates (Figure 6-A-iii, iv; arrows). Leukocyte-platelet aggregates some-

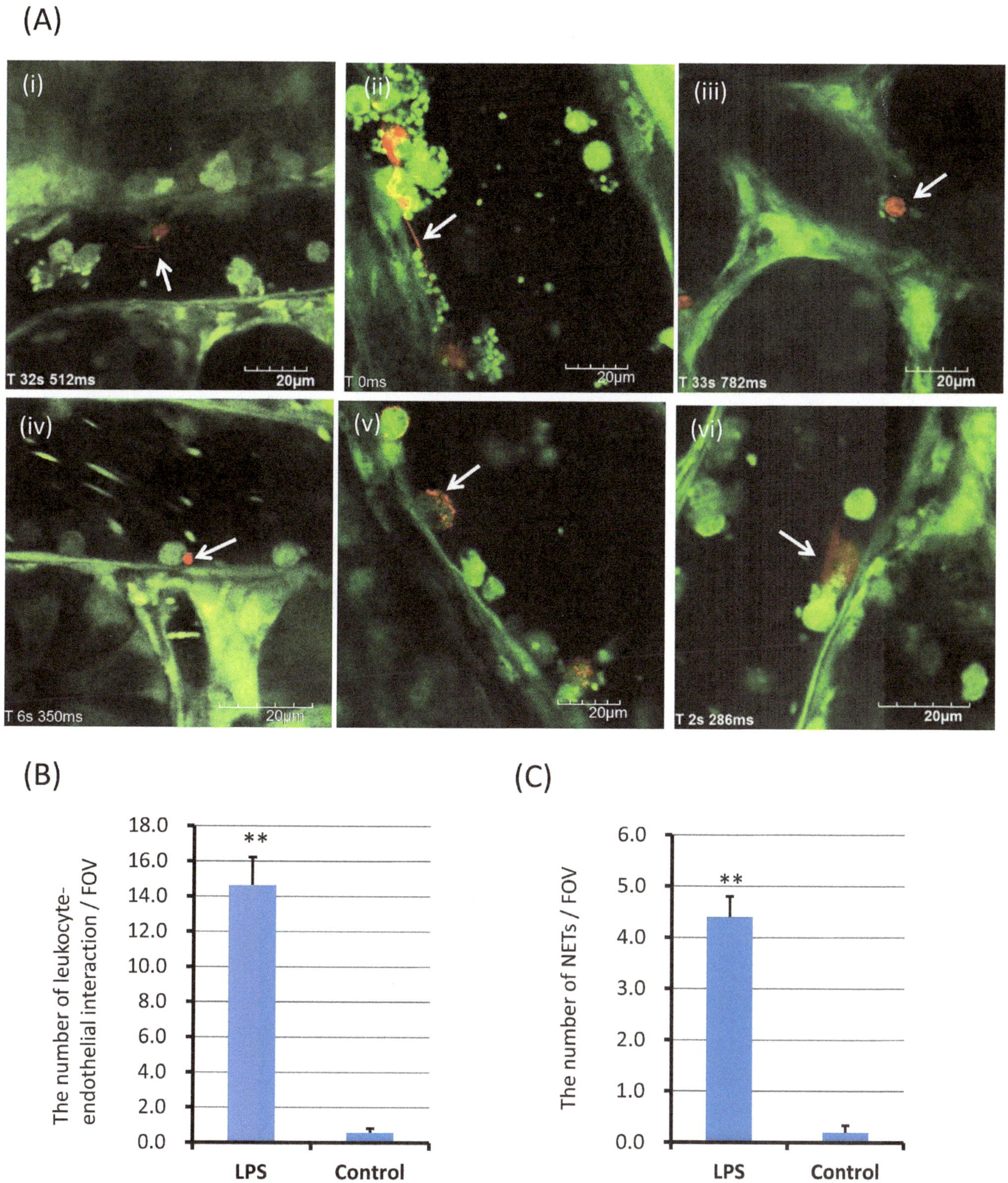

Figure 1. ***In vivo*** **NETs in postcapillary venules of the cecum.** The postcapillary venules of the cecum were observed at 24 h after LPS (20 mg/kg) intraperitoneal administration (n = 10). NETs (red) were detected by SYTOX Orange, Alexa Fluor 594-labeled anti-histone antibody, or Alexa Fluor 594-labeled anti-NE antibody, respectively. NETs were characterized as reticular structures anchored to leukocytes (A-i; Movie S1), reticulolinear structures (A-ii), spot-like structures anchored to leukocytes (A-iii, iv), membranous structures on the surface of leukocytes (A-v) and linear structures anchored to leukocytes (A-vi; Movie S2). The number of leukocyte-endothelial interactions and NETs per FOV was determined as described in materials and methods, respectively. The number of leukocyte-endothelial interactions per FOV (B) were significantly greater in LPS treated mice than control mice (14.6±1.6 vs 0.6±0.2). The number of NETs per FOV (C) was also significantly greater in LPS treated mice than control mice (4.4±0.4 vs 0.2±0.1). Data was presented as mean+standard error. **P<0.01 versus control.

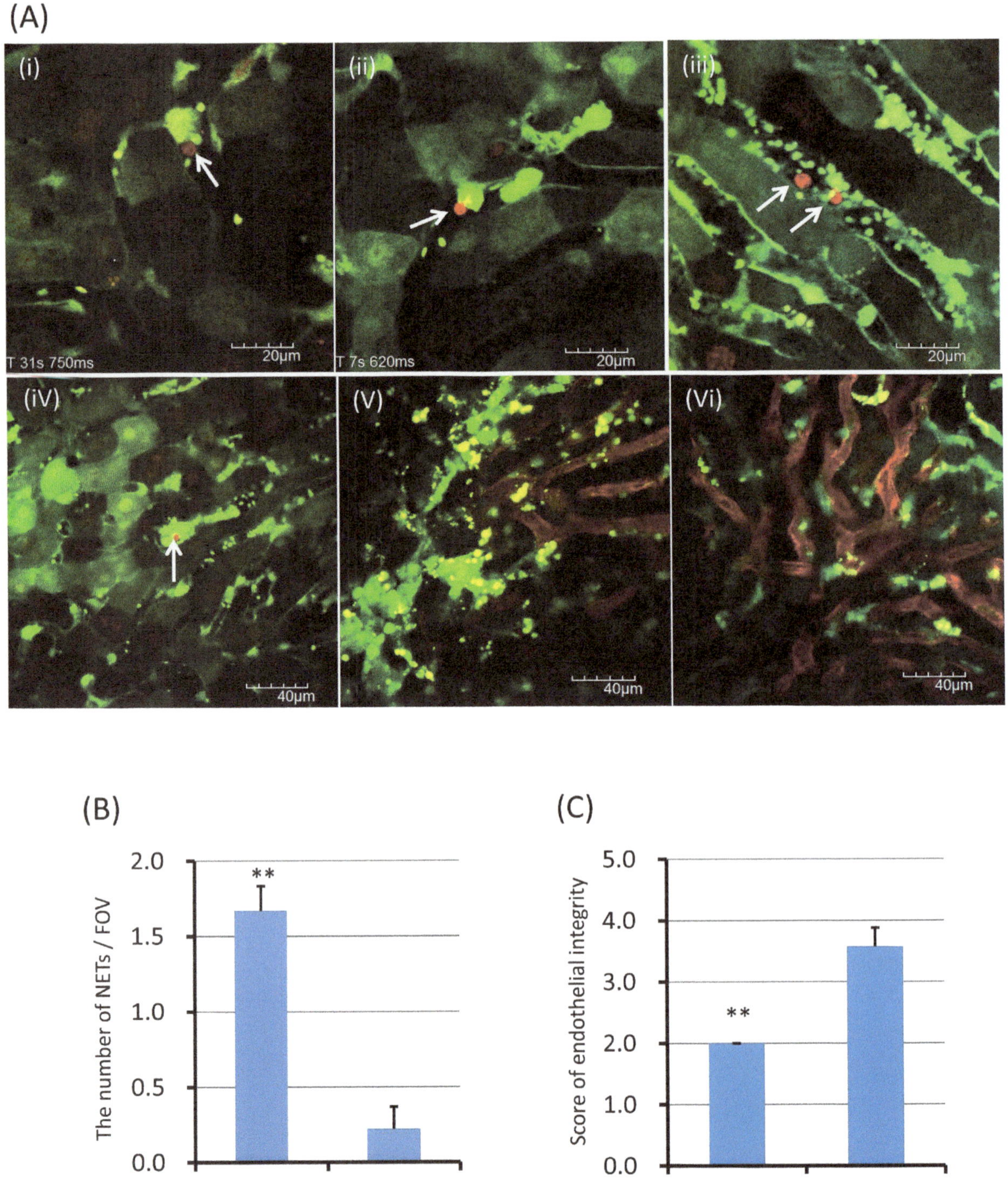

Figure 2. ***In vivo*** **NETs in hepatic sinusoids of the liver.** The hepatic sinusoids were observed at 24 h after LPS (20 mg/kg) intraperitoneal administration (n = 10). NETs (red) were detected by SYTOX Orange, Alexa Fluor 594-labeled anti-histone antibody, or Alexa Fluor 594-labeled anti-NE antibody, respectively. NETs were characterized as spot-like structures anchored to leukocytes (A-i, ii; Movie S3), cell-free DNA fragments (A-iii; Movie S4), and cell-free DNA fragments within platelet aggregates (A-iv). Isolectin GS-IB4 stained hepatic sinusoidal endothelial cells were observed in LPS-treated mice (A-v) and normal mice (A-vi). The number of NETs per FOV and the score of endothelial integrity were determined as described in materials and methods, respectively. The number of NETs per FOV (B) was significantly greater in LPS treated mice than normal control mice (1.7±0.2 vs 0.2±0.1). The score of endothelial integrity (C) was significantly less in LPS treated mice than control mice (.0±0.3 vs 3.6±0.2). Data was presented as mean+standard error. **P<0.01 versus control.

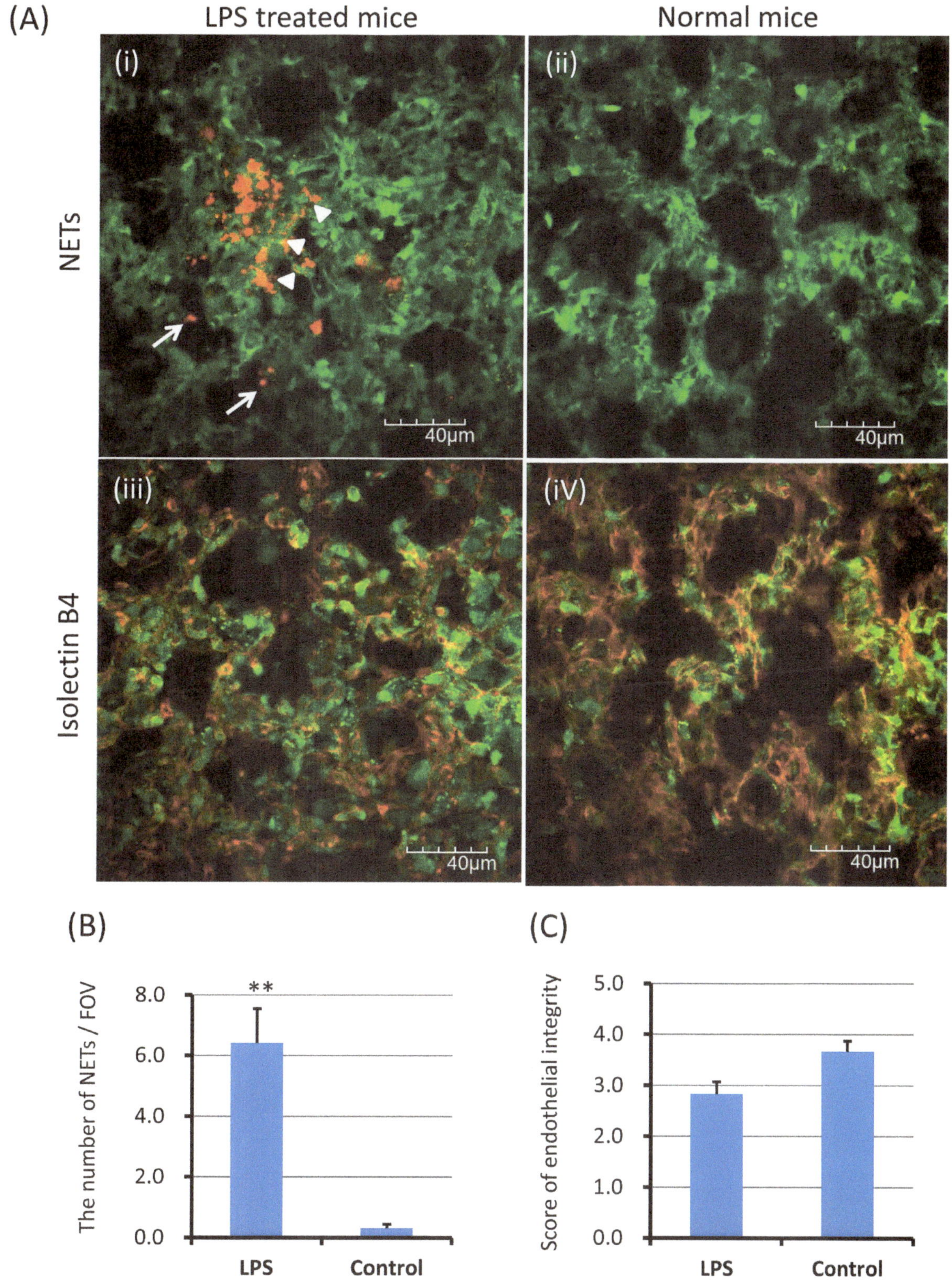

Figure 3. NETs in pulmonary capillaries of the lung. The excised lungs were investigated immediately after intravital imaging of the cecum and liver to evaluate NETs and endothelial injury. NETs (red) were observed in alveolar space (A-i; arrows) and pulmonary capillaries (A-i; arrowheads) of LPS-treated mice. The number of NETs per FOV and the score of endothelial integrity were determined as described in materials and methods, respectively. The number of NETs per FOV was significantly greater in LPS-treated mice than control mice (B; 6.4±1.1 vs 0.3±0.1). The score of endothelial integrity (C) was lower in LPS treated mice than control mice (2.8±0.2 vs 3.7±0.2). Data was presented as mean+standard error. **P<0.01 versus control.

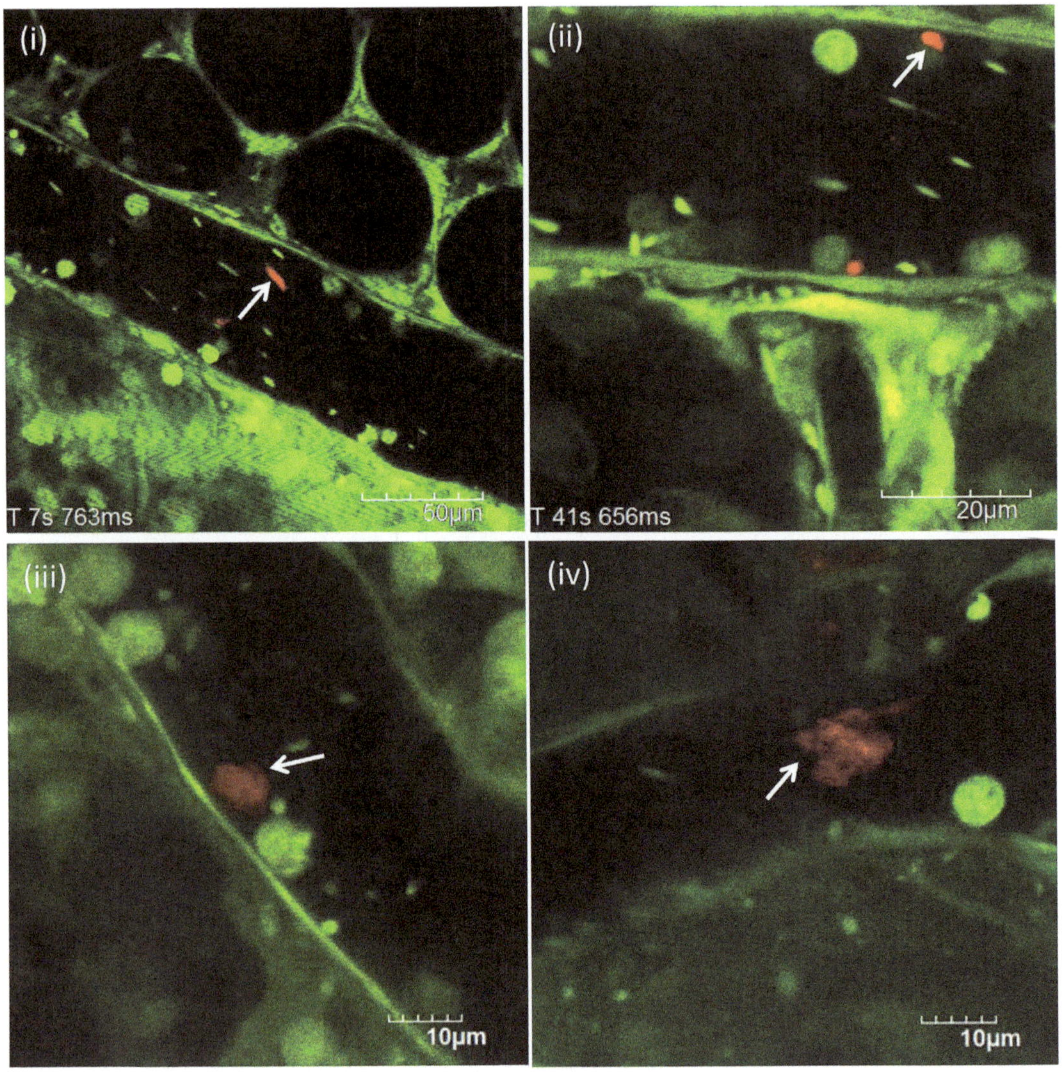

Figure 4. Circulating cell-free NETs. Circulating cell-free NETs (red) were observed in the blood flow of either postcapillary venules of the cesum or hepatic sinusoids of the liver (i, ii) at 24 h after LPS (20 mg/kg) intraperitoneal administration (n = 10). NETs were anchored to the leukocyte adhering to the vascular endothelium (iii; Movie S5). Thereafter, NETs were leaving away from leukocyte, changing shape from solid to cotton-like, and flowing down the vessel. These cotton-like NETs were arrested far away from the leukocyte (iv). They were not observed in control mice.

times included leukocytes with cytoplasmic vacuoles (Figure 6-A-ii; arrowheads).

The blood flow of cecal venules and hepatic sinusoids in LPS-treated mice showed a to-and-fro movement and a heterogeneous flow by location. Furthermore, the blood flow of cecal venules and hepatic sinusoids was impaired earlier than that of arterioles (data not shown). As shown in Figure 6-B, blood flow speeds of arteriole ($p<0.05$), venule ($p<0.01$), and hepatic sinusoid ($p<0.01$) were significantly lower in LPS-treated mice than control, respectively.

The decreased blood flow in microcirculation may be in part caused by heterogeneous microvessel occlusion by platelet aggregates or leukocyte-platelet aggregates. Although several factors are involved in microcirculatory disturbance of a sepsis, the microvessel occlusions with platelet aggregates or leukocyte-platelet aggregates may be also one of the causes of microcirculatory disturbance in a sepsis. In addition, cell-free NETs appeared to be associated with the formation of platelet aggregates or leukocyte-platelet aggregates. However, our observational findings are still insufficient to prove the effect of NETs on microcirculatory disturbances.

Time Course of Change in Nets by Dnase I Treatment *In Vivo*

To examine the time course of change in NETs by DNase I treatment, anchored NETs with optimal size were selected in postcapillary venules of the cecum. Figure 7 shows in vivo NETs before (Figure 7-i, iii) and after (Figure 7-ii, iv) DNase I treatment.

As shown Figure 7-i, ii, NETs were degraded by DNase I treatment with decrease in both its shape and fluorescent intensity within 30 min. Figure 7-iii, iv showed that anchored NETs were disappeared nearly completely without falling apart from neutrophils. No more change in both shape and fluorescent intensity of NETs was found over 30 min in our experimental conditions.

In some cases, massive cell-free NETs were observed in the blood flow after DNase I injection (Figure 7-v; arrow). Since such massive cell-free NETs were not observed in non-DNase I

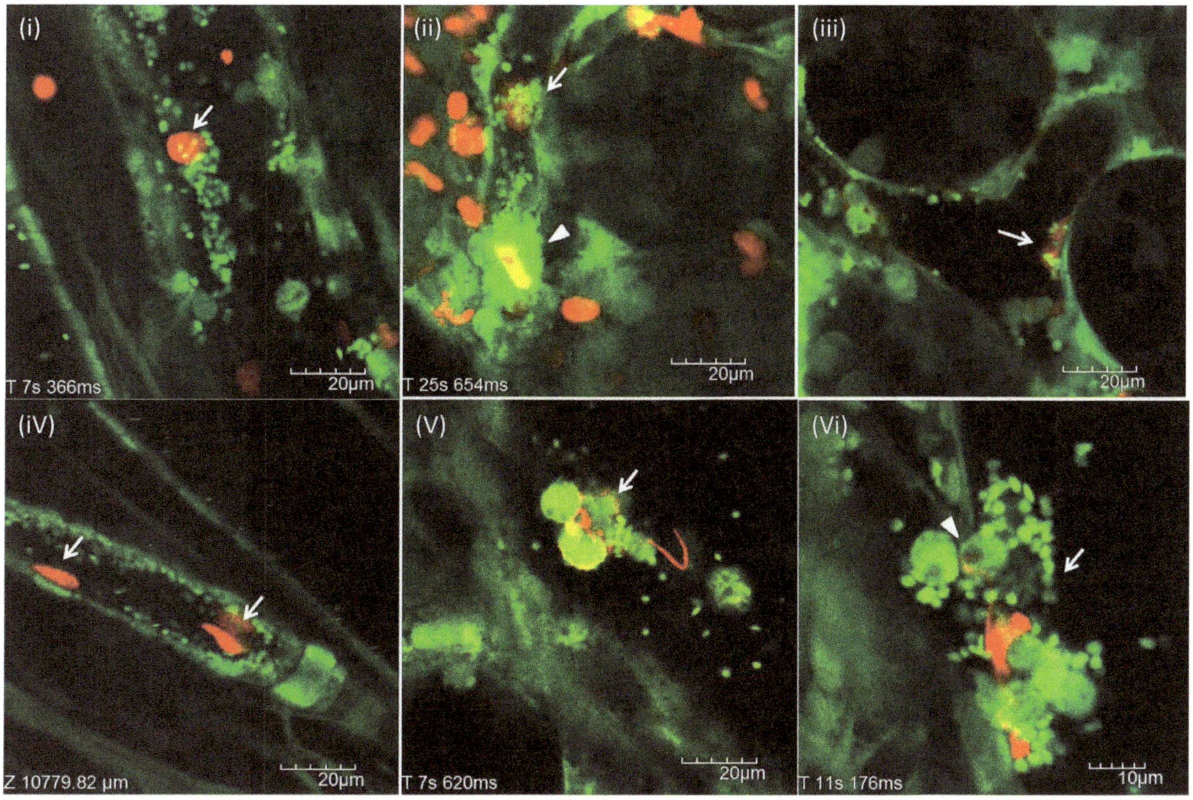

Figure 5. Association between in vivo NETs and platelets, endothelial cells, or leukocyte-platelet aggregates. Interactions of circulating cell-free NETs or anchored NETs with platelets, leukocytes, or vascular endothelium were investigated (n = 10, LPS treated mice). Circulating cell-free NETs (red) were binding to platelet aggregates (i; Movie S6). Platelets were aggregating to cell-free NETs (ii; arrow). Platelet thrombus formation was observed, in which cell-free NETs appeared to be a template for thrombus (ii; arrowhead). Circulating cell-free NETs were also adhering to vascular endothelium in both venule (iii) and arteriole (iv; Movie S7). NETs-leukocyte-platelet aggregates were observed in venules (v, vi; arrow). NETs seemed to be released from the leukocyte with cytoplasmic vacuoles (vi; arrowhead, Movie S8).

treatment group, it was speculated that the upstream anchored NETs may fall apart from neutrophils and may subsequently circulate in the blood.

There was no significant change in both shape and fluorescent intensity of NETs by the injection of the equal amount of PBS (data not shown).

Neutrophil Recruitment and Endothelial Injury in LPS Treated Mice

We also evaluated neutrophil infiltration and endothelial injury in the liver and lung of LPS treated mice by immunohistochemistry as a conventional morphological analysis.

As shown in Figure S5, the number of Gr-1 positive neutrophils was significantly higher in both liver ($p<0.01$) and lung ($p<0.01$) of LPS-treated mice than normal control mice, respectively. The score of endothelial integrity based on the percentage of CD31 positive endothelial cells was significantly lower in the lung ($p<0.05$) than normal control mice. The score of endothelial integrity was lower in the liver than normal control mice, but the difference was not statistically significant ($p = 0.057$).

Discussion

In this study, two forms of NETs were clearly characterized *in vivo*: one form is cell-freeNETs that are released away from neutrophils and circulating in the bloodstream, while the other is anchored NETs that are anchored to neutrophils adhering to the vascular endothelium.

Morphologically, anchored NETs were characterized as linear, reticular, membranous, or spot-like structures. In contrast, cell-free NETs were also characterized as fragmented or cotton-like structures. The association between these morphological features and LPS-induced inflammatory response could not be clarified, because the detection rate of anchored NETs was extremely low as compared with that of leukocyte-endothelial interactions (approximately 3%). Some reports demonstrated that the frequency of NETs might be fairly low even under optimal conditions in vitro. Among one-third of activated neutrophils, less than 10% of them might release NETs [32]. Our results may be consistent with these findings.

In vivo NETs have been characterized morphologically and functionally as previously reported [11,13–15]. McDonald et al demonstrated the LPS induced neutrophil recruitment to the liver and subsequent the production of intravascular NETs (hepatic sinusoids) [13]. They observed that NETs formed large extracellular webs which covered hepatic sinusoids far distant from the nearest neutrophil. Clark et al showed NETs within pulmonary capillaries of an LPS treated mouse [14]. Cools-Lartigue et al also revealed the widespread deposition of NETs within hepatic and pulmonary microvasculature of mice treated with cecal ligation and puncture (CLP) [11]. These all reports show the induction of widespread web-like NETs expanding the entire hepatic sinusoids and pulmonary capillaries by LPS injection or CLP.

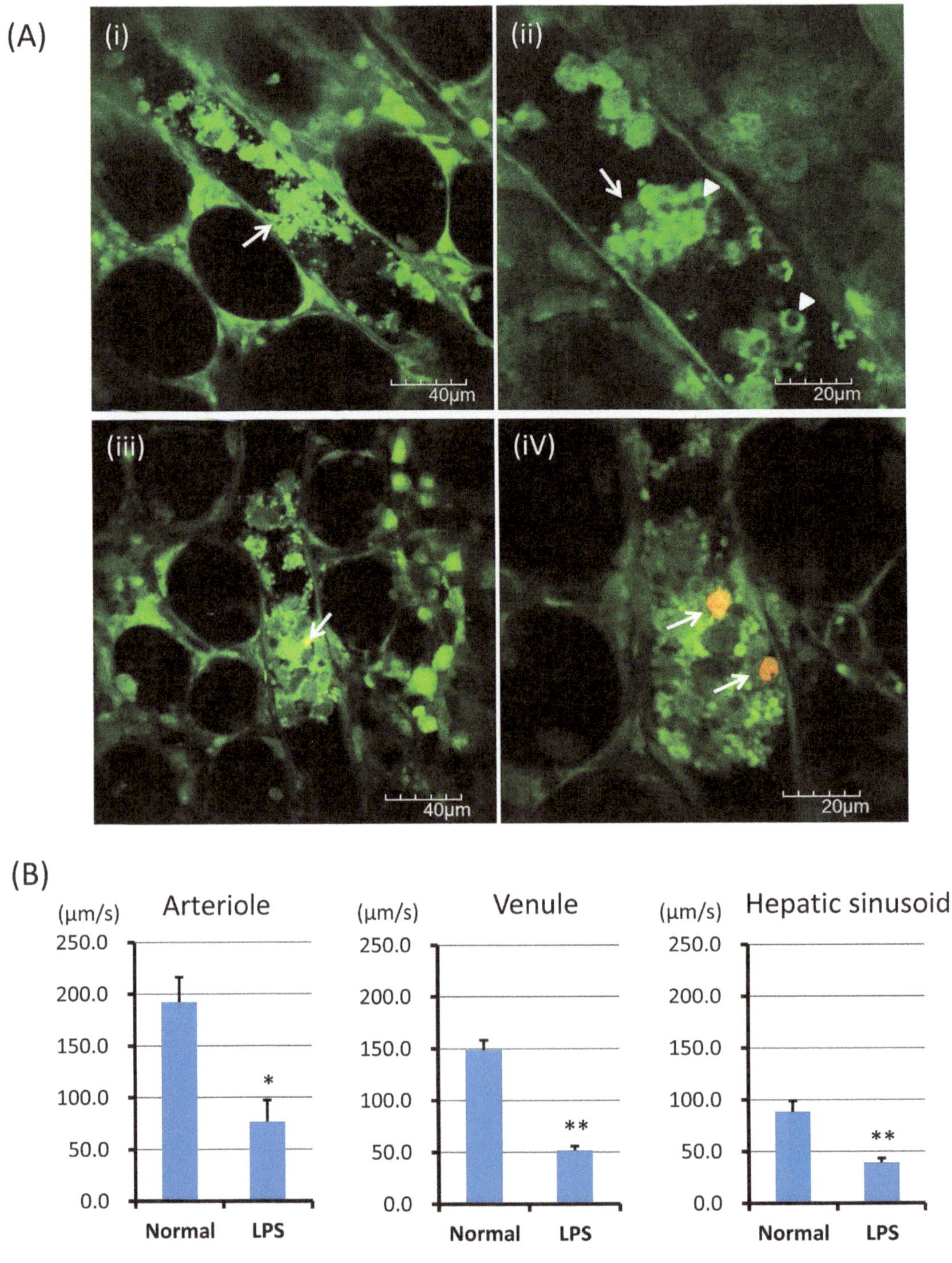

Figure 6. Association between in vivo NETs and microcirculation. Approximately 50% of mice were died from a lethal dose of LPS administration. The survived mice were used as LPS treated mice. In the almost dying mice (n = 10) among the LPS treated mice, microvessels were frequently occluded by platelet aggregates or leukocyte-platelet aggregates (A-i, ii; arrows, Movie S9). In some of them, cell-free NETs (red) appeared to be a template for leukocyte-platelet aggregates (A-iii, iv; arrows). Leukocyte-platelet aggregates sometimes included leukocytes with cytoplasmic vacuoles (A-ii; arrowheads). Blood flow speeds of arteriole, venule, and hepatic sinusoid (B) were significantly lower in LPS-treated mice than control, respectively. Data was presented as mean+standard error. *$P<0.05$, and **$P<0.01$ versus control, respectively.

Since NETs have been reported to be formed from an adherent neutrophil in vitro [14], we firstly observed postcapillary venules where leukocyte-endothelial interactions were frequently initiated and observed to detect in vivo NETs effectively. Unexpectedly, a few NETs (either cell-free or anchored form) were observed in postcapillary venules of the cecum. Contrary to the findings of in vivo NETs in previous reports [11,13,14], a few NETs were observed in both hepatic sinusoids and pulmonary capillaries.

We didn't observed neither the excess production of NETs after excess neutrophil recruitment nor the accumulation of circulating

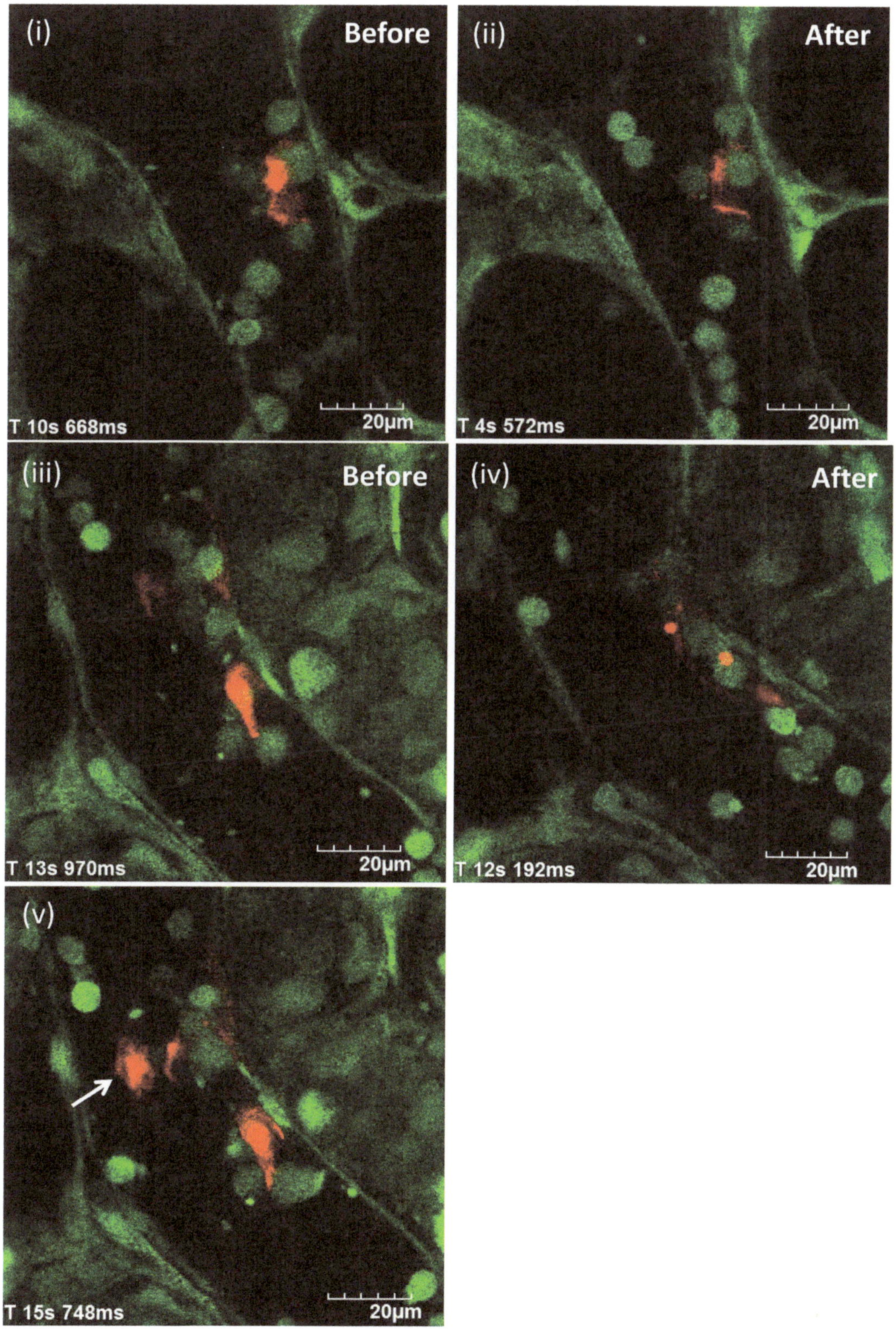

Figure 7. Time course of change in NETs by DNase I treatment *in vivo*. After the identification of in vivo NETs (red) in postcapillary venules of the cecum of LPS treated mice, DNase I at a dose of 1000 U was administered intravenously via a catheter (DNase I treatment group, n = 5). In control group (n = 5), the equal amount of phosphate buffered saline (PBS) was administered after NETs identification. Images were recorded by a method of 30 sec-imaging followed by 90 sec-pause for at least 30 min (at least 15 cycles) to minimize the photobleaching for NETs during the observation. Anchored NETs with optimal size in postcapillary venules of the cecum were selected to examine the time course of change in NETs by DNase I treatment. Figure 7 shows in vivo NETs before (Figure 7-i, iii) and after (Figure 7-ii, iv, v) DNase I treatment.

cell-free NETs in relatively low shear vascular bed such as hepatic sinusoids and pulmonary capillaries. The difference in findings of in vivo NETs between ours and the others [11,13,14] might partly depend on LPS dosage, timing of imaging, and detection method.

Recently, NETs research has focused on its adverse effect on the host [5–12] as well as the distinct function of extracellular trapping and killing pathogens [3,4]. Both nuclear and granular proteins contained in NETs seemed to induce NETs-mediated host cell cytotoxicity [28,29].

In this study, cell-free NETs appeared to interact with platelets, leukocytes, or vascular endothelium of arterioles and venules in the microcirculation of a murine sepsis model. Although we could not yet clarify the direct effect of NETs on these phenomena, our observational findings may support the previous reports about the association between NETs and thrombus formation or endothelial cell damage [5,28,29].

Sepsis is still a life-threatening condition, and defined as a systemic response to infection with the presence of organ dysfunction or failure [30,31].

The almost dying septic mice showed either complete or incomplete microvessel occlusions, which may seem to be caused by platelet aggregates or leukocyte-platelet aggregates. Although several factors are involved in microcirculatory disturbance of a sepsis, the microvessel occlusions with platelet aggregates or leukocyte-platelet aggregates may be also one of the causes of microcirculatory disturbance in a sepsis.

Our observational findings are still insufficient to prove the effect of NETs on microcirculatory disturbances of a sepsis. However, the findings that cell-free NETs appeared to be a template for platelet aggregates or leukocyte-platelet aggregates may suggest the adverse effect of NETs on the host in a sepsis.

We also observed leukocytes showing cytoplasmic vacuoles. Most of them were adhering to the vascular endothelium of postcapillary venules. These leukocytes were considered as NETosis [26,27]. Although we didn't examine the relationship between NETosis and anchored NETs or cell-free NETs, the number of NETosis (leukocytes showing cytoplasmic vacuoles) seemed to be greater than that of anchored NETs (leukocytes attaching NETs). This might be consistent with the results of quantification of cell-free and anchored NETs in vitro.

There are several limitations in our current setting, such as a limited observation area and a limited imaging time [18–23]. The number of interactions of in vivo NETs with platelet, leukocytes, and vascular endothelium observed in our experimental conditions is extremely low even in lethal condition. To proceed the research of NETs-host interactions, it is necessary to modify our experimental conditions.

However, this is the first report that has presented morphological characterization of in vivo NETs and the interactions of in vivo NETs with platelet aggregates, leukocyte-platelet aggregates and vascular endothelium in the microcirculation of a murine sepsis model.

Although further study is needed to clarify the direct effect of NETs on these observations, our results might be useful for the future NETs research.

Supporting Information

Figure S1 Cell-free and anchored NETs *in vitro*. NETs were classified as two forms: NETs that are released away from neutrophils (cell-free NETs), and those that are anchored to neutrophils (anchored NETs). In vitro study, extracellular DNA in culture supernatants was regarded as cell-free NETs, while extracellular DNA on culture wells was regarded as anchored NETs. SYTOX Green detected NETs was significantly higher in culture supernatants than that of control in human (A-i) and murine leukocytes (A-ii). Anchored NETs on culture wells after removal of culture supernatants were significantly higher than that of control wells in human (B-i) and murine leukocytes (B-ii). In fluorescence microscopic examination (C), SYTOX Green stained both extracellular DNAs that were anchored to neutrophils (anchored NETs; green) and nuclei of non-viable neutrophils (green). The data were obtained from representative results of at least three independently repeated experiments, and presented as mean+standard error. *P<0.05, and **P<0.01 versus control, respectively.

Figure S2 Morphological characteristics of NETs *ex vivo*. Murine leukocytes obtained from GFP mice (5×10^5 per well) were seeded onto 16-mm polylysine-coated coverslips in 12-well tissue culture plates. After stimulation with LPS (20 μg/mL) for 6 h, SYTOX Orange (A), Alexa Fluor 594-labeled anti-histone antibody (B), and Alexa Fluor 594-labeled anti-NE antibody (C) was used for the detection of NETs. Ex vivo leukocytes (large, round cells; green), platelets (smaller ones; green), and NETs (red) were observed. Ex vivo NETs were characterized as linear structures (A-i, B-i, and C-i), reticular structures anchored to leukocytes (A-ii, B-ii, and C-ii), reticulolinear structures anchored to leukocytes (A-iii, and B-iii), membranous structures on the surface of leukocytes (C-iii), and spot-like structures anchored to leukocytes (A-iv, B-iv, and C-iv). With regard to the detection of ex vivo NETs, SYTOX Orange, anti-histone antibody, and anti-NE antibody showed nearly same ability to stain NETs, respectively. However, SYTOX orange stained the nuclei of non-viable cells more often than the others.

Figure S3 Plasma cell-free DNA in a murine sepsis model. The intraperitoneal administration of LPS at a dose of 20 mg/kg induced severe septic condition for mice. Heparinized blood was obtained from normal control (n = 5) and LPS-treated mice (5–10 mice at each time point). The concentration of Plasma DNA was quantified using a Quant-iTTM PicoGreen dsDNA Assay Kit. Plasma DNA was significantly increased in LPS-treated mice compared with normal control mice with a peak at 24 h after LPS administration. Data was presented as mean+standard error. *P<0.05 versus control.

Figure S4 Leukocytes showing cytoplasmic vacuoles. Leukocytes showing cytoplasmic vacuoles were observed in LPS-treated mice at the subcellular level (i, ii; arrows). They were more frequently observed in postcapillary venules of the cecum than arterioles or hepatic sinusoids. Some of them released NETs (red) (iii, iv; arrows).

Figure S5 Neutrophil recruitment and endothelial injury in LPS treated mice. Neutrophil infiltration and endothelial injury in the liver and lung of LPS treated mice were evaluated by immunohistochemistry against Gr-1 and CD31, respectively. The number of Gr-1 positive neutrophils was significantly higher in both liver (p<0.01) and lung (p<0.01) of LPS-treated mice than normal control mice, respectively. The score of endothelial integrity based on the percentage of CD31 positive endothelial cells was significantly lower in the lung (p<0.05) than normal control mice. The score of endothelial integrity was lower in the liver than normal control mice, but the difference was not statistically significant (p = 0.057). Data was presented as mean+

standard error. *P<0.05, and **P<0.01 versus control, respectively.

Movie S1 Anchored NETs (reticular form) in postcapillary venules of the cecum.

Movie S2 Anchored NETs (linear form) in postcapillary venules of the cecum.

Movie S3 Anchored NETs (spot-like form) in in hepatic sinusoids of the liver.

Movie S4 Cell-free DNA in in hepatic sinusoids of the liver.

Movie S5 Circulating cell-free DNA (cotton-like form) in postcapillary venules of the cecum.

Movie S6 The binding of platelet aggregates to cell-free NETs in the venules.

Movie S7 The adhesion of cell-free NETs to vascular endothelium in the arterioles.

Movie S8 The leukocyte with cytoplasmic vacuoles and NETs.

Movie S9 Platelet aggregates and leukocyte-platelet aggregates in postcapillary venules.

Author Contributions

Conceived and designed the experiments: KT YK AM MK. Performed the experiments: KT YK TS MO SI. Analyzed the data: YT YO YI TA YM. Contributed reagents/materials/analysis tools: KT KU YM. Contributed to the writing of the manuscript: KT YK AM MK.

References

1. Brinkmann V, Reichard U, Goosmann C, Fauler B, Uhlemann Y, et al. (2004) Neutrophil extracellular traps kill bacteria. Science.303: 1532–1535.
2. Menegazzi R, Decleva E, Dri P. (2012) Killing by neutrophil extracellular traps: fact or folklore? Blood.119: 1214–1216.
3. Brinkmann V, Zychlinsky A. (2012) Neutrophil extracellular traps: is immunity the second function of chromatin? J Cell Biol.198: 773–783.
4. Caudrillier A, Kessenbrock K, Gilliss BM, Nguyen JX, Marques MB, et al. (2012) Platelets induce neutrophil extracellular traps in transfusion-related acute lung injury. J Clin Invest.122: 2661–2671.
5. Fuchs TA, Brill A, Duerschmied D, Schatzberg D, Monestier M, et al. (2010) Extracellular DNA traps promote thrombosis. Proc Natl Acad Sci U S A.107: 15880–15885.
6. Brill A, Fuchs TA, Savchenko AS, Thomas GM, Martinod K, et al. (2012) Neutrophil extracellular traps promote deep vein thrombosis in mice. J Thromb Haemost. 10: 136–144.
7. Döring Y, Manthey HD, Drechsler M, Lievens D, Megens RT, et al. (2012) Auto-antigenic protein-DNA complexes stimulate plasmacytoid dendritic cells to promote atherosclerosis. Circulation. 125: 1673–1683.
8. Megens RT, Vijayan S, Lievens D, Döring Y, van Zandvoort MA, et al. (2012) Presence of luminal neutrophil extracellular traps in atherosclerosis. Thromb Haemost. 107: 597–598.
9. Dubois AV, Gauthier A, Bréa D, Varaigne F, Diot P, et al. (2012) Influence of DNA on the activities and inhibition of neutrophil serine proteases in cystic fibrosis sputum. Am J Respir Cell Mol Biol. 47: 80–86.
10. Villanueva E, Yalavarthi S, Berthier CC, Hodgin JB, Khandpur R, et al. (2011) Netting neutrophils induce endothelial damage, infiltrate tissues, and expose immunostimulatory molecules in systemic lupus erythematosus. J Immunol. 187: 538–552.
11. Cools-Lartigue J, Spicer J, McDonald B, Gowing S, Chow S, et al. (2013) Neutrophil extracellular traps sequester circulating tumor cells and promote metastasis. J Clin Invest. Jul 1. pii: 67484.
12. Demers M, Krause DS, Schatzberg D, Martinod K, Voorhees JR, et al. (2012) Cancers predispose neutrophils to release extracellular DNA traps that contribute to cancer-associated thrombosis. Proc Natl Acad Sci U S A.109: 13076–13081.
13. McDonald B, Urrutia R, Yipp BG, Jenne CN, Kubes P. (2012) Intravascular neutrophil extracellular traps capture bacteria from the bloodstream during sepsis. Cell Host Microbe.12: 324–333.
14. Clark SR, Ma AC, Tavener SA, McDonald B, Goodarzi Z, et al. (2007) Platelet TLR4 activates neutrophil extracellular traps to ensnare bacteria in septic blood. Nat Med. 13: 463–469.
15. Yipp BG, Petri B, Salina D, Jenne CN, Scott BN, et al. (2012) Infection-induced NETosis is a dynamic process involving neutrophil multitasking in vivo. Nat Med.18: 1386–1393.
16. Ustione A, Piston DW. (2011) A simple introduction to multiphoton microscopy. J Microsc.243: 221–226.
17. Pittet MJ, Weissleder R. (2011) Intravital imaging. Cell.147: 983–991.
18. Toiyama Y, Mizoguchi A, Okugawa Y, Koike Y, Morimoto Y, et al. (2010) Intravital imaging of DSS-induced cecal mucosal damage in GFP-transgenic mice using two-photon microscopy. J Gastroenterol.45: 544–553.
19. Koike Y, Tanaka K, Okugawa Y, Morimoto Y, Toiyama Y, et al. (2011) In vivo real-time two-photon microscopic imaging of platelet aggregation induced by selective laser irradiation to the endothelium created in the beta-actin-green fluorescent protein transgenic mice. J Thromb Thrombolysis.32: 138–145.
20. Morimoto Y, Tanaka K, Toiyama Y, Inoue Y, Araki T, et al. (2011) Intravital Three-Dimensional Dynamic Pathology of Experimental Colitis in Living Mice Using Two-Photon Laser Scanning Microscopy. J Gastrointest Surg.15: 1842–1850.
21. Tanaka K, Morimoto Y, Toiyama Y, Okugawa Y, Inoue Y, et al. (2012) Intravital dual-colored visualization of colorectal liver metastasis in living mice using two photon laser scanning microscopy. Microsc Res Tech.75: 307–315.
22. Tanaka K, Okigami M, Toiyama Y, Morimoto Y, Matsushita K, et al. (2012) In vivo real-time imaging of chemotherapy response on the liver metastatic tumor microenvironment using multiphoton microscopy. Oncol Rep.28: 1822–1830.
23. Tanaka K, Toiyama Y, Inoue Y, Uchida K, Araki T, et al. (2013) Intravital imaging of gastrointestinal diseases in preclinical models using two-photon laser scanning microscopy. Surg Today.43: 123–129.
24. Okabe M, Ikawa M, Kominami K, Nakanishi T, Nishimune Y: (1997) 'Green mice' as a source of ubiquitous green cells. FEBS Lett. 407: 313–319.
25. Langer HF, Chavakis T. (2009) Leukocyte-endothelial interactions in inflammation. J Cell Mol Med.13: 1211–1220.
26. Fuchs TA, Abed U, Goosmann C, Hurwitz R, Schulze I, et al. (2007) Novel cell death program leads to neutrophil extracellular traps. J Cell Biol.176: 231–241.
27. Remijsen Q, Kuijpers TW, Wirawan E, Lippens S, Vandenabeele P, et al. (2011) Dying for a cause: NETosis, mechanisms behind an antimicrobial cell death modality. Cell Death Differ.18: 581–588.
28. Saffarzadeh M, Juenemann C, Queisser MA, Lochnit G, Barreto G, et al. (2012) Neutrophil extracellular traps directly induce epithelial and endothelial cell death: a predominant role of histones. PLoS One. 7: e32366.
29. Carmona-Rivera C, Zhao W, Yalavarthi S, Kaplan MJ (2014) Neutrophil extracellular traps induce endothelial dysfunction in systemic lupus erythematosus through the activation of matrix metalloproteinase-2. Feb 25.
30. Meng W, Paunel-Görgülü A, Flohé S, Hoffmann A, Witte I, et al. (2012) Depletion of neutrophil extracellular traps in vivo results in hypersusceptibility to polymicrobial sepsis in mice. Crit Care.16: R137.
31. Pfeiler S, Massberg S, Engelmann B. (2014) Biological basis and pathological relevance of microvascular thrombosis. Thromb Res.Suppl 1: 133 S35–37.
32. Lu T, Kobayashi SD, Quinn MT, Deleo FR. (2012) A NET Outcome. Front Immunol. 5; 3: 365.

Deep Sequencing of HIV-1 near Full-Length Proviral Genomes Identifies High Rates of BF1 Recombinants Including Two Novel Circulating Recombinant Forms (CRF) 70_BF1 and a Disseminating 71_BF1 among Blood Donors in Pernambuco, Brazil

Rodrigo Pessôa[1], Jaqueline Tomoko Watanabe[1], Paula Calabria[1], Alvina Clara Felix[1], Paula Loureiro[2], Ester C. Sabino[3], Michael P. Busch[4], Sabri S. Sanabani[5]* for the International Component of the NHLBI Recipient Epidemiology and Donor Evaluation Study-III (REDS-III)¶

1 Virology Department, São Paulo Institute of Tropical Medicine, University of São Paulo, São Paulo, Brazil, **2** Pernambuco State Center of Hematology and Hemotherapy, Recife, Pernambuco, Brazil, **3** Department of Infectious Disease/Institute of Tropical Medicine, University of São Paulo, São Paulo, Brazil, **4** Blood Systems Research Institute, San Francisco, California, United States of America, **5** Clinical Laboratory, Department of Pathology, Hospital das Clínicas, School of Medicine, University of São Paulo, São Paulo, Brazil

Abstract

Background: The findings of frequent circulation of HIV-1 subclade F1 viruses and the scarcity of BF1 recombinant viruses based on *pol* subgenomic fragment sequencing among blood donors in Pernambuco (PE), Northeast of Brazil, were reported recently. Here, we aimed to determine whether the classification of these strains (n = 26) extends to the whole genome sequences.

Methods: Five overlapping amplicons spanning the HIV near full-length genomes (NFLGs) were PCR amplified from peripheral blood mononuclear cells (PBMCs) of 26 blood donors. The amplicons were molecularly bar-coded, pooled, and sequenced by Illumina paired-end protocol. The prevalence of viral variants containing drug resistant mutations (DRMs) was compared between plasma and PBMCs.

Results: Of the 26 samples studied, 20 NFLGs and 4 partial fragments were *de novo* assembled into contiguous sequences and successfully subtyped. Two distinct BF1 recombinant profiles designated CRF70_BF1 and CRF71_BF1, with 4 samples in profile I and 11 in profile II were detected and thus constitute two novel recombinant forms circulating in PE. Evidence of dual infections was detected in four patients co-infected with distinct HIV-1 subtypes. According to our estimate, the new CRF71_BF1 accounts for 10% of the HIV-1 circulating strains among blood donors in PE. Discordant data between the plasma and PBMCs-virus were found in 15 of 24 donors. Six of these strains displayed major DRMs only in PBMCs and four of which had detectable DRMs changes at prevalence between 1-20% of the sequenced population.

Conclusions: The high percentage of the new RF71_BF1 and other BF1 recombinants found among blood donors in Pernambuco, coupled with high rates of transmitted DRMs and dual infections confirm the need for effective surveillance to monitor the prevalence and distribution of HIV variants in a variety of settings in Brazil.

Editor: Lars Kaderali, Technische Universität Dresden, Medical Faculty, Germany

Funding: This work was supported by grants 2011/11090-5 and 2011/12297-2 from the Fundação de Amparo à Pesquisa do Estado de São Paulo. The study was also supported by the Retrovirus Epidemiology Donor Study-II (HHSN268200417175C) and the Recipient Epidemiology and Donor Outcomes Study-III (HHSN268201100007I) contracts from NHLBI. The funders had no role in study design, data collection and analysis, decision to publish, or preparation of the manuscript.

Competing Interests: The authors have declared that no competing interests exist.

* Email: sabyem_63@yahoo.com

¶ Those responsible for the Recipient Epidemiology and Donor Outcomes Study-III are listed in the acknowledgments.

Introduction

One of the most prominent features of HIV-1 is the remarkable accumulation of genetic diversity in its population during the course of infection. This diversity can be attributed to the high mutation rate of reverse transcriptase (3×10^{-5} substitutions per site per generation) [1], rapid viral turnover (10^8 to 10^9 virions per day) [2], large number of infected cells (10^7 to 10^8 cells) [3], and recombination events that are taking place during replication [4]. Consequently, the HIV-1 population is composed of a swarm of highly genetically related variants, i.e. a *quasispecies*, capable of rapidly adapting to various selective pressures. This diversity has been shown to have an impact not only on viral phenotypes at the level of transmission patterns, pathogenicity and immunology but also in responses to antiretroviral therapy and vaccines [5,6]. Nine distinct genetic subtypes, (A–D, F–H, J and K) are joined in the pandemic today by more than 70 major circulating recombinant forms (CRFs) [http://www.hiv.lanl.gov/content/sequence/HIV/CRFs/CRFs.html] and numerous unique recombinant forms (URFs) have been isolated from individual patients [7]. Recombination between the URFs and CRFs and between the existing CRFs (inter-CRF recombinants) results in emergence of novel second and third generation recombinant forms which would further continue to shape the future of HIV epidemic through the generation of other variants with improved fitness to influence viral transmissibility [8,9]. It has been reported that recombinant viruses including the URFs and CRFs may account for at least 20% of all HIV infections [10]. The existence of recombinant viruses is an evidence of simultaneous infection of multiple viruses during a single transmission event (co-infection) or from the sequential infection of viruses during multiple transmission events (superinfection).

Brazil, the most populous country in the Latin America, is home to about one third of the people living with HIV (608,230) in Central and South America (UNAIDS. 2010–2011 Report on the Brazilian response to HIV/AIDS). HIV-1 subtype B is a major genetic clade circulating in the country but the overall prevalence of non-B strains, particularly URF BF1, C and URF BC, is increasing [11,12,13,14]. Data from recent studies of the viral near full-length genomes (NFLGs) have provided evidence of Brazilian CRF strains designated as CRF28_BF, CRF29_BF, CRF39_BF, CRF40_BF, CRF46_BF and CRF31_BC [12,13,15,16]. Recently, Alencar et al [17] performed a molecular epidemiological survey of HIV-1 in Brazil and analyzed the partial *pol* gene of 341 samples from seropositive blood donors collected between 2007 and 2011 from 4 Brazilian blood centers of the REDS-II (Retrovirus Epidemiological Donor Study) international program. The study reported a relatively high prevalence of subclade F1 (26 [24%] of 110), and only one case of BF1 recombinant among blood donors from Recife, Pernambuco (PE). These findings contrast with those from the previous studies of HIV-1 NFLGs in Brazil [13,18,19,20,21]. We therefore undertook this study to determine whether the classification of these strains extends to the whole genome sequences. Additionally, we aimed to compare the rate of drug resistance mutations (DRMs) in plasma bulk RNA and PBMC massively parallel sequencing (MPS) data to elucidate the differences in resistance profile between both compartments. The results revealed a considerable diversity of BF1 mosaic structures and high percentage of the new RF71_BF1 and other BF1 recombinants among blood donors in PE with high rates of transmitted DRMs and dual infections.

Materials and Methods

Study samples

The 24 peripheral blood mononucleated cells (PBMCs) samples reported in this study were from HIV-1 seropositive blood donors in Recife, capital of Pernambuco in the northeast region of Brazil. The rationale for collection of these samples has been previously reported [17]. No evidence of direct epidemiological linkage could be established. All study subjects provided written informed consent. Ethical approval was obtained from the local ethical review committee of the HEMOPE foundation as well as the Recipient Epidemiology and Donor Evaluation Study-II collaborating centers (Blood Systems Research Institute/University of California San Francisco) and Data Coordinating Center (Westat, Inc.) in the US.

DNA extraction and amplification of the NFLGs

The genomic DNA used for the PCR analyses was extracted using the QIAamp blood kit (Qiagen GmbH, Hilden Germany) according to the manufacturer's instructions. The NFLGs from five overlapping fragments were obtained by PCR using the Platinum *Taq* DNA Polymerase High Fidelity (5 U/µl) (Invitrogen, Life Technologies, Carlsbad, CA) and determined by a previously reported method [12,18]. The amplified DNA fragments from the nested PCR products were separated by gel electrophoresis and purified using Freeze 'N Squeeze DNA Gel Extraction Spin Columns (Bio-Rad, Hercules, CA, USA). Each purified amplicon was quantified using Quant-IT HS reagents (Invitrogen, Life Technologies, Carlsbad, CA), and all five amplicons from a single viral genome were pooled together at equimolar ratios.

Whole viral genome library preparation

Sequencing libraries were prepared as described previously [22]. Briefly, one ng of each sample amplicon pool was used in a fragmentation reaction mix using the Nextera XT DNA sample prep kit according to the manufacturer's protocol (Illumina, San Diego, CA). The tagmentation and fragmentation of each pool were simultaneously performed by incubation for 5 min at 55°C followed by incubation in neutralizing tagment buffer for 5 min at room temperature. After neutralization of the fragmented DNA, a light 12-cycle PCR was performed with Illumina Ready Mix to add Illumina flowcell adaptors, indexes and common adapters for subsequent cluster generation and sequencing. Amplified DNA library was then purified using Agencourt AMPure XP beads (Beckman Coulter), which excluded very short library fragments. Following AMPure purification, the quantity of each library was normalized to ensure equally library representation in our pooled samples. Prior to cluster generation, normalized libraries were further quantified by realtime PCR (qPCR) using the SYBR fast Illumina library quantification kit (KAPA Biosystems) following the instructions of the manufacturer. The qPCR was run on the 7500 Fast Real-Time PCR System (Applied Biosystems). The thermocycling conditions consisted of an initial denaturation step at 95°C for 5 min followed by 35 cycles of 30 s at 95°C and 45 s at 60°C. The final libraries were pooled at equimolar concentration and diluted to 4 nM. To denature the indexed DNA, 5 µL of the 4 nM library were mixed with 5 µL of 0.2 N fresh NaOH and incubated for 5 min at room temperature. 990 µL of chilled Illumina HT1 buffer was added to the denatured DNA and mixed to make a 20 pM library. After this step, 360 µL of the 20 pM library was multiplexed with 6 µL of 12.5 pM denatured PhiX control to increase sequence diversity and then mixed with 234 µL of chilled HT1 buffer to make a 12 pM sequenceable library.

Finally, 600 μL of the prepared library was loaded on an Illumina MiSeq clamshell style cartridge for paired end 250 bp sequencing reads.

Data analysis

Fastq files were generated by the Illumina MiSeq reporter for downstream analysis and validated to evaluate the distribution of quality scores and to ensure that quality scores do not drastically drop over each read. To take the sequencing error rate into account, we only considered variants detected at a frequency higher than 1% and Phred quality score of >30%, i.e., a base call accuracy of 99.9%. Validated fastq files from each viral genome were *de novo* assembled into contiguous sequences and annotated with CLC Genomics Workbench version 5.5 (CLC Bio, Aarhus, Denmark) with default parameters and were additionally assembled using Velvet implemented in the Sequencher program 5.2 (Gene Code Corp., Ann Arbor, MI). The contiguous genomic sequence from each virus strain was extracted from the assembly and used for further analysis. The full designation of samples, according to WHO-proposed nomenclature, is YYBR_PEXXX, where YY stands for the year of study, BR for Brazil, PE for Penambuco, and XXX stands for sample number.

Screening for recombination events and identification of breakpoints

The *de novo* assembled NFLGs and partial consensus sequences were aligned with reference sequences representing subtypes A–D, F–H, J and K obtained from the Los Alamos database (http://hiv-web.lanl.gov) using MAFFT version 7 [23]. Aligned sequences were manually edited and trimmed to the minimal shared length in the BioEdit Sequence Alignment Editor Program. The gap-stripped aligned sequences were screened for the presence of recombination by the bootscan methods and similarity plots implemented in the SIMPLOT program v3.5.1 [24,25]. The following parameters were used in bootscan method: window size, 350 bp; step size, 30 bp; the F84 model of evolution (Maximum likelihood (ML)) as a model to estimate nucleotide substitution; transition\transversion ratio, 2.0; and a bootstrap of 100 trees. In addition, the significant threshold for the bootscan was set at 70%. The jumping profile Hidden Markov Model (jpHMM) [26] was also used to confirm the recombination events and to define the recombination breakpoints according to the HXB2 coordinate system. Recombinant regions of the alignment as determined by the crossover points from the jpHMM and bootscan were analyzed separately by phylogenetic analysis. In further analysis, a network reconstruction was performed for the data set with evidence of recombination using SplitsTree4 version 4.3 [27] using the Neighbor-Net method. The NeighborNet method and the GTR+I+G distance model were used to create the network.

Phylogenetic Analysis

ML phylogenies were constructed using the GTR+I+G substitution model and a BIONJ starting tree. Heuristic tree searches under the ML optimality criterion were performed using the NNI branch-swapping algorithm. The approximate likelihood ratio test (aLRT) based on a Shimodaira-Hasegawa-like procedure was used as a statistical test to calculate branch support. The maximum composite likelihood in MEGA version 6 [28] was used to calculate the genetic distances between and within isolates. All trees were displayed using MEGA version 6.0 software.

Genotyping Analysis

For provirus sequences generated in this study, the MPS reads of partial *pol* gene associated with DRMs in the protease and reverse transcriptase regions of the HIV-1 genome of each sample were aligned to their corresponding consensus sequence using the CLC Genomics Workbench version 5.5 (CLC Bio, Aarhus, Denmark). The minority HIV-1 resistant variants were identified using a threshold of >1.0% of the reads sequenced. Reads with < 1% were discarded to account for potential errors due to the error rate of PCR. Amino acid positions including all listed major mutations and minor mutations associated with drug resistance were identified according to the IAS-USA 2011 and Stanford HIV drug resistance database. Due to the polymorphic nature of most minor protease substitutions, we only considered major mutations as evidence of transmission of drug resistance. The list of the NRTIs resistance related sites **41**, 62, **65**, **67**, **69**, **70**, 71, 74, 75, 77, 115, 116, **151**, **184**, **210**, **215** and **219**; NNRTIs resistance related sites 90, 98, **100**, **101**, **103**, **106**, 108, 138, 179, **181**, **188**, **190**,221, 225, 227, **230**; PIs resistance related sites 10, 16, 11, 20, 24, **30**, **32**, **33**, 35, 36, 43, **46**, **47**, **48**, **50**, 53, **54**, **58**, 60, 62, 63, 64, 69, 71, 73, **74**, **76**, 77, **82**, 83, **84**, 85, **88**, 89, **90** and 93. Bolded numbers are major drug resistance mutation sites.

GenBank accession numbers

All consensus genome assemblies generated in this study were submitted to NCBI's GenBank database (KJ849757 - KJ849783). The two distinct profiles of BF1 identical recombinant structure were registered with the Los Alamos National Database as CRF70_BF1 and CRF71_BF1.

Results

A total of 26 strains preliminarily classified as subclade F1 (n = 25) and BF1 recombinant (n = 1) by sequence analysis of a partial *pol* region in a previous study [17] were corroborated by further phylogenetic analysis of the NFLGs and larger partial fragments. Of note, one BF1 sample (10BR_PE059) was erroneously classified as F1 in our previous study. This sequence was thus corrected in this study and used for further analyses. Sequences were obtained for all five overlapped fragments that cover the NFLGs of 20 participants. Partial sequences were obtained from four fragments derived from 4 samples as shown in **Table 1**. Two samples did not amplify for any fragment. This might be a result of technical difficulties in recovering the provirus, but it is also possible that cells other than PBMCs are infected during the early stages of HIV infection. For the purposes of this report, these 2 samples were not considered further, and the analyses include only the 24 samples whose subtypes were successfully determined.

Analysis of the proviral NFLGs and partial consensus sequences revealed all isolates retain intact reading frames for a majority of their genes and no gross deletions or rearrangements were observed. Recombination analysis from each strain shows two distinct recombinant profiles with 4 samples in profile I and 11 in profile II. The recombinant genomes of both profiles essentially consisted of subclades F1 and subtype B as parental sequences and appeared different from all previously documented CRFs in Brazil and South America. Plausible breakpoints identified in each profile using bootscanning analyses were consistent with those identified using jpHMM (schematically illustrated in Figure 1 and 2). Therefore, the new recombinants strains in profile I and II are now designated CRF70_BF1 and CRF71_BF1, respectively. All of the breakpoints in the two CRFs were mapped and compared. The results revealed great similarity in structure between the two

Table 1. The near full-length genomic (NFLG) and partial fragments subtyping of HIV-from plasma and blood samples.

Sample ID	Sequence Fragment					Subtype		Number of Reads	Av. coverage
	$A_{(546-2598)}$	$B1_{(2157-3791)}$	$B2_{(3236-5220)}$	$C_{(4890-7808)}$	$D_{(7719-9537)}$	Plasma	Provirus		
10BR_PE002	-	+	+	+	+	F	BF1	145757	21.299
10BR_PE004	+	+	+	+	+	F	BF1_CRF70	30843	2625
10BR_PE008	+	+	+	+	+	F	BF1_CRF71	111362	2564
10BR_PE009	+	+	+	+	+	F	BF1_CRF71	23923	5624
10BR_PE016	+	+	+	+	+	F	BF1_CRF70	29409	584
10BR_PE025	+	+	+	+	+	F	BF1_CRF70	84718	2173
10BR_PE026	+	+	-	+	+	F	BF1_CRF71	20503	2635
10BR_PE032	+	+	+	-	+	F	BF1	55741	6084
10BR_PE053	+	+	+	+	+	F	B	78936	3697
10BR_PE059[1]	+	+	+	+	+	F	BF1	30166	2619
10BR_PE064	+	+	+	+	+	F	BF1_CRF71	219755	5608
10BR_PE066	+	+	+	+	+	F	BF1_CRF71	32024	6701
10BR_PE071	+	+	+	+	+	F	BF1_CRF71	98156	5578
10BR_PE073	+	+	+	+	-	F	BF1	47041	1365
10BR_PE084	+	+	+	+	+	F	BF1_CRF71	15195	2034
10BR_PE085	-	-	-	-	-	F		-	-
10BR_PE086	+	+	+	+	+	F	BF1	15348	1106
10BR_PE087	-	-	-	-	-	F		-	-
10BR_PE088	+	+	+	+	+	F	BF1_CRF71	42801	700
10BR_PE090	+	+	+	+	+	F	BF1_CRF71	18052	187
10BR_PE092	+	+	+	+	+	F	BF1_CRF71	4546	201
10BR_PE094	+	+	+	+	+	F	BF1_CRF71	273899	6870
10BR_PE102	+	+	+	+	+	F	BF1	494376	7257
10BR_PE104	+	+	+	+	+	BF1	B/BF1	26901	3324
10BR_PE107	+	+	+	+	+	F	F1	78655	2159
10BR_PE109	+	+	+	+	+	F	BF1_CRF70	165634	6190

[1]Variant was erroneously classified as F1 in our previous study.

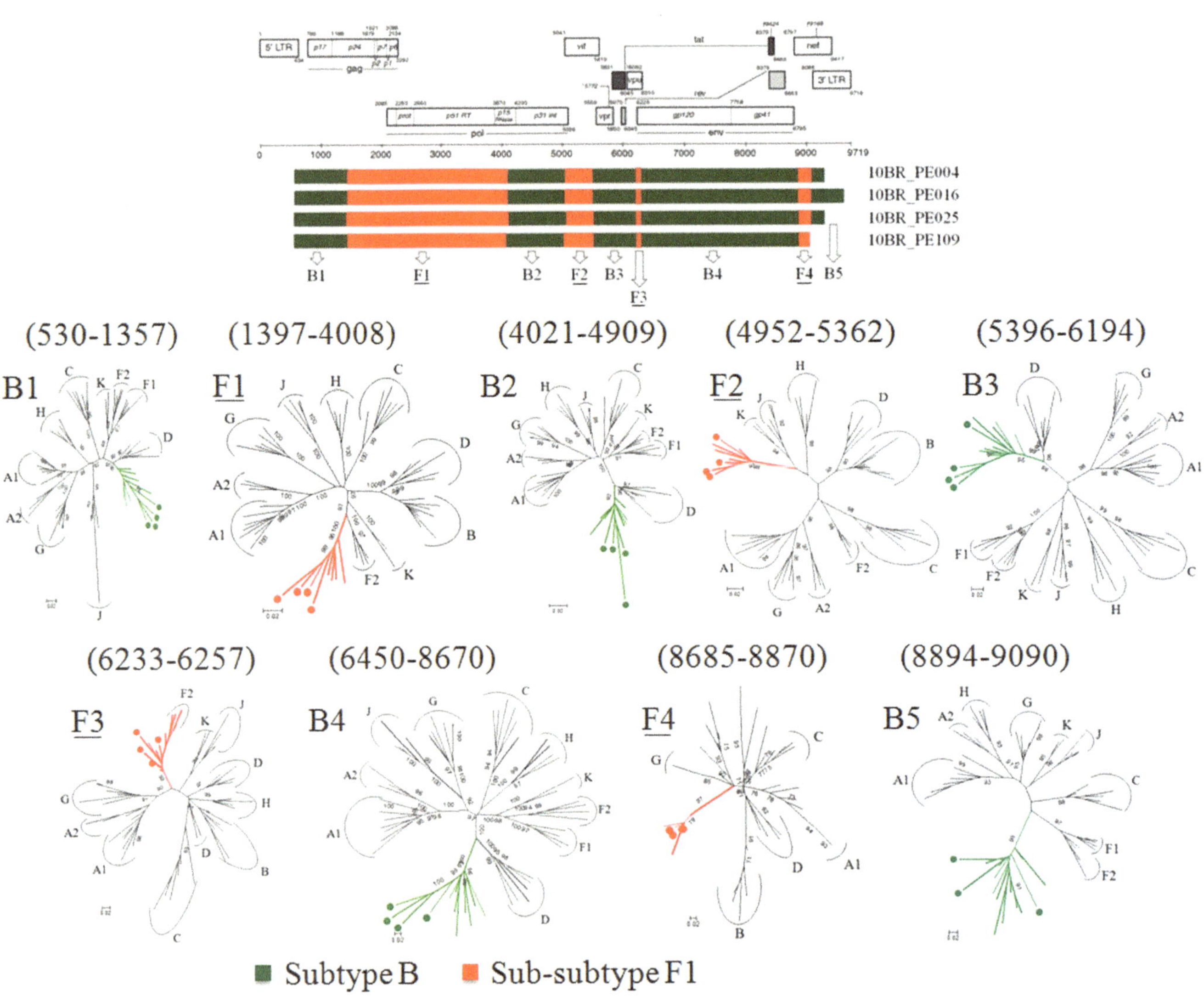

Figure 1. Schematic representation of NFLGs structure and breakpoint profiles with confirmatory phylogenetic trees of the four sequences identified in this study as CRF70_BF1 (colored circles). The phylogenetic trees of the nine mosaic segments defined by jpHMM, similarity plot and bootscan analysis were constructed with PHYML v.3.0. For clarity purposes, the trees were midpoint rooted. The region of subclade F1 and subtypes B are as indicated at the bottom. Positions of breakpoints are numbered relative to the HXB2 numbering system. The approximate likelihood ratio test (aLRT) values of ≥90% are indicated at nodes. The scale bar represents 0.02 nucleotide substitution per site. The results from the ML analysis were sufficiently robust to confirm the structure for the four specimens that were suggested by the recombination analysis.

CRFs. Among the sub-subtype F1 stretches, identified by letter F1 through F4 and F1 through F3 in CRF70_BF1 and CRF71_BF1, respectively (Figure 1 and 2), fragments F1, F2 and F4 appear to be in the same locations. For patient 10BR_PE026, we were unable to amplify fragment designated as B2 in **Table 1** (position 3236–5220) and therefore could not investigate the location of breakpoint at the 5′ of fragment B2 as depicted in Figure 2. Different from CRF71_BF1, CRF70_BF1 appears to contain one too short sub-subtype F1 fragment within the *Vpu* gene (34 bp, nucleotide 6233–6266 according to position in HXB2 GenBank accession no. K03455) interspersed with subtype B. In attempt to find sequences with recombinant structure similar to any of the strains in the two CRFs, multiple sequence alignments including all published BF1 unique NFLGs sequences were built, aligned and subjected to bootscan and automated jpHMM. The results showed that the CRF71_BF1 sequences had a mosaic sequence pattern nearly identical to the previously published Brazilian BF1 isolate 02BR033 (GenBank: DQ358811) in sample collected in 2002 from patient living in São Paulo, Southeast of Brazil [13]. To further test for recombination, ML phylogenetic trees were inferred for the regions of nucleotide sequence on either side of the breakpoints detected by bootscan and jpHMM methods. As shown in Figure 1 and 2, the exploratory tree analysis revealed that each fragment of recombinant virus from each CRF clustered tightly (>90% aLRT) with corresponding fragments of subtype B or F1 reference sequences in agreement with the subtype assigned by recombination analysis. The only disagreement between the recombination and exploratory tree analyses was for a short CRF70_BF1 fragment in the middle of the *Vpu* region (F3 in Figure 2). Despite the fact that F3 fragment in CRF70_BF1 strains have shorter sequences and some group M variants cannot resolve some of the internal nodes, all of the CRF70_BF1 can resolve the terminal nodes and appeared more closely related phylogentically to subclade F1 than the other groups of reference sequences. To

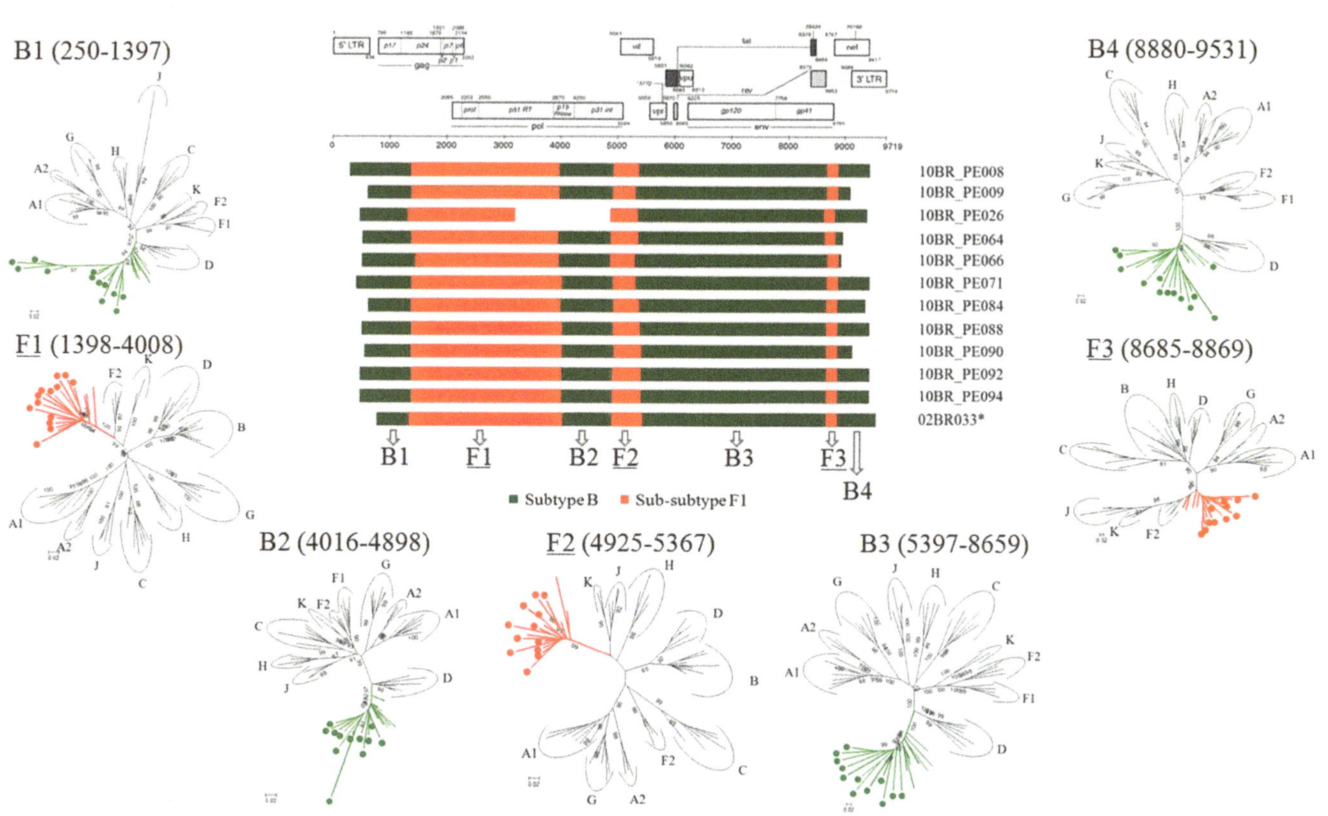

Figure 2. Schematic representation of NFLGs structure and breakpoint profiles with confirmatory phylogenetic trees of the twelve sequences identified in this study as CRF70_BF1 (colored circles). For patient 10BR_PE026, we were unable to amplify fragment designated as B2 and therefore we could not investigate the location of breakpoint at the 5′ of fragment B2. All ML phylogenic trees were constructed using the PHYML v.3.0 package. The region of subclade F1 and subtypes B are indicated at the bottom. Positions of breakpoints are numbered relative to the HXB2 numbering system. For clarity purposes, the trees were midpoint rooted. The approximate likelihood ratio test (aLRT) values of ≥90% are indicated at nodes. The scale bar represents 0.02 nucleotide substitution per site. The results from the ML analysis were sufficiently robust to confirm the structure for the twelve specimens that were suggested by the recombination analysis.

increase the phylogenetic signal, ML trees were performed on concatenated data of discontinuous subtype B and F1 fragment from CRF70_BF1 (Figure 3A and 3B) and CRF71_BF1 (Figure 3A and 3B), which was well confirmed by aLRT values above 90% as shown in Figure 3. Split decomposition was then used to visualize the relationship of the two CRFs (Figure 4). While sequences within each of these two CRF did not group directly with each other, they were present as one group of sequences within a cluster between subtype B and F1. The observed mean intrasubtype genetic distances were 8.2% (range 6.7–10.0%) and 8.7% (range 6.2–9.9%) for CRF70_BF1 and CRF71_BF1 strains, respectively, and closer to the intersubtype distance between both CRFs (8.3%).

Beside the CRFs, in five of the seven strains initially classified as infected with subclade F1, subtype B fragments were detected and appeared to represent URFs strains (Figure 5). The relationships of the viral sequences from patients' PBMCs to the sequences obtained from the corresponding RNA viruses within the same regions were examined for each patient to roughly assess the viral diversity in both compartments (Figure 6). Surprisingly, the intra-individual plasma and proviral sequence variation in four patients (10BR_PE073, 10BR_PE053, 10BR_PE104 and 10BR_PE032) in the partial *pol* regions depicted in Figure 5 (marked with orange boxes) were remarkably high, indicating that the plasma viruses were derived from a population significantly distinct from those of the cellular sources; a result consistent with dual infection with different subtypes (Figure 5 and 6). Except those with dual infections, all the other sequences from both compartments were located close to one another on the same branch and had plasma RNA and proviral DNA variation only ranging between 0.1–0.8% (Figure 4). In the case of subject 10BR_PE104, MPS data revealed a mixture of two distinct consensus sequences, one NFLGs from strain B and a second recombinant of strains B and F1 (4450 bp) almost identical to the plasma virus in the same region. The BF1 segment was present in 7% of MPS reads with a median coverage of 250 reads in the sample from subject 10BR_PE104, while the NFLGs present in 93% of MPS reads with a median coverage of 7250 reads. Thus, the low BF1 copies would not have been detectable using the provirus traditional bulk sequencing approaches. Again, these data confirms that infection in this subject was founded by two genetic lineages. In Figure 5, there were three samples (10BR_PE002 (pro), 10BR_PE032 [17], and 10BR_PE102 [17], which shared one breakpoint at the integrase gene (position 2393–2462 nt), similar to the third breakpoint of the CRF71_BF variants (5′ of fragment F2, Figure 2). This increased prevalence of genetic breakpoints in the integrase region may indicate a possible preference region for recombination to occur.

Three viruses that were classified as BF1 (n = 2; 10BR_PE059, 10BR_PE086) and F1 (10BR_PE107) on partial *pol* analysis were confirmed by NFLGs analysis (Figure 5).

As stated before, the 26 samples selected to this study are derived from 110 blood donors from Recife PE, and all were

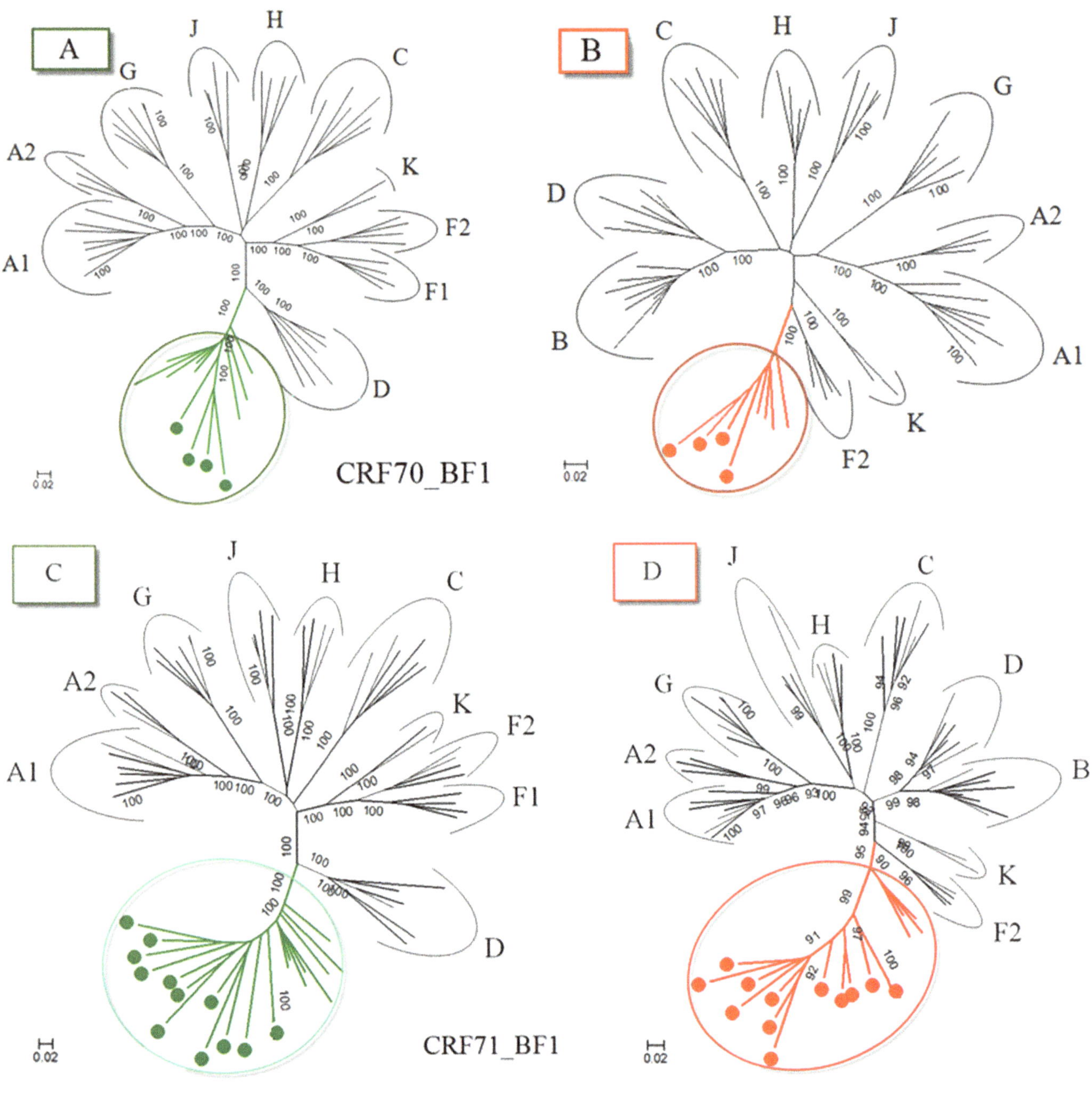

Figure 3. ML phylogenetic tree from concatenated regions assigned as subtype B and F1 from four CRF70_BF1 (3A and 3B) and twelve CRF71_BF1 (3C and 3D) isolates as defined by recombination analysis. Sequences from each region were aligned with reference sequences representing subtypes A–D, F–H, J and K obtained from the Los Alamos database (http://hiv-web.lanl.gov). For clarity purposes, the trees were midpoint rooted. The approximate likelihood ratio test (aLRT) values of ≥90% are indicated at nodes. The scale bar represents 0.02 nucleotide substitution per site. The results from this analysis revealed that each segment of the CRF70_BF1 (3A and 3B) and twelve CRF71_BF1 (3C and 3D) viruses was found to cluster with corresponding segments of subtype B or F1 viruses in agreement with the subtype assigned by recombination analysis.

identified as infected with subclade F1 except two donors who were found to be infected with BF1 recombinant viruses. Genotyping based on NFLGs or long partial fragments of these samples was successful in 24 donors, of whom 11 were infected with CRF71_BF1, 4 with CRF70_BF1, 6 BF1 URF, 1 subtype B, 1 subtype F1, and 1 dually infected with BF1 and B viruses. Based on this analysis, it is evident that non-recombinant subclade F1 accounts for <1% of HIV-1 subtype's circulating in PE and that CRF71_BF1 is responsible for 50% (11/22) of infections caused by BF1 recombinants.

We also aimed in this study to analyze the emergence of proviral HIV DRMs detected by MPS and compare the results with the plasma HIV DRMs detected by previously described plasma bulk sequencing of the same blood donors group to better understand the resistance profile between the two compartments. A summary of these results are provided in **Table 2**. Discordant data between

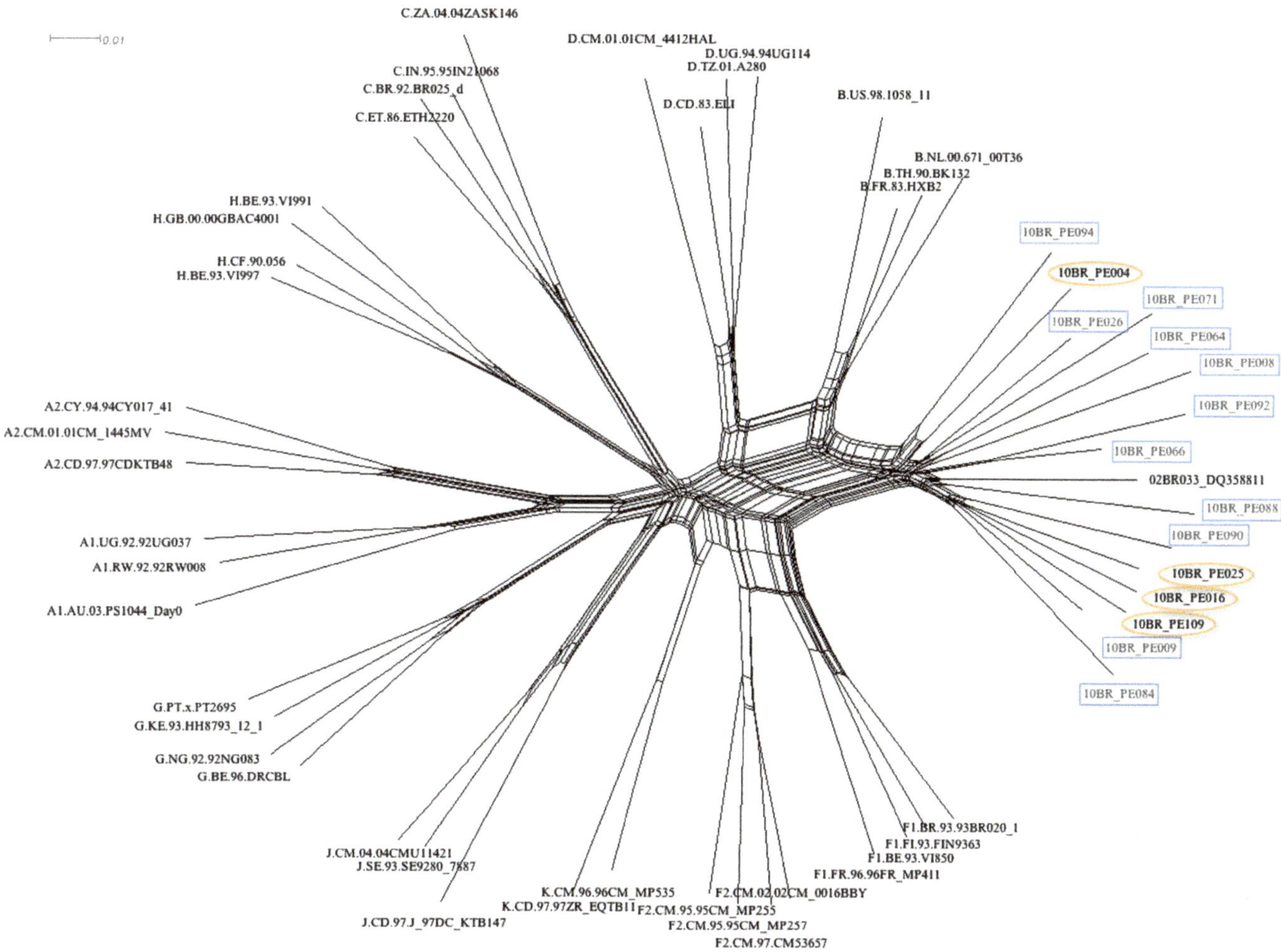

Figure 4. Split networks for four sequences of CRF_70BF1 (marked with orange circles) and eleven CRF_71BF1 (marked with blue boxes) and representatives of HIV subtypes A–K sequences from the Los Alamos database (http://hiv-web.lanl.gov)**.** The splits graphs used distances computed under the GTR+I+G model. The scale bar represents 0.01 nucleotide substitution per site. The results demonstrate that sequences within each of CRF did not group directly with each other, but they were present as one group of sequences within a cluster between subtype B and subclade F1.

the cell free viruses and the PBMC-viruses were found in 15 participants. Six of these strains displayed major amino-acid changes only in the cellular compartment and four of which had detectable major amino-acid changes at prevalence between 1–20% of the sequenced population. Neither major amino-acid changes in the protease nor in the reverse transcriptase coding region were detectable by plasma bulk sequencing. Eleven and two DRMs in the protease and reverse transcriptase regions, respectively, were detected in plasma bulk sequencing but were not observed in MPS data. For the coding region of the protease gene, major PI resistance mutations, namely, M46I, and L33F were detected in four blood donors. As shown in **Table 2**, the overall frequency of minor mutations in both compartments in the protease gene was significantly greater than that detected in reverse transcriptase. Although these mutations were mostly polymorphisms and not directly responsible for drug resistance but they are able to compensate the low protease processivity caused by primary mutations [29]. The proviral DNA MPS analysis in the reverse transcriptase region showed major mutations at the following codons in five patients: M184I, M230I, and E138K. It is well known that HIV-1 harboring the M184I/V mutations has a low viral fitness because of deficient dNTP usage and that the E138K mutation can compensate for the deficit in dNTP usage associated with the M184I/V mutations [30]. The compensatory substitution at codon 230 in motif E contributes to reduced viral replication and has also been shown to confer resistance to all currently available NNRTIs in both phenotypic and biochemical assays [31].

Discussion

This study describes the MPS of proviral NFLGs and larger fragment from 26 well sampled groups of blood donors from PE who had previously been diagnosed as infected with subclade F1 (n = 25) and BF1 recombinant (n = 1) based on *pol* subgenomic fragment from cell free viruses using conventional bulk sequencing. The most remarkable observations in this study are that 23 of the 24 donors in whom genotyping was successful infected with HIV-1 BF1 recombinant variants. Of these, two novel BF1 CRFs with high genetic diversities that exceed >8% difference at both inter- and intra-host level were identified. These results suggest that both CRFs have been in circulation early in the epidemic and have been evolving independently ever since. Based on the similarity of their recombination profile, it is tempting to speculate

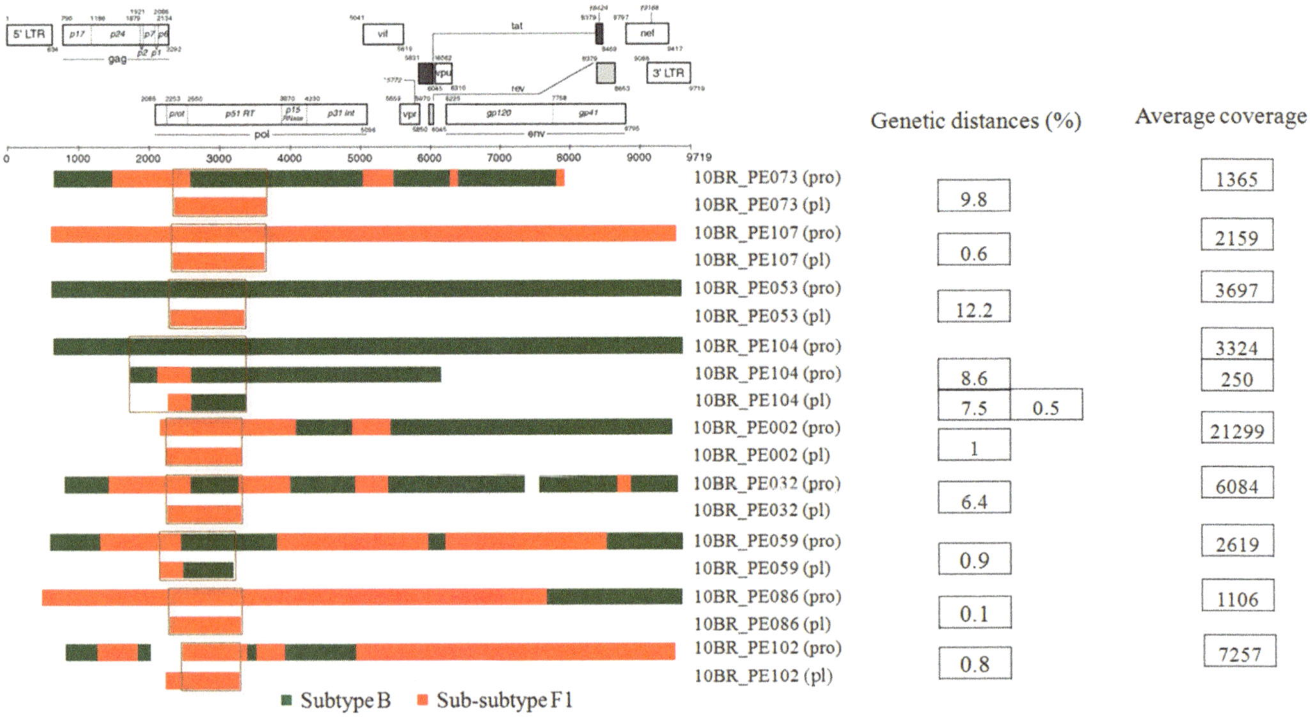

Figure 5. Schematic representation of the NFLGs, partial structure and breakpoint profiles of the BF1 sequences identified in this study from proviral DNA generated by deep sequencing approach and previously published cell free viruses generated by bulk sequencing approach. Sequences were mapped relative to the HXB2 numbering system. Genetic distances of overlapping regions (marked with orange boxes) between sequences from plasma and PBMCs together with the overall mean coverage depth are demonstrated. Distances were computed using the maximum composite likelihood method in MEGA version 6 [28]. As depicted in the figure, the intra-individual plasma and proviral sequence variation in four patients (10BR_PE073, 10BR_PE053, 10BR_PE104 and 10BR_PE032) in the partial *pol* regions (marked with orange boxes) were remarkably high. These results may indicate that the plasma viruses were derived from a population significantly distinct from those of the cellular sources; a result consistent with dual infection with different subtype. In sample 10BR_PE104, MPS data revealed the existence of subtype B NFLGs and a second BF1 recombinant strain (4450 bp) almost identical to the plasma virus in the same region.

that the CRF70_BF1 variants were old "second-generation" recombinants of CRF71_BF1 circulating in PE. Our estimates indicated that the CRF71_BF1 variants are responsible of 50% of infection caused by BF1 recombinants among blood donors in this region of northeast of Brazil. Moreover, if we assume no recombination in the remainder of the genome characterized as subtype B in the previous study, then the prevalence of BF1 recombinant variants is estimated at 20.4% (22/108) and CRF71_BF1 at 10.2% (11/108) of HIV-1 strains circulating among blood donors in PE. Given the high prevalence of CRF71_BF1 observed among the low risk blood donors, it may be suspected that a high prevalence for this variant could be found among other high-risk groups with tight transmission chain and that it has been able to break the transmission barrier from high-risk groups into the general population. Moreover, detection of both CRFs indicates that these variants are actively competing with other BF1 recombinants and other HIV-1 subtypes circulating in this region.

The proportion of BF1 variants described in this study is much greater than the rate reported in 169 individuals recently diagnosed as seropositive for HIV1 (2.8%) in the Metropolitan Region of Recife, Northeastern of Brazil [32] and in other study of 84 patients chronically infected with HIV (3.6%) naïve to antiretroviral treatment [33]. This difference is not surprising, because small fragments from different regions of HIV genomes were characterized in the previous studies while we used larger overlapped fragments to sequence the NFLGs, which is the preferred method for accurate characterization of HIV-1 isolates. Thus, the previous studies are likely to have missed the recombinants samples. Despite the high rate of recombination as estimated using our fairly conservative assumptions, it is probable that our results have underestimated the true rate of infection with BF1 recombinant viruses; particularly our study was limited to donors infected with F1 and BF1 with partially sequenced viral fragments. Thus, it is possible that the BF1 infection in this group will be higher than what was observed if we had sequenced the virus NFLGs in all the 80 subtype B infected donors described in the previous study.

Additional observations of this study are the description of mixed infections with B, F1 and/or BF1recombinants. The use of MPS technology enhanced our power to determine the dual infection of larger fragment of BF1 and genuine NFLGs of subtype B in the PBMCs of patient 10BR_PE104. The BF1 recombination profile was almost identical to the plasma virus in the same region demonstrating an intra-individual plasma and proviral sequence variation of only 0.5%. Thus, it is possible to assume that the primary infected PBMCs harboring the BF1 recombinants in this patient were likely the source of the plasma circulating viral sequences. The observation of an intact NFLGs of subtype B in the PBMCs of patient 10BR_PE104 may argue against the inactivity of this provirus but may agree with assumption that subtype B provirus may be integrated into the chromosome at a site at which its expression is prevented, or it may be transcriptionally inactive by virtue of being extrachromosomal [34]. It is also possible that

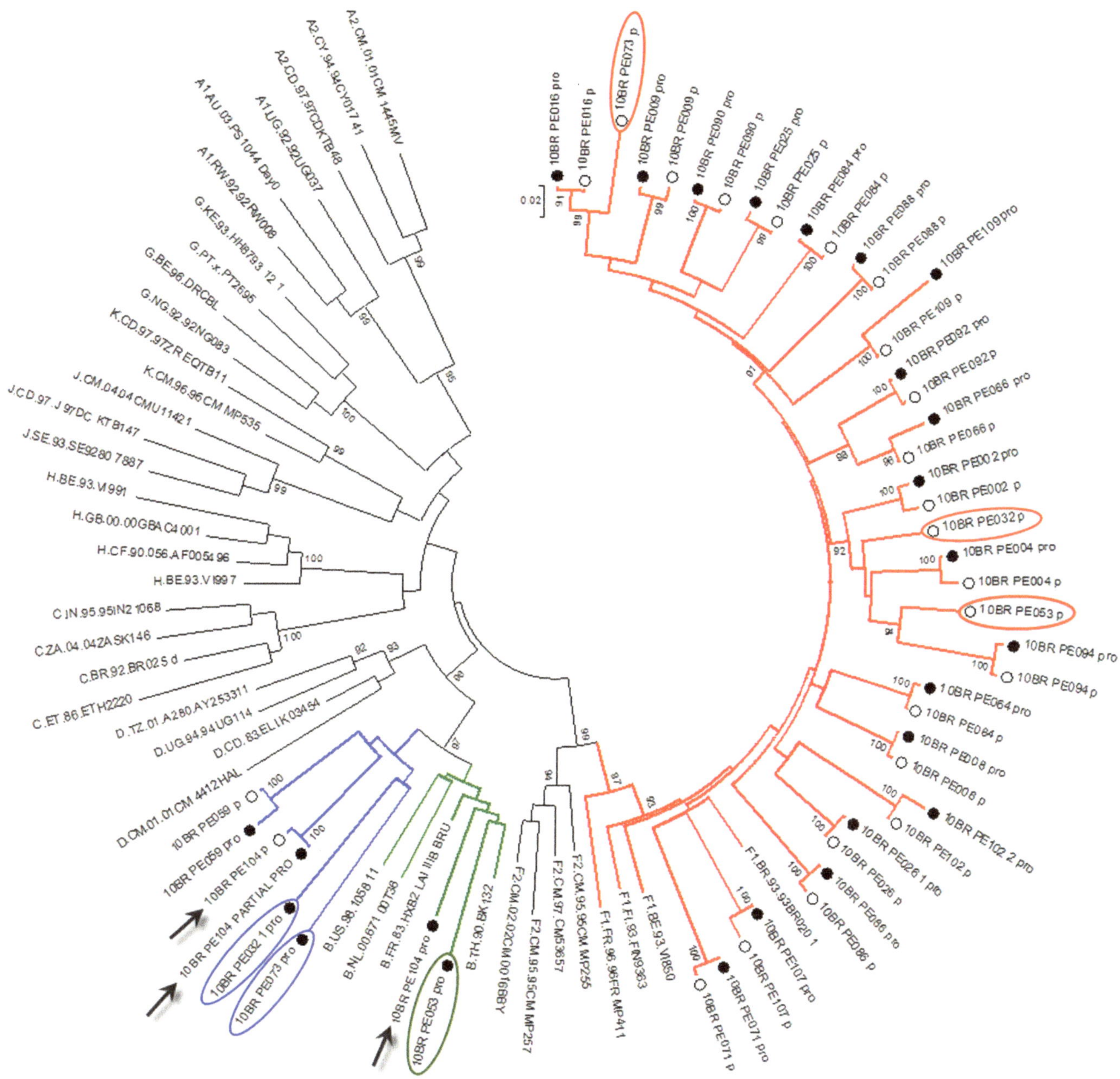

Figure 6. Comparison of phylogenetic clustering profile of sequences from both plasma (empty circles) and provirus (black circles) and other HIV-1 reference sequences from the Los Alamos HIV-1 database representing 11 genetic subtypes. Viral sequences from both compartments were aligned with the complete set of reference sequences obtained from the Los Alamos database (http://hiv-web.lanl.gov). Green, blue and red colored branches represent subtype B, BF1 recombinants, and subclade F1, respectively. Sequence with discordant results between PBMCs and plasma are marked with blue and red oval circles, respectively. For purposes of clarity, the tree was midpoint rooted. The approximate likelihood ratio test (aLRT) values of $\geq$90% are indicated at nodes. The scale bar represents 0.02 nucleotide substitutions per site. Except subjects 10BR_PE073, 10BR_PE053, 10BR_PE104 and 10BR_PE032, each patient forms a tight cluster and is distinct from other subjects with aLRT SH-like supports >95% for all inter-subject clusters. The results from the ML analysis added further support to the results depicted in figure and were sufficiently robust to confirm the event of dual infection with different subtype. In case 10BR_PE104 (indicated by black arrow), MPS data revealed the existence of subtype B NFLGs and a second BF1 recombinant strain almost identical to the plasma virus in the same region.

the adaptation of the B strains to the PBMC in this patient allows them to avoid competitive exclusion by the dominant strain in plasma. In the other three samples with dual infections, subtype F1 seen in the plasma were completely absent in the PBMCs. Discordances in the HIV subtypes in both compartments may suggest differential sources of infecting viruses. It is also conceivable that the discordances in the HIV subtypes in PBMCs and plasma are likely due to low-level minority strains present as B/BF1 variants that are not detected with bulk plasma sequencing or that the F1 viruses shed in the plasma were more fit. The evidence of dual infections in this study adds support to previous studies [35,36,37,38,39], as this event is far more common in

Table 2. Drug resistance mutations detected with bulk sequencing (plasma) and deep sequencing (PBMCs).

Sample ID	Protease gene coding region		Reverse transcriptase gene coding region(nRTIs)		Reverse transcriptase gene coding region (NNRTIs)	
	PLASMA (Bulk sequencing)	**PBMC (Deep sequencing)**	**PLASMA (Bulk secuencing)**	**PBMC (Deep sequencing)**	**PLASMA (Bulk secuencing)**	**PBMC (Deep sequencing)**
10BR_PE002•	M36I, V77I¶, L89M	M36I,_V82I_, L89M		**_M184I*_**		**_M230I*_**
10BR_PE004•	M36I, V77I, L89M	M36I,**_M46I_**,V77I, L89M			V106I¶	
10BR_PE008•	M36I, D60E, L89M	M36I, D60E, L89M				_V106I_
10BR_PE009•	L10V, M36I, L89M	L10V, M36I, L89M		_F77L*_[1], **_M184I*_**		**_M230I*_**
10BR_PE016•	L10V, M36I, L89M	L10V, _G16E_, M36I, L89M				
10BR_PE025	L10V, K20R, M36I, L89M	L10V, K20R, M36I, L89M				
10BR_PE026	M36L, L89M	M36I, L89M				
10BR_PE032•	L10V, M36I, L89M	L10V, **_L33F*_**, M36I, L89M		**_M184I*_**		_V108I_, **_M230I*_**
10BR_PE053•	M36I¶, L89M¶	_V77I_				
10BR_PE059	L10I, M36I, L89M	L10I, M36I, L89M				
10BR_PE064	M36I, L89M	M36I, L89M				
10BR_PE066•	L10V, K20R¶, M36I, D60E¶, I62V, L63P, L89M, I93L	L10V, M36I, D60E, I62V, L89M, I93L				
10BR_PE071•	M36I	M36I		_F77L*_[1]		
10BR_PE073	M36I, I64M	M36I, I64M				
10BR_PE084	L10V, M36I, I64M, L89M	L10V, M36I, I64M, L89M				
10BR_PE086•	L10I¶, K20R, M36I, I62V, L89M, I93L	K20R, M36I, I62V, L89M, I93L				
10BR_PE088	M36I, V82I, L89M	M36I, V82I, L89M			V106I	V106I
10BR_PE090•	L10I, M36I, L89M	L10I,M36I, **_M46I*_**, L89M		**_M184I*_**		
10BR_PE092	M36I, D60E, I62V, I64M, L89M	M36I, D60E, I62V, I64M, L89M				
10BR_PE094	K20R, M36I, L89M	K20R, M36I, L89M				
10BR_PE102•	L10I¶, M36I¶, I64L¶					
10BR_PE104•	K20R¶, M36I	M36I, _L63P_, _V77I_, _I93L_				
10BR_PE107•	M36I, I62V, L63P¶, L89M	M36I, I62V, L89M			V108I¶	
10BR_PE109•	K20M, M36I, D60E, L63P, L89M	K20M, M36I, **_M46I*_**, D60E, L63P, L89M		_F77L*_[1]		_E138K_

Samples displayed discordant genotypic data between the cell free viruses and the PBMC-viruses are marked by black dots, Major mutations are marked in boldface type, Major drug resistance mutations at prevalence >20% of the sequenced population are underlined, Major drug resistance mutations at prevalence <20% of the sequenced population are marked by star symbol, Mutations detect only in PBMCs are marked in italic face type.
[1]Transmitted drug resistance mutation, Mutations detect only in plasma are marked by pilcrow symbol.

Brazil where these subtypes co-circulate. Furthermore, these data agree with the consensus that the presence of two or more HIV-1 subtypes within an infected individual is relatively frequent [40,41]. It is unclear from this study whether the occurrence of HIV multiple distinct strains was the result of superinfection with a second variant at a later time, or whether simultaneous infection with multiple viral strains occurred during a single transmission event. However, the circulation of multiple subtypes in Brazil fortifies the possibility of both scenarios. The overall results indicate that the rate of HIV-1 mixed infections within this Brazilian group is higher than 16%. From these results, we believed that the use of PBMC DNA in addition to plasma RNA is expected to provide highest sensitivity to detect mixed infection via population MPS. Whether dual infection and/or recombination had an impact on the clinical outcomes of the blood donors in this study was unknown, since the available clinical data resulted from one assessment that seek to understand risk exposures and motivations to donate blood.

Other important observation of this study is the underestimation of transmitted resistance obtained by routine plasma analysis that is revealed by the examination of the MPS populations of the archived proviruses in PBMCs. In this study, comparing both sources would have detected 11 DNA provirus disclosed DRMs by MPS not detected by routine plasma bulk analysis. In this study, eleven DNA provirus sequence had detectable DRMs previously missed by plasma bulk analysis. Six of these strains had 17 DRMs only in the PBMCs and four of which had detectable major DRMs at prevalence between 1–20% of the MPS population. These results support the previous observations that standard bulk sequencing cannot fully access the spectrum of viral variants archived in the proviral DNA [42]. The relatively higher proportion of recently infected donors carried low-abundance resistance mutations leads us to believe that the rate of the current transmitted DRMs is underestimated. It is well known that conventional Sanger sequencing of bulk PCR products are limited to the detection of high-frequency variants that present in greater than 20% of the sequenced viral population [43,44]. However, we were able to detect additional DRMs at prevalence higher than 20% of the MPS provirus variants that had not been identified using plasma bulk sequencing. This result probably indicates that MPS approach permit characterization of considerable heterogeneity in the diversity and frequency variations in the proviral DNA [45]. Since the time of infection is unknown, it possible that some of the transmitted mutants in cell free viruses may disappear over time while persisting in cellular HIV-1 DNA [46,47,48]. All together, these results justify the inclusion of proviral DNA from PMBCs as a valuable source for resistance analysis, which is in agreement with previous reports [49,50]. On the other hand, we expected that our MPS approach would detect the entire mutations spectrum from the amplified and sequenced viral population that was displayed by conventional sequencing of the cell free viruses, but this does not hold true for some mutations. Seven patient samples with some detectable DRMs by bulk sequencing approach were not observed in PBMCs reads obtained through the MPS approach. One possible explanation beside the limiting factors intrinsic to PCR is that our MPS approach of the amplified fragments is not sufficiently sensitive to detect all DRMs. It is also possible that the discordant genotypes in these patients are due to dual infection. This was confirmed in patients 10BR_PE053 and 10BR_PE104 who displayed two phylogenetically distinct populations in the sequenced regions.

Apart from small sample size, the present study was limited by the investigation of only the HIV-1 proviruses. Although plasma HIV-1 RNA remains the material of choice for the determination of drug-resistant mutations and guiding therapeutic decisions [51,52] the proviral PBMC DNA sequence can contain a variety of multiple DRMs that are not present in plasma [47,53]. This, combined with the stability of DNA compared with RNA [54], and the fact that HIV DNA recovered from the proviral compartment can reliably be used for the determination of DRMs in treatment naïve patients [55] influenced our decision to use proviral DNA in this study.

Finally, needless to say, HIV phylogenetic analysis based on the complete genome sequences is more reliable than that of the *pol* or other small partial fragment alone. The high percentage of the new CRF71_BF1 and other BF1 recombinants found among blood donors in Pernambuco, coupled with high rates of transmitted DRMs and dual infections confirm the need for effective surveillance to monitor the prevalence and distribution of HIV variants in a variety of settings in Brazil.

Acknowledgments

The Recipient Epidemiology and Donor Outcomes Study-III is the responsibility of the following persons:

Cesar de Almeida Neto[1], Alfredo Mendrone-Junior[1], Anna Bárbara Carneiro-Proietti[2], Divaldo de Almeida Sampaio[3], Paula Loureiro[3], Clarisse Lobo[4] Maria Esther Lopes[4], Ester Cerdeira Sabino[5], Ligia Capuani[5], João Eduardo Ferreira[5], Pedro Losco Takecian[5], Cláudia Di Lorenzo Oliveira[6], Brian Custer[7], Michael P. Busch[7*], Thelma T. Gonçalez[7], Donald brambilla[8], Christopher McClure[8], Simone A. Glynn[9]

[1]Fundação Pró-Sangue Hemocentro de São Paulo, SP, Brazil.

[2]Fundação Hemominas, Belo Horizonte, MG, Brazil.

[3]Fundação Hemope, Recife, PE, Brazil.

[4]Hemorio, Rio de Janeiro, RJ, Brazil.

[5]University of São João Del-Rei, MG, Brazil

[6]University of São Paulo, SP, Brazil.

[7]Blood Systems Research Institute, San Francisco, CA, USA/University of California, San Francisco, San Francisco CA, USA

[8]RTI international

[9]National Heart, Lung, and Blood Institute, NIH

*Group leader:

Michael P. Busch, M.D., Ph.D.

Blood Systems Research Institute

270 Masonic Avenue

San Francisco, CA 94118-4417

mbusch@bloodsystems.org

Author Contributions

Conceived and designed the experiments: SSS. Performed the experiments: RP JTW PC SSS. Analyzed the data: RP JTW PC ACF SSS. Contributed reagents/materials/analysis tools: PL ECS MPB. Contributed to the writing of the manuscript: MPB SSS.

References

1. Mansky LM, Temin HM (1995) Lower in vivo mutation rate of human immunodeficiency virus type 1 than that predicted from the fidelity of purified reverse transcriptase. J Virol 69: 5087–5094.
2. Wei X, Ghosh SK, Taylor ME, Johnson VA, Emini EA, et al. (1995) Viral dynamics in human immunodeficiency virus type 1 infection. Nature 373: 117–122.
3. Chun TW, Carruth L, Finzi D, Shen X, DiGiuseppe JA, et al. (1997) Quantification of latent tissue reservoirs and total body viral load in HIV-1 infection. Nature 387: 183–188.
4. Sabino EC, Shpaer EG, Morgado MG, Korber BT, Diaz RS, et al. (1994) Identification of human immunodeficiency virus type 1 envelope genes recombinant between subtypes B and F in two epidemiologically linked individuals from Brazil. J Virol 68: 6340–6346.
5. Spira S, Wainberg MA, Loemba H, Turner D, Brenner BG (2003) Impact of clade diversity on HIV-1 virulence, antiretroviral drug sensitivity and drug resistance. J Antimicrob Chemother 51: 229–240.
6. Rambaut A, Posada D, Crandall KA, Holmes EC (2004) The causes and consequences of HIV evolution. Nat Rev Genet 5: 52–61.
7. Peeters M, Toure-Kane C, Nkengasong JN (2003) Genetic diversity of HIV in Africa: impact on diagnosis, treatment, vaccine development and trials. AIDS 17: 2547–2560.
8. Thomson MM, Perez-Alvarez L, Najera R (2002) Molecular epidemiology of HIV-1 genetic forms and its significance for vaccine development and therapy. Lancet Infect Dis 2: 461–471.
9. Konings FA, Haman GR, Xue Y, Urbanski MM, Hertzmark K, et al. (2006) Genetic analysis of HIV-1 strains in rural eastern Cameroon indicates the evolution of second-generation recombinants to circulating recombinant forms. J Acquir Immune Defic Syndr 42: 331–341.
10. Arien KK, Vanham G, Arts EJ (2007) Is HIV-1 evolving to a less virulent form in humans? Nat Rev Microbiol 5: 141–151.
11. Barreto CC, Nishyia A, Araujo LV, Ferreira JE, Busch MP, et al. (2006) Trends in antiretroviral drug resistance and clade distributions among HIV-1–infected blood donors in Sao Paulo, Brazil. J Acquir Immune Defic Syndr 41: 338–341.
12. Sanabani S, Neto WK, de Sa Filho DJ, Diaz RS, Munerato P, et al. (2006) Full-length genome analysis of human immunodeficiency virus type 1 subtype C in Brazil. AIDS Res Hum Retroviruses 22: 171–176.
13. Sanabani S, Kleine Neto W, Kalmar EM, Diaz RS, Janini LM, et al. (2006) Analysis of the near full length genomes of HIV-1 subtypes B, F and BF recombinant from a cohort of 14 patients in Sao Paulo, Brazil. Infect Genet Evol 6: 368–377.
14. Passaes CP, Guimaraes ML, Bello G, Morgado MG (2009) Near full-length genome characterization of HIV type 1 unique BC recombinant forms from Southern Brazil. AIDS Res Hum Retroviruses 25: 1339–1344.
15. Guimaraes ML, Eyer-Silva WA, Couto-Fernandez JC, Morgado MG (2008) Identification of two new CRF_BF in Rio de Janeiro State, Brazil. AIDS 22: 433–435.
16. Santos AF, Sousa TM, Soares EA, Sanabani S, Martinez AM, et al. (2006) Characterization of a new circulating recombinant form comprising HIV-1 subtypes C and B in southern Brazil. AIDS 20: 2011–2019.
17. Alencar CS, Sabino EC, Carvalho SM, Leao SC, Carneiro-Proietti AB, et al. (2013) HIV genotypes and primary drug resistance among HIV-seropositive blood donors in Brazil: role of infected blood donors as sentinel populations for molecular surveillance of HIV. J Acquir Immune Defic Syndr 63: 387–392.
18. Sanabani SS, Pastena ER, da Costa AC, Martinez VP, Kleine-Neto W, et al. (2011) Characterization of partial and near full-length genomes of HIV-1 strains sampled from recently infected individuals in Sao Paulo, Brazil. PLoS One 6: e25869.
19. Sanabani SS, Pastena ER, Neto WK, Martinez VP, Sabino EC (2010) Characterization and frequency of a newly identified HIV-1 BF1 intersubtype circulating recombinant form in Sao Paulo, Brazil. Virol J 7: 74.

20. Sanabani SS, Pastena ER, Kleine Neto W, Barreto CC, Ferrari KT, et al. (2009) Near full-length genome analysis of low prevalent human immunodeficiency virus type 1 subclade F1 in Sao Paulo, Brazil. Virol J 6: 78.
21. Thomson MM, Sierra M, Tanuri A, May S, Casado G, et al. (2004) Analysis of near full-length genome sequences of HIV type 1 BF intersubtype recombinant viruses from Brazil reveals their independent origins and their lack of relationship to CRF12_BF. AIDS Res Hum Retroviruses 20: 1126–1133.
22. Pessoa R, Watanabe JT, Nukui Y, Pereira J, Kasseb J, et al. (2014) Molecular characterization of human T-cell lymphotropic virus type 1 full and partial genomes by illumina massively parallel sequencing technology. PLoS One 9: e93374.
23. Katoh K, Misawa K, Kuma K, Miyata T (2002) MAFFT: a novel method for rapid multiple sequence alignment based on fast Fourier transform. Nucleic Acids Res 30: 3059–3066.
24. Salminen MO, Carr JK, Burke DS, McCutchan FE (1995) Identification of breakpoints in intergenotypic recombinants of HIV type 1 by bootscanning. AIDS Res Hum Retroviruses 11: 1423–1425.
25. Lole KS, Bollinger RC, Paranjape RS, Gadkari D, Kulkarni SS, et al. (1999) Full-length human immunodeficiency virus type 1 genomes from subtype C-infected seroconverters in India, with evidence of intersubtype recombination. J Virol 73: 152–160.
26. Schultz AK, Zhang M, Leitner T, Kuiken C, Korber B, et al. (2006) A jumping profile Hidden Markov Model and applications to recombination sites in HIV and HCV genomes. BMC Bioinformatics 7: 265.
27. Huson DH, Bryant D (2006) Application of phylogenetic networks in evolutionary studies. Mol Biol Evol 23: 254–267.
28. Tamura K, Stecher G, Peterson D, Filipski A, Kumar S (2013) MEGA6: Molecular Evolutionary Genetics Analysis version 6.0. Mol Biol Evol 30: 2725–2729.
29. Nijhuis M, Schuurman R, de Jong D, Erickson J, Gustchina E, et al. (1999) Increased fitness of drug resistant HIV-1 protease as a result of acquisition of compensatory mutations during suboptimal therapy. AIDS 13: 2349–2359.
30. Xu HT, Oliveira M, Quashie PK, McCallum M, Han Y, et al. (2012) Subunit-selective mutational analysis and tissue culture evaluations of the interactions of the E138K and M184I mutations in HIV-1 reverse transcriptase. J Virol 86: 8422–8431.
31. Xu HT, Quan Y, Schader SM, Oliveira M, Bar-Magen T, et al. (2010) The M230L nonnucleoside reverse transcriptase inhibitor resistance mutation in HIV-1 reverse transcriptase impairs enzymatic function and viral replicative capacity. Antimicrob Agents Chemother 54: 2401–2408.
32. Cavalcanti AM, Brito AM, Salustiano DM, Lima KO, Silva SP, et al. (2012) Recent HIV infection rates among HIV positive patients seeking voluntary counseling and testing centers in the metropolitan region of Recife - PE, Brazil. Braz J Infect Dis 16: 157–163.
33. de Medeiros LB, Lacerda HR, Cavalcanti AM, de Albuquerque Mde F (2006) Primary resistance of human immunodeficiency virus type 1 in a reference center in Recife, Pernambuco, Brazil. Mem Inst Oswaldo Cruz 101: 845–849.
34. Simmonds P, Balfe P, Peutherer JF, Ludlam CA, Bishop JO, et al. (1990) Human immunodeficiency virus-infected individuals contain provirus in small numbers of peripheral mononuclear cells and at low copy numbers. J Virol 64: 864–872.
35. Soares de Oliveira AC, Pessoa de Farias R, da Costa AC, Sauer MM, Bassichetto KC, et al. (2012) Frequency of subtype B and F1 dual infection in HIV-1 positive, Brazilian men who have sex with men. Virol J 9: 223.
36. Sanabani SS, Pessoa R, Soares de Oliveira AC, Martinez VP, Giret MT, et al. (2013) Variability of HIV-1 genomes among children and adolescents from Sao Paulo, Brazil. PLoS One 8: e62552.
37. Ramos A, Tanuri A, Schechter M, Rayfield MA, Hu DJ, et al. (1999) Dual and recombinant infections: an integral part of the HIV-1 epidemic in Brazil. Emerg Infect Dis 5: 65–74.
38. Diaz RS, Sabino EC, Mayer A, Mosley JW, Busch MP (1995) Dual human immunodeficiency virus type 1 infection and recombination in a dually exposed transfusion recipient. The Transfusion Safety Study Group. J Virol 69: 3273–3281.
39. Blackard JT, Mayer KH (2004) HIV superinfection in the era of increased sexual risk-taking. Sex Transm Dis 31: 201–204.
40. Redd AD, Mullis CE, Serwadda D, Kong X, Martens C, et al. (2012) The rates of HIV superinfection and primary HIV incidence in a general population in Rakai, Uganda. J Infect Dis 206: 267–274.
41. Cornelissen M, Pasternak AO, Grijsen ML, Zorgdrager F, Bakker M, et al. (2012) HIV-1 dual infection is associated with faster CD4+ T-cell decline in a cohort of men with primary HIV infection. Clin Infect Dis 54: 539–547.
42. Wirden M, Soulie C, Valantin MA, Fourati S, Simon A, et al. (2011) Historical HIV-RNA resistance test results are more informative than proviral DNA genotyping in cases of suppressed or residual viraemia. J Antimicrob Chemother 66: 709–712.
43. Van Laethem K, Van Vaerenbergh K, Schmit JC, Sprecher S, Hermans P, et al. (1999) Phenotypic assays and sequencing are less sensitive than point mutation assays for detection of resistance in mixed HIV-1 genotypic populations. J Acquir Immune Defic Syndr 22: 107–118.
44. Gunthard HF, Wong JK, Ignacio CC, Havlir DV, Richman DD (1998) Comparative performance of high-density oligonucleotide sequencing and dideoxynucleotide sequencing of HIV type 1 pol from clinical samples. AIDS Res Hum Retroviruses 14: 869–876.
45. Bansode V, McCormack GP, Crampin AC, Ngwira B, Shrestha RK, et al. (2013) Characterizing the emergence and persistence of drug resistant mutations in HIV-1 subtype C infections using 454 ultra deep pyrosequencing. BMC Infect Dis 13: 52.
46. Geretti AM, Fox Z, Johnson JA, Booth C, Lipscomb J, et al. (2013) Sensitive assessment of the virologic outcomes of stopping and restarting non-nucleoside reverse transcriptase inhibitor-based antiretroviral therapy. PLoS One 8: e69266.
47. Bon I, Gibellini D, Borderi M, Alessandrini F, Vitone F, et al. (2007) Genotypic resistance in plasma and peripheral blood lymphocytes in a group of naive HIV-1 patients. J Clin Virol 38: 313–320.
48. Parisi SG, Boldrin C, Cruciani M, Nicolini G, Cerbaro I, et al. (2007) Both human immunodeficiency virus cellular DNA sequencing and plasma RNA sequencing are useful for detection of drug resistance mutations in blood samples from antiretroviral-drug-naive patients. J Clin Microbiol 45: 1783–1788.
49. Jakobsen MR, Tolstrup M, Sogaard OS, Jorgensen LB, Gorry PR, et al. (2010) Transmission of HIV-1 drug-resistant variants: prevalence and effect on treatment outcome. Clin Infect Dis 50: 566–573.
50. Bon I, Alessandrini F, Borderi M, Gorini R, Re MC (2007) Analysis of HIV-1 drug-resistant variants in plasma and peripheral blood mononuclear cells from untreated individuals: implications for clinical management. New Microbiol 30: 313–317.
51. Bi X, Gatanaga H, Ida S, Tsuchiya K, Matsuoka-Aizawa S, et al. (2003) Emergence of protease inhibitor resistance-associated mutations in plasma HIV-1 precedes that in proviruses of peripheral blood mononuclear cells by more than a year. J Acquir Immune Defic Syndr 34: 1–6.
52. Kaye S, Comber E, Tenant-Flowers M, Loveday C (1995) The appearance of drug resistance-associated point mutations in HIV type 1 plasma RNA precedes their appearance in proviral DNA. AIDS Res Hum Retroviruses 11: 1221–1225.
53. Riva E, Pistello M, Narciso P, D'Offizi G, Isola P, et al. (2001) Decay of HIV type 1 DNA and development of drug-resistant mutants in patients with primary HIV type 1 infection receiving highly active antiretroviral therapy. AIDS Res Hum Retroviruses 17: 1599–1604.
54. Banks L, Gholamin S, White E, Zijenah L, Katzenstein DA (2012) Comparing Peripheral Blood Mononuclear Cell DNA and Circulating Plasma viral RNA pol Genotypes of Subtype C HIV-1. J AIDS Clin Res 3: 141–147.
55. Chew CB, Potter SJ, Wang B, Wang YM, Shaw CO, et al. (2005) Assessment of drug resistance mutations in plasma and peripheral blood mononuclear cells at different plasma viral loads in patients receiving HAART. J Clin Virol 33: 206–216.

A Real Time PCR Platform for the Simultaneous Quantification of Total and Extrachromosomal HIV DNA Forms in Blood of HIV-1 Infected Patients

Anna Casabianca[1*], Chiara Orlandi[1], Benedetta Canovari[2], Maddalena Scotti[1], Marcello Acetoso[2], Massimo Valentini[2], Enzo Petrelli[2], Mauro Magnani[1]

1 Department of Biomolecular Sciences, University of Urbino "Carlo Bo", Urbino (PU), Italy, **2** Azienda Ospedaliera Ospedali Riuniti Marche Nord - Presidio Ospedaliero San Salvatore, Pesaro (PU), Italy

Abstract

Background: The quantitative measurement of various HIV-1 DNA forms including total, unintegrated and integrated provirus play an increasingly important role in HIV-1 infection monitoring and treatment-related research. We report the development and validation of a SYBR Green real time PCR (*TotUFsys* platform) for the simultaneous quantification of total and extrachromosomal HIV-1 DNA forms in patients. This innovative technique makes it possible to obtain both measurements in a single PCR run starting from frozen blood employing the same primers and standard curve. Moreover, due to identical amplification efficiency, it allows indirect estimation of integrated level. To specifically detect 2-LTR a qPCR method was also developed.

Methodology/Findings: Primers used for total HIV-1 DNA quantification spanning a highly conserved region were selected and found to detect all HIV-1 clades of group M and the unintegrated forms of the same. A total of 195 samples from HIV-1 patients in a wide range of clinical conditions were analyzed with a 100% success rate, even in patients with suppressed plasma viremia, regardless of CD4+ or therapy. No significant correlation was observed between the two current prognostic markers, CD4+ and plasma viremia, while a moderate or high inverse correlation was found between CD4+ and total HIV DNA, with strong values for unintegrated HIV DNA.

Conclusions/Significance: Taken together, the results support the use of HIV DNA as another tool, in addition to traditional assays, which can be used to estimate the state of viral infection, the risk of disease progression and to monitor the effects of ART. The *TotUFsys* platform allowed us to obtain a final result, expressed as the total and unintegrated HIV DNA copy number per microgram of DNA or 10^4 CD4+, for 12 patients within two working days.

Editor: Yuntao Wu, George Mason University, United States of America

Funding: This work was supported by Gilead Science Srl. The funder had no role in study design, data collection and analysis, decision to publish, or preparation of the manuscript.

Competing Interests: The work was supported by "Fellowship Program 2011" of Gilead Science Srl. The funders had no role in study design, data collection and analysis, decision to publish, or preparation of the manuscript. The authors have declared that no competing interests exist.

* Email: anna.casabianca@uniurb.it

These authors contributed equally to this work.

Introduction

HIV infection has been transformed over the past two decades from a lethal disease to a manageable chronic condition thanks to the advent of combination antiretroviral therapy (ART). Nevertheless, virus persistence in reservoirs prevents complete virus eradication in patients treated with current therapies [1–3]. In recent years, *a)* the introduction of new drugs (e.g. viral integrase inhibitors, co-receptor antagonists), in addition to the classic inhibitors of reverse transcriptase and protease, which interfere with other steps in the virus life cycle, and/or new therapeutic vaccinations, *b)* efforts to gain a greater understanding of the nature and role of the reservoir in AIDS pathogenesis and *c)* low-level persistent viremia despite clinically successful antiretroviral therapy have encouraged a careful analysis of the kinetics and relative contributions of the viral DNA to HIV-1 replication and latency during disease progression and ART treatment.

Total cell-associated HIV-1 DNA (total HIV DNA) is present in infected cells in three major forms that reflect the different stages and fates of development during viral replication: integrated proviral DNA (IDNA) and unintegrated (extrachromosomal) forms (UF) including both linear and circular DNA (1-LTR and 2-LTR). Several authors have shown the presence of small amounts (1% or more) of the aberrant circular forms. HIV-1 infection *in vitro* and *in vivo* results in an abundance of UF, regardless of cell type and

Workflow:
Time required

1. Defrost 3-4 ml of twelve whole blood samples, mix well and transfer into a 15 ml tube

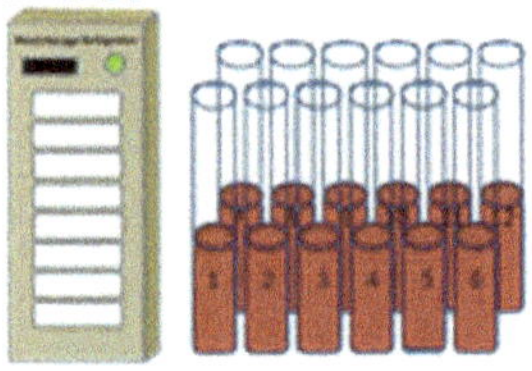

00:15:00

2. Wash with 10 ml of physiological solution containing 0.1% NP-40

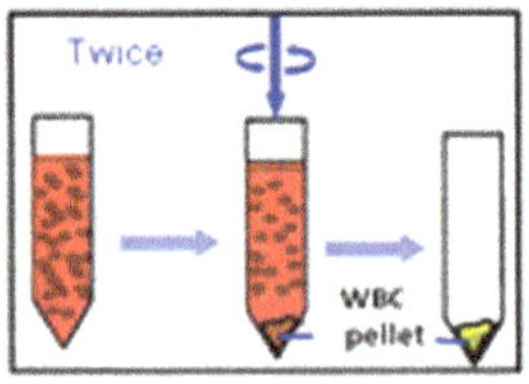

01:15:00

✓ Centrifuge 10 min at 3750 rpm at room temperature
✓ Discard the liquid without disturbing the pellet
✓ Wash the WBC pellet and centrifuge again
✓ Discard the liquid and incubate the WBC for 45 min at 37 °C in 6-8 ml of lysis buffer

3. Purify the DNA by phenol extraction following ethanol precipitation and RNase digestion

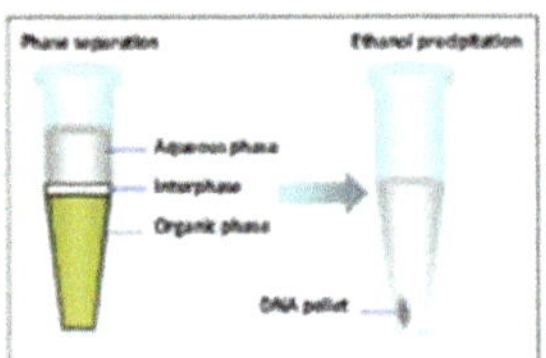

02:00:00

4. Quantify by NanoDrop ND-1000 Spectrophotometer

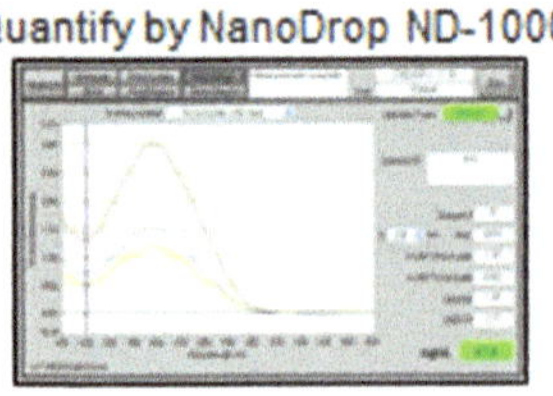

00:15:00

5. Sample preparation for total HIV DNA quantification
✓Mix 10 μg of DNA with 1.5 volume of Hydrogen peroxide solution
✓Incubate at 37°C for 30 min
✓Precipitate by ethanol
✓Quantify again by NanoDrop ND-1000

01:15:00

6. Sample preparation for Unintegrated HIV DNA quantification

Resuspension		Alkaline Lysis		Neutralization		Centrifuge
Resuspended 5 μg of DNA in Buffer P1 (250 μl of total volume)	→	Add 250 μl Buffer P2 and mix gently	→	Add 350 μl Buffer N3 and mix gently	→	Centrifuge at 12500 rpm 10 min

Loading to column	Centrifuge	Washing	Centrifuge	Washing	Centrifuge	Column drying	Elution	Centrifuge
Transfer supernatant to column (600 μl, 70.58% of processed DNA)	1 min; Discard flow through	Add 500 μl Buffer PB	1 min; Discard flow through	Add 750 μl Buffer PB	1 min; Discard flow through	1 min	Trasfer column to a new microcentrifuge tube. Add 106 μl pre-heated Buffer EB (70°C). Stand for 20 min at 50°C.	1 min; Store unintegrated HIV DNA at 4°C or -20°C.

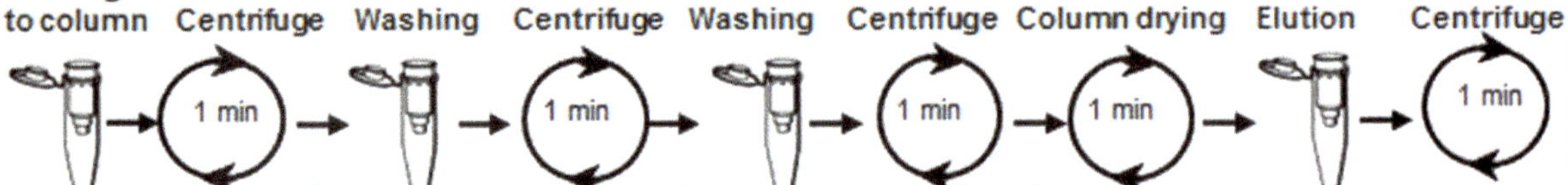

01:00:00

7. Set up a 96-well reaction plate arranging unknown samples and standards as in the layout shown. Each sample is tested in two replicates of 0.5 μg and one replicate of 1 μg of cellular DNA or LMW fraction DNA.

02:00:00

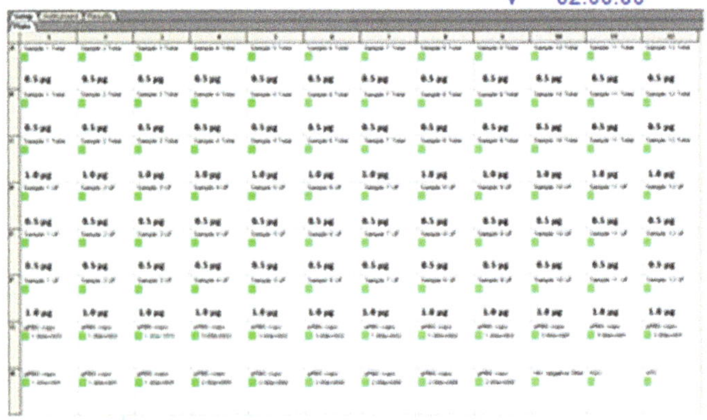

8. Load the *TotUFsys* Plate into the 7500 Real Time PCR System and start the run setting the following thermal cycling conditions (dissociation stage is added)

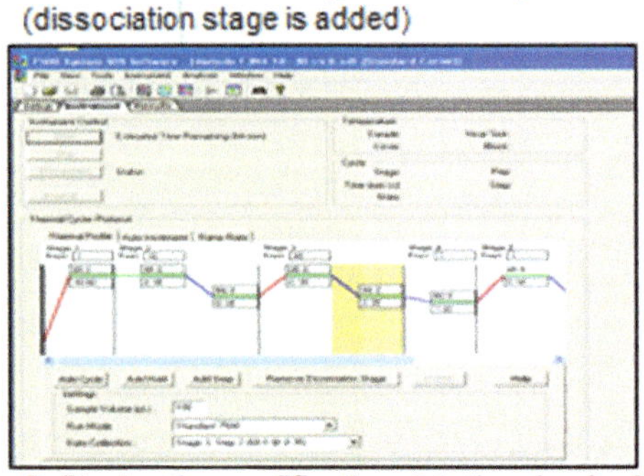

01:45:00

9. Display the amplification plot, the standard curve and export the extrapolated quantity of total and unintegrated HIV DNA

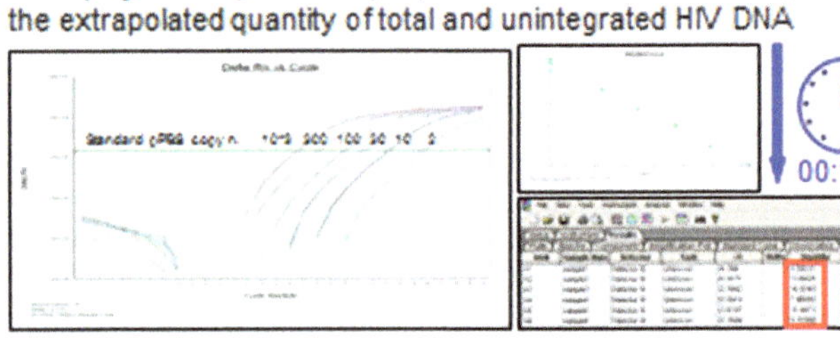

00:15:00

10. Data analysis. Details are reported in section "*Data analysis of quantification of total, unintegrated (TotUFsys platform) and 2-LTR HIV DNA forms*". For each sample, total and unintegrated HIV DNA forms are expressed as:
HIV DNA copy number/μg DNA or LMW fraction DNA or
HIV DNA copy number/10^4 CD4+

Total time: 10/14 h

Figure 1. Complete workflow of the whole procedure for the quantification of total and unintegrated HIV DNA forms in 12 samples, from frozen blood until data analysis.

activation status [4–7]. Blood, lymphoid tissue and brain tissue show a ratio of extrachromosomal to integrated forms of 99:1, while the ratio linear/1-LTR/2-LTR is 20:9:1 [1,8,9]. Regarding stability, the following order was found: integrated DNA>circular DNA (1-LTR and 2-LTR)>linear DNA. The detection of high levels of unintegrated DNA in the brain has been associated with the development of AIDS dementia [9]. In particular, 2-LTR circles, have been suggested as a possible marker of recent infection due to their labile nature, although stable unintegrated forms have been shown to exist, and hence their utility as a clinical marker of recent infection is questionable. 2-LTR circles are often viewed as overall markers of all unintegrated forms, although they are present at relatively low levels compared to other HIV DNA species. The extrachromosomal forms are biologically active: they produce functional viral proteins, are toxic to the cell and can trigger the apoptotic cascade [7,10–12].

Currently, HIV-1 RNA levels and CD4+ T lymphocyte counts are the standard markers used in clinical practice for the management and the monitoring of HIV-1 infected patients. CD4+ T cell counts yield information on the patient's immunological status and the HIV-RNA load provides information on the extent of viral replication at the time of the assay. At present, antiretroviral protocols use drugs that suppress the replicative ability of HIV-1 to the point that circulating virus in plasma becomes undetectable using the standard commercial viral RNA detection assays (20–50 copies/ml). However, low levels of free virus can still be detected in a majority of patients on ART using ultrasensitive assays. After several years of therapy, this residual viremia reaches a plateau of 1–10 copies/ml and does not appear to decline any further [13]. Hence, in this scenario, it would be useful to have additional virological markers for monitoring and predicting therapy responses and for measuring the degree of HIV-1 persistence in patients on ART. Assays that quantify viral DNA have been already developed and are taking an important role in HIV cure-related research. Total HIV DNA has been used for a number of years and is currently the most feasible tool available for large-scale clinical trials and cohort studies [14–20]. Several reports have investigated the prognostic value of HIV DNA measurement as a marker of disease progression and treatment efficacy [21–27]. HIV DNA provides essential information on the reservoir and dynamics of the HIV-1 infection, especially in patients with undetectable plasma viremia, in whom HIV DNA could represent the only biomarker of viral activity that can be easily detected.

The aim of this work was to evaluate the reliability and usefulness of the simultaneous quantification of total and all unintegrated HIV DNA forms (linear+1- and 2-LTR circles) in a wide range of clinical situations. We used a high performance workflow and a PCR plate layout (*TotUFsys* platform), starting from a single cellular DNA recovered once from whole blood of HIV-1 infected patients. These patients reported to the reference hospital for routine clinical tests. Based on a previously developed strategy [28], we improved the whole blood leukocyte assay (pbs-rtPCR) in terms of robustness for total HIV DNA quantification and also developed a new SYBR Green qPCR, which was optimized and validated for quantifying all unintegrated forms. For a further comprehensive analysis of the clinical samples, we also developed a SYBR Green qPCR based method to specifically detect 2-LTR circles in the same cellular DNA samples used for the quantification of total and unintegrated HIV DNA. Both the *TotUFsys* platform and the 2-LTR assay were developed analyzing the Guidelines for the Validation of Analytical Procedures (http://www.ich.org). An appropriate exogenous control was added to monitor the various steps of the procedure, and negative controls were also tested. The complete workflow of the whole procedure for the quantification of total and unintegrated HIV DNA forms is illustrated in Figure 1.

Results

Patient characteristics

Clinical characteristics of patients and their different clinical pictures are summarized in Table 1.

Primer and diagnostic specificity

Primer specificity for HIV-1 clades in group M was confirmed *in silico* by BLAST (Figure S1) [29], and also by real time PCR using different HIV-1 subtypes and HIV-2 ROD complete proviral sequences [28]. No cross-reactivity with retroviral endogenous sequences (HERV) [30] was detected in 100 HIV-1 negative blood donors using real time PCR [28]. Moreover, an additional 150 HIV-1 negative samples were checked. Samples showing only a very weak peak, consistently below 2 copies (Ct mean value±SD: 26.60±0.87, n = 35), were considered as nonspecific PCR signals (Figure 2, panel A and Table S1).

Standard curve, sensitivity and reproducibility of the assay (*TotUFsys* platform)

For HIV DNA quantification, the pPBS standard curve was constructed with half-log plasmid serial dilutions from 10^3 to 10 copies and 2 copies. The quantification limit (QL) was set at 2 copies/PCR reaction. The standard was analyzed in the presence or absence of 0.5 µg of HIV-1 negative DNA (background DNA, bk DNA). The two curves revealed no differences in their linear range of quantification or PCR efficiency (Δslope<0.1, Applied Biosystems User Bulletin No. 2 http://www3.appliedbiosystems.com/cms/groups/mcb_support/documents/generaldocuments/cms_040980.pdf, 1997). Moreover, in the presence of 0.5 µg of bk DNA no inhibitory effect was detected (2-copy Ct value: 25.47±0.89 and 25.35±0.59 with or no bk DNA, respectively, Table S2). Hence, the standard without bk DNA was used for total and unintegrated HIV DNA measurements (Figure 2, panel B and Table S3). The method's reproducibility was calculated by the percentage of coefficient variation for Ct values (CV_{Ct}) and for copy numbers (CV_{Cn}). The CV_{Ct} and CV_{Cn} mean values of pPBSstd were 1.32% and 20%, respectively (Table S4). These data were confirmed assaying the reproducibility of some samples as inter and intra-assay variations (Table S5).

Unintegrated HIV DNA separation from high molecular weight DNA

The selective separation of extrachromosomal HIV DNA from high molecular weight (HMW) genomic DNA, which could harbor integrated HIV-1 provirus, was performed adapting a plasmid DNA purification through column chromatography on silica gel procedure. This strategy was reported for the first time by Sharkey *et al.* [6] for the selective detection of 2-LTR circles and by others [15,31] using a PBMC pellet of about ~2–6×10^7 cells. In the present investigation, the possible use of a small amount of

Table 1. Clinical characteristics of the patients.

Characteristic	Value
Male	39 (66%)
Female	20 (34%)
Age, median years (range)	44 (27–70)
CD4+ T cell count at nadir, median cells/μl (range)	250 (2–1200)
HIV-1 RNA load at nadir, median copies/ml (range)	10^5 (<50-10^6)
Years since diagnosis, median years (range)	4 (<1–28)
Treatment-naïve	11 (19%), 32 blood samples
ART-experienced	48 (81%), 163 blood samples
Years on ART, median years (range), n = 48	2.5 (<1–19)
Multidrug resistant HIV-1 infection (MDR)	21 (36%), 85 blood samples
HCV, HBV, Syphilis, TBC co-infected	23 (39%)

cellular DNA (5 μg) was evaluated. This DNA was obtained by the phenol extraction procedure able to ensure an HMW of typically ~100–200 Kb [32] and non degraded DNA. The genomic DNA extracted using commercial kits (<50 kb) could be co-purified in the eluate fraction. To assess the performance of this approach, 5 μg of an HMW DNA sample and an equal amount of the molecular weight Marker II (Lambda DNA/HindIII), used as a procedure monitor, were processed in columns and the eluate fractions were analyzed by agarose gel electrophoresis. The results showed the absence of HMW DNA>10 Kb and a slight degradation of the DNA sample, demonstrating the ability of the procedure to selectively recover the DNA which approximates the genome length of HIV-1 (Figure S2). To assess the extent of DNA degradation, the β-actin housekeeping gene was amplified and quantified on ACTstd. The percentage was estimated at 5.0±1.3% (mean±SD, n = 20), revealing the presence of a negligible amount of HMW DNA fragments co-purified in the low molecular weight (LMW) DNA fraction, containing unintegrated HIV DNA (Table S6). Clearly, this drawback was intrinsic in the spin-column method itself, and did not affect the final results. To measure the actual recovery of unintegrated forms, the 13 Kb pEXg plasmid, which simulates the HIV-1 genome length,

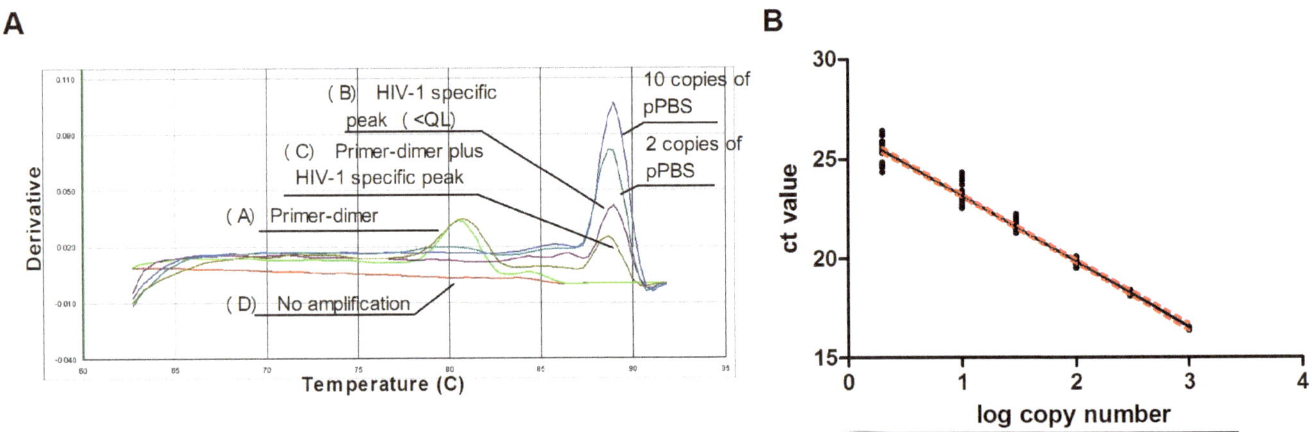

Table	n	%
Primer-dimer (A)	54	36
HIV-1 specific peak (B)	35	23
Primer -dimer plus HIV-1 specific peak (C)	24	16
No amplification (D)	37	25
Total	150	100

Best-fit values	
Slope	-3.295 ± 0.05379
Y-intercept when X=0.0	26.44 ± 0.08511
X-intercept when Y=0.0	8.026
1/slope	-0.3035
95% Confidence Intervals	
Slope	-3.402 to -3.188
Y-intercept when X=0.0	26.27 to 26.61
X-intercept when Y=0.0	7.814 to 8.252
Goodness of Fit	
r^2	0.9766

Figure 2. Post-PCR melt curve analysis and standard curve. (A) Different dissociation curves that are shown in percentages of their relative amounts in the analysis of 150 HIV-1 negative DNA samples. Only 10 and 2 copies of standard are displayed. (B) Mean standard curve obtained in the *TotUFsys* PCR experiments (n = 8).

was included at the beginning of the column separation procedure as an exogenous standard. A typical experiment involved the addition of known amounts of the pEXg (10^2 or 10^3 copies) to 5 μg of cellular DNA, followed by the evaluation of the recovered quantity by qPCR. Repeated experiments showed high levels of recovery (94%–98%, Table S7). We used 10^2 and 10^3 plasmid copies because the expected copies/PCR were 10 and 100 respectively, reflecting the HIV DNA content found in HIV-1 positive patients (range from 2 to 108 in 73 samples) [28].

Quantification of total and unintegrated HIV DNA forms in blood samples

In order to confirm that the *TotUFsys* was able to detect and quantify the different HIV DNA forms in a range of clinical pictures, a total of 195 HIV-1 positive blood samples were tested. The samples were collected from ART-experienced subjects (163, 84%) and from treatment-naïve patients (32, 16%). To enhance precision and sensitivity, HIV DNA copy numbers were measured in a replicate of 0.5–1.0 μg of DNA or LMW fraction DNA from 2 to 8 and normalized to 1 μg of cellular DNA. Table 2 shows the quantifications of the total and unintegrated HIV DNA of 5 representative samples and how the final data were calculated and normalized.

For 100% of the analyzed samples we were able to give a final result as the total, unintegrated and integrated provirus HIV DNA copy number, regardless of plasma viremia, CD4+ T cell count or therapy (Table S8). Provirus was obtained by subtracting unintegrated from total HIV DNA. For total HIV DNA, the highest percentage (95%) of quantified samples (QL, 2 copies) was found in samples with a CD4+ T cell count <350, whereas the lowest percentage (81%) was found in samples with plasma viremia >50 copies/ml and in ART–naïve samples, although it should also be noted that these two groups were smaller than the other groups. For unintegrated HIV DNA, the highest value was found in samples with plasma viremia >50 copies/ml and in ART–naïve samples (75%). Of note, although the differences are small, there were more samples with undetectable integrated HIV DNA in patients under treatment, with suppressed plasma viremia and higher CD4+ T cell counts. The median total HIV DNA was 17 (range: <2–923, IQR: 5–40) and 693 copies (range: 12–30044, IQR: 180–1584) per μg of DNA or ml of whole blood, respectively; the median unintegrated HIV DNA was 5 (range: <2–238, IQR: <2–14) and 192 copies (range: 12–6931, IQR: 76–549). The integrated HIV DNA revealed a median of 9 (range: <2–802, IQR: <2–26) and 355 (range: 12–26105, IQR: 72–1016) per μg of DNA or ml of whole blood, respectively. In Figure 3 are reported the percentages of copy number distribution of the total, unintegrated and integrated HIV DNA forms. We evidenced that 65% of sample quantifications of the various forms were in the range 2–60 copies, supporting the use of the half-log dilution standard curve to enhance precision of the data. To account for the variation in the number of CD4+ T cells in different samples, the results were further normalized by the CD4+ percentage of total WBC and expressed as copies/10^4 CD4+. This normalization is based on the assumption that most of the HIV DNA is in the CD4+ T cells [33,34] and on our statistical analysis which showed an average of 10867 CD4+ analyzed per μg of DNA (median, range: 8632, 158–34869). Median HIV DNA was 21 (range: <2–2407, IQR: 6–50) and 6 (range: 1–1457, IQR: 2–17) copies per 10^4 CD4+ for total and unintegrated forms, respectively. The integrated form showed a median of 10 (range: 0–950, IQR: 3–32) copies per 10^4 CD4+. Table 3 shows the differences in HIV DNA load in some samples according to the normalization procedure that was chosen. Individuals with quite similar data trends regarding total HIV DNA copies/μg (or ml of blood) recorded in two sequential visits (patients 9–35), actually show at least a two-fold decrease in the content of HIV DNA copies/μg or even a nearly 20-fold decrease, considering the same data expressed for 10^4 CD4+ T cells. This decrease correlates with the increase in equal measure of the percentage of CD4+ T cells. The decrease in HIV DNA content is actually much more evident considering the data normalized for 10^4 CD4+, a nearly five-fold decrease (patients 41, 26, 22). Likewise, an apparent two- to five-fold increase (patients 33, 52, 56) results in no change in the HIV DNA load for 10^4 CD4+. Due to the impact of the normalization procedure on the quantification of HIV DNA, we decided henceforth to conduct each type of subsequent analyses comparing the data obtained by qPCR (copy number/μg DNA) to those expressed for 10^4 CD4+ T cells, considering these data to be more informative than HIV DNA per ml of blood.

Correlations between study parameters in blood samples

The correlations between the amount of HIV DNA and plasma viremia or CD4+ T cell counts and between HIV-1 RNA and CD4+ were examined using Spearman's rank test. Most correlations were found when the data were expressed for 10^4 CD4+ (Table S9). When all 195 samples were analyzed together, no significant correlation was observed between plasma viremia and CD4+ ($r = -0.14$, $p = 0.05$) and there was a marginal positive correlation between plasma viremia and the amount of unintegrated HIV DNA ($r = 0.31$, $p < 0.0001$). However, there was a moderate inverse correlation between CD4+ T cell counts and both total ($r = -0.48$, $p < 0.0001$) and UF HIV DNA ($r = -0.52$, $p < 0.0001$). Due to the wide range of clinical situations within our cohort of samples, correlations were evaluated in different subsets, dividing them into six groups according to various criteria. Two groups were defined according to evidence of resistance: MDR (Multidrug resistant HIV-1 infection) and non-MDR. Three groups were identified on the basis of therapy: ART, under RAL, and without therapy (Naïve). Finally, a sixth group was defined according to measurable plasma viremia (HIV-1 RNA> 50 copies/ml). There was an inverse moderate correlation between viral load and CD4+ T cell counts only in the treatment-naïve group ($r = -0.57$, $p < 0.005$). Plasma viremia showed a weak positive correlation with HIV DNA (total and UF) in the non-MDR group ($r \geq 0.31$, $p < 0.005$), it correlated strongly with HIV DNA in the treatment-naïve group ($r \geq 0.66$, $p < 0.0001$) and in the samples with measurable plasma viremia ($r \geq 0.40$, $p \leq 0.005$). Each of these correlations was stronger when the UF were considered. Interestingly, there was consistently a significant inverse correlation between CD4+ and HIV DNA in all the groups examined (r within −0.40 and −0.77, $p < 0.0001$). Such inverse correlations were stronger for UF (Figure 4). We selected 45 subjects for whom at least two sequential samples were available, to compare samples from an arbitrary time zero (START, first sampling available) to those taken at the end of the observation period (STOP, last sampling available) and the following groups were analyzed: treatment-naïve, under ART, ART-subjects under RAL intensification and a last group was formed by combining the latter two groups (Table S10). It should be noted that for the 45 patients, while a modest correlation between plasma viremia and CD4+ ($r = -0.29$, $p = 0.06$) or HIV DNA ($r \geq 0.40$, $p \geq 0.01$) is reduced to insignificant values from the beginning to the end of the observation period, the higher inverse correlation between CD4+ and HIV DNA observed at the beginning ($r \leq -0.67$, $p < 0.0001$) remained moderate at the end of the observation period ($r = -0.53$, $p < 0.005$). In the treatment-naïve group, there were no statistically significant correlations (p≥

Table 2. Quantification of total and unintegrated (UF) HIV DNA copy number in five different samples.

Run	Sample 1		Sample 2		Sample 3		Sample 4		Sample 5	
	Total HIV DNA	UF HIV DNA	Total HIV DNA	UF HIV DNA	Total HIV DNA	UF HIV DNA	Total HIV DNA	UF HIV DNA	Total HIV DNA	UF HIV DNA
1st qPCR	15	5	14	5	19	7	21	16	39	17
1st qPCR	14	2	10	3	24	10	22	12	50	17
2nd qPCR	11	2	11	5	24	10	28	18	43	22
2nd qPCR	12	3	16	5	20	11	24	13	46	16
2nd qPCR	13	6	13	5	23	12	20	11	50	22
2nd qPCR	11	4	12	8	24	7	23	14	45	20
2nd qPCR	20	3	17	5	22	11	25	12	41	20
2nd qPCR	15	3	10	4	21	12	25	16	43	17
Coefficient of variation	21.25%	40.41%	20.52%	28.28%	8.86%	20.00%	10.91%	17.50%	8.88%	12.80%
Lower 95% CI of mean	11	2	11	4	20	8	21	12	41	17
Upper 95% CI of mean	16	5	15	6	24	12	26	16	48	21
Sum	110	29	101	39	176	81	189	113	358	149
[a]Copies/μg	28	7	25	10	44	20	47	28	89	37
[b]Copies/ml of blood	780	195	1309	524	2667	1212	1846	1100	4124	1715
[c]Copies/10^4 CD4+	13	3	55	22	24	11	48	29	104	43

[a]The results were obtained dividing the sum of the copy number from a total of eight replicates (two 0.5 μg replicates in the 1st qPCR and six 0.5 μg replicates in the 2nd qPCR) by 4 and expressed as HIV DNA copy number/μg of DNA.

[b]Taking into account the WBC number, the results can be reported as copies/ml of blood with the formula: (copies/μg DNA)×WBC no. per ml/142857 cells, assuming that 142857 cells are present in one μg of DNA. WBC counts/μl are 3980 (sample 1), 7480 (sample 2), 8660 (sample 3), 5610 (sample 4), and 6620 (sample 5).

[c]Taking into account %CD4+, the results can be reported as copies/10^4 CD4+ with the formula: [(copies/μg DNA)/(CD4+/WBC×142857 WBC)]×10^4. The %CD4+ are: 15.0% (sample 1), 3.2% (sample 2), 12.9% (sample 3), 6.8% (sample 4), and 6.0% (sample 5).

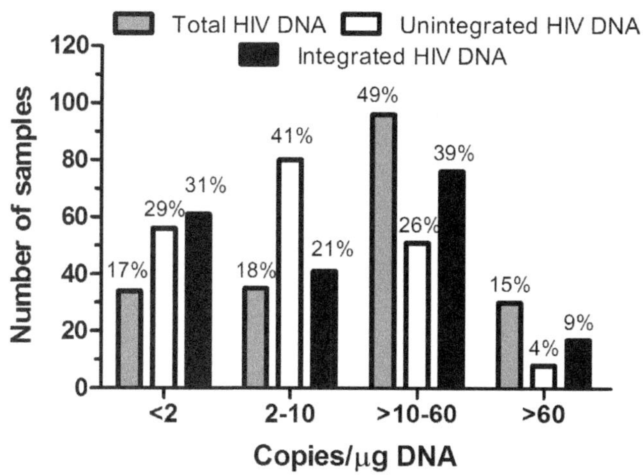

Figure 3. Distribution of total, unintegrated and integrated HIV DNA copy number in four range: very low (<2 copies), low (2–10), medium (>10–60) and high (<60) for 195 blood samples.

0.23). This may be due to the small number of patients. For patients under the ART regimen, significant initial moderate inverse correlations were observed between CD4+ T cell counts and both plasma viremia ($r = -0.53$, $p = 0.02$) and total HIV DNA ($r = -0.62$, $p = 0.01$), and a stronger correlation was found with UF ($r = -0.73$, $p<0.005$). At the end of the observation period, the only correlation that is was still evident, although not statistically significant, was between CD4+ and UF ($r = -0.42$, $p = 0.09$). In the under RAL group, there was a significant moderate inverse correlation between plasma viremia and CD4+ only at the end of the observation period ($r = -0.53$, $p = 0.03$). The higher correlation between plasma viremia and the amount of HIV DNA ($r \geq 0.61$, $p = 0.01$) became nearly insignificant by the end of the observation period. On the contrary, the moderate inverse correlation between CD4+ and HIV DNA ($r \leq -0.57$, $p \leq 0.02$) strengthened during the observation period becoming a strong inverse correlation ($r \leq -0.75$, $p \leq 0.005$). In the ART & under RAL group, the only correlation that remained moderate throughout the observation period was between CD4+ and HIV DNA ($r \leq -0.53$, $p \leq 0.005$), while the correlation between HIV-1 RNA and CD4+ or HIV DNA was reduced at the end of the study to lower values, which were not always statistically significant.

Development and validation of 2-LTR circles in blood samples

To specifically detect 2-LTR circles in blood samples we designed a SYBR Green qPCR using primers flanking the dual-repeat cassette within the circular form, which is formed after end-to-end 5′ and 3′ LTR ligation. The primers were specific to the sequences of the M group reported in HIV Sequence Compendium 2013 [29]. Moreover, they were tested in 50 HIV-1 negative DNA samples showing no amplification in 86% of the samples ($n = 43$) and nonspecific amplification in the remaining 14% ($n = 7$). The amplification of the 2-LTR junction was linear over a 5-log range, and sensitivity allowed the detection of two copies per reaction (Ct mean value±SD: 27.37±1.11), even in the presence of 0.5 μg of bk DNA. The p2LTR standard showed a mean curve of $y = -3.3287x+28.37$ ($n = 8$), with an efficiency of 98–100%, and a linear correlation of $R^2 = 0.99$. The reproducibility assayed by %CV of copy number of the standard curve was 19% in the 10^5 to 2 copy number range. 2-LTR were measured in replicates of 0.5 μg of cellular DNA from 2 to 8 and normalized to 1 μg of DNA and to 10^4 CD4+. To validate 2-LTR assay some randomly selected blood samples were tested (Table 4). Most of the samples (16 of 30, 53%) had very low levels of 2-LTR (<2 copies/μg DNA), while the remaining samples showed between 2 and 10 copies/μg DNA. No significant differences were found in the three groups analyzed on the basis of therapy: treatment-naïve, ART and under RAL ($p = 0.379$ and $p = 0.770$ for normalization per μg of DNA or per 10^4 CD4+, respectively, Kruskal-Wallis test). Likewise, no significant differences were found between MDR and non-MDR groups ($p = 0.741$ and $p = 0.207$ for normalization per μg DNA or per 10^4 CD4+ respectively, Mann-Whitney test). Due to similar PCR efficiencies for unintegrated and 2-LTR circles, we provide data regarding the 1-LTR circles and, if present, linear HIV DNA, subtracting the level of 2-LTR from all unintegrated forms.

Discussion

Total cell-associated HIV-1 DNA consists of unintegrated linear and circular 1-LTR and 2-LTR forms and integrated proviral DNA. Recent reports suggest that transcription from unintegrated HIV DNA appears to be a normal early step in HIV replication pointing to a potential role for unintegrated viral DNA in HIV-1 pathogenesis. High levels of UF can be detected *in vivo* and it is the most prevalent form of HIV DNA (2 log more than IDNA) in resting and activated CD4+ T cells [35,36].

QPCR-based methods are now available to accurately quantify HIV DNA forms and they are widely used to explore the pathogenetic role of reservoirs, viral persistence and to monitor the effectiveness of antiviral therapy. Some of these assays have a throughput which is too low (up to 40 replicates for just a single sample) [37] and too expensive for use in large clinical trials or in routine clinical practice to complement CD4+ T cell counts and HIV-1 RNA, which are routinely used in the management of HIV-1 infected patients. Some authors have performed a concurrent measurement of total and integrated HIV DNA [16–18]. However, no methodology has been developed for assaying total HIV DNA and all unintegrated forms in a relatively simple manner. The aim of this work was to evaluate the reliability and usefulness of the simultaneous quantification of total and unintegrated HIV DNA forms (*TotUFsys* platform) in HIV-1 blood samples. The novelty of the strategy lies in the fact that for each sample, both measurements are obtained in a single PCR run starting from a single DNA isolated from a small amount of frozen blood, omitting the PBMC separation on ficoll-hypaque gradient. The assay uses specific primers spanning the highly conserved PBS region and its flanking sequences [28] and is unaffected by the location of the HIV-1 integration site, unlike the *Alu*-assay [17,37]. Employing the same primers and using a single standard curve, the identical amplification efficiency and sensitivity allowed us to accurately compare the data. Moreover, it appears that the integrated level can be calculated indirectly as the difference between the total and unintegrated HIV DNA. Unlike other published reports, for the first time, the UF were separated from HMW DNA through column chromatography on silica gel, starting from a small amount of cellular DNA (5 μg) and then quantified in the LMW fraction. The phenol-chloroform DNA extraction procedure ensured a not degraded, HMW DNA, and only a slight cross-contamination of genomic DNA fragments in the LMW fraction were observed. Other faster or automated DNA extraction procedures may also be used, first thoroughly assessing genomic DNA contamination in the eluate fraction. The high rate of recovery demonstrates the feasibility of the separation method

Table 3. The effect of the data normalization procedure on the quantification of HIV DNA in blood samples from HIV-1 positive subjects.

Patient	Time point	WBC cell count/μl	CD4+ T cell count/μl	% CD4+	Fold change	Total HIV DNA copy no.					
						per μg of DNA	Fold change	per ml of blood	Fold change	per 10^4 CD4+	Fold change
9	1	5100	340	6.7	2.6	106	1.1	3784	1.2	111	2.4
	4	3940	683	17.3		115		3172		46	
10	1	4890	110	2.2	2.4	62	1.1	2122	1.6	193	2.2
	7	7130	389	5.5		68		3394		87	
16	1	6890	326	4.7	1.8	15	1.0	723	1.7	22	1.8
	9	4160	354	8.5		15		437		12	
18	1	5200	470	9.0	2.2	63	0.9	2293	1.1	49	2.3
	2	6030	1190	19.7		59		2490		21	
19	1	7690	100	1.3	1.8	39	1.0	2099	1.2	210	1.9
	2	6320	150	2.4		38		1681		112	
30	1	8970	40	0.4	6.9	18	0.9	1130	1.1	283	7.4
	6	8490	263	3.1		17		1010		38	
35	1	1810	2	0.1	17.0	38	0.9	481	2.8	2407	18.0
	2	5420	102	1.9		36		1366		134	
41	1	2370	42	1.8	4.4	10	2.0	166	1.1	40	10.0
	3	5130	400	7.8		5		180		4	
26	1	12100	40	0.3	4.3	21	5.3	1779	15.6	445	22.3
	5	4060	58	1.4		4		114		20	
22	1	4880	120	2.5	4.5	170	7.4	5807	8.3	484	34.6
	6	4340	477	11.0		23		699		14	
33	1	7400	157	2.1	2.0	14	1.9	725	1.7	46	1.0
	4	6390	273	4.3		27		1208		44	
52	1	3210	45	1.4	3.5	23	3.0	517	3.1	115	0.8
	2	3300	163	4.9		69		1594		97	
56	1	9540	70	0.7	6.9	20	5.4	1336	2.5	186	0.8
	3	4500	227	5.0		107		3371		148	

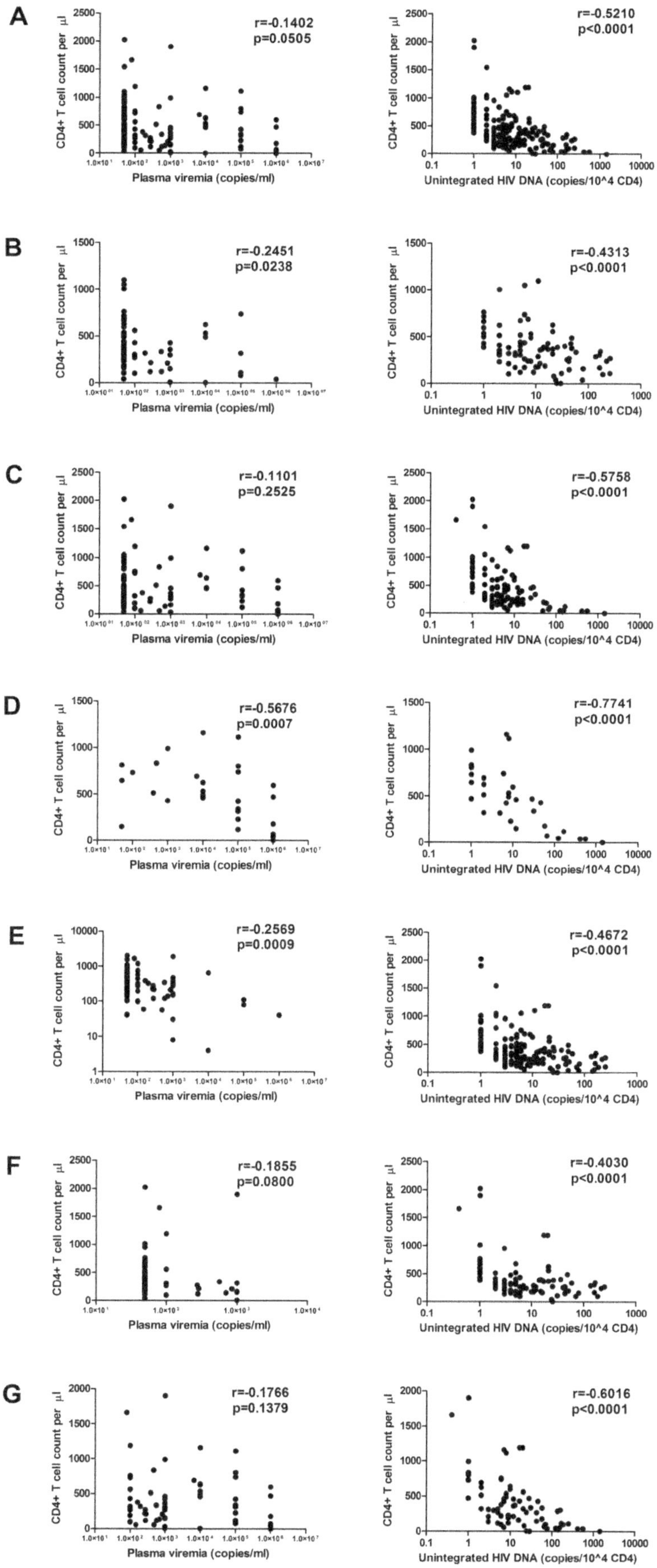
A
r=-0.1402
p=0.0505
r=-0.5210
p<0.0001
B
r=-0.2451
p=0.0238
r=-0.4313
p<0.0001
C
r=-0.1101
p=0.2525
r=-0.5758
p<0.0001
D
r=-0.5676
p=0.0007
r=-0.7741
p<0.0001
E
r=-0.2569
p=0.0009
r=-0.4672
p<0.0001
F
r=-0.1855
p=0.0800
r=-0.4030
p<0.0001
G
r=-0.1766
p=0.1379
r=-0.6016
p<0.0001
CD4+ T cell count per µl
Plasma viremia (copies/ml)
Unintegrated HIV DNA (copies/10^4 CD4)

Figure 4. Correlations between study parameters in blood samples. Correlations between plasma viremia and CD4+ T cell counts (left panel) and between unintegrated HIV DNA and CD4+ T cell counts (right panel) in (A) a total of 195 blood samples, (B) 85 blood samples collected from patients with multidrug-resistant HIV-1 infection, (C) 110 blood samples collected from patients who had no evidence of resistance, (D) 32 treatment-naïve samples, (E) 163 ART samples, (F) 90 under RAL samples and (G) 72 samples with HIV-1 RNA loads above 50 copies/ml of plasma. Only the correlation between CD4+ and unintegrated HIV DNA is shown because it is stronger than the correlation between CD4+ and total HIV DNA.

starting with DNA to measure extrachromosomal forms in HIV patients. A qPCR to specifically detect 2-LTR circles in the same DNA sample used for the quantification of total and UF HIV DNA was also developed. Due to the unique nature of the LTR-LTR junction, which can be readily assayed by PCR [8], the 2-LTR circles are often recognized as overall markers of all unintegrated forms and it has been suggested that could be a surrogate marker of HIV-1 replication, although their use remains debatable, primarily due to controversy regarding their half-life. Because of this ongoing dispute and the low 2-LTR levels (also confirmed in our group of samples), the quantification of all the unintegrated forms seemed a more correct approach to reduce the percentage of samples near the low quantification limit (from 53% to 29%). However, the method is a useful tool for the quantification of 2-LTR in DNA samples from *in vitro* experiments involving the use of purified CD4+ T cells, PBMC or macrophages, where a higher content of these forms is expected. The decision to develop both the 2-LTR and *TotUFsys* assays based on SYBR Green instead of fluorogenic probes stems from the high LTR-LTR junction sequence heterogeneity [38], and the fact that the presence of even just a single mismatched base at the 5′ end of the probe can fail to detect the target sequence and/or affect the quantifications with the risk of "false negative" results. High sensitivity (2 copies), high amplification efficiency and specificity across different clades within group M were demonstrated. In addition, no cross-reactivity with HERV, which are highly similar in terms of DNA sequence to HIV-1, was revealed in HIV-negative samples, confirming the absence of interference in very low HIV DNA copy quantification and a realistic diagnostic specificity. The accuracy of the results was improved by a standard of half-log plasmid dilutions in the low range of quantification. Reproducibility was realistic over the experimentally determined standard curve dynamic range, showing the reliability of the technical set-up over time. Moreover, to maximize assay precision in the samples with a low HIV DNA level (copy number ≤30), repetitive sampling (8 replicates) allowed us to report standard deviation, coefficient of variation and confidence interval. Reliable, simultaneous quantification of total and unintegrated HIV DNA was obtained for 195 blood samples collected from HIV-1 patients in a wide range of clinical pictures during routine laboratory monitoring. A high success rate was obtained for all the samples, even those from patients with suppressed plasma viremia, regardless of CD4+ T cell counts, or therapy. We conducted each type of analysis by considering normalization per μg of DNA as well as per 10^4 CD4+ since they harbour most of the HIV-1 genomes detectable in blood, highlighting that inappropriate normalization may induce misleading effects and conclusion regarding the real state of patient health. Moreover, when the amount of HIV DNA is expressed for CD4+, the results could have greater relevance.

If we consider all the samples together, while there was only a marginal positive correlation between plasma viremia and the amount of HIV DNA, both total HIV DNA and unintegrated forms inversely correlated with CD4+ T cell counts. However, no significant correlation was observed between the two currently most frequently used prognostic markers: plasma viremia and CD4+ count. Within the cohort of patients, correlations were evaluated in six different clinical situations. There was consistently a significant inverse correlation between CD4+ and HIV DNA in all subsets, reaching the highest value between CD4+ and unintegrated HIV DNA and no significant correlation was found between HIV-1 RNA and CD4+, except for the treatment-naïve group. Forty-five subjects monitored for an observation period, showed the strongest correlation between CD4+ and HIV DNA and this was the only correlation that remains over time. The same conclusion could be drawn even when considering separately subjects under ART, subjects under RAL intensification or the combination of these. In particular, from moderate to very strong correlations were observed frequently between CD4+ and total HIV DNA, and almost always between CD4+ and unintegrated HIV DNA. These analyses highlight the limited correlation between CD4+ and plasma viremia in patients under classical ART or/and ART plus an integrase inhibitor agent such as Raltegravir and show that the correlation is often lost after effective ART. In general, we found that in our cohort of patients representing different clinical situations, there was a weak or no correlation between CD4+ and viremia. However, we found a high inverse correlation between CD4+ and HIV DNA with the strongest correlations for unintegrated forms.

Conclusions

The use of a distinctive and well-performing workflow and a layout of PCR plates (*TotUFsys* platform), allowed us to obtain in less than two working days, HIV DNA copy number per μg of DNA or 10^4 CD4+ for 12 HIV-1 patients. We developed a practical method able to simultaneously measure total and unintegrated HIV DNA as well as indirectly integrated provirus, in a wide range of clinical situations typical of HIV-1 infection, such as treatment-naive, under effective/suboptimal ART, new drug regimes, MDR and or co-infected patients. Because the assay makes use of frozen whole blood specimens, it has broad applications and is well-suited for a large series of sequential samples collected within clinical trials/vaccination protocols. A careful choice of the most suitable DNA extraction method makes it possible to easily adapt our assay to alternative sample types such as tissue biopsies, purified CD4+ T cells, PBMC or macrophages from *in vitro* experiments, and on the same specimen collected for routine plasma viremia determination, after removal of the plasma for the HIV-RNA assay. Our findings support the quantification of total and unintegrated HIV DNA as an additional or alternative tool to traditional assays to estimate the state of viral infection, the risk of disease progression and to monitor the effects of therapy (suppressive or new treatments), providing useful data that could influence decisions whether to initiate, change, intensify or simplify the ART. Moreover, the newly developed *TotUFsys* platform is relatively fast and less labor intensive than other already existing quantification assays.

Materials and Methods

The essential steps of the procedure for the quantification of total and unintegrated HIV DNA forms in 12 samples, from frozen blood until data analysis is illustrated in Figure 1.

Table 4. Quantification of 2-LTR circles in blood samples.

Sample	CD4+T cell count/μl	HIV-1 RNA (copies/ml)	CD4+ present in one μg of DNA	2-LTR linear	UF HIV DNA	[a]1-LTR +	2-LTR	UF HIV DNA	1-LTR + linear	[b]MDR/non-MDR
				(copies/μg DNA)			(copies/10^4 CD4+)			
1	739	10^5	21199	10	13	3	5	6	1	MDR
2	426	10^5	15685	7	11	4	4	7	3	non-MDR
3	180	10^6	6785	<2	40	39	1	59	58	non-MDR
4	320	10^5	9564	<2	2	1	1	2	1	MDR
5	70	10^6	1048	<2	7	6	10	67	57	non-MDR
6	513	396	14286	<2	3	2	1	2	1	non-MDR
7	317	10^5	14799	<2	8	7	1	5	4	non-MDR
8	596	10^6	17131	<2	18	17	1	10	9	non-MDR
Naive, n = 8		median, IQR		<2, <2–6	10, 4–17	5, 2–15	1, 1–5	7, 3–47	4, 1–45	
9	487	<50	12184	7	8	1	6	7	1	non-MDR
10	926	<50	20541	2	3	1	1	1	0	non-MDR
11	959	<50	14528	4	4	0	3	3	0	non-MDR
12	835	<50	25060	8	9	1	3	4	1	non-MDR
13	639	10^4	16157	3	17	14	2	10	8	non-MDR
14	321	100	13527	2	3	1	1	2	1	non-MDR
15	105	<50	5396	<2	<2	0	2	2	0	non-MDR
16	272	10^3	9547	<2	5	4	1	5	4	non-MDR
17	192	100	5108	<2	5	4	2	9	7	non-MDR
18	227	<50	7206	8	9	1	11	13	2	non-MDR
19	462	10^3	16709	<2	11	10	1	7	6	non-MDR
20	146	<50	3685	2	<2	0	5	3	0	non-MDR
ART, n = 12		median, IQR		2, <2–6	5, 3–9	1, 0–4	2, 1–5	5, 2–9	1, 0–6	
21	764	<50	16241	<2	<2	0	1	1	0	MDR
22	291	<50	4874	6	5	0	12	11	0	MDR
23	263	<50	4425	3	3	0	7	6	0	MDR
24	306	<50	6063	3	3	0	5	5	0	MDR
25	178	<50	2913	<2	3	2	3	10	7	MDR
26	430	<50	10519	<2	<2	0	1	1	0	MDR
27	951	<50	21195	4	7	3	2	3	1	non-MDR
28	163	10^3	7056	<2	11	10	1	16	15	non-MDR
29	1,900	10^3	28692	<2	<2	0	0	0	0	non-MDR
30	1,011	<50	28154	<2	3	2	0	1	1	non-MDR
Under RAL, n = 10		median, IQR		<2, <2–3	3, 1–6	0, 0–2	2, 1–6	4, 1–10	0, 0–3	

Table 4. Cont.

Sample	CD4+T cell count/µl	HIV-1 RNA (copies/ml)	CD4+ present in one µg of DNA	2-LTR linear	UF HIV DNA	[a]1-LTR +	2-LTR	UF HIV DNA	1-LTR + linear
[b]MDR/non-MDR									
				(copies/µg DNA)			(copies/10^4 CD4+)		
Kruskal-Wallis test				0.379	0.056	0.019	0.770	0.408	0.048
Mann-Whitney test				0.741	0.069	0.018	0.207	0.672	0.040

[a]Determined subtracting the level of 2-LTR from all unintegrated HIV DNA forms, taking into account the similar PCR efficiencies of 2-LTR and UF.
[b]The median (IQR) value for 2-LTR/µg DNA was 2 (<2–5) and <2 (<2–4) for MDR and non-MDR group, respectively; for 2-LTR/10^4 CD4+ was 4 (1–7) and 2 (1–3) for the MDR and non-MDR group, respectively.
The median (IQR) value for UF HIV DNA/µg DNA was 3 (<2–5) and 7 (3–11) for the MDR and non-MDR groups, respectively; for UF HIV DNA/10^4 CD4+ was 6 (1–9) and 5 (2–10) for the MDR and non-MDR group, respectively.
The median (IQR) value for 1-LTR + linear forms/µg DNA was 0 (0–2) and 3 (1–8) for the MDR and non-MDR group, respectively; for 1-LTR + linear forms/10^4 CD4+ was 0 (0–1) and 2 (1–7) for the MDR and non-MDR group, respectively.

The methods were carefully developed following the validation parameters (specificity, limit of quantification (QL) and detection (DL), linear range of quantification, reproducibility and repeatability) specified in the Guidelines for the Validation of Analytical Procedures (http://www.ich.org/fileadmin/Public_Web_Site/ICH_Products/Guidelines/Quality/Q2_R1/Step4/Q2_R1__Guideline.pdf).

Patients and blood samples

Fifty-nine adult HIV-1 positive patients, who reported to the reference hospital (Azienda Ospedaliera Ospedali Riuniti Marche Nord - Presidio Ospedaliero San Salvatore, Pesaro, Italy) from January 2009 until May 2011 for routine blood tests, provided from a single sample to nine blood samples for a total of 195 specimens. All subjects were asked to sign a written informed consent for the collection and storage of their blood samples for research purposes, according to Declaration of Helsinki principles. The study was approved by the San Salvatore Hospital ethics committee.

Quantification of plasma viremia and CD4+ T cell counts

Plasma obtained from blood samples in EDTA was frozen at −80°C until tested.

The viral load in plasma was quantified using the Artus HI Virus-1 QS-RGQ Kit. The kit is a ready-to-use system for the detection of HIV-1 RNA using PCR on Rotor-Gene Q Instruments. Sample preparation and assay setup make use of the QIAsymphony SP/AS instruments (Qiagen), according to the manufacturer's instructions.

Lymphocyte surface phenotypes and CD4+ lymphocyte counts were determined using flow cytometry analysis by Immunotech-Beckman Coulter (Marseille, France).

Nucleic acid extraction

For each sample, the cellular DNA was isolated from leukocytes (WBC) from 3 or 4 ml of peripheral blood according to the previously described method [28]. Briefly, after incubation of the WBC pellet for 45 min at 37°C in a lysis buffer, the DNA was purified by phenol extraction followed by ethanol precipitation and RNase treatment. Isolated DNAs were quantified by NanoDrop ND-1000 Spectrophotometer (NanoDrop Technologies, Wilmington, DE, USA) and the absorbance ratios of 260/280 and 260/230 were used to control the purity of the samples: all samples had a ratio of about 1.8 and 2.0 respectively, and are accepted as "pure" DNA. A mean DNA recovery of 20±7 µg/ml of blood was obtained for a total of 60 or 80 µg of DNA/blood sample, more than adequate for the quantification of all HIV DNA forms. One aliquot of HIV-1 negative blood was extracted in each experiment, together with the clinical samples to monitor extraction procedure. Ten µg of DNA were mixed with 1.5 volume of hydrogen peroxide solution and incubated at 37°C for 30 min prior to ethanol precipitation and re-suspension to obtain a theoretical concentration of 100 ng/µl. The DNA were then quantified again. This step was performed to improve low copy detection of the total HIV DNA and 2-LTR circles on a consistent background of high molecular weight DNA in PCR experiments (up to 1 µg/PCR).

Isolation of unintegrated HIV DNA

The extrachromosomal HIV DNA was purified from 5 µg of cellular DNA using the QIAprep miniprep kit (Qiagen) according to the manufacturer's instructions and the recommended modifications were used for the isolation of low-copy number plasmids. Moreover, we made some further changes in the amount of the supernatant loaded in each column (600 μl of 850 μl total, corresponding to 71% of the processed DNA, 3529 ng) and the volume of elution (106 μl of buffer EB). Two separate purifications were performed for each sample and the eluate fractions containing extrachromosomal forms (low molecular weight, LMW fraction DNA), were combined at the end of the procedure. To monitor for cross-contamination, one sample of H_2O in place of DNA and one HIV-1 negative DNA were processed every twelve samples.

Oligonucleotide primers

The primers were selected and analyzed using the Oligo Primer Analysis software (version 6.65; Cascade, CO, USA). The forward primer PBSf (5′-TAGCAGTGGCGCCCGA-3′) and the reverse primer PBSr (5′-TCTCTCTCCTTCTAGCCTCCGC-3′); the forward primer 2LTRf (5′-TAGTGTGTGCCCGTCTGT-3′) and the reverse primer 2LTRr (5′-TGTGTAGTTCTGCCAAT-CAG-3′); the forward primer EXgf (5′-CCGCTGTATCA-CAAGGGCTGGTACC-3′) and the reverse primer EXgr (5′-GGAGCCCGTGTAGAGCATGACGATC-3′); the forward primer ACTf (5′-CCGCCCGTCCACACCC-3′) and the reverse primer ACTr (5′-CTGACCCATGCCCACCATCA-3′) were purchased from Sigma-Genosys and maintained at −20°C at a concentration of 100 μM in TE 10-1 mM, pH 8.0, in single-use aliquots.

Construction of plasmid and standard curves

The use of the pPBS plasmid (161 bp-PBS fragment derived from HIV-1 PNL4-3 vector cloned into the pGEM-T vector) as a reference standard was previously validated [28].

The 2-LTR plasmid (p2LTR) was obtained by cloning a 176 bp of LTR-LTR junction within the circular form in a pGEM-T vector.

The 13 Kb exogenous plasmid (pEXg) was obtained by cloning a 225 bp fragment of a plant gene (GenBank accession no. U16123) in an appropriate plasmid (PINCO: 12889 bp) [39].

The cloned fragment sequences were confirmed using the automatic sequencer ABI Prism 310 Genetic Analyzer (Applied Biosystems, Foster City, CA, USA).

To determine the exact copy number, the linearized plasmids were accurately quantified with the NanoDrop ND-1000 Spectrophotometer. Standard curves (pPBSstd, p2LTRstd and pEXgstd) were constructed with 10-fold and half-log plasmid serial dilutions, in a range from 10^5 to 10, including 2 molecules. Dilutions in TE buffer were freshly prepared for each experiment from aliquots of 10^9 copies stored at −80°C. The standard curve (ACTstd) used for the quantification of a 177 bp fragment of the β-actin housekeeping gene (ACT, GenBank accession no. NM_001101.3), was made freshly for each experiment with 10- and 2-fold serial dilutions of a reference genomic DNA ranging from 1000 to 0.01 ng.

SYBR Green I real time PCR

The organization of the *TotUFsys* platform for the quantification of HIV DNA forms (total and unintegrated) is described in the paragraph below. QPCR of various targets was set up in a final volume of 100 μl using 96-well plates. 0.5–1.0 μg of cellular DNA or the equivalent quantity in μl of LMW fraction DNA was added to the mixture containing 50 μl of 2× master mix Hot-Rescue Real Time PCR Kit-SG (Diatheva srl, Fano, Italy) and 100 nM of each primer. For the pEXg and β-actin, a variable quantity of DNA was assayed on the basis of the specific PCR experiment. The amplification profile for total HIV DNA, unintegrated HIV DNA, pEXg and β-actin was as follows: one cycle of 10 min at 95°C to activate the Hot-Rescue DNA polymerase followed by 40 cycles in two steps, consisting of 15 sec at 95°C and 35 sec at 68°C, while for 2-LTR circles one cycle of 15 min at 95°C followed by 40 cycles of three steps consisting of 95°C for 15 sec, annealing at 60°C for 20 sec and extension at 72°C for 35 sec. The fluorescence intensity of the products was measured at the end of each cycle and post-PCR melt curve analysis was performed to detect primer-dimers or other non-specific products and to confirm the specificity of the target. Amplification, data acquisition and analysis were carried out using an Applied Biosystems 7500 Real-Time PCR instrument with the Sequence Detection System software package (version 1.4.0). Three (for copy numbers ≥10) or six replicates (for copy numbers below 10) of standard scalar dilutions were included in each plate. Standard curves were created automatically and accepted when the slopes were between −3.40 and −3.26 (97–100% efficiency) and the minimum value of the correlation coefficient (R^2) was 0.98. The percentage of amplification efficiency was calculated as (10^(−1/slope)−1)×100. In all experiments, negative controls containing water (NTC) or HIV-1 negative DNA were tested.

Data analysis of quantification of total, unintegrated (*TotUFsys* platform) and 2-LTR HIV DNA forms

The *TotUFsys* platform was performed essentially exploiting the whole blood leukocyte pbs-rtPCR assay [28] with the following improvements:

a) a more precise standard of half-log serial dilutions in the low range of quantification (from 10^3 to 10, and 2-copy dilution) rather than the broad dynamic range that is normally used, unless otherwise specified.

b) Each clinical sample was analyzed in triplicate. The first PCR (1st qPCR) consisted of two wells containing 0.5 μg each plus one well containing 1.0 μg of DNA or the equivalent quantity in μl of the LMW fraction DNA. The amount of 0.5 μg was increased by doubling to 1.0 μg to ensure the detection of the target even in the low copy number (near the QL). The copy number measured for each replicate was obtained by interpolation of the Ct value from the standard and if this was quantified over 30 copies/PCR determination (coefficient of variation 21%), the result for each sample was given adding up the copy number from the two 0.5 μg replicates and expressed as HIV DNA copy number/μg of DNA or LMW fraction DNA.

c) A second PCR (2nd qPCR) performed for an HIV DNA datum quantified below 30 copies/PCR determination, and consisting of:

c.1) six 0.5 μg (for a total of 3 μg) replicates for samples which in the 1st qPCR had been quantified in the range between 30 to 2 copies/PCR determination. The result was given dividing by 4 the sum of the copy number from a total of eight replicates (two 0.5 μg replicates in the 1st qPCR+six 0.5 μg replicates in the 2nd qPCR) and expressed as HIV DNA copy number/μg of DNA or LMW fraction DNA;

c.2) three 0.5 μg (for a total of 1.5 μg) replicates and three 1.0 μg (for a total of 3.0 μg) replicates for samples which in the 1st qPCR had been quantified near or detected below the QL (<2 copies/PCR replicate). After excluding the presence of inhibitors adding 2 or 10 pPBS standard copies in a spike-PCR, the result was given by adding copy numbers from the quantifiable replicates for a total of 6.5 μg (~10^6 WBC, assuming 7.0 pg of DNA content per human diploid genome as conversion factor [40]) of DNA or LMW fraction DNA processed (two 0.5 μg replicates plus one 1.0 μg replicate in the 1st qPCR+three 0.5 μg replicates plus three 1.0 μg replicates in the 2nd qPCR) and expressed as HIV DNA copy number/6.5 μg of DNA or LMW fraction DNA. For subsequent analysis these data were then expressed to one μg of DNA or LMW DNA fraction.

d) HIV DNA copy number was also expressed as copies/10^4 CD4+ T cells, assuming that 142857 cells are present in one μg of DNA. The following formula was used for each sample:

$$[(\text{copies}/\mu\text{g DNA})/(\text{CD4}+/\text{WBC}\times 142857\ \text{WBC})]\times 10^4.$$

Taking into account WBC number/ml of whole blood, the result can be reported as the HIV DNA copy number/ml of whole blood, with the formula: HIV DNA copy no. per μg DNA×WBC no. per ml/142857 cells [28].

e) The number of PCR cycles was reduced from 45 to 40, and the data collection of the first ten cycles is omitted (the Ct value is in the range 1 to 30) for a more accurate threshold set up.

Quantification of integrated HIV DNA measurement

Integrated HIV DNA was obtained indirectly, subtracting the unintegrated HIV DNA determined directly in the LMW fraction from total HIV DNA which was also determined directly in total cellular DNA with the formula: total HIV DNA copy number/μg DNA – UF copy number/μg of LMW fraction DNA. Integrated HIV DNA was then normalized to 10^4 CD4+ T cells. We also included examples of indirect calculation of integrated proviral DNA showing the feasibility of this approach.

Statistical analysis

The Ct values of the standard dilutions were exported to a Microsoft Excel worksheet for the calculation of averages, standard deviations (SD) and coefficients of variation (CV%) in order to evaluate the method's accuracy.

The data are presented as medians, range (minimum to maximum) and interquartile range (IQR, 25th to 75th percentile). All comparisons between two different groups were performed using the nonparametric Mann-Whitney U test for unpaired data or the nonparametric Kruskal-Wallis test for comparison between more than two groups. The correlation between two parameters was determined using Spearman's correlation coefficient. For samples below the limit of quantification (QL), an imputed value corresponding to ½ QL was used for statistical analysis [41]. Statistical significance was accepted for p values below 0.05.

Supporting Information

Figure S1 Primer specificity for HIV-1 group M http://www.hiv.lanl.gov/content/sequence/HIV/COMPENDIUM/2013compendium.html.

Figure S2 Gel electrophoresis analysis of HMW DNA and Marker II eluate fractions using QIAprep miniprep kit (Qiagen).

Table S1 Diagnostic specificity.

Table S2 pPBS standard curve in assence or presence of HIV-1 negative human DNA.

Table S3 Ct value and copy number.

Table S4 Method reproducibility calculated by the percentage of the coefficient of variation for Ct value (A) and for copy number (B).

Table S5 Quantification of total HIV DNA copy number in three different samples tested in three separate experiments.

Table S6 Cross-contamination level of HMW DNA measured in eluate fraction by qPCR of β-actin house-keeping gene.

Table S7 Recovery test of extrachromosomal forms.

Table S8 Characteristics of total, unintegrated and integrated HIV DNA measurements in samples.

Table S9 Correlations between study parameters in blood samples.

Table 10 Correlation between study parameters in patients at the beginning and the end of the observation period.

Acknowledgments

The authors would like to thank Dr. Debora Libetti for her valuable contributions to the laboratory experiments. The English in this manuscript was revised by Timothy C. Bloom, a native English speaker with extensive experience in scientific editing.

Author Contributions

Conceived and designed the experiments: AC CO. Performed the experiments: CO AC MS. Analyzed the data: AC CO. Wrote the paper: AC CO. Collected samples: BC EP MA MV. Managed the patients: BC EP MA MV. Reviewed the manuscript: BC EP MA MV. Performed statistical analysis: CO. Prepared figures: CO. Coordinated and supervised the whole study: MM.

References

1. Chun TW, Carruth L, Finzi D, Shen X, DiGiuseppe JA, et al. (1997) Quantification of latent tissue reservoirs and total body viral load in HIV-1 infection. Nature 387: 183–188.
2. Chun TW, Engel D, Berrey MM, Shea T, Corey L, et al. (1998) Early establishment of a pool of latently infected, resting CD4(+) T cells during primary HIV-1 infection. Proc Natl Acad Sci U S A 95: 8869–8873.
3. Finzi D, Hermankova M, Pierson T, Carruth LM, Buck C, et al. (1997) Identification of a reservoir for HIV-1 in patients on highly active antiretroviral therapy. Science 278: 1295–1300.
4. Bell P, Montaner LJ, Maul GG (2001) Accumulation and intranuclear distribution of unintegrated human immunodeficiency virus type 1 DNA. J Virol 75: 7683–7691.

5. Kelly J, Beddall MH, Yu D, Iyer SR, Marsh JW, et al. (2008) Human macrophages support persistent transcription from unintegrated HIV-1 DNA. Virology 372: 300–312.
6. Sharkey ME, Teo I, Greenough T, Sharova N, Luzuriaga K, et al. (2000) Persistence of episomal HIV-1 infection intermediates in patients on highly active anti-retroviral therapy. Nat Med 6: 76–81.
7. Sloan RD, Wainberg MA (2011) The role of unintegrated DNA in HIV infection. Retrovirology 8: 52.
8. Butler SL, Hansen MS, Bushman FD (2001) A quantitative assay for HIV DNA integration in vivo. Nat Med 7: 631–634.
9. Teo I, Veryard C, Barnes H, An SF, Jones M, et al. (1997) Circular forms of unintegrated human immunodeficiency virus type 1 DNA and high levels of viral protein expression: association with dementia and multinucleated giant cells in the brains of patients with AIDS. J Virol 71: 2928–2933.
10. Brussel A, Mathez D, Broche-Pierre S, Lancar R, Calvez T et al. (2003) Longitudinal monitoring of 2-long terminal repeat circles in peripheral blood mononuclear cells from patients with chronic HIV-1 infection. AIDS 17: 645–652.
11. Munir S, Thierry S, Subra F, Deprez E, Delelis O (2013) Quantitative analysis of the time-course of viral DNA forms during the HIV-1 life cycle. Retrovirology 10: 87.
12. Wu Y (2004) HIV-1 gene expression: lessons from provirus and non-integrated DNA. Retrovirology 1: 13.
13. Palmer S, Maldarelli F, Wiegand A, Bernstein B, Hanna GJ, et al. (2008) Low-level viremia persists for at least 7 years in patients on suppressive antiretroviral therapy. Proc Natl Acad Sci U S A 105: 3879–3884.
14. Agosto LM, Liszewski MK, Mexas A, Graf E, Pace M, et al. (2011) Patients on HAART often have an excess of unintegrated HIV DNA: implications for monitoring reservoirs. Virology 409: 46–53.
15. Brussel A, Sonigo P (2003) Analysis of early human immunodeficiency virus type 1 DNA synthesis by use of a new sensitive assay for quantifying integrated provirus. J Virol 77: 10119–10124.
16. Carr JM, Cheney KM, Coolen C, Davis A, Shaw D, et al. (2007) Development of methods for coordinate measurement of total cell-associated and integrated human immunodeficiency virus type 1 (HIV-1) DNA forms in routine clinical samples: levels are not associated with clinical parameters, but low levels of integrated HIV-1 DNA may be prognostic for continued successful therapy. J Clin Microbiol 45: 1288–1297.
17. Koelsch KK, Liu L, Haubrich R, May S, Havlir D, et al. (2008) Dynamics of total, linear nonintegrated, and integrated HIV-1 DNA in vivo and in vitro. J Infect Dis 197: 411–419.
18. Mexas AM, Graf EH, Pace MJ, Yu JJ, Papasavvas E, et al. (2012) Concurrent measures of total and integrated HIV DNA monitor reservoirs and ongoing replication in eradication trials. AIDS 26: 2295–2306.
19. Avettand-Fenoel V, Chaix ML, Blanche S, Burgard M, Floch C, et al. (2009) LTR real-time PCR for HIV-1 DNA quantitation in blood cells for early diagnosis in infants born to seropositive mothers treated in HAART area (ANRS CO 01). J Med Virol 81: 217–223.
20. Yu JJ, Wu TL, Liszewski MK, Dai J, Swiggard WJ, et al. (2008) A more precise HIV integration assay designed to detect small differences finds lower levels of integrated DNA in HAART treated patients. Virology 379: 78–86.
21. Katzenstein TL, Oliveri RS, Benfield T, Eugen-Olsen J, Nielsen C, et al. (2002) Cell-associated HIV DNA measured early during infection has prognostic value independent of serum HIV RNA measured concomitantly. Scand J Infect Dis 34: 529–533.
22. Kostrikis LG, Touloumi G, Karanicolas R, Pantazis N, Anastassopoulou C, et al. (2002) Quantitation of human immunodeficiency virus type 1 DNA forms with the second template switch in peripheral blood cells predicts disease progression independently of plasma RNA load. J Virol 76: 10099–10108.
23. Lewin SR, Murray JM, Solomon A, Wightman F, Cameron PU, et al. (2008) Virologic determinants of success after structured treatment interruptions of antiretrovirals in acute HIV-1 infection. J Acquir Immune Defic Syndr 47: 140–147.
24. Morand-Joubert L, Marcellin F, Launay O, Guiramand-Hugon S, Gerard L, et al. (2005) Contribution of cellular HIV-1 DNA quantification to the efficacy analysis of antiretroviral therapy: a randomized comparison of 2 regimens, including 3 drugs from 2 or 3 classes (TRIANON, ANRS 081). J Acquir Immune Defic Syndr 38: 268–276.
25. Parisi SG, Andreis S, Mengoli C, Scaggiante R, Ferretto R, et al. (2012) Baseline cellular HIV DNA load predicts HIV DNA decline and residual HIV plasma levels during effective antiretroviral therapy. J Clin Microbiol 50: 258–263.
26. Rouzioux C, Hubert JB, Burgard M, Deveau C, Goujard C, et al. (2005) Early levels of HIV-1 DNA in peripheral blood mononuclear cells are predictive of disease progression independently of HIV-1 RNA levels and CD4+ T cell counts. J Infect Dis 192: 46–55.
27. Viard JP, Burgard M, Hubert JB, Aaron L, Rabian C, et al. (2004) Impact of 5 years of maximally successful highly active antiretroviral therapy on CD4 cell count and HIV-1 DNA level. AIDS 18: 45–49.
28. Casabianca A, Gori C, Orlandi C, Forbici F, Federico PC, et al. (2007) Fast and sensitive quantitative detection of HIV DNA in whole blood leucocytes by SYBR green I real-time PCR assay. Mol Cell Probes 21: 368–378.
29. Foley BT, Leitner T, Apetrei C, Hahn B, Mizrachi I, et al. (2013) HIV Sequence Compendium 2013. 13–17. Available: http://www.hiv.lanl.gov/content/sequence/HIV/COMPENDIUM/2013compendium.html. Accessed 2014 Oct 13.
30. Griffiths DJ (2001) Endogenous retroviruses in the human genome sequence. Genome Biol 2: REVIEWS1017.
31. Buzon MJ, Massanella M, Llibre JM, Esteve A, Dahl V, et al. (2010) HIV-1 replication and immune dynamics are affected by raltegravir intensification of HAART-suppressed subjects. Nat Med 16: 460–465.
32. Sambrook J, Russell DW (2001) Molecular Cloning: A Laboratory Manual. Cold Spring Harbour Laboratory Press. 6.4 p
33. Eriksson S, Graf EH, Dahl V, Strain MC, Yukl SA, et al. (2013) Comparative analysis of measures of viral reservoirs in HIV-1 eradication studies. PLoS Pathog 9: e1003174.
34. Finzi D, Blankson J, Siliciano JD, Margolick JB, Chadwick K, et al. (1999) Latent infection of CD4+ T cells provides a mechanism for lifelong persistence of HIV-1, even in patients on effective combination therapy. Nat Med 5: 512–517.
35. Brussel A, Sonigo P (2004) Evidence for gene expression by unintegrated human immunodeficiency virus type 1 DNA species. J Virol 78: 11263–11271.
36. Wu Y, Marsh JW (2003) Early transcription from nonintegrated DNA in human immunodeficiency virus infection. J Virol 77: 10376–10382.
37. O'Doherty U, Swiggard WJ, Jeyakumar D, McGain D, Malim MH (2002) A sensitive, quantitative assay for human immunodeficiency virus type 1 integration. J Virol 76: 10942–10950.
38. Jurriaans S, de RA, Dekker J, Goudsmit J, Cornelissen M (1992) Analysis of human immunodeficiency virus type 1 LTR-LTR junctions in peripheral blood mononuclear cells of infected individuals. J Gen Virol 73 (Pt 6): 1537–1541.
39. Grignani F, Kinsella T, Mencarelli A, Valtieri M, Riganelli D, et al. (1998) High-efficiency gene transfer and selection of human hematopoietic progenitor cells with a hybrid EBV/retroviral vector expressing the green fluorescence protein. Cancer Res 58: 14–19.
40. Gregory TR (2014) Animal genome size databases. Available: http://www.genomesize.com. Accessed 2014 Oct 13.
41. Helsel DR (2005) More than obvious: better methods for interpreting nondetect data. Environ Sci Technol 39: 419A–423A.

Late-Onset of Spinal Neurodegeneration in Knock-In Mice Expressing a Mutant BiP

Hisayo Jin[1], Naoya Mimura[2], Makiko Kashio[1], Haruhiko Koseki[3], Tomohiko Aoe[1,4]*

1 Department of Anesthesiology, Chiba University Graduate School of Medicine, Chiba City, Chiba, Japan, 2 Department of Medicine and Clinical Oncology, Chiba University Graduate School of Medicine, Chiba City, Chiba, Japan, 3 Laboratory for Developmental Genetics, RIKEN Research Center for Allergy and Immunology, Yokohama, Japan, 4 Department of Anesthesiology, Tokyo Women's Medical University, Yachiyo Medical, Center, Yachiyo, Chiba, Japan

Abstract

Most human neurodegenerative diseases are sporadic, and appear later in life. While the underlying mechanisms of the progression of those diseases are still unclear, investigations into the familial forms of comparable diseases suggest that endoplasmic reticulum (ER) stress is involved in the pathogenesis. Binding immunoglobulin protein (BiP) is an ER chaperone that is central to ER function. We produced knock-in mice expressing a mutant BiP that lacked the retrieval sequence in order to evaluate the effect of a functional defect in an ER chaperone in multi-cellular organisms. Here we report that heterozygous mutant BiP mice revealed motor disabilities in aging. We found a degeneration of some motoneurons in the spinal cord accompanied by accumulations of ubiquitinated proteins. The defect in retrieval of BiP by the KDEL receptor leads to impaired activities in quality control and autophagy, suggesting that functional defects in the ER chaperones may contribute to the late onset of neurodegenerative diseases.

Editor: Hiroyasu Nakano, Toho University School of Medicine, Japan

Funding: Grants-in-Aids for Science Research from the Ministry of Education, Culture, Sports, Science and Technology of Japan to T.A. (20059008, http://www.mext.go.jp/english/) The funders had no role in study design, data collection and analysis, decision to publish, or preparation of the manuscript.

Competing Interests: The authors have declared that no competing interests exist.

* Email: taoe@faculty.chiba-u.jp

Introduction

Proteins destined for the secretory pathway are inserted into the ER cotranslationally and subjected to quality control [1]. ER molecular chaperones and folding enzymes such as BiP, calnexin, and protein disulfide isomerase facilitate the correct folding or degradation of these newly synthesized proteins as well as of misfolded proteins [2]. The accumulation of misfolded proteins in the ER beyond the capacity of quality control causes ER stress and induces the unfolded protein response (UPR) [3]. Further ER stress can cause cellular dysfunction and cell death, resulting in diverse human disorders such as neurodegenerative diseases [4].

Mammalian ER luminal chaperones have a carboxyl terminal Lys-Asp-Glu-Leu (KDEL) amino acid sequence, which is recognized by the KDEL receptor in post-ER compartments [5]. ER chaperones and the KDEL receptor are sorted into the transport vesicles coated with coat protein (COP) I complex and retrieved to the ER [6]. Yeast BiP (Kar2p) is essential for survival, while the deletion of the retrieval sequence (in yeast: His-Asp-Glu-Leu, HDEL) is dispensable because the UPR is activated and the loss of the chaperone in the ER is compensated for [7]. The complete depletion of BiP also has lethal effects on mammalian early embryonic cells [8].

In order to elucidate the physiological processes that are sensitive to the retrieval of BiP during development and adulthood in multi-cellular organisms, we previously produced knock-in mice expressing a mutant BiP in which the retrieval sequence was deleted by homologous recombination. The homozygous mutant BiP mice died within several hours after birth due to respiratory failure with impaired biosynthesis of the pulmonary surfactant, especially surfactant protein C, by alveolar type II cells [9]. The heterozygous mutant BiP mice grew up to be apparently normal adults. However, vulnerability to ER stress may exist in the mutant BiP mice, leading to chronic organ injuries. Indeed, some of them displayed motor disabilities in aging. We found a degeneration of some motoneurons in the spinal cord accompanied by accumulations of ubiquitinated proteins. The accumulation of misfolded proteins is one of the most common features in neurodegenerative diseases. Functional defects in the ER chaperones may contribute to the late onset of neurodegenerative diseases.

Results

The mutant BiP mice revealed motor disabilities in aging

The heterozygous mutant BiP mice live as long as the wild type mice (Figure 1A). We could not detect a significant motor disability during their young period, using the Rotarod performance test. At very advanced ages, some of the mutant BiP mice displayed paralysis and tremors after they were more than one year old, although a few wild-type mice show partial paresis (Figure 1B). Some of aged mutant BiP mice displayed loss of righting reflex and suffered from paralysis (Figure 1C, D, and Video S1). The ratio of motor disabilities is significantly higher in the heterozygous mutant BiP mice.

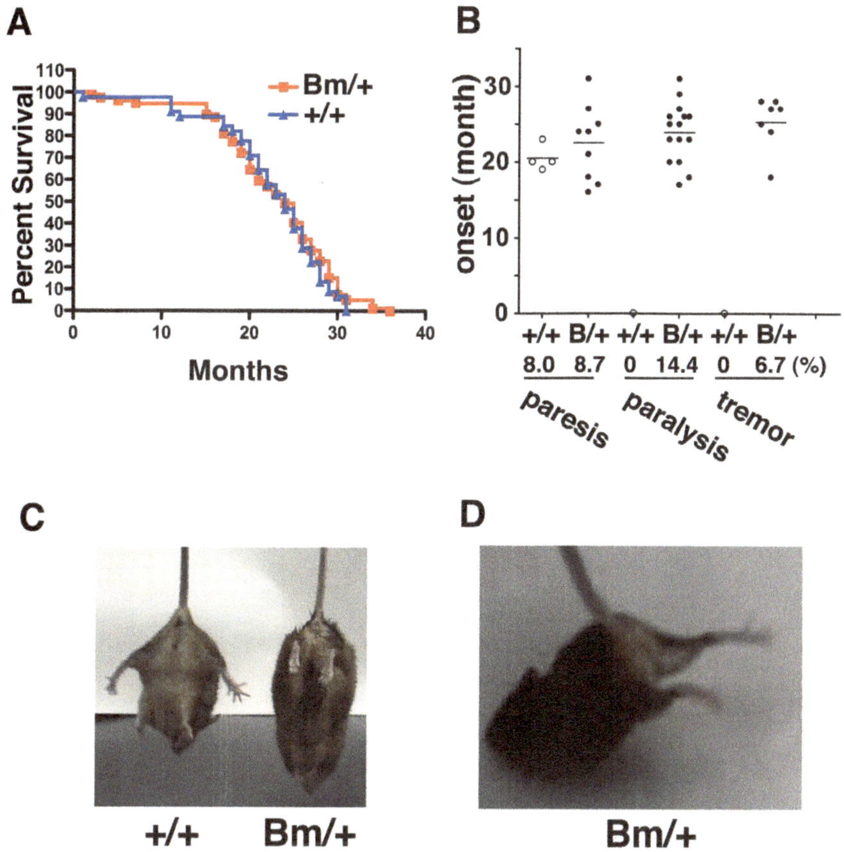

Figure 1. The mutant BiP mice revealed motor disabilities in aging. (A) Kaplan-Meier plots demonstrate that the heterozygous mutant BiP mice (Bm/+, n = 80) live as long as the wild-type mice (+/+, n = 45). (B) Some of the mutant BiP mice displayed paralysis and tremors after they were more than one year old. Heterozygous mutant BiP mice (Bm/+, n = 104) and wild type mice (n = 50) more than 10 months old were observed. No sign of weakness; +/+ 46/50, Bm/+ 73/104, tremor; +/+ 0/50, Bm/+ 9/104, paresis of one hindlimb; +/+ 4/50, Bm/+ 9/104, paralysis of one or both hindlimbs; +/+ 0/50, Bm/+ 15/104. To compare values between two groups, Chi-square and Fisher's exact test was done. Statistical significance was found. P value is 0.0033. (C) A seventeen month-old mutant BiP mouse displayed paralysis and loss of righting reflex. (D) A seventeen month-old mutant BiP mouse displayed paralysis (Video S1).

Motoneurons at the anterior horn of spinal cords of aged mutant BiP mice suffer from ER stress

In order to investigate whether defective retrieval of the mutant BiP may contribute to the pathogenesis of motor disability, we examined the spinal cords of both the wild type and mutant BiP mice. By staining with an anti-KDEL antibody, we found that some large cells expressed BiP and other KDEL-containing chaperones highly at the anterior horn of the spinal cords of 6 month-old mice of both types. Those cells were also stained with an anti-choline acetyltransferase antibody, suggesting that motoneurons at the anterior horn expressed ER chaperones highly (Figure 2A). Then we examined much older mutant BiP mice with motor disability. Motoneurons at the anterior horn of the spinal cord stained with an anti-choline acetyltransferase antibody in a 29 month-old mutant BiP mouse were less than those in the wild type mice (Figure 2B). We found that some large cells at the anterior horn of the spinal cord of the 29 month-old mutant BiP mouse expressed CHOP, a cell death related transcriptional factor during ER stress. The expression of CHOP was less obvious in the wild type littermate (Figure 2C). In accordance with these findings, terminal deoxynucleotidyl transferase dUTP nick end labeling (TUNEL) staining revealed that some apoptotic cells existed in the mutant spinal cord, accompanied by an enhanced gliosis stained with an anti-glial fibrillary acidic protein (GFAP) antibody (Figure 3A and B). It was difficult to find a TUNEL positive cell in the wild type spinal cord. We counted cells in Figure 3B. The ratio of GFAP positive cells was significantly higher in the mutant BiP spinal cord (Bm/+, 17 m) compared to that in the wild type (+/+, 16 m).

These data suggest that motoneurons at the anterior horn of spinal cords of aged mutant BiP mice suffer from ER stress, resulting in cell death.

Some motoneurons in the spinal cord revealed a degeneration accompanied by accumulations of protein aggregations

Protein aggregation and neuronal cell death are hallmarks of various neurodegenerative diseases [10]. We examined protein aggregation in the mutant spinal cord by staining it with an anti-ubiquitin antibody, which revealed cytoplasmic aggregations in the large cells at the anterior horn of the aged mutant BiP mouse (Figure 3C). One possible candidate for the aggregated proteins is superoxide dismutase (SOD) 1 [11]. Point mutations of the human SOD 1 gene are associated with a familial motoneuron disease (amyotrophic lateral sclerosis, ALS) [12]. While we observed fuzzy perinuclear staining with an anti-SOD1 antibody in large cells at the anterior horn of the spinal cords of wild type mice,

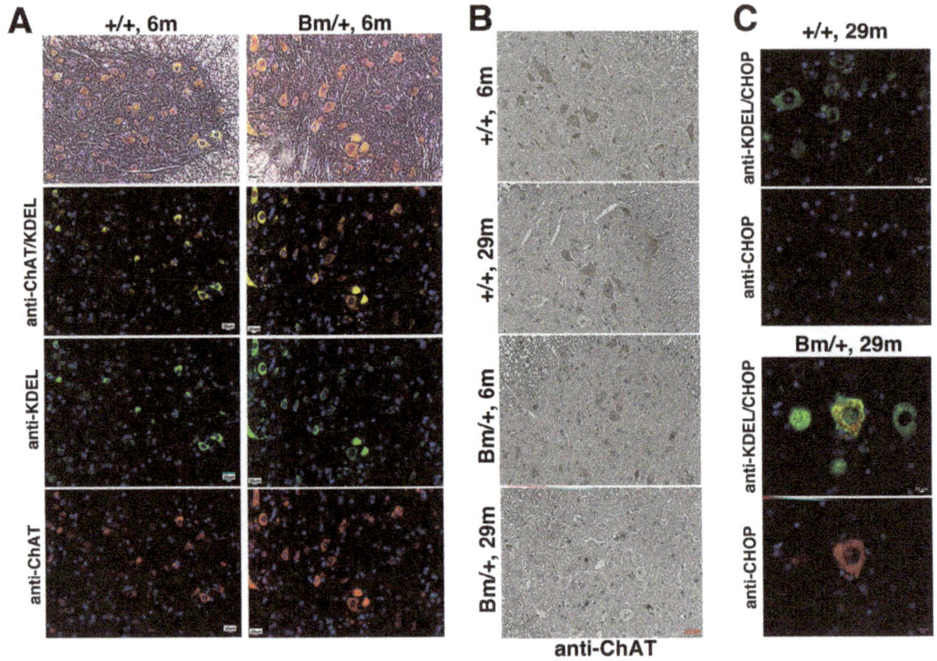

Figure 2. Motoneurons at the anterior horn of spinal cords of aged mutant BiP mice suffer from ER stress. (A) Motoneurons stained by an anti-choline acetyltransferase antibody (red) at the anterior horn in the spinal cord of both a 6 month-old wild type (+/+, 6 m) and a 6 month-old mutant BiP mouse (Bm/+, 6 m) express ER chaperones as well (green). Scale bars, 20 um. (B) The immunoreactivity with an anti-choline acetyltransferase antibody at the anterior horn is reduced in the aged 29 month-old mutant spinal cord (Bm/+, 29 m). Scale bars, 20 um. (C) Large cells at the anterior horn of the aged 29 month-old mutant spinal cord (Bm/+, 29 m) express ER chaperones as well as CHOP. Scale bars, 10 um. The nuclei were stained with Hoechst 33258 (blue, A and C).

aggregations were found instead in the cells of the mutant BiP mice. Those aggregations were much more obvious in the aged 26 month-old mutant BiP mouse (Figure 4, Bm/+, 26 m).

We examined the expression of BiP and the mutant BiP in the brain and spinal cord of the mutant BiP mice by Western blotting in Figure 5. The expression of GRP94, another ER chaperone, seemed to be increased in the aged mutant BiP brain and spinal cord. We also found an accumulation of SOD1 aggregates in the aged mutant BiP spinal cord, which corresponds to the finding in Figure 4.

Deletion of the retrieval signal from BiP may cause aberrant quality control

We examined the effect of ER stress on the distribution of BiP, an endogenous ligand of the KDEL receptor, in the secretory pathway by sucrose gradient analysis in Hela cells (Figure 6A). While most BiP was found in the ER in the resting state, a significant amount could be detected in the post-ER fractions in these cells during ER stress when treated with tunicamycin (2.5 ug/ml for 24 h) which disrupts protein glycosylation in the ER, thereby inducing the UPR (Figure 6B). Then, we examined the effect of deletion of the retrieval signal from BiP. A myc-tagged mutant BiP with the KDEL sequence deleted was transiently expressed in HeLa cells. While some of the mutant BiP were localized in the ER, significant amounts were also found in the post-ER fractions (Figure 6C), suggesting that a certain fraction of BiP was transported from the ER and retrieved from the post-ER by the KDEL receptor [13]. Thus, the deletion of the retrieval signal from BiP may results in mis-sortings of cargo proteins to the secretory pathway out of the ER.

Loss of the retrieval signal may also cause a failure of the activation of the KDEL receptor. Since KDEL receptor activation has been reported to promote autophagy and removal of aggregated proteins, including SOD1 [14], we examined whether autophagy induced in the mutant BiP cells (Figure 6D). We found ER stress caused by tunicamycin treatment induced the expression of BiP in the wild type mouse embryonic cells (MEF) as well as that of the mutant BiP in the mutant MEF, while autophagy was induced only in the wild type MEF accompanying the accumulation of light chain 3AII (LC3AII).

If the lack of the KDEL sequence from BiP affects autophagy, cytosolic aggregates might be accumulated in the homozygous mutant BiP MEF. We over-expressed SOD1-GFP in the wild type and the homozygous mutant BiP MEF. While SOD1 distributed through the cytoplasm in the wild type MEF, it accumulated in the perinuclear space and some aggregations were found in the cytoplasm of the mutant BiP MEF (Figure 7).

Thus, lack of the KDEL sequence from BiP may lead to some functional defects of the ER chaperone in quality control and autophagy, resulting in the late onset of neurodegenerative diseases.

Discussion

Some of the mutant BiP mice revealed motor disabilities in aging. We found a degeneration of some motoneurons in the spinal cord accompanied by the accumulation of ubiquitinated proteins. BiP, also called the 78-kD glucose-regulated protein (GRP78), is a member of the heat shock protein 70 family of proteins and is one of the most abundant ER chaperones, assisting in protein translocation, folding, and degradation [15]. Quality control in the early secretory pathway is a ubiquitous mechanism

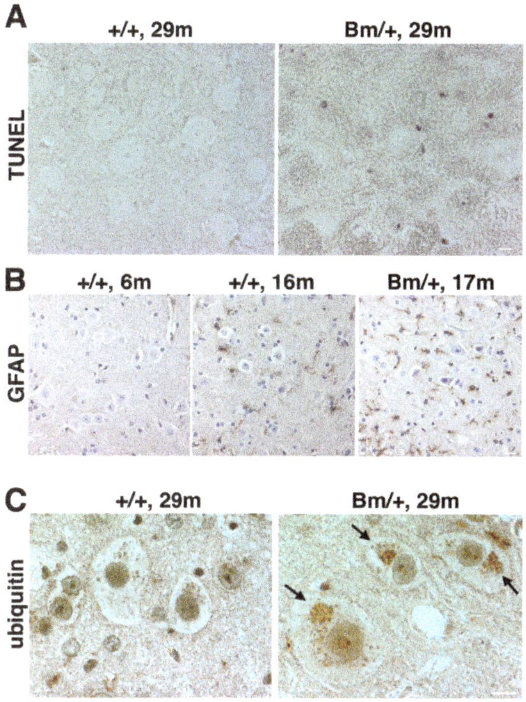

Figure 3. Some motoneurons in the spinal cord revealed a degeneration accompanied by accumulations of ubiquitinated proteins. (A) TUNEL staining revealed some apoptotic cells at the anterior horn in the spinal cord of a 29 month-old mutant BiP mouse (Bm/+, 29 m). Scale bars, 10 um. (B) The immunoreactivity with an anti-GFAP antibody at the anterior horn is increased in a 17 month-old mutant spinal cord (Bm/+, 17 m). Scale bars, 20 um. GFAP positive cells are counted (five fields in each mouse, GFAP positive cells/the number of nucleus). +/+, 16 m; 33/199, 35/174, 34/192, 40/181, 42/207, Bm/+, 17 m; 42/132, 50/140, 59/147, 39/154, 58/143 +/+, 6 m; 5/143, 4/131, 4/141, 0/95, 0/107. The ratio of GFAP positive cells is significantly higher in the mutant BiP spinal cord (Bm/+, 17 m) compared to that in the wild type (+/+, 16 m) by t test (p value is 0.0009). (C) The aggregations were stained by an anti-ubiquitin antibody in the large cells at the anterior horn of the 29 month-old mutant spinal cord (Bm/+, 29 m, arrowheads). Scale bars, 10 um.

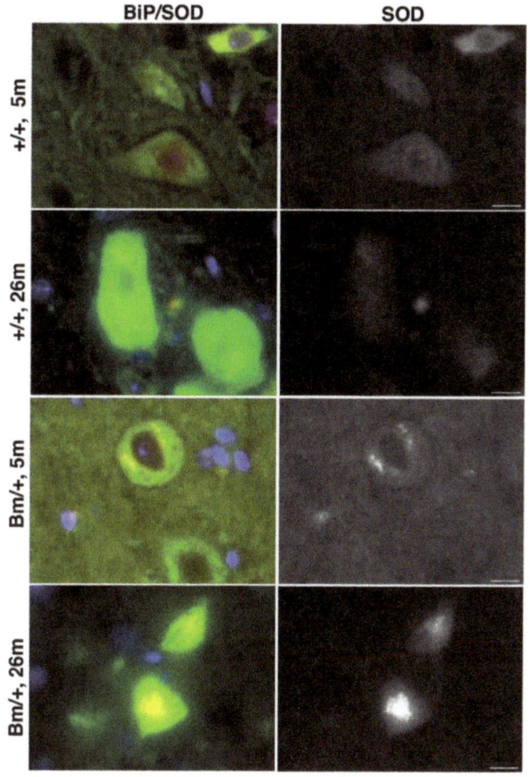

Figure 4. Aggregations were obvious in the aged mutant BiP mouse. The aggregations were evaluated by immunofluorescence microscopy with double labeling by using a rabbit anti-SOD1 antibody (red) and a mouse anti-KDEL mAb for the wild type BiP and other ER chaperones (green, +/+, 5 and 26 month-old), or by using a rabbit anti-SOD1 antibody (red) and a mouse anti-HA mAb (15E6) for the mutant BiP (green, Bm/+, 5 and 26 month-old). Scale bars, 10 um. Aggregations were observed in large cells at the anterior horn of a 26-month-old mutant spinal cord (Bm/+, 26 m).

for adapting to ER stress, and the KDEL receptor and BiP are essential components of this system [13]. Proper ER-to-Golgi transport, and the subsequent retrieval of proteins and lipids to the ER, are thought to contribute to quality control [13,16]. Deletion of the retrieval sequence from the BiP, and the consequent lack of mutant BiP recycling by the KDEL receptor, could have possible effects on protein folding in the ER and post-ER.

Mutant BiP were mostly localized to the ER, and the expression was enhanced by tunicamycin in the mutant BiP MEF [9]. A significant fraction of the mutant BiP was secreted from the cells even in the resting state, reflecting a deletion of the KDEL sequence and an impaired retrieval of mutant BiP [9]. The KDEL proteins are ER chaperones; therefore, their expression is induced extensively upon ER stress, which may cause the saturation of the KDEL receptor-mediated retrieval. A fraction of the wild-type BiP was also secreted into the medium upon ER stress caused by the tunicamycin treatment, indicating that retrieval by the KDEL receptor is saturable [9].

The homozygous mutant BiP mice have defects in some professional secretory cells. They survive only several hours after birth due to impaired pulmonary surfactant biosynthesis by alveolar type II epithelial cells causing respiratory failure [9]. They also have cortical dysplasia in the brain due to impaired synthesis of reelin by Cajal-Retzius cells. Thus, the retrieval function of BiP is essential in vivo. However, mouse embryonic fibroblasts from the homozygous mutant BiP mice are viable. Therefore, living as a whole animal may suffer from various insults from the environment.

The accumulation of misfolded proteins is one of the most common features in neurodegenerative diseases. One possible explanation for the late onset of sporadic forms of neurodegeneration is a decline, with aging, of the cellular machinery to cope with protein overload in the ER. The expression level of BiP decreases, and its chaperone function is progressively reduced due to age-related oxidization reported in rodents [10,17]. The mutant BiP with impaired retrieval seemed to fail the induction of autophagy, which might further limit the capacity of ER quality control.

The heterozygous mutant BiP mice grew up to be adults and showed apparently normal organ development. However, vulnerability to ER stress may exist, and that vulnerability could result in chronic organ injuries with aging such as renal tubular-interstitial injury, as described in our previous work [18]. We are also interested in the relationship between ER stress and neural degeneration due to aging, such as Alzheimer's disease [19], Parkinson's disease [20], and amyotrophic lateral sclerosis [11]. The involvement of impaired BiP function in neurodegenerative

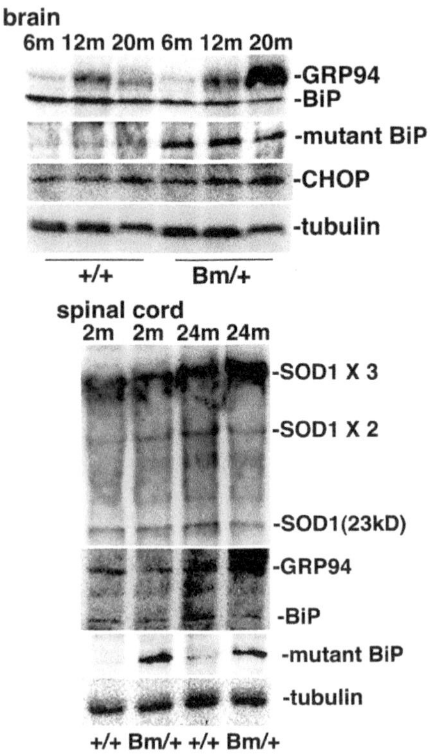

Figure 5. The expressions of chaperones in the mutant BiP mice. The heterozygous mutant BiP mice and the litter mate wild type mice were anesthetized by pentobarbital, and the brains and spinal cords were removed. They were subjected to Western blot analysis with an anti-KDEL mouse mAb for BiP and GRP94, an anti-HA mouse mAb for mutant BiP, an anti-CHOP rabbit antiserum, and an anti-SOD1 rabbit antiserum.

diseases has been reported in a mouse model where the disruption of SIL1, a co-chaperone of BiP, causes protein accumulation and neurodegeneration [21].

Interestingly, we previously found disordered layer formation in the cerebral cortex and cerebellum in the homozygous mutant BiP neonates. Among proteins involved in corticogenesis, we found that the expression of reelin, secreted by Cajal-Retzius cells [22] was markedly reduced in the mutant brain [23]. Several studies have suggested the possible role of reelin in the pathogenesis of human mental disorders such as schizophrenia, autism, bipolar disorder, and Alzheimer's disease [24,25]. Reelin and ApoE share ApoER2 on the cortical neurons [26], and ApoE inhibits reelin signaling by competing for binding to ApoER2. The E4 allele of ApoE increases the risk of developing sporadic forms of Alzheimer's disease. Because reelin signaling through ApoER2 in adult brains modulates synaptic plasticity and memory formation [27], a defective reelin signaling pathway may contribute to the pathogenesis of adult mental disorders. Thus, reelin signaling and ER quality control may be related to the pathogenesis of adult mental disorders, as seen in the reeler mutant-like cerebral malformation in the homozygous mutant BiP neonates [23].

The administration of chemical chaperones that promote protein folding in the ER has been reported to be effective in treating type2 diabetes, which has been shown, in experiments using a mouse model, to be connected to ER stress [28]. We have also shown that a chemical chaperone prevented the development of morphine tolerance caused by ER stress [29]. Our present study suggests that ER chaperones would be promising therapeutic targets in the treatment of chronic neurodegenerative diseases.

Methods

Cells and reagents

Mouse embryonic fibroblasts (MEFs) were prepared from 13.5-day-old embryos [9]. MEFs and HeLa cells were grown in a complete medium that consisted of Dulbecco's modified Eagle's medium (DMEM; Sigma Chemical Co., Irvine, UK) with 10% fetal bovine serum, 2 mM glutamine, 50 µg/ml streptomycin and 50 U/ml penicillin G at 37°C in a 5% CO_2 incubator.

The following antibodies were used: rabbit antiserum against CHOP/GADD153, rabbit antiserum against ubiquitin, rabbit antiserum against superoxide dismutase 1 (Santa Cruz Biotechnology), rabbit antiserum against choline acetyltransferase (Millipore), rabbit antiserum against glial fibrillary acidic protein (GFAP, DakoCytomation), rabbit antiserum against Derlin-1 (MBL), mouse mAb 9E10 against the myc epitope (ATCC), mouse mAb against g-tubulin, mouse mAb against Golgi p58 (Sigma Chemical), mouse mAb SPA-827 against BiP (KDEL sequence, Stressgen), mouse mAb AF8 against calnexin (kindly provided by MM. Brenner, Boston, MA), mouse mAb 15E6 against HA tag (kindly provided by VW Hsu, Boston, MA). rabbit polyclonal antiserum against light chain (LC) 3A (Cell Signaling), Cy-2-conjugated donkey antibody against rabbit IgG, Cy-3-conjugated donkey antibody against rabbit IgG and Cy-3-conjugated donkey antibody against mouse IgG (Jackson Immunoresearch Laboratories). Tunicamycin was purchased from Nacali tasque. Hoechst 33258 was purchased from Invitrogen. Chloroquine was purchased from Sigma-Aldrich.

Plasmids and transfection

A cDNA for the BiP deleted with the KDEL sequence was obtained by inserting a stop codon into a rat BiP cDNA (a gift from Dr. H.R.B. Pelham, MRC Laboratory of Molecular Biology, UK) just before the region encoding the carboxyl terminal KDEL sequence with a PCR reaction. The PCR product was subcloned into a pcDNA3.1 myc-His vector (Invitrogen). A PCR-generated fragment corresponding to the wild-type human SOD1 cDNA from human cDNA library was cloned into the plasmid pGFP vector (Clontech). The DNA sequences were verified using the Applied Biosystems ABI Prism 310 genetic analyzer. Transfection was performed with Fugene 6 (Roche, Basel, Switzerland).

Mutant BiP mice

All animal experimental procedures were in accordance with a protocol approved by the Institutional Animal Care Committee of Chiba University, Chiba, Japan. A rat BiP cDNA was used as a probe to isolate a genomic clone containing the whole exon of the BiP gene from the 129/SvJ mouse genomic library in lFIXII (Stratagene). A targeting vector was used for electroporation into R1 EScells. We used homologous recombination to establish knock-in mice expressing BiP lacking the carboxyl-terminal KDEL sequence [9]. The missing KDEL sequence was replaced by a hemagglutinin (HA) tag. The resulting male chimeras were mated to C57BL/6 females. The mutant-BiP mice were investigated on the compound genetic background between the 129/SvJ derived from R1 ES cells and C57BL/6J. The heterozygotes were intercrossed to generate homozygous mutants. This hybrid line was maintained by brother-sister mating for at least ten generations.

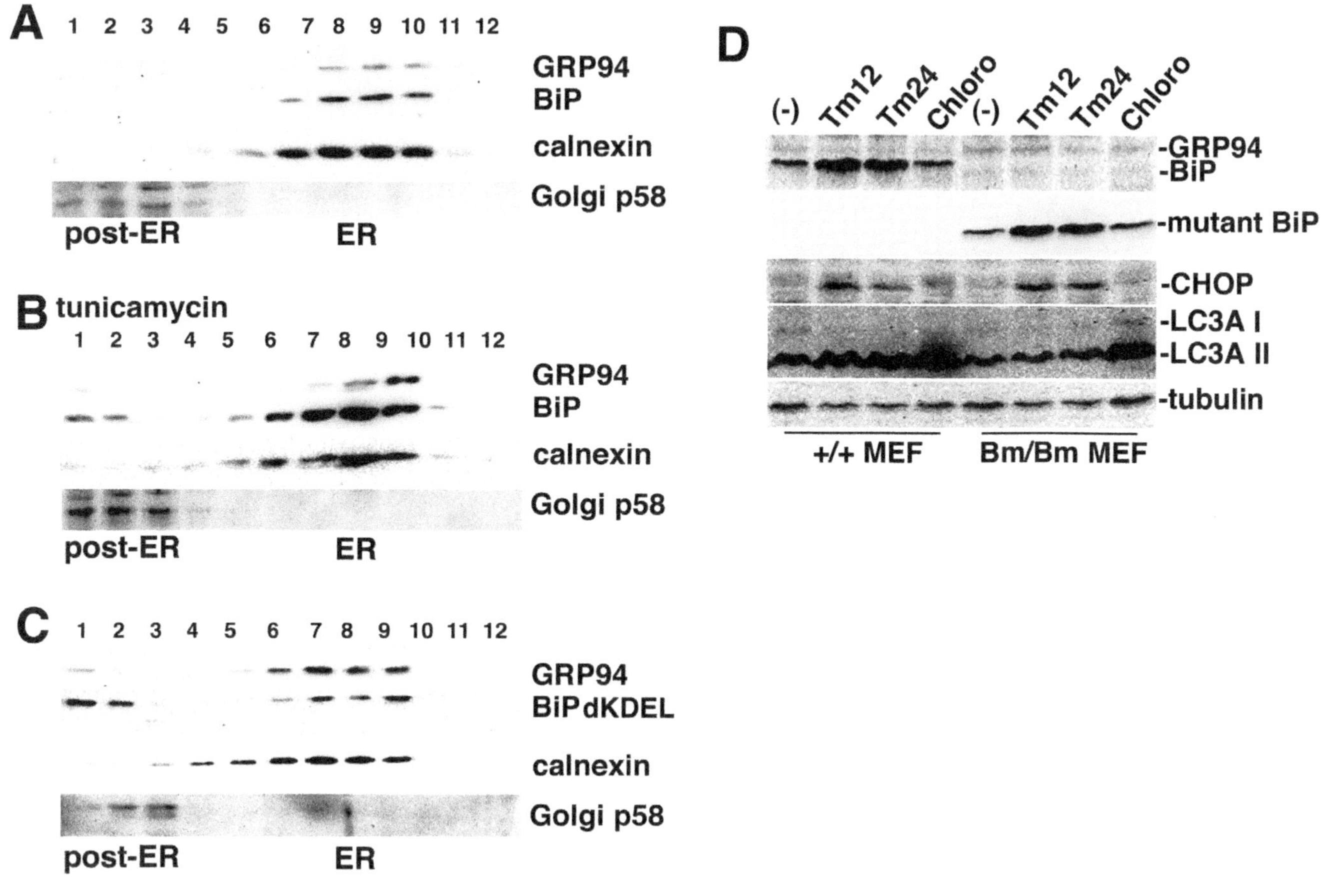

Figure 6. Lack of the KDEL sequence from BiP may lead to some functional defects of the ER chaperone in quality control and autophagy. (A, B) A fraction of BiP is secreted from the ER under stressed conditions. The postnuclear supernatants (PNS) from HeLa cells with (B) or without (A) treatment by tunicamycin 2.5 ug ml^{-1} for 24 h were separated on a continuous sucrose gradient (20% to 50%, fraction 1; top, fraction 12; bottom). An aliquot of each fraction was analyzed by SDS-PAGE. The distributions of GRP94, BiP, Golgi p58 and calnexin were determined by Western blotting. (C) HeLa cells transiently expressing the mutant BiP with the KDEL sequence deleted were collected and homogenized. The PNS from those cells were separated on a continuous sucrose gradient (20% to 50%, fraction 1; top, fraction 12; bottom). An aliquot of each fraction was analyzed by SDS-PAGE. The distributions of the GRP94, myc-tagged mutant BiP, Golgi p58 and calnexin were determined by Western blotting. (D) Wild-type MEFs and BiP MEFs were treated with tunicamycin (2.5 ug ml^{-1} for 12, 24 h) or chloroquine (50 uM for 12 h). Cells were subjected to Western blot analysis with an anti-KDEL mouse mAb for BiP, an anti-HA mouse mAb for mutant BiP, an anti-CHOP rabbit antiserum, an anti-LC3A antiserum, and an anti-tubulin mAb.

Western blotting

Cultured cells were washed twice with ice-cold PBS and then homogenized in a buffer containing 0.4% (w/v) Nonidet P-40, 0.2% N-lauroylsarcosine, 30 mM Tris/HCl pH 8.0, 1 mM EDTA, 10 µg/ml aprotinin, 10 µg/ml leupeptin, 30 µg/ml N-acetyl-L-leucinal-L-lecinal-L-norleucinal (ALLN, Sigma Chemical). The mice were deeply anesthetized with pentobarbital (Dainippon Sumitomo Pharma). Brains and spinal cords were homogenized by sonication (UR-20P, TOMY, Tokyo, Japan) in a buffer containing 0.4% (w/v) Nonidet P-40, 0.2% N-lauroylsarcosine, 30 mM Tris/HCl pH 8.0, 1 mM EDTA, 10 µg/ml aprotinin, 10 µg/ml leupeptin, 30 µg/ml ALLN.

The lysates were centrifuged, and the supernatants were resuspended in SDS-PAGE sample buffer and then separated by SDS-PAGE under reducing conditions. The proteins were transferred from the gels to polyvinylidene fluoride membranes (Immobilon-P, Millipore Corp.), and Western blotting was done as previously described [30]. Imaging was obtained by LAS-1000 and Image Gauge software (Fuji Photo Film Co. Ltd.).

Sucrose gradient experiment

A postnuclear supernatant was obtained and loaded on a continuous sucrose gradient (20–50%), as described previously [13]. Twelve fractions were obtained from each sample. An aliquot of each fraction was separated by SDS-PAGE under reducing conditions, and the distribution of each protein was determined by Western blotting, developed by chemiluminescence (ECL, Amersham Pharmacia Biotech). Imaging was obtained by LAS1000 and Image Gauge software (Fuji Photo Film Co. Ltd., Tokyo, Japan).

Immunohistochemistry

The mice were deeply anesthetized with pentobarbital and fixed by transcardiac perfusion with 4% paraformaldehyde in phosphate-buffered saline (PBS). The spinal cords were further immersion-fixed for 12 h in 4% paraformaldehyde at 4°C. After fixation, they were dehydrated in increasing concentrations of ethanol and embedded in paraffin wax. For the immunofluorescence, the sections (8 µm) were incubated with 10% normal goat or bovine serum in PBS for 30 min to block nonspecific antibody

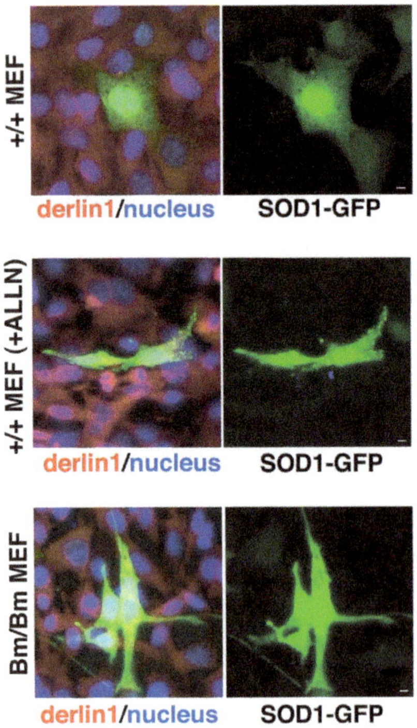

Figure 7. Aggregations were obvious in the mutant BiP MEF. The aggregations by transient expressions of SOD1-GFP were evaluated by immunofluorescence microscopy with labeling by using a rabbit anti-Derlin1 antibody for the ER staining (red) and SOD1-GFP (green) in wild type (+/+) and the homozygous mutant (Bm/Bm) MEF with Hoechst 33342 for nuclear staining. Scale bars, 10 um. Aggregations of SOD1were observed in the mutant BiP MEF as well as in the wild type MEF treated with a proteasome inhibitor, ALLN (10 ug/ml), at 37°C for 12 h.

binding, and then incubated with a primary antibody in PBS for 1 h at room temperature. The sections were rinsed with PBS and then incubated with a mixture of Cy3-conjugated anti-rabbit IgG and Cy2-conjugated anti-mouse IgG in PBS for 1 h at room temperature. Then, the sections were rinsed with PBS and mounted on glass slides with Perma Fluor (Immunon). Immunolocalization was observed with a fluorescence microscope using FITC/rhodamine filters and a Plan-Neofluar 20× and 40× NA 0.75 objective (Axiovert 200 M, Carl Zeiss). The brightness and contrast were optimized by AxioVision 4.4 software (Carl Zeiss), and the immunofluorescence images were captured with a digital camera (AxioCam MRm, Carl Zeiss). For the immunohistochemistry, the spinal cord sections were incubated with 10% normal goat or bovine serum in PBS for 30 min to block nonspecific antibody binding, and then incubated with a primary antibody in PBS for 12 h at 4°C. The sections were rinsed with PBS, incubated with a secondary antibody in PBS for 2 h at room temperature, and then visualized using the VECTASTAIN Elite ABC kit (Vector Laboratories) with diaminobenzidine (Sigma).

TUNEL staining

The mice were deeply anesthetized with pentobarbital (Dainippon Sumitomo Pharma). The spinal cords were isolated, and apoptotic cells were visualized by TUNEL assay based on the manufacturer's protocol (Roche) as previously described [30]. The TUNEL staining was observed with a microscope using a N-Achroplan 40× NA 0.65 objective (Axio Imager A1, Carl Zeiss). The brightness and contrast were optimized by AxioVision Rel.4.7 software (Carl Zeiss), and the images were captured with a digital camera (AxioCam MRc, Carl Zeiss).

Statistical analysis

To compare values between groups, Chi-square and Fisher's exact test (Figure. 1) and t-test (Figure 3B) were used (GraphPad Prism 4.0, GraphPad Software, San Diego, CA). Statistical significance was accepted at $P < 0.05$.

Supporting Information

Video S1 A seventeen month-old heterozygous mutant BiP mouse displayed paralysis.

Acknowledgments

We thank Dr. Shigemasa Goto (National hospital organization Chiba medical center) and Dr. Keita Kimura for helpful aids and critical comments.

Author Contributions

Conceived and designed the experiments: TA HK. Performed the experiments: HJ NM MK HK TA. Analyzed the data: TA. Contributed reagents/materials/analysis tools: TA HJ. Wrote the paper: TA.

References

1. Ellgaard L, Helenius A (2003) Quality control in the endoplasmic reticulum. Nat Rev Mol Cell Biol 4: 181–191.
2. Pfaffenbach KT, Lee AS (2011) The critical role of GRP78 in physiologic and pathologic stress. Curr Opin Cell Biol 23: 150–156.
3. Ron D, Walter P (2007) Signal integration in the endoplasmic reticulum unfolded protein response. Nat Rev Mol Cell Biol 8: 519–529.
4. Roussel BD, Kruppa AJ, Miranda E, Crowther DC, Lomas DA, et al. (2013)Endoplasmic reticulum dysfunction in neurological disease. Lancet Neurol 12: 105–118.
5. Lewis MJ, Pelham HR (1992) Ligand-induced redistribution of a human KDEL receptor from the Golgi complex to the endoplasmic reticulum. Cell 68: 353–364.
6. Orci L, Stamnes M, Ravazzola M, Amherdt M, Perrelet A, et al. (1997) Bidirectional transport by distinct populations of COPI-coated vesicles. Cell 90: 335–349.
7. Beh CT, Rose MD (1995) Two redundant systems maintain levels of resident proteins within the yeast endoplasmic reticulum. Proc Natl Acad Sci U S A 92: 9820–9823.
8. Luo S, Mao C, Lee B, Lee AS (2006) GRP78/BiP is required for cell proliferation and protecting the inner cell mass from apoptosis during early mouse embryonic development. Mol Cell Biol 26: 5688–5697.
9. Mimura N, Hamada H, Kashio M, Jin H, Toyama Y, et al. (2007) Aberrant quality control in the endoplasmic reticulum impairs the biosynthesis of pulmonary surfactant in mice expressing mutant BiP. Cell Death Differ 14: 1475–1485.
10. Gorbatyuk MS, Gorbatyuk OS (2013) The Molecular Chaperone GRP78/BiP as a Therapeutic Target for Neurodegenerative Disorders: A Mini Review. J Genet Syndr Gene Ther 4.
11. Nishitoh H, Kadowaki H, Nagai A, Maruyama T, Yokota T, et al. (2008) ALS-linked mutant SOD1 induces ER stress- and ASK1-dependent motor neuron death by targeting Derlin-1. Genes Dev 22: 1451–1464.
12. Gurney ME, Pu H, Chiu AY, Dal Canto MC, Polchow CY, et al. (1994) Motor neuron degeneration in mice that express a human Cu, Zn superoxide dismutase mutation. Science 264: 1772–1775.
13. Yamamoto K, Fujii R, Toyofuku Y, Saito T, Koseki H, et al. (2001) The KDEL receptor mediates a retrieval mechanism that contributes to quality control at the endoplasmic reticulum. Embo J 20: 3082–3091.
14. Wang P, Li B, Zhou L, Fei E, Wang G (2011) The KDEL receptor induces autophagy to promote the clearance of neurodegenerative disease-related proteins. Neuroscience 190: 43–55.

15. Munro S, Pelham HR (1986) An Hsp70-like protein in the ER: identity with the 78 kd glucose- regulated protein and immunoglobulin heavy chain binding protein. Cell 46: 291–300.
16. Hammond C, Helenius A (1994) Quality control in the secretory pathway: retention of a misfolded viral membrane glycoprotein involves cycling between the ER, intermediate compartment, and Golgi apparatus. J Cell Biol 126: 41–52.
17. Brown MK, Naidoo N (2012) The endoplasmic reticulum stress response in aging and age-related diseases. Front Physiol 3: 263.
18. Kimura K, Jin H, Ogawa M, Aoe T (2008) Dysfunction of the ER chaperone BiP accelerates the renal tubular injury. Biochem Biophys Res Commun 366: 1048–1053.
19. Katayama T, Imaizumi K, Sato N, Miyoshi K, Kudo T, et al. (1999) Presenilin-1 mutations downregulate the signalling pathway of the unfolded-protein response. Nat Cell Biol 1: 479–485.
20. Imai Y, Soda M, Inoue H, Hattori N, Mizuno Y, et al. (2001) An unfolded putative transmembrane polypeptide, which can lead to endoplasmic reticulum stress, is a substrate of Parkin. Cell 105: 891–902.
21. Zhao L, Longo-Guess C, Harris BS, Lee JW, Ackerman SL (2005) Protein accumulation and neurodegeneration in the woozy mutant mouse is caused by disruption of SIL1, a cochaperone of BiP. Nat Genet 37: 974–979.
22. D'Arcangelo G, Miao GG, Chen SC, Soares HD, Morgan JI, et al. (1995) A protein related to extracellular matrix proteins deleted in the mouse mutant reeler. Nature 374: 719–723.
23. Mimura N, Yuasa S, Soma M, Jin H, Kimura K, et al. (2008) Altered quality control in the endoplasmic reticulum causes cortical dysplasia in knock-in mice expressing a mutant BiP. Mol Cell Biol 28: 293–301.
24. Tissir F, Goffinet AM (2003) Reelin and brain development. Nat Rev Neurosci 4: 496–505.
25. Fatemi SH (2005) Reelin glycoprotein: structure, biology and roles in health and disease. Mol Psychiatry 10: 251–257.
26. D'Arcangelo G, Homayouni R, Keshvara L, Rice DS, Sheldon M, et al. (1999) Reelin is a ligand for lipoprotein receptors. Neuron 24: 471–479.
27. Beffert U, Weeber EJ, Durudas A, Qiu S, Masiulis I, et al. (2005) Modulation of synaptic plasticity and memory by Reelin involves differential splicing of the lipoprotein receptor Apoer2. Neuron 47: 567–579.
28. Ozcan U, Yilmaz E, Ozcan L, Furuhashi M, Vaillancourt E, et al. (2006) Chemical chaperones reduce ER stress and restore glucose homeostasis in a mouse model of type 2 diabetes. Science 313: 1137–1140.
29. Dobashi T, Tanabe S, Jin H, Mimura N, Yamamoto T, et al. (2010) BiP, an endoplasmic reticulum chaperone, modulates the development of morphine antinociceptive tolerance. J Cell Mol Med 14: 2816–2826.
30. Hamada H, Suzuki M, Yuasa S, Mimura N, Shinozuka N, et al. (2004) Dilated cardiomyopathy caused by aberrant endoplasmic reticulum quality control in mutant KDEL receptor transgenic mice. Mol Cell Biol 24: 8007–8017.

18

Hypoxia in Vascular Networks: A Complex System Approach to Unravel the Diabetic Paradox

Yérali Gandica[1], Tobias Schwarz[1,2], Orlando Oliveira[1], Rui D. M. Travasso[1,3]*

1 Center for Computational Physics, Department of Physics, University of Coimbra, Coimbra, Portugal, **2** Heinz-Brandt-Schule, Berlin, Germany, **3** Center of Ophthalmology and Vision Sciences(COCV), Institute for Biomedical Imaging and Life Sciences (IBILI), Faculty of Medicine, University of Coimbra, Coimbra, Portugal

Abstract

In this work we model the extent of hypoxia in the diabetic retina as a function of the area affected by vessel disruption. We find two regimes that differ on the ratio between the area of disrupted vasculature and the area of tissue in hypoxia. In the first regime the hypoxia is *localized* in the vicinity of the vascular disruption, while in the second regime there is a *generalized* hypoxia in the affected tissue. The transition between these two regimes occurs when the tissue area affected by individual sites of vessel damage is on the order of the square of the characteristic irrigation length in the tissue (the maximum distance that an irrigated point in the tissue is from an existing vessel). We observe that very high levels of hypoxia are correlated with the rupture of larger vessels in the retina, and with smaller radii of individual sites of vessel damage. Based on this property of vascular networks, we propose a novel mechanism for the transition between the nonproliferative and the proliferative stages in diabetic retinopathy.

Editor: Timothy W. Secomb, University of Arizona, United States of America

Funding: Y.G., T.S. and R.D.M.T. acknowledge financial support from Fundos FEDER through Programa Operacional Factores de Competitividade – COMPETE and by Fundação para a Ciência e Tecnologia, through project FCOMP-01-0124-FEDER-015708. The authors acknowledge support from Fundação para a Ciência e Tecnologia through project PEst-OE/FIS/UI0405/2014. R.D.M.T. acknowledges financial support from Fundação para a Ciência e Tecnologia through the Investigador FCT program. The funders had no role in study design, data collection and analysis, decision to publish, or preparation of the manuscript.

Competing Interests: The authors have declared that no competing interests exist.

* Email: rui@teor.fis.uc.pt

Introduction

Diabetes occurs when the pancreas does not secrete enough insulin or the body is unable to process it properly [1]. High levels (and/or wide fluctuations) of glucose concentration in the blood can lead to a number of complications, including an increased risk of cardio-vascular disease, kidney disease (nephropathy), neural damage (neuropathy), and retinal disease (diabetic retinopathy, DR) [2]. The number of deaths attributed to diabetes is about 9% of the global total of deaths [3].

Diabetic retinas suffer extensive blood vessel disruption (e.g. the formation of defects such as micro-aneurisms, and dramatic vessel proliferation increase, leading to the formation of small blood lakes and to loss of vessel function) [4] which stems from the inflammatory environment that is associated with high levels of methilglyoxal [5], and lead to the production of several proteins that have a vascular destabilization action. An example is the angiopoietin-2 (Ang-2) [6] that binds the receptors Tie-2 at the membrane of the vessels' endothelial cells, thus preventing the mediation of angiopoietin-1 in the maturation of the capillaries. Therefore, in the absence of pro-angiogenic factors, high levels of Ang-2 induce an increase of vessel permeability, with the consequence of a deficient tissue irrigation [7] (note, however, that the loosening of the Tie-2 junctions between endothelial cells is also an important step of the angiogenic process, and therefore, Ang-2 is able to promote angiogenesis depending on the presence of pro-angiogenic factors). It has been shown experimentally in mice that retinal vascular network damage is able to drive neo-vascularization characteristic of the later stages of DR [8,9].

A large body of work has been done to understand the pathogenesis of diabetic microvasculopathy [10,11]. Most of these efforts have been centered in the mechanisms related to specific signaling pathways [12,13]. Nevertheless, we argue in the present work that the spatial distribution of areas with deficient irrigation, i.e. in hypoxia, also play an important role in the determining the progression of the disease. In these regions, the lack of oxygen leads to higher levels of angiogenic factors that promote the remodeling of the vasculature as well as the growth of neo-vessels, both hallmarks of DR [14]. In consequence, the study of how the distribution of hypoxic regions depends on vascular damage is essential for the understanding of DR's progression. In this work we will focus on the changes in irrigation after events of vessel blockage, inspired by the effect of factors such as Ang-2, that are present in high levels in a DR setting, and that have the potential to drive extensive vessel damage rendering the smaller vessels non-functional. This study is closely related with the analysis of resilience in spatial complex networks, where is investigated the effect of a particular amount of damage in the nodes and/or links on the integrity of the complex network.

The resilience of complex networks to damage has attracted a great deal of attention in the past years [15–23]. Most of the studies on this topic link the random or selected removal of nodes to the alteration in the structural properties of networks and have important applications. For example, the study of the percolation properties of a network of social relations upon node removal can be applied directly to viral epidemics. In this case, random node removal gives information about the amount of agents to immunize in order to prevent the propagation of the epidemics

[24]. Also, the consequences of the breakdown of power lines resultant from a natural hazard, for example, is a problem that can be formulated in terms of the failure of interconnected networks, see e.g. [25,26].

Networks are studied by defining the nodes of the system and the connectivity between them by means of edges or bonds. Other specific characteristics can be added according to the system that is modeled, such as bond weights, directionality, etc [15–17]. Typically, when structural and dynamic characteristics of a network are determined solely by their connectivity, it can be considered to be embedded in an abstract "network space" [27]. However, when networks have the role of delivering energy, water or nutrients, the physical space constraints are important. In these networks, resilience after the rupture of bonds at a particular location is connected to the lack of goods, energy, water or nutrients in spatial regions, and not to the number of nodes and bonds affected per se [28]. Not surprisingly, the applications of the study of the resilience in spatial networks are vast, however most previous studies in resilience of complex networks have not considered spatial constraints [27].

Vascular networks are a particular type of spatial network constituted by two different topologies of connections that fulfill different functions [29]. Larger vessels, arterioles and venules form *specific* fractal tree-like networks [30–33] that are responsible for blood transport [34]. In these structures, alterations in the branching pattern [35], branching lengths [36,37], fractal dimension [32,38] among others, are often an indication of a pathology. On the other hand, nutrient and oxygen diffusion is carried out mainly by capillaries which are laid down in space approximately in a lattice-like structure [29,39,40]. Vascular networks are dynamic, since they can adapt to the nutrient requirements of the tissue they irrigate [41]. Therefore, spatial constraints, such as the nutrient and protein diffusion, affect not only the tissue cells survival, but also the structure of the vascular network itself.

Earlier studies on the hypoxia in damaged vascular networks showed a localized decrease in irrigation after specific targeting of blood vessels. Blinder et al. [30] studying robustness of distribution of blood in rodent neocortex to occlusion experiments found that removing 15% of the connections in the backbone isolates 5% of the cortex from perfusion. More recently, the same authors investigated experimentally the volume of micro-infarctions in the rat brain, resultant of the occlusion of specific arterioles [42], demonstrating that even small volumes of low irrigation have important cognitive consequences.

Our aim is to relate the different stages of DR with the distribution of tissue irrigation decrease after a total loss of vascular function in localised regions in the retina. This article is organized as follows. In the next section the retina vessel network is described, together with the details of calculation of the tissue irrigation. In the Simulation and Results section we investigate how the affected irrigation changes with the damaged vasculature. In the Discussion section the results are analyzed and its physio-pathological implications to the development of DR are discussed. Finally, in the last section we summarize and conclude.

Materials and Methods

The aim of this work is to propose a mechanism relating the evolution of the proliferative stage of DR with the patterns of hypoxia in the retinal tissue after damage of its vascular network. Therefore, we start with a vascular network that mimics the retinal vasculature. The top layer of the vasculature at the retina is almost two dimensional [43], so that its approximate structure can be obtained from the digitalization of an angiography. In this work we used an angiography of a human retina (with 1684×1192 lattice units, equivalent to 9.4×6.6 mm; each lattice unit corresponds to 5.6 μm), obtained from a patient in the early stages of diabetic retinopathy (left panel in Fig. 1). Patients at Coimbra's University Hospitals routinely perform angiographies to assess the progress of different diseases (normally DR or age related macular degeneracy). This results in an image where the deficiencies of the retinal vascular network can be clearly visualized. The hospital stores several of these images obtained from anonymous patients as example of the different stages of relevant pathologies. We chose one image from that set corresponding to a very early stage of DR, where the pathology-driven vasculature alteration was the least perceptible. No human tissues or cells were used in this study.

A closed vascular network is obtained extending manually the thinner arterial vessels to intercept the thinner veins (see Fig. 1 center). Taking into account the thickness and contrast in the original angiography, we are able to manually identify the sites where the vessels overlap without establishing bifurcations. Even missing the thinnest capillaries, this network provides the basic structure of in-vivo retinal networks. The measured number of bifurcations between the main vessel (artery or vein) and the furthermost capillary is 35. This number is of the same order of magnitude as the number of successive vessel bifurcations observed in higher organisms [44].

The blood flow in the network (right panel in Fig. 1) is approximated by assuming Poiseuille flow in all vessels, i.e., that they have cylindrical symmetry and that the blood viscosity is high enough to neglect turbulence and inertial effects [44]. For the human body, this is a good approximation, except for the larger arteries and veins [44]. At every bifurcation in the vessel network we apply blood flow conservation, i.e. the sum of incoming flows to a node matches the sum of the outgoing flows. In all calculations we also disregard the alterations in blood viscosity due to the Fahreus-Lindqvist effect and the viscoelasticity of the blood (in the Text S1 we demonstrate that the inclusion of the Fahreus-Lindqvist effect does not affect in a significant way our results).

Our analysis is based on a steady state study, and therefore we do not take into account the pressure and radii variation at the larger vessels due to the heart beat. Also, given that most of the flow in the retinal vessels is laminar, solving the full Navier-Stokes equation can only change the pressure at the vessels for a small amount, leaving essentially unchanged the calculated hypoxia regions after vessel suppression.

Very high levels of Ang-2 increase the vessel permeability, and, in the limit, render them incapable of irrigating the tissue. In this work we take this limit, and consider the total loss of function of individual thin vessels in the regions affected by vessel damage. We use a simplified method to estimate the effects of vascular disruptions on tissue oxygen levels. In reality, the oxygen level declines nonlinearly with the distance along each vessel, depending on the flow rate, the oxygen consumption rate, and on the nonlinear oxygen binding characteristics of hemoglobin. For simplicity, we here use intravascular hydrostatic pressure as an index of position along each flow pathway, and assume a linear dependence of the oxygen concentration on pressure, setting the levels of oxygen at the retinal artery equal to 1 and the concentration at the veins equal to 0. Since the model used is linear in the levels of oxygen in the tissue, the profile of hypoxia observed is independent of the values of the oxygen levels at the arteries and veins, if the critical oxygen concentration for hypoxia in the tissue is altered accordingly. In fact, we expect that the observed hypoxic regions after vessel suppression will depend

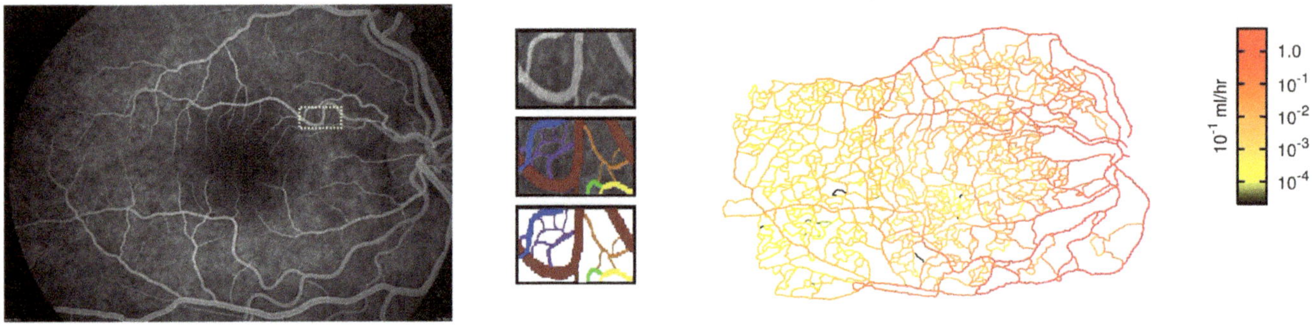

Figure 1. Characterization of the vascular network. Left panel: The original angiography of the retina that was digitalized. Identified with a small rectangle is the area that is amplified in the central panel. Center panel: Zoom of detail in angiography: original detail (top); manual identification of vessels with different colors indicating joined vessels of similar caliber (center); geometry that is digitalized to obtain the reconstructed network (bottom). Right panel: The blood flow in the reconstructed network. The color gradient indicates the flow intensity.

mainly on the diffusion of oxygen in the tissue (and in particular on the characteristic irrigation length, i.e. the maximum distance that an irrigated point in the tissue is from a vessel, function of the oxygen diffusion length, the oxygen consumption rate and the critical oxygen concentration for hypoxia), and not on the details of how the oxygen levels at the vessels are calculated (see below and Text S1).

The transport of oxygen to the tissues occurs via a diffusive process. We consider that the oxygen consumption rate in the tissue is constant and, therefore, the time-independent concentration of oxygen c_O can be obtained from the Poisson equation

$$L^2 \nabla^2 c_O = c_O, \qquad (1)$$

where L is the tissue oxygen diffusion length. In this equation, we linearize the Michaelis-Menten kinetics normally used for the consumption of oxygen by the tissue [45,46], since the regions of hypoxia that are analyzed in this work are determined by the characteristic irrigation length (see below and Text S1), i.e. by the levels of oxygen far from the immediate vicinity of the capillaries, which is where the non-linear behavior of the Michaelis-Menten is relevant.

Equation (1) is solved in a large rectangular domain that includes the totality of vessel network. We use the successive over-relaxation method setting the concentration of oxygen to zero at the borders of the domain, and having as boundary condition the concentration of oxygen at the vessels that are able to irrigate. The capillary endothelium is highly specialized to permit the exchange of oxygen between the blood and the tissue. In contrast, main arteries and veins have the function of transporting the blood to and from the capillaries [34] and have thick walls that often require their proper irrigation to be oxygenated. For this reason, we consider that only the thinner vessels (venules, arterioles and capillaries) with flow larger than zero can irrigate (in the model we assign this function to vessels with diameter smaller than 24 μm so that most of the vessels in the simulation participate actively in irrigation of the tissue). Therefore, when equation (1) is solved for every point in the tissue, the concentration of oxygen is fixed as boundary condition at the smaller vessels (with diameter smaller than 24 μm) if their flow is larger than zero.

If c_O falls below a critical value, C_m, the tissue cells will enter in hypoxia. In Fig. 2 we show the maximum value for C_m such that all the tissue region highlighted in the inset (inside the turquoise dashed rectangle) is in normoxia as a function of L (since a site is in normoxia if $c_O > C_m$, the plot corresponds to the minimum value of c_O inside the highlighted region as a function of L). In order to avoid the irregular boundary of the network, we will focus on the rectangular region highlighted in the inset of Fig. 2 in the rest of the work. The lower the value L, the faster equation (1) is solved numerically. We chose $L = 20$ lattice units (112μm) and $C_m = 0.06$ (corresponding to a point on the beginning of the rising part of the curve in Fig. 2) for faster run times and we have found that our results are independent of this particular choice for L (see also Text S1).

Results

To simulate the effect of localized vascular loss of function of the thinner vessels, we consider small circular regions of radius R in the vascular network where the vessel damage occurs. Inside these regions, we block all vessels with diameter smaller than a cutoff, Λ. These circular regions are distributed randomly within the highlighted area in the inset of Fig. 2. The area fraction covered by these blocking regions will be deemed A_{blk}. In what follows we will take $\Lambda = 4.35$ lattice units, i.e. 24 μm, the average of the

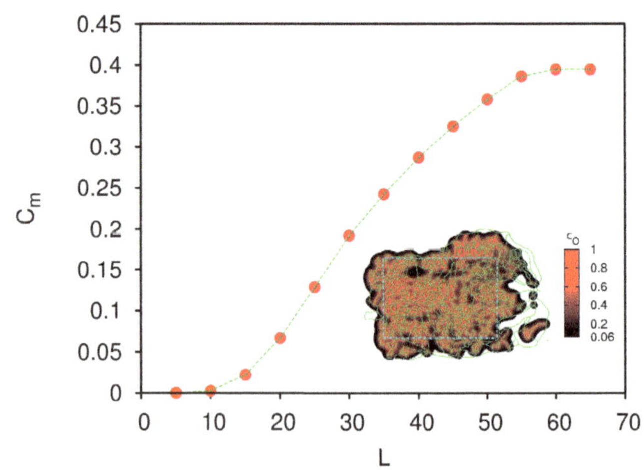

Figure 2. Plot of the C_m required for the normoxia of all tissue inside the rectangle (inset) as a function of the diffusion length of oxygen, L. Inset: In this diagram we represent the vascular network analyzed (in green), the c_O in the retina (in the gradient black-red) for $L = 20$ lattice units and $C_m = 0.06$, and the boundary of the region of the retina analyzed in this work (in turquoise).

diameters of the vessels in our network. The results will be compared to those using a larger cutoff $\Lambda = 8$ lattice units, i.e. 45 μm. Physiologically, taking larger values of Λ means considering also the suppression of thicker vessels.

Once the vessels are blocked, the blood flow will be altered (i.e. we re-calculate the flow, now in the altered vessel network), the irrigation of the retina will be lower and this may lead to new regions in hypoxia. We measure how the total area in hypoxia changes with A_{blk}, the area where the thin vessels are blocked.

Fig. 3 depicts the average area in hypoxia, A_H, for only one blocking circular area of radius R. The data in the plot are the average over 500 random realisations of the blocking sites. The picture shows the results for different values of diffusion length L and two different cutoffs Λ. Interestingly, for all these different parameters there is a single critical value of the radius ($R_c \approx 50$) below which only one blocking circle does not induce an appreciable change in the irrigation of the network. It is therefore necessary a minimal size of the blocking target to produce an area in hypoxia. We observe that this characteristic distance in the system does not depend on the value of L or Λ, but on the maximum distance that a point is from a capillary vessel in the analyzed network (see Text S1). Hence, R_c will be designated by the characteristic irrigation length.

We proceed by increasing the number of damaged circular neighborhoods, which are distributed randomly (they may overlap). We calculate the fraction of area in hypoxia, A_H, as a function of the area fraction of retina affected by the vessel disrupting proteins, A_{blk}, see Fig. 4. Each curve corresponds to vessel damaged regions built with blocking circles with the same radius R. The radii are indicated in lattice units. For equal blocked areas the hypoxia can be considerably different, depending on the radii of the blocking regions.

We observe a monotonic increase of A_H with A_{blk} for all the values of R. In general, for large blocked areas, a larger R corresponds to a smaller area in hypoxia. However, for small values of A_{blk} we found a different behavior depending if R is larger or lower than the characteristic irrigation length, $R_c \approx 50$. Above this radius (Fig. 4 left), at blocking areas below a critical area $A_c \approx 0.47$, and contrary to what happens for $A_{blk} > A_c$, a

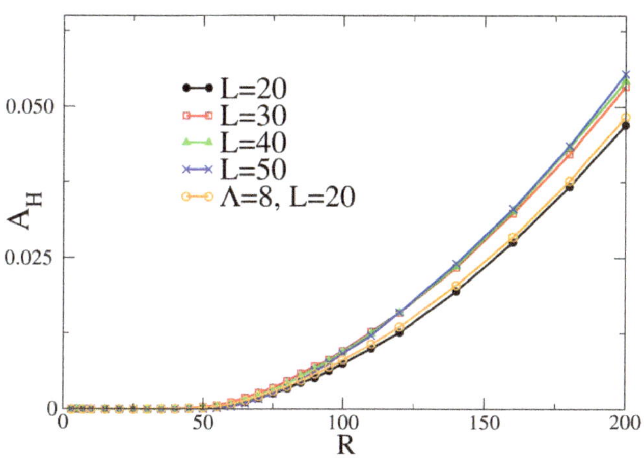

Figure 3. Resulting area in hypoxia for one blocking spot of radius R. Each curve has a different diffusion length, $L = 20$, 30, 40 and 50 (each point in the graphic represents the average of 500 runs). Also shown are the results for $L = 20$ with $\Lambda = 8$. The curves for different Λ and $L = 20$ are, essentially, undistinguishable. In all cases the radius of the circle necessary for an average hypoxia region larger than zero is $R_c \approx 50$.

larger R corresponds to a larger area in hypoxia. On the other hand, for $R < R_c$ (Fig. 4 right) the area in hypoxia is independent of the radius for very low A_{blk}, i.e. all the curves collapse into a single curve at low A_{blk} (the section of the curve where this collapse occurs depends on the value of R, with a larger overlap region for larger values of R). Besides, for $R < R_c$, the value of A_{blk} at which the transition to the large area regime occurs is lower than $A_c \approx 0.47$ and strongly dependent on the radius, in opposition to the situation where $R > R_c$. This transition for $R < R_c$ is associated with a very steep increase in A_H. The slope of this increase is larger for smaller values of R.

Discussion

Damage and Hypoxia

To understand the dependence of the A_H on A_{blk} and R, we will start by analyzing how hypoxia regions are formed after vessel blockage in this system.

The blockage induced by a single circular region with radius larger than the characteristic irrigation length produces an area in hypoxia which is smaller than the blocked region (Fig. 5a). Points inside the blocking region that are at a distance larger than the characteristic irrigation length R_c from the circumference of the region, are in hypoxia. Hence, for blocking circles with $R > R_c$, the area that is still irrigated is approximately equal to $2\pi R R_c$, i.e. it grows linearly with R and not with R^2. Therefore, for larger blocking circles, the areas inside each circle that are still irrigated are proportionally smaller. Consequently, for $R > R_c$, for a small number of these regions and for the same covered area, we observe that higher values of R will correspond to a higher hypoxic area (see Fig. 4 left).

As the number of blocked areas gets larger, A_{blk} increases until the system reaches a regime in which regions are not irrigated, in spite of not having their vessels blocked. This is the consequence of being surrounded by the circular blocking areas (Fig. 5b)). In this regime, the number of such oxygen deprived regions will be larger if R is smaller, since for smaller R the number of circular blocking areas is higher, for the same A_{blk}. With a higher number of circular regions becomes easier to surround not affected areas, blocking the required vessels to deprive those regions of irrigation. Therefore, if $A_{blk} > A_c$, smaller R will correspond to larger A_H, in opposition to what is observed for $A_{blk} < A_c$.

A completely different scenerio occurs for $R < R_c$, i.e. when we are covering the network with targets smaller than its characteristic irrigation length. In this regime the effect of covering areas loses its local nature, because a single blocking region can not create hypoxia (as seen in Fig. 3). Hypoxia can only be reached with the cooperating effect of many blocking regions. This can be clearly seen in Fig. 5c, where the few hypoxic areas are the result of the particular disposition of various neighboring blocking spots.

As the number of blocking spots increases, there will be a density at which these spots have a high probability for blocking vessels separated by R_c. Above this density, that corresponds to a critical area A^*_{blk}, hypoxia will occur everywhere in the tissue. An example of such a situation is in Fig. 5d. We expect a sharp transition between $A_H \approx 0$ and almost total hypoxia at this particular density of blocking sites. For A^*_{blk} the area in hypoxia will be dramatically larger than A_{blk}. This effect can be clearly seen in the steep slope of the curves in right panel of Fig. 4.

It is possible to obtain the dependence of the critical area A^*_{blk} on R for very small R, disregarding overlap between the circles. Consider a blocking region of radius R much smaller than R_c. To have hypoxia, circles have to block vessels that are located at least at a distance $2R_c$. One of these circles blocks a given vessel, if its

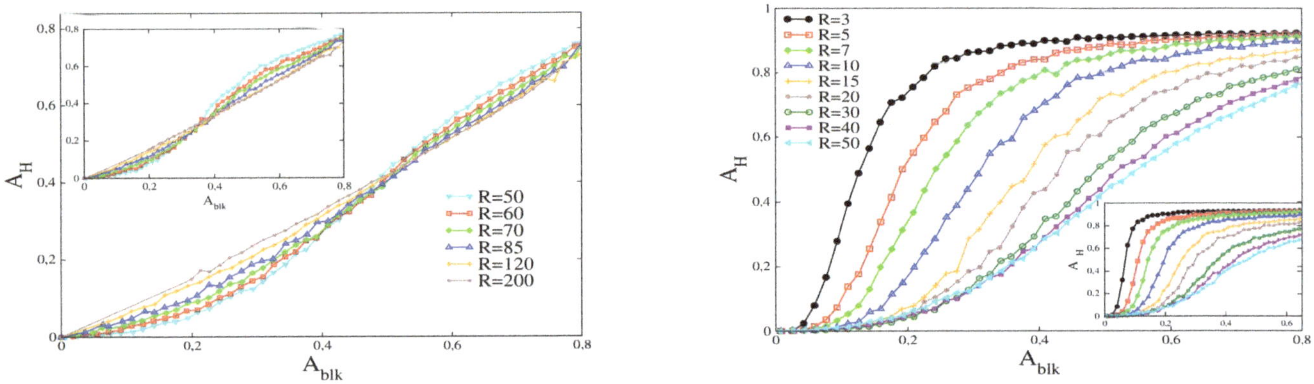

Figure 4. Fraction of area in hypoxia (A_H) versus fraction of area vessel disruption in the retina (A_{blk}). Left panel: Plots for $\Lambda = 4.35$ and radii of each blocking circular neighborhood larger than 50 lattice units. The inset corresponds to $\Lambda = 8$, i.e. when vessels with diameter smaller than 8 lattice units are compromised. Right panel: Same as in the left panel, but for radii smaller than 50.

center is closer to the vessel than a distance R. The associated probability for cutting the vessel is then of the order $p \sim \frac{R}{R_c}$. On the other hand, in 2D the number of blocking regions in a square of side $2R_c$ will be $4\rho R_c^2$, where ρ is the number of blocking circles per unit area. In order to have hypoxia everywhere, the critical A^*_{blk} should be such that is able to block the vessels, i.e. the probability of blocking a vessel is on the order of unity. Hence, the minimum density of points required, ρ^* obeys

$$4\rho^* R_c^2 \frac{R}{R_c} = 4\rho^* R_c R \sim 1 \ .$$

We approximate $\rho^* \approx \frac{A^*_{blk}}{\pi R^2}$, obtaining finally that $A^*_{blk} \sim \frac{\pi R}{4R_c} \sim R$, i.e. the blocking area at the steepest slope in the right panel of Fig. 4 has a linear dependence with R.

For $R > R_c$ to have a large hypoxic region, the distance between the blocked centers should be on the order of the blocking circles radius, i.e. $\sqrt{1/\rho^*} \sim 2R$. Then, $\frac{\pi R^2}{A^*_{blk}} \sim 4R^2$ and for $R > R_c$, $A^*_{blk} \equiv A_c \sim O(1)$ is independent of R.

In Fig. 6 we show the log-log graph of the inflexion points for the curves plotted in Fig. 4. The inflexion points are obtained through a fit of the curves to an hyperbolic tangent function superimposed on a linear function. The error bars correspond to the statistical error of the non-linear fit. We associate the inflexion points to the transition values for A^*_{blk}. We can see that the dependence of A^*_{blk} is linear for R much smaller than R_c, becoming independent of R for $R > R_c$, in good agreement with the predictions discussed above.

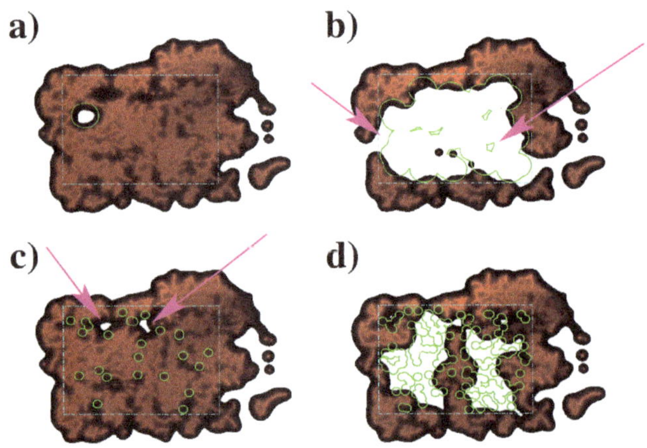

Figure 5. Irrigation, i.e. the density plot of c_O, in different scenarios. a) one blocking circle with $R = 80$, b) 50 blocking circles with $R = 80$ (arrows signal sites with no irrigation or vessel damage), c) 24 blocking circles with $R = 25$ (arrows signal areas in hypoxia resultant from the combined action of several blocking sites) and d) 153 blocking circles with $R = 25$. For each plot, the blocked regions are in green, the local irrigation are represented by the color gradient, from black (lower) to red (higher) and the areas in white inside rectangle of interest have $c_O < C_m$, and are in hypoxia.

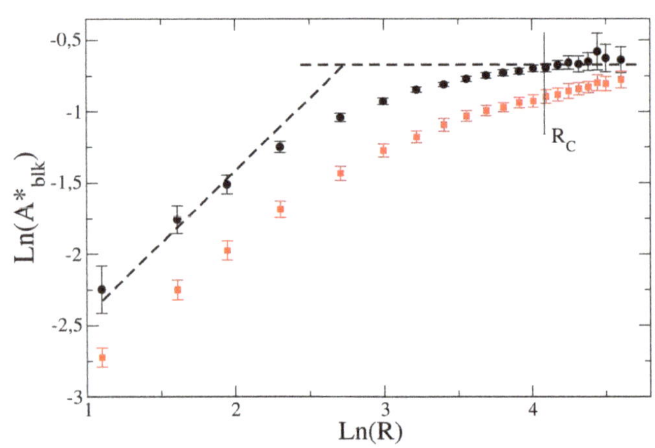

Figure 6. In black circles, the logarithm of inflexion points, from curves showed in Fig. 4, versus the logarithm of R. We compare to two straight dashed lines with slope 1 and 0. We observe that the transition points follow $A^*_{blk} \sim R$ for R much smaller than R_c and $A^*_{blk} \sim O(1)$ for $R > R_c$. In red squares the same for $\Lambda = 8$ lattice units.

For $R > R_c$ the size of the blocking circles are larger than any characteristic scale in the underlining network, and the irrigation of the tissue will be blocked only when the blocking circles percolate the system. We also verify the non-dependence of A^*_{blk} on R which is characteristic of the circular blocking neighborhoods percolation (see Text S1). Therefore in this regime the transition does not depend on the underlining network.

Consequences for DR progression

We observed that the complex effects of covering areas with targets smaller than the lattice parameter produces hypoxic regions that can grow easily larger than the affected area for $R < R_c$. This regime can have important consequences in the progression of the disease.

It is a known fact that DR can be divided in two main stages with different phenotypes. The earliest stage of DR is nonproliferative diabetic retinopathy (NPDR). Though this stage can be itself divided in different sub-stages [1,2], it is characterized by the presence of micro-aneurisms (swellings in capillaries and arterioles), a variable degree of vessel blockage and the consequent deprivation of irrigation in some regions of the retina. The most advanced stage of DR, the proliferative diabetic retinopathy, PDR, is characterized by neovascularization, the growth of abnormal (fragile and leaky) new blood vessels, which may lead to blindness through hemorrhage and scarring [47]. This pathological retinal angiogenesis generates randomly orientated and physiologically deficient vessels that do not conform to neuronal histology [14].

The creation of this abnormal and dense structures is rooted in the following paradox (often referred in the literature as the diabetic paradox [48,49]): if the prevalent action in DR is the regression, disruption and blockage of blood vessels, then how does the hallmark of the most advanced stage of the disease is a very high vascular density? Does the fact that the vascular disruption sites in DR are extremely small and localized [50,51] play an important role in the progression of the disease?

According to our study, the blockage of vessels, akin to what happens in DR, leads to a deficient irrigation of the tissue, and to an increase of hypoxia in the retina. However, a tissue in hypoxia leads to an increase in the production of the HIF-1 (Hypoxia Inducible Factor) transcription factor, which has angiogenic factors, such as VEGF, as targets. The consequence is the triggering of neovascularization in the tissue [52–54]. We expect that when this neovascularization occurs repeatedly in regions where vessel regression and blockage occurred, the increase in VEGF levels will occur locally, balancing the effects of the antiangiogenic factors that led to the vessel disruption. The result will be a vasculature with the same physiological density and caliber but with possible local malformations [55]. In these situations we expect to find a NPDR phenotype.

However, when the disruptions of the vasculature lead to hypoxia in regions with little or no vessel regression, the neovascularization resultant from the high VEGF levels in these regions will not counterbalance the original disruption. Therefore, the process of angiogenesis would lead to a denser vasculature. In these situations we expect to find a PDR phenotype.

As we mentioned, in the right panel of Fig. 4 we observe a regime where the area in hypoxia is larger than the affected area. In this regime, associated with low values of R and large A_{blk}, we clearly have areas that will be producing very high levels of VEGF, since they are in hypoxia, and still have functional vessels. This setting suggests a high vessel density as consequence, and we can associate this effect with a PDR phenotype.

Therefore, we predict that the PDR phenotype occurs when $R < R_c$ as the density of affected points increases, i.e. as the disease progresses. This will happen in sections where a fraction of the retina larger than A^*_{blk} is affected. Besides, the existence of very small and localized sites of vascular disruption in DR in vivo is in agreement with the hypothesis of $R < R_c$ being required for PDR to develop [50,51].

However, we found that there is a possibility to decrease A^*_{blk} and to obtain the PDR regime at lower affected areas. In the insets of Fig. 4 we show A_H as a function of A_{blk}, but now we change the cutoff of the system to $\Lambda = 8$ lattice units. In this case in each blocking region all vessels with radius smaller than 8 units will be compromised, i.e. thicker vessels may also be affected. In spite that, in this case the minimum radius R_c of a blocking circles that can induce hypoxia is still the same as it is shown in Fig. 3. Accordingly, we still observe in the inset of Fig. 4 left and in Fig. 6 the approximately constant value for A^*_{blk} for $R > R_c$. Of course that, as R grows, the value of A^*_{blk} should reach $A_c \approx 0.47$, the value associated with the percolation of the blocking circles in this system. However for $R > R_c$ the increase of A_{blk} is extremely slow (Fig. 6).

For all values of R we observe that the values of A^*_{blk} are much lower when the thick vessels are also affected. Even for the largest R in the left panel of Fig. 4 the value $A^*_{blk} \approx 0.4$ is lower than the case where only the capillaries are affected. This is consequence of the specific structure of the retina network. The largest vessels are few in number but have the important role of distributing the blood through all the network. Cutting these vessels lead to a larger loss in irrigation than cutting only the small capillaries. The consequence is a lower value for the critical A_{blk}.

In what concerns the progression of DR, we anticipate that the PDR phenotype can dominate in two scenarios: either the affected area increases, or the type of vessels affected is altered and larger vessels are also compromised. In both situations the phenotype is most severe when the radius of each focus of damage is smaller, for the same affected area.

Conclusion

We analyzed the effect of vessel damage in the retina irrigation, consequent of the high levels of vessel destabilizing proteins, such as Ang-2, in a diabetic environment. In this study we modelled blood flow and the oxygen concentration in the tissue. Although more exhaustive methods exist to describe oxygen pressure dynamics [45,56–59] and the flow in vascular networks [60], the present model captures the main ingredients of the processes involved. However, when more subtle vessel disruption events are considered, (e.g. increases in the permeability of the capillaries that do not compromise the vessel viability, partial blockage of vessels), a more complete description of oxygen transport needs to be implemented, including how the oxygen levels decline nonlinearly with distance along each vessel as a function of the flow rate, and how it is consumed in the tissue according to a Michaelis-Menten kinetics [45,58,59]. The study of oxygen levels in these situations complement the work presented, and will be the subject of a future study.

Having access to the basic topology of the vascular network of a human retina, we found two regimes delimited by a critical size of blocking spots radius. This critical radius corresponds to the characteristic irrigation length in the network. Furthermore, these results suggest that the prevalent phenotype of the pathology can be a direct consequence of the distribution of disrupted and hypoxic regions in the tissue. We associate the situation where the hypoxia occurs prevalently in the region of vessel disruption with the non-proliferative diabetic retinopathy phenotype. On the other hand, if the extensive regions of hypoxia occur outside the region of vessel disruption we expect a proliferative diabetic retinopathy phenotype.

Our results suggest that disrupting the vessels in the retina with targets of radius lower than the characteristic irrigation length in the tissue (typical in DR [50,51]), may lead to large hypoxia levels with relatively low values of vessel destabilizing areas. These areas will be even lower if the vessel destabilizing environment is able to rupture thicker vessels. These results convey a new way of thinking about the diabetic paradox [48,49]: allowing the possibility that localized vessel disruption points lead to the formation of large regions in hypoxia, which have the ability to drive neovascularization [52,53], excessive angiogenesis is able to occur in pathologies that are driven by regression and blockage of blood vessels.

These conclusions on the mechanisms for the early development of the two phenotypes of DR may be of high importance in the definition of prevention strategies for the development of DR is risk patients.

Supporting Information

Text S1 In this text we discuss several details of our model. We focus on the relation between the characteristic irrigation length and the geometry of the network, on the relevance of modeling the Fahreus-Lindqvist effect, and on the relation between the percolation transition and the transition from the non proliferative phenotype to the proliferative phenotype.

Acknowledgments

The authors thank fruitful discussions with João Carvalho, Jaime Silva, Rui Bernardes, Conceição Lobo, Rosa Fernandes and the Henrique Girão's group. The authors would also like to thank the editor and the anonymous referees for their comments and helpful discussions which contributed to improve the final version of the text.

Author Contributions

Conceived and designed the experiments: TS OO RDMT. Performed the experiments: YG TS RDMT. Analyzed the data: YG TS RDMT. Contributed reagents/materials/analysis tools: TS RDMT. Wrote the paper: YG OO RDMT.

References

1. Yun WL, Acharya R, Venkatesh YV, Chee C, Min L C, et al. (2008) Identification of different stages of diabetic retinopathy. Information Sciences 178: 106–121.
2. Bearse MA Jr, Adams AJ, Han Y, Schneck ME, Ng J, et al. (2006) A Multifocal Electroretinogram Model Predicting the Development of Diabetic Retinopathy. Prog Retin Eye Res 25: 425–448.
3. World Health Organization. Media Centre. Available: http://www.who.int/mediacentre/factsheets/fs236/en/. Accessed: 2014 October 28.
4. Barber AJ, Antonetti DA (2003) Mapping the blood vessels with paracellular permeability in the retinas of diabetic rats. Invest Ophthal & Vis Sci, 44: 5410–5416.
5. Bento CF, Fernandes R, Matafome P, Sena C, Seiça R, et al. (2010) Methylglyoxal-induced imbalance in the ratio VEGF/Ang-2 secreted by retinal pigment epithelial cells leads to endothelial dysfunction. Exp Physiol 95: 955–970.
6. Hammes HP, Lin J, Wagner P, Feng Y, Vom Hagen F, et al. (2004) Angiopoietin-2 causes pericyte dropout in the normal retina: evidence for involvement in diabetic retinopathy. Diabetes 53: 1104–1110.
7. Maisonpierre PC, Suri C, Jones PF, Bartunkova S, Wiegand SJ, et al. (1997) Angiopoietin-2, a natural antagonist for Tie2 that disrupts in-vivo angiogenesis. Science 277: 55–60.
8. Smith LE, Wesolowski E, McLellan A, Kostyk SK, D'amato R, et al. (1994) Oxygen-induced retinopathy in the mouse. Investigative Ophthalmology & Visual Science 35: 101–111.
9. Connor KM, Krah NM, Dennison RJ, Aderman CM, Chen J, et al. (2009) Quantification of oxygen-induced retinopathy in the mouse: a model of vessel loss, vessel regrowth and pathological angiogenesis. Nature Protocols 4:1565–1573.
10. Davis S, Gale NW, Rudge JS, Wiegand SJ, Holash J (2000) Vascular-specific growth factors and blood vessel formation. Nature 407: 242–248.
11. Acharya UR, Ng EYK, Tan JH, Sree SV, Ng KH (2012) An Integrated Index for the Identification of Diabetic Retinopathy Stages Using Texture Parameters. J Med Syst 36: 2011–2020.
12. Reiter C, Sandirasegarane L, Wu XH, Nakamura M, Barber AJ, et al. (2005) The retinal insulin receptor, signaling pathway is impaired by diabetes: A potential mechanism contributing to diabetic retinopathy. Diabetes 54: A222.
13. Jun JI, Lau LF (2011) Taking aim at the extracellular matrix: CCN proteins as emerging therapeutic targets. Nature Reviews Drug Discovery 10: 945–963.
14. Gariano RF, Gardner TW (2005) Retinal angiogenesis in development and disease. Nature 438: 960–6.
15. Newman M, Barabási A-L, Watts D (2006) Structure and Dynamics of Networks. Princeton, NJ: Princeton University Press.
16. Barrat A, Barthèlemy M, Vespignani A (2008) Dynamical Processes on Complex Networks. Cambridge: Cambridge University Press.
17. Paul G, Sreenivasan S, Stanley HE (2005) Resilience of complex networks to random breakdown, Phys Rev E 72: 056130.
18. Albert R, Jeong H, Barabási AL (2000) Error and attack tolerance of Complex Networks. Nature 406: 378–382.
19. Callaway DS, Newman MEJ, Strogatz SH, Watts DJ (2000) Network robustness and fragility: Percolation on random graphs. Phys Rev Lett 85: 5468–5471.
20. Cohen R, Erez K, Ben-Avraham D, Havlin S (2000) Resilience of the Internet to random breakdowns. Phys Rev Lett 85: 4626–4628.
21. Cohen R, Erez K, Ben-Avraham D, Havlin S (2001) Breakdown of the Internet under Intentional Attack. Phys Rev Lett 86: 3682–3685.
22. Dall'Asta L, Barrat A, Barthelemy M, Vespignani A (2006) Vulnerability of weighted networks. J Stat Mech P04006.
23. Paul G, Tanizawa T, Havlin S, Stanley HE (2004) Optimization of robustness of complex networks. The European Physical Journal B-Condensed Matter and Complex Systems 38: 187–191.
24. Pastor-Satorras R, Vespignani A (2002) Immunization of complex networks. Phys Rev E 65: 036104.
25. Vespignani A (2010) Complex networks: The fragility of interdependency. Nature 464: 984–985.
26. Buldyrev SV, Parshani R, Paul G, Stanley HE, Havlin S (2010) Catastrophic cascade of failures in interdependent networks. Nature 464: 1025–1028.
27. Gastner MT, Newman MEJ (2006) The spatial structure of networks. Eur. Phys. J. B 49:247–252.
28. Barthélemy M (2011) Spatial networks. Physics Reports 499: 1–101.
29. Secomb TW, Alberding JP, Hsu R, Dewhirst MW, Pries AR (2013) Angiogenesis: An Adaptive Dynamic Biological Patterning Problem. PLoS Computational Biology 9: e1002983.
30. Blinder P, Shih AY, Rafie C, Kleinfeld D (2010) Topological basis for the robust distribution of blood to rodent neocortex. Proc Natl Acad Sci USA 107: 12670–12675.
31. Guibert R, Fonta C, Plouraboué F (2010) A New Approach to Model Confined Suspensions Flows in Complex Networks: Application to Blood Flow. Transp Porous Med 83: 171–194.
32. Masters BR (2004) Fractal analysis of the vascular tree in the human retina. Annual Review of Biomedical Engineering 6: 427–552.
33. Avakian A, Kalina RE, Sage H, Rambhia AH, Elliott KE, et al. (2002) Fractal analysis of region-based vascular change in the normal and non-proliferative diabetic retina. Current Eye Research 24: 274–280.
34. Flores J, Corvera Poiré E, del Río JA, López de Haro M (2010) A plausible explanation for heart rates in mammals. J Theor Biol 265: 599–603.
35. Murray CD (1926) The Physiological Principle of Minimum Work: I. The Vascular System and the Cost of Blood Volume. Proc Natl Acad Sci USA 12: 207–214.
36. West GB (1999) The Origin of Universal Scaling Laws in Biology. Physica A 263: 104–113.
37. Herman AB, Savage VM, West GB (2011) A Quantitative Theory of Solid Tumor Growth, Metabolic Rate and Vascularization. Plos One 6: e22973.
38. Daxer A (1993) Characterisation of the neovascularisation process in diabetic refinopathy by means of fractal geometry: diagnostic implications. Graefe's Arch Clin Exp Ophthalmol 231: 681–686.
39. Blinder P, Tsai PS, Kaufhold JP, Knutsen PM, Suhl H, et al. (2013) The cortical angiome: an interconnected vascular network with noncolumnar patterns of blood flow. Nature Neuroscience 16: 889–897.
40. Owen MR, Alarcón T, Maini PK, Byrne HM (2009) Angiogenesis and vascular remodelling in normal and cancerous tissues. J Math Biol 58: 689–721.
41. Travasso RDM, Corvera Poiré E, Castro M, Rodríguez-Manzaneque JC, Hernández-Machado A (2011) Tumor angiogenesis and vascular patterning: a mathematical model. PLoS One 6: e19989.

42. Shih AY, Blinder P, Tsai PS, Friedman B, Stanley G, et al. (2012) The smallest stroke: occlusion of one penetrating vessel leads to infarction and a cognitive deficit. Nature Neuroscience 16: 55–63.
43. Milde F, Lauw S, Koumoutsakos P, Iruela-Arispe ML (2013) The mouse retina in 3D: quantification of vascular growth and remodeling. Integrative Biology 5: 1426–1438.
44. Flores J, Romero AM, Travasso RDM, Corvera Poiré EC (2013) Flow and anastomosis in vascular networks, J Theor Biol 317: 257–270.
45. Secomb TW, Hsu R, Park EY, Dewhirst MW (2004) Green's function methods for analysis of oxygen delivery to tissue by microvascular networks. Annals of Biomedical Engineering 32: 1519–1529.
46. Secomb TW, Alberding JP, Hsu R, Dewhirst MW, Pries AR (2013) Angiogenesis: An Adaptive Dynamic Biological Patterning Problem. PLoS Computational Biology 9: e1002983.
47. Sivakumar R, Ravindran G, Muthayya M, Lakshminarayanan S, Velmurughendran CU (2005) Diabetic Retinopathy Analysis. Journal of Biomedicine and Biotechnology 2005: 20–27.
48. Fadini GP, Sartore S, Baesso I, Lenzi M, Agostini C, et al. (2006) Endothelial progenitor cells and the diabetic paradox. Diabetes Care 29: 714–716.
49. Costa C (2011) Vasculogenesis in Diabetes-Associated Diseases: Unraveling the Diabetic Paradox. In: Simionescu DT, Simionescu A, editors. Vasculogenesis and Angiogenesis - from Embryonic Development to Regenerative Medicine. Rijeka: InTech open. pp 107–130.
50. Vinores SA, McGehee R, Lee A, Gadegbeku C, Campochiaro PA (1990) Ultrastructural localization of blood-retinal barrier breakdown in diabetic and galactosemic rats. Journal of Histochemistry & Cytochemistry 38: 1341–1352.
51. Vinores SA, Gadegbeku C, Campochiaro PA, Green WR (1989) Immunohistochemical localization of blood-retinal barrier breakdown in human diabetics. The American Journal of Pathology 134: 231–235.
52. Shweiki D, Itin A, Soffer D, Keshet E (1992) Vascular endothelial growth factor induced by hypoxia may mediate hypoxia-initiated angiogenesis. Nature 359: 843–845.
53. Pugh CW, Ratcliffe PJ (2003) Regulation of angiogenesis by hypoxia: role of the HIF system. Nature Medicine 9: 677–684.
54. Treins C, Giorgetti-Peraldi S, Murdaca J, Monthouël-Kartmann MN, Van Obberghen E (2005) Regulation of hypoxia-inducible factor (HIF)-1 activity and expression of HIF hydroxylases in response to insulin-like growth factor I. Molecular Endocrinology19: 1304–1317.
55. Jain RK (2005) Normalization of tumor vasculature: an emerging concept in antiangiogenic therapy. Science 307: 58–62.
56. Hellums JD, Nair PK, Huang NS, Ohshima N (1996) Simulation of intraluminal gas transport processes in the microcirculation. Ann Biomed Eng 24: 1–24.
57. Pittman RN (2011) Regulation of tissue oxygenation. Marston Gate: Morgan & Claypool Life Sciences.
58. Goldman D (2008) Theoretical models of microvascular oxygen transport to tissue. Microcirculation 15: 795–811.
59. Popel AS (1989) Theory of oxygen transport to tissue. Crit Rev Biomed Eng 17: 257–321.
60. Formaggia L, Lamponi D, Tuveri M, Veneziani A (2006) Numerical modeling of 1D arterial networks coupled with a lumped parameters description of the heart. Computer Methods in Biomechanics and Biomedical Engineering 9: 273–288.

A Polymeric Prodrug of 5-Fluorouracil-1-Acetic Acid Using a Multi-Hydroxyl Polyethylene Glycol Derivative as the Drug Carrier

Man Li[◔], Zhen Liang[◔], Xun Sun, Tao Gong*, Zhirong Zhang*

Key Laboratory of Drug Targeting and Drug Delivery Systems, Ministry of Education, West China School of Pharmacy, Sichuan University, Chengdu, Sichuan, PR China

Abstract

Purpose: Macromolecular prodrugs obtained by covalently conjugating small molecular drugs with polymeric carriers were proven to accomplish controlled and sustained release of the therapeutic agents *In vitro* and *in vivo*. Polyethylene glycol (PEG) has been extensively used due to its low toxicity, low immunogenicity and high biocompatibility. However, for linear PEG macromolecules, the number of available hydroxyl groups for drug coupling does not change with the length of polymeric chain, which limits the application of PEG for drug conjugation purposes. To increase the drug loading and prolong the retention time of 5-fluorouracil (5-Fu), a macromolecular prodrug of 5-Fu, 5-fluorouracil-1 acid-PAE derivative (5-FA-PAE) was synthesized and tested for the antitumor activity *in vivo*.

Methods: PEG with a molecular weight of 38 kDa was selected to synthesize the *multi-hydroxyl polyethylene glycol* derivative (PAE) through an addition reaction. 5-fluorouracil-1 acetic acid (5-FA), a 5-Fu derivative was coupled with PEG derivatives via ester bond to form a macromolecular prodrug, 5-FA-PAE. The *in vitro* drug release, pharmacokinetics, *in vivo* distribution and antitumor effect of the prodrug were investigated, respectively.

Results: The PEG-based prodrug obtained in this study possessed an exceedingly high 5-FA loading efficiency of 10.58%, much higher than the maximum drug loading efficiency of unmodified PEG with the same molecular weight, which was 0.98% theoretically. Furthermore, 5-FA-PAE exhibited suitable sustained release in tumors.

Conclusion: This study provides a new approach for the development of the delivery to tumors of anticancer agents with PEG derivatives.

Editor: Ronald Hancock, Laval University Cancer Research Centre, Canada

Funding: The authors acknowledge the financial support from the National Natural Science Foundation of China (no. 30873167) and the National Basic Research Program of China (973 program, No: 2013CB932504). The funders had no role in study design, data collection and analysis, decision to publish, or preparation of the manuscript.

Competing Interests: The authors have declared that no competing interests exist.

* Email: gongtaoy@126.com (TG); zrzzl@vip.sina.com (ZZ)

◔ These authors contributed equally to this work.

Introduction

Cancer is one of the most life-threatening diseases worldwide, which seriously endangers human health and survival [1,2]. Surgery, radiotherapy, chemical medication, biological immunization therapies are the major treatment strategies, among which chemotherapy plays an important role in the treatment of cancer [3–9]. Regarding chemotherapies, 5-fluorouracil (5-Fu) is one of the most widely used antimetabolites in clinic [10], which shows significant inhibitory effect against a broad spectrum of solid tumors [11–13]. Traditional chemotherapies such as 5-Fu are cytotoxic agents that inhibit rapidly proliferating cancer cells. Due to its low specificity, side effects such as myelosuppression, mucositis, dermatitis and diarrhea are commonly observed during the clinical application of 5-Fu [14–16]. Additionally, 5-Fu has a very short half life of about 20 minutes and is rapidly eliminated after administration. The irregular oral absorption and the low bioavailability often results in poor clinical therapeutic outcome [17–19].

To address the aforementioned problems, researchers have tried various methods to improve the efficacy and to reduce the toxicity of 5-Fu, including modification of the chemical structure, formulation strategies and novel delivery systems. Several small molecular prodrugs of 5-Fu were developed, such as 5-fluoro-2′-deoxyuridine, 1-(2-tetrahydrofuryl)-5-fluorouracil and 3, 5-dioctanoyl 5-fluoro-2-deoxyuridine [20–22]. Various delivery systems have been developed for the targeted delivery of 5-Fu [23]. Menei *et al* developed biodegradable microspheres to obtain sustained delivery of 5-Fu for the treatment of glioblastoma [24]. Liposomes have been used as a sustained delivery system for 5-Fu [25]. In recent years, macromolecular carrier/delivery systems have been studied extensively. Macromolecular prodrugs obtained by combining small molecular drugs with polymeric carriers could slowly release the therapeutic agents *in vivo* with an improved half-life [26–31]. Moreover, the enhanced permeability and retention (EPR) effect may contribute to the accumulation of macromolecular prodrugs within the solid tumor, which would lead to a tumor-targeted drug delivery and reduced toxicity to normal tissues [32–34]. Moreover, the EPR effect has been regarded as the "golden rule" in the design of antitumor drugs. Based on the EPR effect, numerous tumor-targeted drug delivery systems were developed using macromolecules such as albumin (65 kDa), transferrin (90 kDa), IgG (immunoglobulin, 150 kDa), α2-macroglobulin (240 kDa) and ovomucoid of chicken eggwhite (29 kDa, highly glycosylated protein), and some have entered clinical trials [35].

In addition to the aforementioned macromolecular materials, polyethylene glycol (PEG) has become a material of great interests due to its low toxicity, low immunogenicity and high biocompatibility [36–38]. The molecular weight of PEG used in forming macromolecular prodrugs would impact the *in vivo* behaviors of the conjugates because the retention time of the prodrugs increased with the molecular weight of the carriers [30]. Prolonged retention of the prodrug is critical to the tumor accumulation of the therapeutic agents loaded. However, for linear PEG macromolecules, the number of available hydroxyl groups for drug coupling does not change with the length of the polymeric chain, which limits the application of PEG for drug conjugation purposes. Therefore,the development of new PEG derivatives to improve its drug loading efficiency has become a hot topic in material science and is of great significance to the tumor-targeted delivery of small molecular agents and 4-arm PEG derivatives were thus developed [39], and the 4-arm PEG based prodrugs have entered clinical trials with promising results [40–44]. For small molecular drugs such as 5-Fu, treatment requires a high therapeutic concentration, while the macromolecular based prodrugs have a relatively low drug loading efficiency. Thus, the modification of linear PEG creates derivatives with high drug loading efficiency which will have great significance for anticancer drug development [45].

In this study, a macromolecular prodrug, 5-fluorouracil-1 acid-PAE derivative (5-FA-PAE), was designed and synthesized to increase the drug loading efficiency, achieve delivery to the tumor and prolong the retention time. PEG with a molecular weight of 38 kDa was selected as the starting material to obtain the multi-hydroxyl PEG derivative, which was then coupled with 5-fluorouracil-1 acetic acid (5-FA), to afford the prodrug. The *in vitro* drug release, pharmacokinetics, *in vivo* distribution and antitumor effect of the prodrug were investigated, respectively.

Materials and Methods

Materials

Polyethylene glycol (PEG, average molecular weight ~38 kDa), allyl glycidyl ether (AGE), mercaptoethanol, 1-(3-dimethylaminopropyl)-3-ethylcarbodiimide hydrochloride (EDC·HCl) and N-hydroxysuccinimide (NHS) were purchased from Sigma-Aldrich (USA). Sodium hydride (NaH) was supplied by Damao Chemical Reagent Factory (Tianjin, China). 5-Fluorouracil (USP29) was purchased from Nantong Jinghua Pharmaceuticals Co., Ltd (Jiangsu, China). All other chemicals used were of reagent grade.

Synthesis of multi-hydroxyl polyethylene glycol derivative (polyethylene glycol-allyl glycidyl ether-mercaptoethanol, PAE)

Polyethylene glycol-allyl glycidyl ether (PA) was synthesized as described before [46,47] with some modifications. Briefly, 10.0 g of PEG was melted in an oil bath at 120°C with stirring under vacuum for about 3 h to remove the adsorbed moisture before adding 120 mg of NaH. The mixture was stirred for 4 h at 120°C, and 2.0 ml of AGE was added. The product was recrystallized with isopropanol to remove the micromolecular materials.

Synthesis of 5-FA-PAE prodrug

5-FA was synthesized as previously described [48,49] with some modification. Briefly, 6.5 g of 5-Fu was dissolved in 25 ml of aqueous solution of potassium hydroxide (4 M), then 15 ml of aqueous solution of chloroacetic acid (5 M) was added dropwise with stirring. The pH value of the reaction mixture was monitored and kept at 10 by adding an aqueous solution of potassium hydroxide (10 M) during the addition of chloroacetic acid and throughout the whole course of the reaction. The mixture was heated to 50°C in an oil bath with stirring for 8 h, and then acidified by HCl to obtain 5-FA.

A solution of 5-FA (0.496 g) in 1 ml of dimethylformamide was added dropwise to a solution of 0.5 g of PAE in 20 ml of dimethylformamide, then 0.196 g (1.7 mmol) of NHS and 0.4 g (2.09 mmol) of EDC·HCl were added sequentially. After a further 16 h of incubation at room temperature away from light, the mixture was precipitated with 150 ml of isopropanol. The obtained residue was recrystallized by isopropanol several times until the reagents and uncoupled 5-FA were totally removed (monitored by TLC and HPLC), then dried in vacuum at 40°C overnight.

HPLC analysis

HPLC assay was established for the determination of 5-FA in PBS, plasma or tissues homogenates, which was performed using Shimadzu instruments (Chiyoda-Ku, Japan) consisting of a CTO-10A column thermostat, two LC-10AT pumps and a SPD-10A UV detector. A Scienhome ODS column (5 μm, 150×4.6 mm, Tianjin, China) was used to separate samples. Phosphate buffer (0.05 M, pH 2.5) was used as the mobile phase at a flow rate of 1 ml/min. The temperature of the column was kept at 35°C and the effluent was detected at 270 nm. Studies showed that the precision, accuracy, and recovery of this HPLC method all met the measurement requirements.

Safety evaluation

All animal experiments were approved by the Institutional Animal Care and Ethic Committee of Sichuan University (Approved No. SYXK2013-185). All animals were fed on a light and dark cycle and allowed free access to standard chow and water. Temperature and relative humidity were kept at 25°C and 50%, respectively. After experiment, mice were sacrificed by neck dislocation, and all efforts were made to minimize suffering. Myelosuppression is one of the major side effects of 5-Fu [14]. To assess the suppression level, 60 male Kunming mice (20–25 g, purchased from Laboratory Animal Center of Sichuan University) were randomly divided into 5 groups (n = 12) and were intravenously administered with 5-Fu (27.66 mg/kg), 5-FA (40 mg/kg), PAE (338 mg/kg) or 5-FA-PAE (378 mg/kg) (equivalent to 0.213 mmol/kg 5-FA). The control group was given physiological saline (0.009 g/ml). Zero point one mL blood samples were collected at prearranged time intervals (one day before injection and 1, 4, 7, and 10 days post injection). The white blood cells (WBC) and the blood platelets number were counted by MEK-6318K Automated Hematology Analyzer (Nihonkohden, Shinjuku-ku, Japan) as an index of myelosuppression.

In vitro drug release

The *in vitro* drug release of 5-FA-PAE was investigated in physiological saline (0.009 g/ml), PBS with various pH values, 50% mouse plasma (diluted with PBS, pH 7.4, v/v) and 50% mouse tumor homogenate which was obtained from the H22 tumor loaded mice (homogenized and diluted with physiological saline). An aqueous solution of 5-FA-PAE (100 μl) was added to 4 ml of preheated release medium (physiological saline or PBS with pH = 3.04, 4.51, 6.02, 7.41, 8.99). The mixture was maintained in a water bath at 37°C under continuously stirring, and 100 μl of each sample was collected at fixed time intervals (i.e. 0.25, 1, 3, 6, 10, 24, 48, 72, 96 h). The samples from physiological saline and PBS was acidified by 100 μl hydrochloric acid (1 M), diluted with 300 μl mobile phase and analyzed by HPLC. The samples from mouse plasma and tumor homogenate were obtained in duplicate at each time point (100 μl each). For hydrolysis, samples were mixed with 50 μl of aqueous solution of 5-bromouracil (96 μg/ml, 50 μl) as the internal standard, and then supplemented with 100 μl sodium hydroxide (1 M) and acidified by 100 μl hydrochloric acid (1 M), and extracted by 3.3 ml of ethyl ester for 15 min. After centrifugation at 10,000 rpm for 5 min, 2.7 ml of the ethyl ester portion was collected, concentrated in a nitrogen gas flow, redissolved in 100 μl of the mobile phase and centrifuged at 10,000 rpm for 10 min before HPLC analysis. The other group was not subjected to hydrolysis by substituting sodium hydroxide solution with saline and acidifying with 50 μl hydrochloric acid. The differences of 5-FA in the two groups at the same time point was the unreleased 5-FA in each sample. The decrement method was used to calculate the release rate. All experiments were conducted in triplicate.

Pharmacokinetics study

Male Wistar rats were purchased from The laboratory Animal Center of Sichuan University. 12 Wistar rats (body weight: 200 g±20 g) were divided into two groups randomly (n = 6). The control group and the test group were administered intravenously with 20 mg/kg of 5-FA and 189 mg/kg 5-FA-PAE (equivalent to 20 mg/kg of 5-FA) dissolved in physiological saline, respectively. The blood samples were collected into heparinized centrifuge tubes at predetermined intervals (see Table S2 in file SI) by retro-orbital puncture, and the plasma was separated by centrifugation. Each plasma sample of the test groups was divided into two portions. They were treated as hydrolyzed and unhydrolyzed as described in the "*In vitro* drug release" section. The two portions of the samples were analyzed by HPLC to determine the plasma concentrations of released 5-FA and total 5-FA of the conjugate whereas the plasma samples of the control group were treated as unhydrolyzed samples.

In vivo distribution

Murine H22 hepatocarcinoma cells (purchased from Type Culture Collection of Chinese Academy of Sciences) were maintained in RPMI 1640 medium supplemented with 2 mM L-glutamine and 10% fetal bovine serum (FBS) at 37°C with 5% CO_2, and were passaged every 2 or 3 days. The tumor-bearing animal model was established by subcutaneous injection of H22 cells (1×10^7 cells/ml, in 0.2 ml saline) into the right axillary region of Kunming mice. The sizes of tumors were monitored 7 days after inoculation and the tumor volumes were calculated as described in the "*Antitumor activity in tumor-bearing mice*" section. The mice with tumor volumes between 0.35 cm^3 and 0.65 cm^3 were randomized into two groups (n = 30). The control group and the test groups were administered intravenously with 20 mg/kg of 5-FA or 189 mg/kg 5-FA-PAE (equivalent to 20 mg/kg of 5-FA) dissolved in physiological saline (0.009 g/ml), respectively. The mice were exsanguinated and sacrificed by neck dislocation at predetermined time points. Tissues including heart, liver, spleen, lung, kidney, brain and tumor were collected, washed with physiological saline, weighed and homogenized with two fold concentrated physiological saline. The samples of the test group were treated as hydrolyzed samples as described in the section "*In vitro* drug release", whereas those of the control group were treated as unhydrolyzed samples. All data are presented as the concentration of 5-FA.

Antitumor activity in tumor-bearing mice

The tumor-bearing mice model was established as previously described in the "*In vivo distribution*" section. 72 h after inoculation, mice with no signs of tumor growth were exclude from this experiment. 48 tumor-bearing mice were randomly divided into 4 groups (n = 12). The control group was administered intravenously with 20 ml/kg of physiological saline. The other groups were administered intravenously with 30 mg/kg (0.160 mmol/kg) of 5-FA or 284 mg/kg 5-FA-PAE (equivalent to 0.160 mmol/kg 5-FA) dissolved in physiological saline. 5-Fu (20.47 mg/kg, 0.160 mmol/kg) was administered as a control. All animals were administered once on day 3, 5, 7, 9, 11, 13, 15 after the inoculation of H22 cells and sacrificed on day 20. Tumors and organs (heart, liver, spleen, lung, kidney, brain and thymus) were removed and weighed. The tumor volume and tumor control rate were evaluated. The tumor volume, organ/body weight index and tumor control rate were calculated as follows:

$$\text{Tumor volume (mm}^3) = 0.5 \times \text{Width}^2 \times \text{Length}$$

$$\textit{Organ/body weight index} = \textit{weight of each organ (tumor)}/\textit{weight of mouse} \times 100$$

$$\textit{Tumor control rate}\ (\%) = \left(\begin{array}{l}\textit{average tumor weight of control group} -\\ \textit{average tumor weight of test group}\end{array}\right) \Big/ \begin{array}{l}\textit{average tumor weight}\\ \textit{of control group}\end{array}$$

Data analysis

The data of pharmacokinetics and *in vivo* distribution study were processed using the Drug and Statistics Software 2.0 (DAS 2.0, Shanghai, China). The statistical analysis of the samples was performed by using one-way ANOVA and Student's *t*-test. p-values <0.05 were considered as statistically different.

Results and Discussion

Synthesis and characterization of 5-FA-PAE prodrug

As a polyether macromolecule, PEG is widely used for its suitable solubility and bioavailability in developing drug delivery systems [50–53]. However, as a drug carrier, the loading efficiency of prodrugs based on PEG is significantly constrained due to the limited positions for drug conjugation, *i.e.*, two hydroxy groups in the linear PEG molecule [45]. Thus, the modification of PEG to create derivatives with higher drug loading efficiency is greatly needed. PEG with a molecular weight of 38 kDa was selected as the starting material to synthesize the derivative (Fig. 1A). Allyl glycidyl ether was coupled to both ends of PEG under the catalysis of sodium hydride to form an intermediate, namely PA, with multi-double bonds on the side chains. PA was further reacted with small molecules through the addition reaction of the double bonds and the thiol group to afford various PEG derivatives with multi-hydroxyl groups. ^{1}H-NMR showed that the double bonds disappeared completely in PAE (Figure S1 in file SI). The GPC analysis demonstrated that PA and PAE had similar molecular weight distribution as the starting material PEG (Table 1). As a common drug carrier, the molecular weight of PEG greatly influenced the *in vivo* behaviors of prodrugs [54]. As the molecular weight increases, the *in vivo* clearance rate decreases. Thus, PEG with a higher Mw is likely to prolong the retention time of prodrugs and increase the drug accumulation in a tumor. It is suggested that the Mw of PEG should be no less than 30 kD to prevent the prodrug from quick elimination from kidney [55]. Accordingly, PEG of 38 kD was used as the starting material.

However, 5-Fu could not be directly coupled with the carriers due to the lack of available hydroxyl groups in the structure. The derivative of 5-Fu, 5-fluorouracil-1-acetic acid (5-FA), was synthesized first. The macromolecular prodrug multi-hydroxyl polyethylene glycol-5-fluorouracil-1-acetic acid (5-FA-PAE) was obtained by covalently conjugating 5-FA with the PEG derivative under the catalysis of carbodiimide condensing agents (Figure 1B). The successful synthesis of the 5-fluorouracil derivative and the prodrug was confirmed by ^{1}H-NMR (Figure S1 in file SI). A higher molecular weight (Mw) and polydispersity (PDI) of 5-FA-PAE were observed compared with those of PAE (Table 1). HPLC analysis indicated that after the double bond-thiol addition reaction, multiple hydroxyl groups were introduced on the PEG backbone thus making it capable of loading more drugs. The drug loading efficiency of 5-FA-PAE was determined as 10.58%, much higher than the maximum drug loading efficiency of PEG with the same molecular weight, which was calculated as 0.98% theoretically. The drug loading efficiency of 5-FA-PAE was improved by

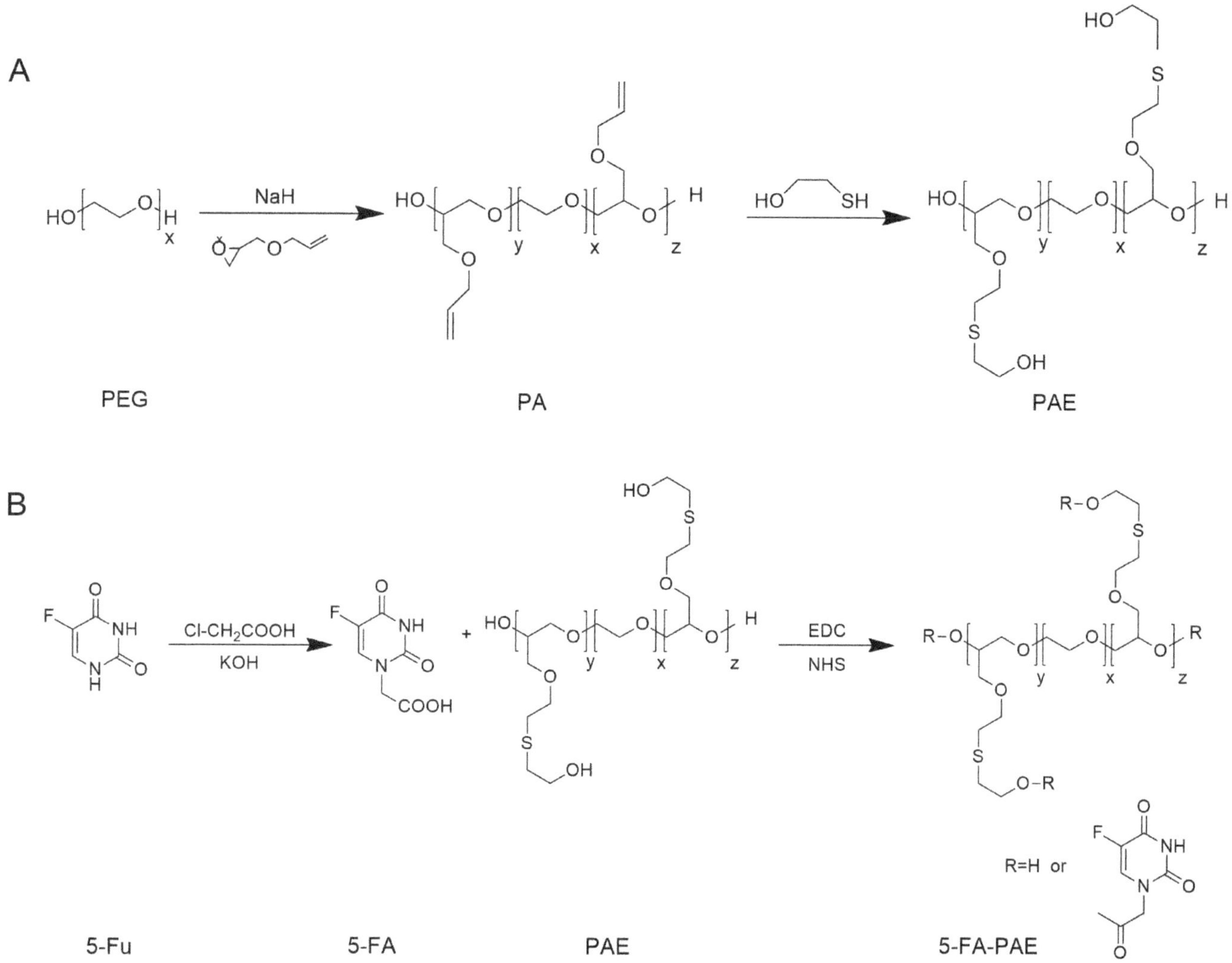

Figure 1. Synthesis routes of PAE (A) and 5-FA-PAE conjugates (B). (A) PA was synthesized by adding NaH to PEG and the mixture was stirred for 4 h at 120°C. Then PAE was obtained by adding AGE to the mixture. (B) 5-FA was added dropwise to PAE in dimethylformamide, then NHS and EDC·HCl were added. After incubation, the mixture was precipitated with isopropanol. The obtained residue was recrystallized by isopropanol several times and dried in vacuum at 40°C overnight to produce 5-FA-PAE.

Table 1. The molecular weight of the polymeric carrier (PEG, PA, PAE) and the prodrug (5-FA-PAE).

Compound	MP (Da)	Mw (Da)	Mn (Da)	PDI
PEG	38914	38045	27596	1.38
PA	33984	36039	21322	1.69
PAE	34282	36628	20842	1.76
5-FA-PAE	35413	44629	19998	2.23

PDI: polydispersity.

10.8-fold compared to that of 5-FA. The significant enhancement in drug loading efficiency would greatly increase the drug concentration within a tumor via the EPR effect.

Safety evaluation

To investigate the myelosuppression levels after 5-FA or 5-FA-PAE treatment, hematological parameters (i.e. the number of white blood cells and blood platelets) were measured at different time points after drug administration. Changes in these parameters presumably reflect the occurrence of myelosuppression and abnormality in the immune system. As shown in Table 2, the WBC count decreased after intravenous injection of 5-Fu, 5-FA and 5-FA-PAE. Only the group of 5-Fu exhibited significant reduction of WBC ($5.39\pm2.17\times10^9$/L one day after injection, $p<0.05$). Then the WBC level increased gradually. Notably, the increase of WBC in the 5-Fu group was slower, leading to a lower WBC level at day 10 ($8.59\pm2.39\times10^9$/L) compared with the level before administration ($9.55\pm1.28\times10^9$/L), while the WBC level of other groups recovered within 4 days. Another major indicator of myelosuppression is the change in blood platelets number. Table S1 in file SI shows that though the platelets number of 5-Fu decreased 1 day after injection, the blood platelets of all groups didn't exhibit any significant changes, indicating that both 5-FA and 5-FA-PAE hardly affect the platelets level at such doses. Taken together, these results indicated that the prodrug of 5-Fu, 5-FA-PAE, showed a lower toxicity than 5-Fu.

In vitro drug release

The *in vitro* drug release behavior of 5-FA-PAE was investigated using phosphate buffered saline (PBS) of various pH values, physiological saline, mouse plasma and tumor homogenate as the release media. The release rate of 5-FA-PAE was pH-dependent. As the pH increased, the release rate increased significantly, reaching 94.1%±5.88% at 96 h when the pH was 8.99 (Figure 2A). This is mostly likely due to the hydrolysis of ester bonds under basic conditions. However, if the conjugation with the PEG derivative increased the retention time in plasma, this would possibly enhance the drug accumulation in a tumor (Figure 2B). The release rate of prodrug 5-FA-PAE in plasma was 89.46%±6.36% at 10 h, and reached 98.15%±1.96% at 24 h, while the rate was 55.9%±0.61% in tumor homogenate at 24 h, suggesting that the ester bond can be easily degraded by easterases in plasma.

Pharmacokinetics study

A major drawback of 5-Fu is the relatively short half-life, which results in poor patient compliance and side effects. 5-FA, the derivative of 5-Fu, shows the same metabolism and clearance rate as 5-Fu. Moreover, after conjugation with PEG, the retention time in plasma was greatly prolonged, which might enhance tumor accumulation. After administration intravenously, 5-FA was rapidly eliminated from the blood circulation, which led to a complete removal at 6~8 h after administration, whereas the elimination rate of 5-FA-PAE was much lower than that of 5-FA, and the blood retention time of this macromolecular prodrug reached more than 96 h (Figure 3). The detailed plasma concentration of 5-FA and 5-FA-PAE at different time points are shown in Table S2 in file SI. Some pharmacokinetic parameters, such as the area under the curve (AUC), the mean retention time (MRT) and the elimination half-life ($t_{1/2}$) of 5-FA-PAE were much higher than those of 5-FA, *i.e.*, 25.6 times for AUC (546.6±36.7 μg/ml ·h vs 21.37±4.36 μg/ml ·h), 11.7 times for MRT (7.962±0.400 h vs 0.679±0.142 h) and 14.4 times for $t_{1/2}$ (22.10±5.92 h vs 1.538±0.419 h), indicating a much longer blood circulation times and a remarkably enhanced bioavailability of the macromolecular prodrug (Table 3). Meanwhile, the amount of 5-FA released from 5-FA-PAE in rat plasma was determined. Although the total amount of 5-FA-PAE in rat plasma was significantly higher than that of 5-FA, the concentration of released 5-FA from 5-FA-PAE was not as much as 5-FA. It was lower than the 5-FA group within 30 min after administration and then increased slightly afterwards (Table S2 in file SI). This may

Table 2. The number of white blood cells in mice administered with saline, 5-Fu, 5-FA, PAE or 5-FA-PAE ($\times10^9$/L).

	1 day before injection	1 day after injection	4 days after injection	7 days after injection	10 days after injection
saline	9.77±1.99	8.86±2.79	11.19±6.78	12.24±4.37	12.06±7.58
5-FA-PAE	9.35±1.39	8.73±1.90	11.73±5.44	12.00±2.02	12.52±3.78
5-FA	9.13±2.23	8.99±1.86	10.32±5.71	10.24±4.50	11.55±3.62
PAE	9.54±1.64	8.46±1.85	9.85±3.09	10.74±5.13	11.93±3.40
5-Fu	9.55±1.28	5.39±2.17*	6.84±5.76	7.34±2.82	8.59±2.39

Each value represents the mean ± SD (n = 12).
*$p<0.05$ vs. 5-Fu,1 day before injection.

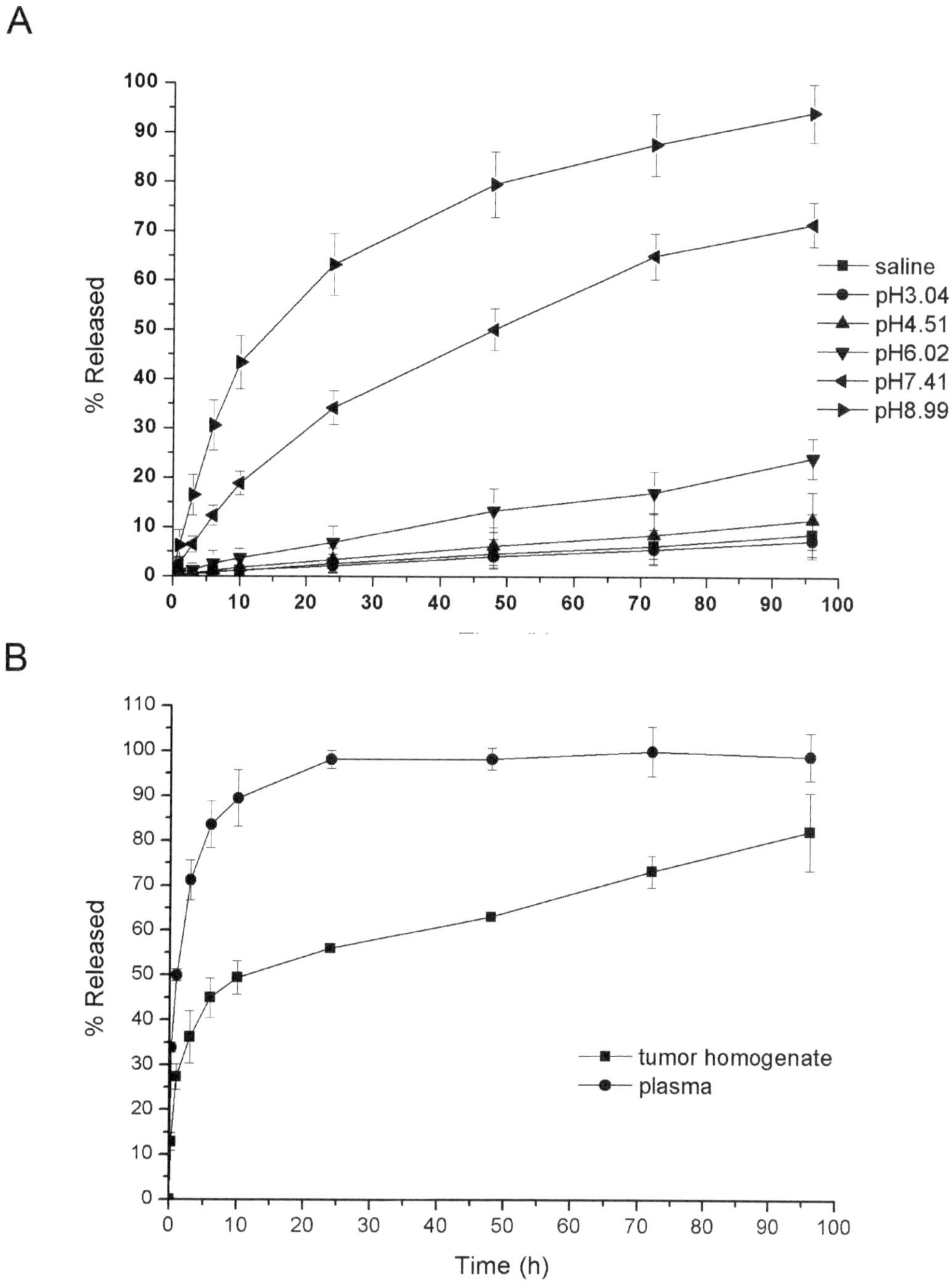

Figure 2. *In vitro* drug release of 5-FA-PAE. (A) Drug release profiles of 5-FA-PAE in PBS and saline. 100 μl 5-PA-PAE was added to preheated release media (PBS of different pH values or saline) and incubated at 37°C with stirring. Samples were collected at fixed time intervals, acidified by hydrochloric acid (1 M) and analyzed by HPLC. (B) Drug release profiles of 5-FA-PAE in murine tumor homogenate and plasma. The samples from mouse plasma and tumor homogenate were obtained in duplicate at each time point (100 μl each). For hydrolysis, 100 μl sodium hydroxide (1 M) were added to samples followed by 100 μl hydrochloric acid (1 M). The other group was not subjected to hydrolysis by substituting sodium hydroxide solution with saline and acidifying with 50 μl hydrochloric acid. The differences of 5-FA in the two groups at the same time point was the unreleased 5-FA in each sample. Each value represents the mean ± SD (n = 3).

have an impact on the antitumor efficacy of 5-FA-PAE, but could avoid certain possible side effects.

Due to the obvious discrepancy of retention time between 5-FA and 5-FA-PAE, two sets of different time points were adopted to fully describe the *in vivo* fate of 5-FA and 5-FA-PAE. The first time point for 5-FA and 5-FA-PAE was 1 min and 5 min after administration, respectively.

In the *in vitro* release study, about 98% of 5-FA was released from 5-FA-PAE in plasma at 24 h, in other words, 2% 5-FA-PAE remained intact, while in the pharmacokinetics study, the concentration of unreleased 5-FA-PAE was 228.276±5.441 μg/ml 5 min after administration (the difference between total concentration of 5-FA-PAE and free 5-FA released from 5-FA-PAE), and decreased to 2.439±0.258 at 24 h (about 1.1% of the

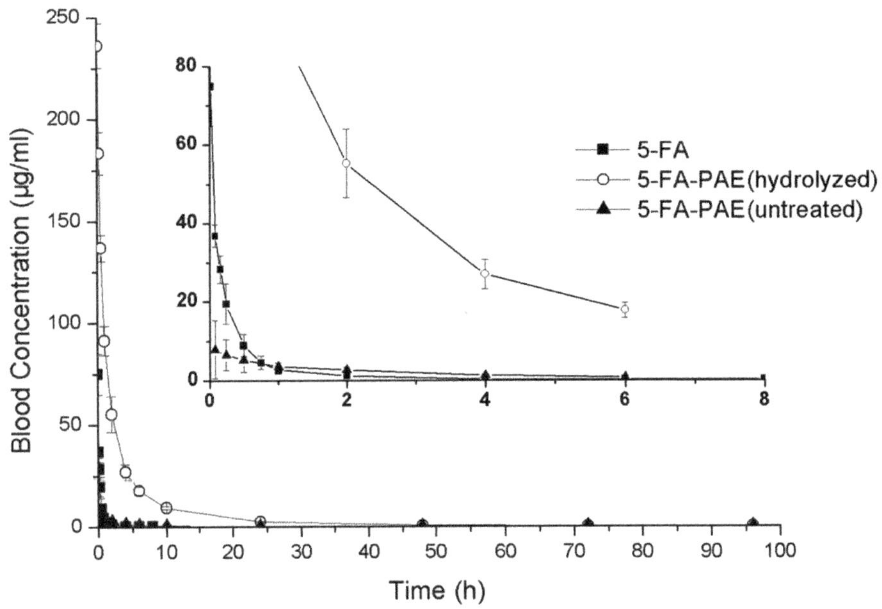

Figure 3. Pharmacokinetics of 5-FA and 5-FA-PAE after *i.v.* injection. The control group and the test groups were administered intravenously with 20 mg/kg of 5-FA or 189 mg/kg of 5-FA-PAE (equivalent to 20 mg/kg of 5-FA) dissolved in physiological saline, respectively. Each plasma sample of the 5-FA-PAE group was divided into two portions (treated as hydrolyzed and unhydrolyzed), which were analyzed by HPLC to determine the plasma concentrations of released 5-FA and total 5-FA of the conjugate whereas the plasma samples of the control group were treated as unhydrolyzed samples. Each value represents the mean ± standard deviation (n = 6).

concentration at 5 min), which is consistent with the previous *in vitro* release study. Comparing the concentration of the free 5-FA of unhydrolyzed and hydrolyzed 5-FA-PAE group, it can be concluded that the unreleased 5-FA-PAE was intact in the blood circulation, which could accumulate in tumor tissue in the form of prodrug and then slowly release 5-FA at the tumor site to achieve antitumor effect. 5-FA was shown to be rapidly eliminated from blood, while after conjugation with PAE, the retention time was significantly prolonged, which may be attributed to a protective role of PEG. Thus, the prolonged retention time of 5-FA not only extended the duration time and enhanced the bioavailability, but also improved the delivery of macromolecular drugs to a tumor.

In vivo distribution

Small molecular drugs eliminate quickly after intravenous administration, which could distribute them to normal tissues through capillaries nonspecifically. To analyze the *in vivo* biodistribution of 5-FA-PAE, the murine hepatic cancer cell line (H22) was used to establish the tumor-bearing animal model. The hepatoma H22 model has been widely use as a tumor model in the study of antitumor drugs and its mechanism. Generally, it is believed that the orthotopic tumor can better simulate the pathologic process of tumor development. However, due to the high mortality rate of animals and the complexity of operation, we

Table 3. Pharmacokinetic parameters of 5-FA and 5-FA-PAE after i.v. injection in rats.

Parameters	Unit	5-FA	5-FA-PAE
AUC $_{0\text{-}t}$	μg/ml·h	21.37±4.36	546.6±36.7
AUC $_{0\text{-}\infty}$	μg/ml·h	21.63±4.47	551.5±35.0
MRT $_{0\text{-}t}$	h	0.679±0.142	7.962±0.400
MRT $_{0\text{-}\infty}$	h	0.795±0.240	9.072±0.513
VRT $_{0\text{-}t}$	h^2	1.519±0.326	190.2±19.7
VRT $_{0\text{-}\infty}$	h^2	2.703±1.558	335.8±79.4
$t_{1/2}$	h	1.538±0.419	22.10±5.92
T_{max}	h	0.0167±0	0.097±0.034
V	ml/g	2.107±0.620	1.172±0.358
Cl	ml/g/h	0.967±0.259	0.036±0.002
C_{max}	μg/ml	74.92±10.16	232.4±13.5

AUC, area under the plasma concentration−time curve; MRT, mean residence time; VRT, variance of mean residence time; $t_{1/2}$: elimination half life; T_{max}, time of maximum concentration; V, apparent volume of distribution; CL, clearance; Cmax, the maximum of 5-FA concentration in plasma.
Each value represents the mean ± SD (n = 5).

A

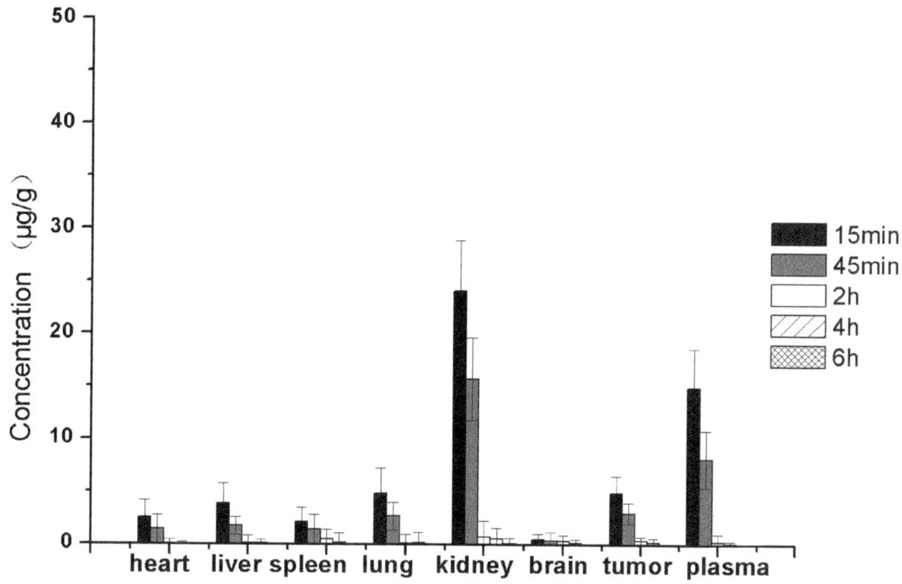

B

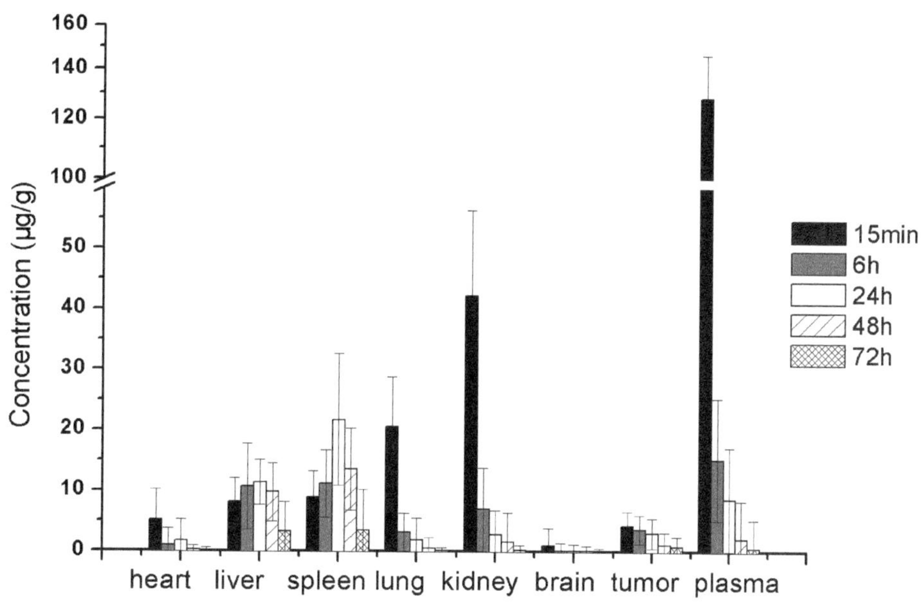

Figure 4. Biodistribution of 5-FA (A) and 5-FA-PAE (B) after *i.v.* injection. The tumor-bearing animal model was established by subcutaneous injection of H22 cells into Kunming mice. The control group and the test groups were administered intravenously with 20 mg/kg of 5-FA or 5-FA-PAE (equivalent to 20 mg/kg of 5-FA), respectively. The mice were exsanguinated and sacrificed at predetermined time points. Tissues (heart, liver, spleen, lung, kidney, brain and tumor) were collected, weighed and homogenized with two fold concentrated physiological saline. The samples of the test group were treated as hydrolyzed samples, whereas those of the control group were treated as unhydrolyzed samples. All data are presented as the concentration of 5-FA. Each value represents the mean ± standard deviation (n = 6).

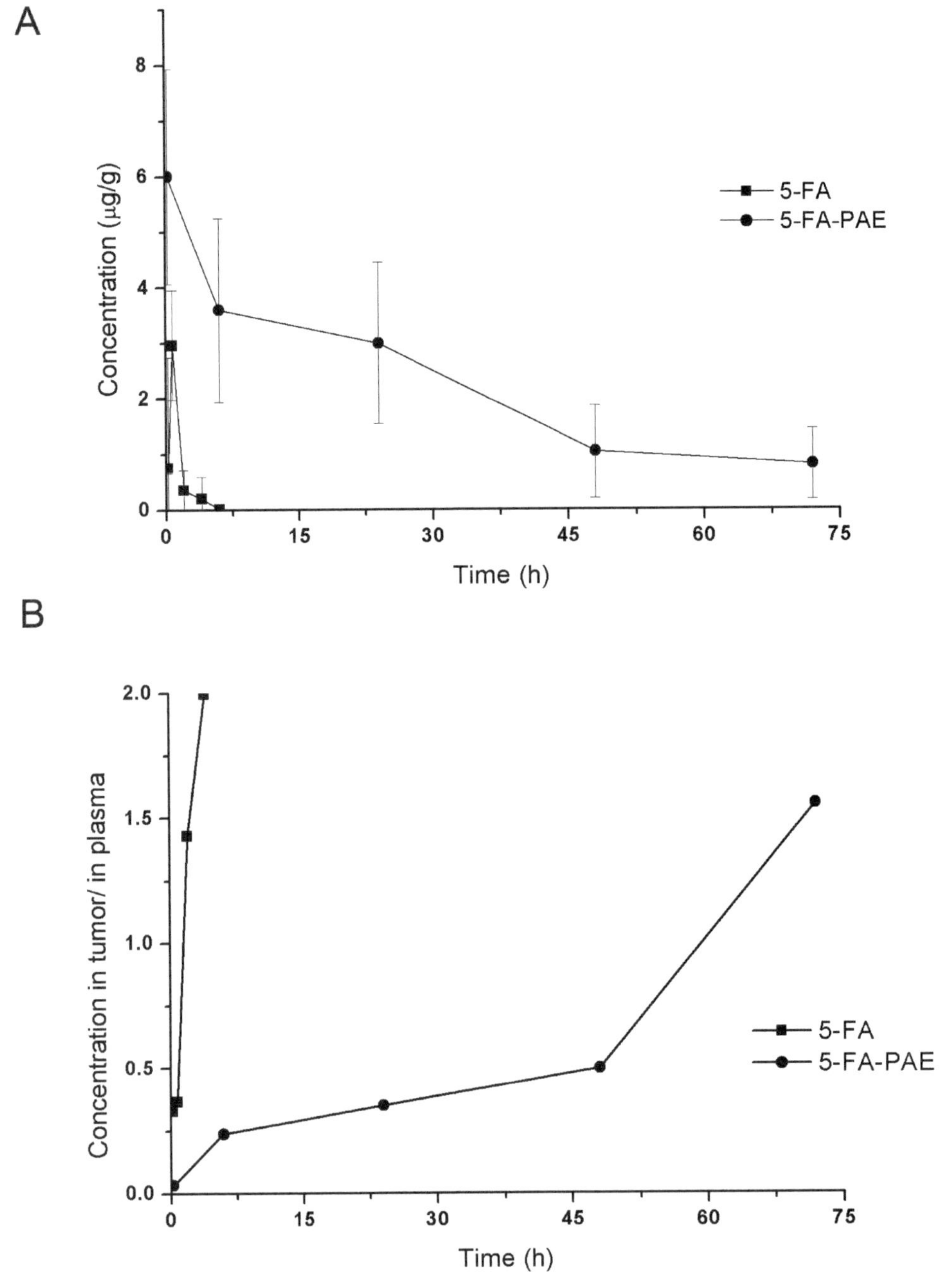

Figure 5. Drug concentration in tumor and plasma. The tumor-bearing mice model was described in the "*In vivo* biodistribution" section. The control group and the test groups were administered intravenously with 20 mg/kg of 5-FA and 5-FA-PAE (equivalent to 20 mg/kg of 5-FA), respectively. (A) Drug concentration of 5-FA and conjugated 5-FA-PAE in tumor at different time points. (B) Ratio of drug concentration in tumor vs. that in plasma of 5-FA and conjugated 5-FA-PAE.

adopted the ectopic model. After intravenous injection, at all time points, the concentration of 5-FA in kidney was significantly higher than other organs and in the tumor, suggesting that renal excretion was the major pathway of 5-FA elimination from the body. Other than kidney, 5-FA did not show any specificity in distribution with similar drug concentrations in heart, liver, spleen, lung and tumor. 15 min after the intravenous injection of 5-FA-PAE, the plasma concentration was the highest of all samples (128.1±18.3 μg/g). However, as the time increased, the plasma concentration of 5-FA-PAE decreased rapidly, dropping to 8,57±3.33 μg/g at 24 h, while the concentration in liver and spleen increased gradually and peaked at 24 h (11.35±3.78 μg/g in liver and 21.68±10.83 μg/g in spleen). 5-FA-PAE was detectable in all organs and tumor at 72 h after injection (consistent with the pharmacokinetics study), indicating that the retention time of 5-FA-PAE was longer than 5-FA (Fig. 4A and 4B).

The concentration of 5-FA and 5-FA-PAE in tumor is shown in Fig 5A. The concentration of 5-FA decreased rapidly after administration and was undetectable after 6 h. Though the

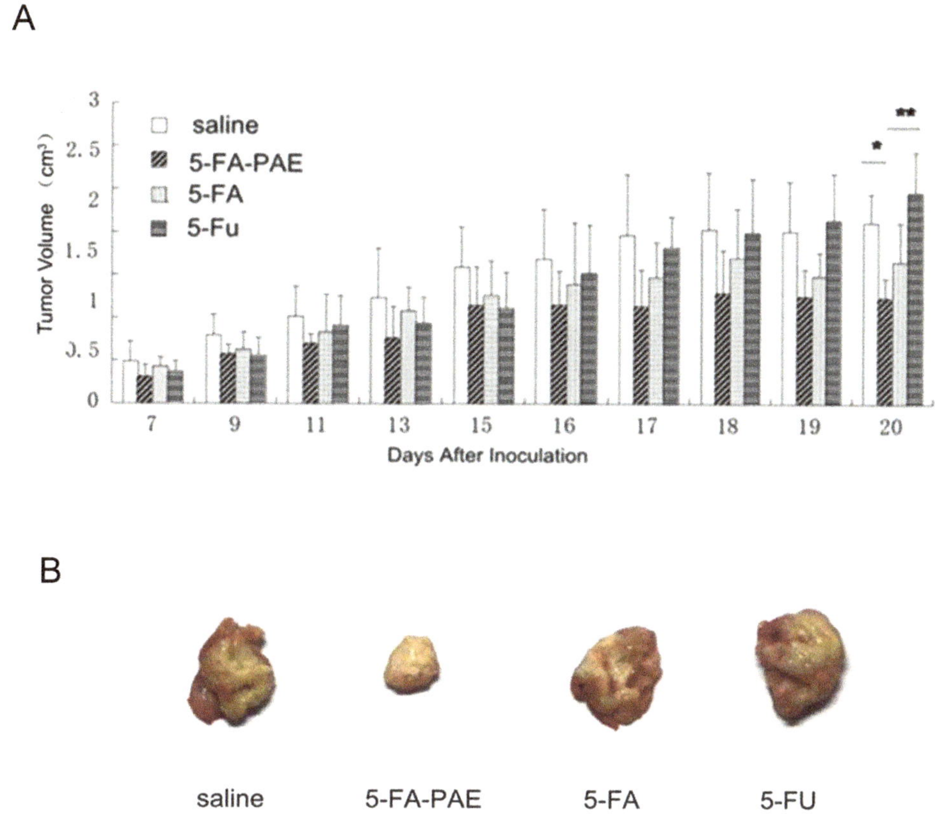

Figure 6. The antitumor effects on tumor-bearing mice. Mice were i.v injected with saline (20 mg/kg, 0.160 mmol/kg), 5-FA-PAE (284 mg/kg, 0.160 mmol/kg), 5-FA (30 mg/kg, 0.160 mmol/kg) or 5-Fu (20.47 mg/kg, 0.160 mmol/kg) on day 3, 5, 7, 9, 11, 13 and 15 after inoculation of H22 cells. On day 20, mice were sacrificed. Tumors and organs were removed and weighed. (A) The tumor volumes after inoculation (n = 6–12). * $p<0.05$, ** $p<0.01$. (B) Images of tumors in tumor-bearing mice on day 20 after inoculation of tumor cells (n = 6).

maximum concentration of 5-FA-PAE was slightly lower than 5-FA at 15 min after injection (4.22±2.3 μg/g for 5-FA-PAE and 4.86±1.62 μg/g for 5-FA), the concentration of 5-FA-PAE remained at a relatively high level and lasted for 72 h, indicating that 5-FA-PAE could slowly release 5-FA in the tumor and exert an antitumor effect. The concentration in the tumor vs. those in plasma of 5-FA-PAE and 5-FA is displayed in Fig. 5B. 45 min after administration, the concentration of 5-FA in tumor was lower than that in plasma, and then increased rapidly afterwards. 4 h after injection, the ratio of tumor/plasma concentration reached 1.99, suggesting that 5-FA could distribute from plasma to tumor within a short time, and that the clearance rate of 5-FA in plasma was higher than that in the tumor. 6 h after administration, the 5-FA concentration was almost undetectable in both plasma and tumor. The ratio of tumor/plasma concentration of 5-FA-PAE increased steadily within 48 h after injection and was lower than 0.5. Between 48 h to 72 h, the ratio increased quickly and reached 1.56 at 72 h, indicating that the clearance of 5-FA-PAE from tumor was much lower than that from the plasma. These results indicated that the amount of 5-FA-PAE in tumor lasted longer compared with that of 5-FA, exhibiting a sustained-release profile.

Table 4. Tumor weight and tumor control rate of mice administrated with saline, 5-Fu, 5-FA or 5-FA-PAE.

Treatment	Tumor weight (g)	Tumor control rate (%)
saline	2.229±0.521	-
5-FA-PAE	1.072±0.249 **	51.9±11.2$^{\Delta}$
5-FA	1.449±0.392 *	35.0±17.6$^{\Delta}$
5-Fu	2.383±0.841	−6.9±37.7

*$p<0.05$ vs. saline group.
**$p<0.01$ vs. saline group.
$^{\Delta}p<0.05$ vs. 5-Fu group.
Each value represents the mean ± SD (n = 6).

Table 5. The organ/body weight index of mice administrated with saline, 5-Fu, 5-FA or 5-FA-PAE.

Tissue	saline	5-FA-PAE	5-FA	5-Fu
Heart	0.440±0.047	0.431±0.042	0.443±0.031	0.424±0.038
Liver	5.643±0.291	6.255±1.023	5.737±1.068	5.601±0.897
Spleen	1.226±0.390	1.360±0.543	1.398±0.478	1.264±0.694
Lung	0.978±0.236	0.955±0.141	1.068±0.407	0.900±0.109
Kidney	1.368±0.131	1.377±0.083	1.426±0.113	1.298±0.089
Brain	1.355±0.110	1.317±0.203	1.421±0.302	1.452±0.308
Thymus	0.192±0.097	0.261±0.070	0.221±0.155	0.167±0.086
Tumor	7.088±1.961	3.381±1.224*$^{\Delta}$	4.957±2.336	8.816±3.578

*$p<0.05$ vs. saline group.
$^{\Delta}p<0.05$ vs. 5-Fu group.
Each value represents the mean ± SD (n=6).

Though the initial concentration and tumor/blood concentration ratio of 5-FA were higher than 5-FA-PAE, a high elimination rate of 5-FA severely limited its therapeutic effect in clinic. In comparison, the concentration of 5-FA-PAE in the tumor could be maintained at a relatively high level, which lasted for more than 70 h, despite the large variation (probably due to inter-individual difference). Similarly, the tumor/blood concentration ratio of 5-FA-PAE showed a gradually increasing trend.

Antitumor effect in tumor-bearing mice

5-Fu is the first-choice antimetabolite in the treatment of colon cancer and colorectal cancer. 5-FA, a derivative of 5-Fu, has been reported to be effective and safe [56–59]. To address the antitumor activity of the prodrug, 5-FA and 5-Fu were both used as controls. In the pharmacokinetics studies of anticancer drugs, two dosing regimens are commonly used. One is the preventive administration strategy in which drugs are administered at the beginning of the tumor growth. The other one is the therapeutic administration with drugs administered when the tumor growth reached a certain size. Since the relatively high mortality rate of the H22 tumor model in the later period of this experiment, we adopted a prophylactic administration scheme, i.e. 72 h after inoculation, mice with no signs of tumor growth were excluded from this experiment. Based on the pharmacokinetics and biodistribution results, we administered the drugs every other day (from day 3 to day 15 after inoculation). The antitumor effect of 5-FA-PAE was assessed by analyzing tumor volume, tumor control rate and the organ/body weight index of tumor-bearing mice. From the beginning of administration, the tumor volume of 5-FA-PAE group was smaller than that of the saline group, showing the highest antitumor activity (Figure 6A and 6B). The 5-FA and 5-Fu groups also displayed some antitumor effect. However, after the last administration on day 15, the tumor volume of these two groups increased obviously, while the tumor size of the 5-FA-PAE group did not, which suggested that the antitumor activity of 5-FA-PAE could last for a longer time. This is compatible with the pharmacokinetics results in which 5-FA-PAE showed a much longer retention time than that of 5-FA. 20 days after inoculation, the average tumor volume of 5-FA-PAE group was significantly smaller than that of the 5-Fu and saline groups ($p<0.01$). However, no significant differences were observed between the 5-FA and 5-FA-PAE groups. This may be due to the large variation of the 5-FA group.

Though the tumor control rates of the 5-FA-PAE and 5-FA groups were not significantly different ($p>0.05$), the tumor control rates of the 5-FA-PAE group (51.9±11.2%) and the 5-FA group (35.0±17.6%) were significantly higher than that of the 5-Fu and saline groups (Table 4). Since the tumor growth can affect the weight of normal organs, the organ/body weight index was used to assess the impact. The tumor/body index of the 5-FA-PAE (3.381±1.224) group was much lower than those of the 5-Fu (8.816±3.578) and saline groups (7.088±1.961, $p<0.05$, Table 5). No significant differences were observed in other organ/body indices.

Owing to the conjugation with PEG, 5-FA-PAE exhibited a longer retention time, which led to a long-lasting antitumor effect. Notably, during the administration period, the death rate in the tumor-bearing mice of the 5-FA-PAE group is relatively high. This is probably due to the tumor growth and the toxicity of 5-FA-PAE, which is also a drawback of our present regimen and needs further refinement. However, after administration of all doses, no more deaths were observed in the 5-FA-PAE group, indicating that the toxicity caused by repeated administration of 5-FA-PAE was reversible. While in the 5-FA and 5-Fu groups, large number of animal deaths were observed after all administrations, suggesting a shorter duration of their antitumor effect.

Conclusion

To solve the paradox of drug loading and the molecular weight of PEG, we synthesized a PEG multi-hydroxyl derivative (PAE). PAE was coupled with 5-FA via ester bonds to afford 5-FA-PAE, and the drug loading efficiency was shown to be 10.8-fold higher than using unmodified PEG. Besides, the retention time and bioavailability of 5-FA-PAE were greatly improved compared to 5-FA, showing a prolonged half-life and improved antitumor efficacy *in vivo*. Owing to the improved drug loading efficiency and prolonged half-life, the multi-hydroxyl PEG derivative PAE proves to be an efficient carrier for 5-Fu. Future study should focus on further improving the tumor-targeting efficiency and the antitumor effect of 5-FA-PAE while reducing its toxicity. This paper provides some insights for the future development of antitumor drugs using PEG as a drug carrier.

Supporting Information

File S1 Supporting files. Figure S1, Identification of different polymers. The ^{1}H-NMR spectra of 5-Fu (A), 5-FA (B), PEG (C), the polymeric carrier PAE (D) and the prodrug 5-FA-PAE (E). **Table S1**, The number of blood platelets in mice administered with saline, 5-Fu, 5-FA, PAE or 5-FA-PAE. ($\times 10^9$/L). **Table S2**, Plasma concentration of 5-FA and 5-FA-PAE at different time points.

Author Contributions

Conceived and designed the experiments: ZL XS TG ZZ. Performed the experiments: ZL. Analyzed the data: ML. Wrote the paper: ML.

References

1. Sarkar FH (2010) Recent trends in anti-cancer drug discovery. Mini Rev Med Chem 10: 357–358.
2. Na Y (2009) Recent cancer drug development with xanthone structures. J Pharm Pharmacol 61: 707–712.
3. Meada H (2001) SMANCS and polymer-conjugates macromolecular drug: advantages in cancer chemotherapy. Adv Drug Deliv Rev 46: 169–185.
4. Dang CT (2006) Drug treatments for adjuvant chemotherapy in breast cancer: recent trials and future directions. Expert Rev Anticancer Ther 6: 427–436.
5. Thompson N, Lyons J (2005) Recent progress in targeting the Raf/MEK/ERK pathway with inhibitors in cancer drug discovery. Curr Opin Pharmacol 5: 350–356.
6. Kelloff GJ, Boone CW, Malone W, Steele V (1993) Recent results in preclinical and clinical drug development of chemopreventive agents at the National Cancer Institute. Basic Life Sci 61: 373–386.
7. Sartor O, Halstead M, Katz L (2010) Improving outcomes with recent advances in chemotherapy for castrate-resistant prostate cancer. Clin Genitourin Cancer 8: 23–28.
8. Deeken JF, Figg WD, Bates SE, Sparreboom A (2007) Toward individualized treatment: prediction of anticancer drug disposition and toxicity with pharmacogenetics. Anti-cancer Drugs 18: 111–126.
9. Kintzel PE, Dorr RT (1995) Anticancer drug renal toxicity and elimination: dosing guidelines for altered renal function. Cancer Treat Rev 21: 33–64.
10. Duschinsky R, Pleven E, Heidelberger C (1957) The synthesis of 5-fluoropyrimidines. J Chem Soc 79: 4559–4560.
11. Ogiso T, Noda N, Asai N, Kato Y (1976) Antitumor agents. I. Effect of 5-fluorouracil and cyclophosphamide on liver microsomes and thymus of rat. Jpn J Pharmacol 26: 445–453.
12. Ogiso T, Noda N, Masuda H, Kato Y (1978) Antitumor agents. II. Effect of 5-fluorouracil and cyclophosphamide on immunological parameters and liver microsomes of tumor-bearing rats. Jpn J Pharmacol 28: 175–183.
13. Parker WB, Cheng YC (1990) Metabolism and mechanism of action of 5-fluorouracil. Pharmacol Ther 48: 381–395.
14. Macdonald JS (1999) Toxicity of 5-fluorouracil. Oncology 13: 33–34.
15. Shuey DL, Setzer RW, Lau C, Zucker RM, Elstein KH, et al. (1995) Biological modeling of 5-fluorouracil developmental toxicity. Toxicology 102: 207–213.
16. Van Kuilenburg AB, Meinsma R, Van Gennip AH (2004) Pyrimidine degradation defects and severe 5-fluorouracil toxicity. Nucleosides, Nucleotides and Nucleic Acids 23: 1371–1375.
17. Iyer L, Ratain MJ (1999) 5-fluorouracil pharmacokinetics: causes for variability and strategies for modulation in cancer chemotherapy. Cancer Invest 17: 494–506.
18. Milano G, Chamorey AL (2002) Clinical pharmacokinetics of 5-fluorouracil with consideration of chronopharmacokinetics. Chronobiol Int 19: 177–189.
19. Schalhorn A, Kühl M (1992) Clinical pharmacokinetics of fluorouracil and folinic acid. Semin Oncol 19: 82–92.
20. Pazdur R, Hoff PM, Medgyesy D, Royce M, Brito R (1998) The oral fluorouracil prodrugs. Oncology 12: 48–51.
21. Malet-Martino M, Martino R (2002) Clinical studies of three oral prodrugs of 5-fluorouracil (capecitabine, UFT, S-1): a review. Oncologist 7: 288–323.
22. Wang JX, Sun X, Zhang ZR (2002) Enhanced brain targeting by synthesis of 3′,5′-dioctanoyl-5-fluoro-2′-deoxyuridine and incorporation into solid lipid nanoparticles. Eur J Pharm Biopharm 54: 285–290.
23. Arias JL (2008) Novel strategies to improve the anticancer action of 5-fluorouracil by using drug delivery systems. Molecules 13: 2340–2369.
24. Menei P (1999) Local and sustained delivery of 5-Fluorouracil from biodegradable microspheres for the radiosensitization of glioblastoma. Cancer 86: 325–330.
25. Gupta Y, Jain A, Jain P, Jain SK (2007) Design and development of folate appended liposomes for enhanced delivery of 5-FU to tumor cells. J.Drug Targeting 15: 231–240.
26. Azori M (1987) Polymeric prodrugs. Crit Rev Ther Drug Carrier Syst 4: 39–65.
27. Hoste K, De Winne K, Schacht E (2004) Polymeric prodrugs. Int J Pharm 277: 119–131.
28. D'Souza AJM, Topp EM (2004) Release from polymeric prodrugs: linkages and their degradation. J Pharm Sci 93: 1962–1979.
29. Takakura Y, Hashida M (1995) Macromolecular drug carrier systems in cancer chemotherapy: macromolecular prodrugs. Crit Rev Oncol Hematol 18: 207–231.
30. Onishi H, Machida Y (2008) In vitro and in vivo evaluation of microparticulate drug delivery systems composed of macromolecular prodrugs. Molecules 13: 2136–2155.
31. Huang Y, Park YS, Wang J, Moon C, Kwon YM, et al (2010) ATTEMPTS system: a macromolecular prodrug strategy for cancer drug delivery. Curr Pharm Des 16: 2369–2376.
32. Goh PP, Sze DM, Roufogalis BD (2007) Molecular and cellular regulators of cancer angiogenesis. Curr Cancer Drug Targets 7: 743–758.
33. Maeda H, Fang J, Inutsuka T, Kitamono Y (2003) Vascular permeability enhancement in solid tumor: various factors, mechanisms involved and its implications. Int Immunopharmacol 3: 319–328.
34. Maeda H, Wu J, Sawa T, Matsumura Y, Hori K (2000) Tumor vascular permeability and the EPR effect in macromolecular therapeutics: a review. J Control Release 65: 271–284.
35. Maeda H, Bharate GY, Daruwalla J (2009) Polymeric drugs for efficient tumor-targeted drug delivery based on EPR-effect. Eur J Pharm Biopharm 71: 409–419.
36. Sawa T, Wu J, Akaike T, Maeda H (2000) Tumor-targeting chemotherapy by a xanthine oxidase-polymer conjugate that generates oxygen-free radicals in tumor tissue. Cancer Res 60: 666–671.
37. Pasut G, Veronese FM (2007) Polymer-drug conjugation, recent achievements and general strategies. Prog Polym Sci 32: 933–961.
38. Veronese FM, Harris JM (2002) Theme issue on "Peptide and Protein Pegylation I". Adv Drug Deliv Rev 54: 453–606.
39. Zhao H, Rubio B, Sapra P, Wu D, Reddy P, et al (2008) Novel prodrugs of SN38 using multiarm poly(ethylene glycol) linkers. Bioconjug Chem 19: 849–859.
40. Rowinsky EK, Rizzo J, Ochoa L, Takimoto CH, Forouzesh B, et al. (2003) A phase I and pharmacokinetic study of pegylated camptothecin as a 1-hour infusion every 3 weeks in pantients with advanced solid malignancies. J Clin Oncol 21: 148–157.
41. Guo Z, Wheler JJ, Naing A, Mani S, Goel S, et al. (2008) Clinical pharmacokinetics (PK) of EZN-2208, a novel anticancer agent, in patients (pts) with advanced malignancies: a phase I, first-in-human, dose-escalation study. J Clin Oncol 26: 2556.
42. Ton NC, Parker GJ, Jackson A, Mullamitha S, Buonaccorsi GA, et al. (2007) Phase I evaluation of CDP791, a PEGylated di-Fab' conjugate that binds vascular endothelial growth factor receptor 2. Clin Cancer Res 13: 7113–7118.
43. Michallet M, Maloisel F, Delain M, Hellmann A, Rosas A, et al. (2004) Pegylated recombinant interferon-a lpha-2b vs recombinant interferon-alpha-2b for the initial treatment of chronic-phase chronic myelogenous leukemia: a phase III study. Leukemia 18: 309–315.
44. Hwu WJ, Panageas KS, Menell JH, Lamb LA, Aird S, et al. (2006) Phase II study of temozolomide plus pegylated interferon-alpha-2b for metastatic melanoma. Cancer 106: 2445–2451.
45. Pasut G, Veronese FM (2009) PEG conjugates in clinical development or use as anticancer agents: an overview. Adv Drug Deliv Rev 61: 1177–1188.
46. Koyama Y, Umehara M, Mizuno A, Itaba M, Yasukouchi T, et al. (1996) Synthesis of novel poly(ethylene glycol) derivatives having pendant amino groups and aggregating behavior of its mixture with fatty acid in water. Bioconjug Chem 7: 298–301.
47. Burton SC, Harding DRK (1998) Preparation of chromatographic matrices by free radical addition ligand attachment to allyl groups. J Chromatogr A 796: 273–282.
48. Hao AJ, Deng YJ, Li TF, Suo XB,Cao YH, et al. (2006) Degradation kinetics of fluorouracil-acetic-acid-dextran conjugate in aqueous solution. Drug Dev Ind Pharm 32: 757–763.
49. Udo K, Hokonohara K, Motoyama K, Arima H, Hirayama F, et al. (2010) 5-Fluorouracil acetic acid/beta-cyclodextrin conjugates: drug release behavior in enzymatic and rat cecal media. Int J Pharm 388: 95–100.
50. Smyth HF Jr Carpenter CP, Weil CS (1950) The toxicology of the polyethylene glycols. J Am Pharm Assoc 39: 349–354.
51. Richter AW, Akerblom E (1983) Antibodies against polyethylene glycol produced in animals by immunization with monomethoxy polyethylene glycol modified proteins. Int Arch Allergy Appl Immunol 70: 124–131.
52. Zalipsky S, Gilon C, Zilkha A (1983) Attachment of drugs to polyethylene glycols. Eur Polym J 19: 1177–1183.
53. Sheridan W, Menchaca D (1998) Overview of the safety and biologic effects of PEG-rHuMGDF in clinical trials. Stem Cells 16: 193–198.
54. Riebeseel K, Biedermann E, Löser R, Breiter N, Hanselmann R, et al. (2002) Polyethylene glycol conjugates of methotrexate varying in their molecular weight from MW 750 to MW 40000: synthesis, characterization, and structure-activity relationships in vitro and in vivo. Bioconjug Chem 13: 773–785.

55. Greenwald RB, Gilbert CW, Pendri A, Conover CD, Xia J, et al. (1996) Drug delivery systems: water soluble taxol 2'-poly(ethylene glycol) ester prodrugs-design and in vivo effectiveness. Med Chem 39: 424–431.
56. Chung SM, Yoon EJ, Kim SH, Lee MG, Heejoo L, et al. (1991) Pharmacokinetics of 5-fluorouracil after intravenous infusion of 5-fluorouracil-acetic acid-human serum albumin conjugates to rabbits. Int J Pharm 68: 61–68.
57. Zuo D, Jiang T, Guan H, Wang KQ, Qi X, et al. (2001) Synthesis, Structure and Antitumor Activity of Dibutyltin Oxide Complexes with 5-Fluorouracil Derivatives. Crystal Structure of [(5-Fluorouracil)-1-$CH_2CH_2COOSn(n\text{-}Bu)_2]_4O_2$. Molecules 6: 647–654.
58. Kang NI, Lee SM, Maeda M, Ha CS, Cho WJ (2002) Synthesis, antitumour and DNA replication activities of polymers containing vinyl-(5-fluorouracil)-ethanoate. Polym Int 51: 443–449.
59. Yang ZY, Wang LF, Yang XP, Wang DW, Li YM (2000) Pharmacological study on antitumor activity of 5-fluorouracil-1-acetic acid and its rare earth complexes. J Rare Earth 18: 140–143.

20

Mean Platelet Volume (MPV) Predicts Middle Distance Running Performance

Giuseppe Lippi[1]*, Gian Luca Salvagno[2], Elisa Danese[2], Spyros Skafidas[3], Cantor Tarperi[4], Gian Cesare Guidi[2], Federico Schena[4]

1 Laboratory of Clinical Chemistry and Hematology, Academic Hospital of Parma, Parma, Italy, **2** Laboratory of Clinical Biochemistry, Department of Life and Reproduction Sciences, University of Verona, Verona, Italy, **3** CeRiSM (Centre for Mountain Sport and Health), Rovereto (TN), Italy, **4** Department of Neurological, Neuropsychological, Morphological and Movement Sciences, University of Verona, Verona, Italy

Abstract

Background: Running economy and performance in middle distance running depend on several physiological factors, which include anthropometric variables, functional characteristics, training volume and intensity. Since little information is available about hematological predictors of middle distance running time, we investigated whether some hematological parameters may be associated with middle distance running performance in a large sample of recreational runners.

Methods: The study population consisted in 43 amateur runners (15 females, 28 males; median age 47 years), who successfully concluded a 21.1 km half-marathon at 75–85% of their maximal aerobic power (VO_2max). Whole blood was collected 10 min before the run started and immediately thereafter, and hematological testing was completed within 2 hours after sample collection.

Results: The values of lymphocytes and eosinophils exhibited a significant decrease compared to pre-run values, whereas those of mean corpuscular volume (MCV), platelets, mean platelet volume (MPV), white blood cells (WBCs), neutrophils and monocytes were significantly increased after the run. In univariate analysis, significant associations with running time were found for pre-run values of hematocrit, hemoglobin, mean corpuscular hemoglobin (MCH), red blood cell distribution width (RDW), MPV, reticulocyte hemoglobin concentration (RetCHR), and post-run values of MCH, RDW, MPV, monocytes and RetCHR. In multivariate analysis, in which running time was entered as dependent variable whereas age, sex, blood lactate, body mass index, VO_2max, mean training regimen and the hematological parameters significantly associated with running performance in univariate analysis were entered as independent variables, only MPV values before and after the trial remained significantly associated with running time. After adjustment for platelet count, the MPV value before the run ($p = 0.042$), but not thereafter ($p = 0.247$), remained significantly associated with running performance.

Conclusion: The significant association between baseline MPV and running time suggest that hyperactive platelets may exert some pleiotropic effects on endurance performance.

Editor: Pedro Tauler, University of the Balearic Islands, Spain

Funding: The authors have no support or funding to report.

Competing Interests: The authors have declared that no competing interests exist.

* Email: glippi@ao.pr.it

Introduction

According to a recent on-line survey, recreational running is the most popular leisure sport activity, followed by lifting weights, biking, hiking and other outdoor activities [1]. More specifically, 75% of adults aged 24 to 44 years are engaged in outdoor running activities at least once a week in the US [2]. The typical middle distance runner is a "normal" trained adult subject, with few previous experiences in competitive sport and without special functional characteristics. The broad popularity of middle distance is mostly attributable to a variety of reasons, which include no need of special talent or highly-specialized and expensive equipment, and the remarkable benefits on health, fitness, stress reduction and weight control [2]. It is also noteworthy that the practice of habitual running has been associated with a significantly reduced risk of obesity, hypertension, diabetes, cardiovascular disease, cancer, osteoporosis, depression and several other chronic conditions, thus resulting in an overall 20% to 40% lower risk of mortality [3].

Both running economy and overall performance in middle distance running depend on a number of physiological factors, which are partially different from those required for short and long distance running [4,5]. The published research on half-marathon runners has mainly focused on a number of specific anthropometric variables (i.e., midaxillary skinfold, body mass index, percent body fat), functional characteristics (i.e., maximal aerobic power [VO_2max)], body core temperature), volume and intensity in training [6–8]. Despite the well-established relationship existing between packed cell volume, VO_2max, aerobic performance and maximal exercise capacity [9–11], a fact that has also contributed to the increase use of blood doping in sports during the past decades [12], there is little information about the association between hematological variables and middle distance running performance. As such, the aim of this study was to investigate whether some hematological parameters may predict half-marathon running time in a large sample of recreational runners.

Materials and Methods

The study was performed during a specific event called "Run For Science", held in Verona (Italy) in April 2014, with the purpose of analyzing the normal response of adult person to middle distance running. Forty three amateur runners were recruited (15 females and 28 males; median age 47 years and IQR 42–50 years; median body mass index 23 kg/m^2 and IQR, 22–25 kg/m^2), who successfully concluded a 21.1 km half-marathon at 75–85% of their VO_2max. All athletes were members of a non professional team, were habitually involved in recreational running (mean training regimen 222 min/week and IQR 191–253 min/week; maximal oxygen uptake 50 mL/kg/min and IQR 46–55 mL/kg/min), and had rested for not less than 36 hours before the trial. Maximal aerobic capacity was individually measured in the last two weeks before the event by a running test on a treadmill using a breath by breath ergospirometric system (Quark B2, Cosmed Italy). After appropriate familiarization, each runner underwent a progressive incremental test, starting from habitual running pace and increasing speed of 0.5 km/h every min till reaching the volitional exhaustion. None of the subjects were taking medications known to alter erythrocyte or platelet metabolism, including antiplatelet or antihypertensive drugs and erythropoiesis stimulating substances. The trial started at 9.30 AM and the 21.1 km distance was covered on a relatively flat route near Verona (35 m vertical gain, with maximal slope of 1.8%), in a partially sunny day with temperatures between 12–19°C and humidity between 55–75%. Participants were free to drink *ad libitum* during the run. Blood was drawn in primary blood tubes containing K_2EDTA (Terumo Europe N.V., Leuven, Belgium) 10 min before the start of the run and immediately thereafter (i.e., within 15 min after conclusion). The whole blood samples were immediately transported to the local laboratory under controlled conditions of temperature and humidity, where a complete blood cell count (CBC) was performed on Advia 2120 (Siemens Healthcare Diagnostics, Tarrytown NY, USA), which included measurement of hematocrit, hemoglobin, red blood cell (RBC) count, mean corpuscular volume (MCV), mean corpuscular hemoglobin (MCH), mean corpuscular hemoglobin concentration (MCHC), RBC distribution width (RDW), platelet count, mean platelet volume (MPV), white blood cell (WBC) count and differential, reticulocyte count and reticulocyte hemoglobin concentration (RetCHR). The analysis of blood specimens was concluded within 2 hours after sample collection and all results were finally expressed as median and interquartile range (IQR). Differences of pre-run and post-run values were analyzed with Wilcoxon's test for paired samples. Univariate (i.e., Spearman's correlation) and multivariate analysis (with adjustment for age, sex, blood lactate, body mass index, VO_2max, mean training regimen and CBC parameters significantly associated with running time in univariate correlation) were performed, in order to identify potential predictors of running performance. The statistical analysis was performed with Analyse-it (Analyse-it Software Ltd, Leeds, UK) for Microsoft Excel (Microsoft Corporation, Redmond, WA, USA). All subjects gave a written consent for being enrolled in this investigation. The study was approved by the local ethical committee (Department of Neurological, Neuropsychological, Morphological and Movement Sciences, University of Verona) and performed in accord with the Helsinki Declaration of 1975 (additional information can be downloaded from the institutional Website: http://www.dsnm.univr.it/?ent=iniziativa&id=5382, Last accessed, 10 October 2014).

Results

The 43 amateur runners completed the run in a median time of 113 min (IQR, 105–121 min). As predictable, the median running performance of the 28 male athletes (100 min and IQR 101–118 min) was significantly better than that of the 15 females athletes (120 min and IQR 113–123 min; $p<0.001$). The median body weight decreased by 2.2% after the run (from 73.1 to 71.5 kg; $p<0.001$). The median lactate value measured in capillary blood at the end of the run was 4.0 mmol/L (IQR, 3.0–4.9 mmol/L). The variation of the CBC parameters after the run is shown in table 1. The values of lymphocytes and eosinophils exhibited a significant decrease compared to pre-run values, whereas those of MCV, platelets, MPV, WBC, neutrophils and monocytes were found to be significantly increased after the run. In univariate analysis, significant predictors of finishing time were the pre-run values of hematocrit, hemoglobin, MCH, RDW, MPV, RetCHR, whereas the post-run values of MCH, RDW, MPV, monocytes and RetCHR were also associated with running performance (Table 2). The VO_2max was the best overall predictor of running time ($r=-0.601$; $p<0.001$), whereas neither body mass index or blood lactate at the end of the half-marathon were significantly associated with running performance (Table 2). In multivariate analysis, in which running time was entered as dependent variable whereas age, sex, blood lactate, body mass index, VO_2max, mean training regimen and the CBC parameters significantly associated with running performance in univariate analysis were entered as independent variables, only MPV values before and after the trial remained significantly associated with running time (Table 3). After adjustment for the platelet count, the MPV value before the run ($p=0.042$), but not thereafter ($p=0.247$), remained significantly associated with running performance (Fig. 1). Neither the platelet count ($r=-0.210$; $p=0.303$) or the MPV ($r=0.039$; $p=0.851$) were significantly associated with VO_2max in univariate analysis.

Discussion

Due to the increasing popularity of recreational running as a form of leisure activity and health-promoting behavior, a large number of studies have been performed over the past decades to identify the most reliable predictors of running economy and performance. The large majority of these investigations focused on anthropometric variables, functional characteristics, as well as volume and intensity of training [13]. With the notable exception of hemoglobin and packed cell volume, little information is available on other hematological parameters that may predict middle distance running performance [14]. This investigation was hence specifically planned to establish whether some hematological parameters comprised within the CBC may be significantly associated with half-marathon running time.

The leukocytes variations recorded in this study are not new, since an increase of total leukocyte, neutrophil and monocyte counts along with a decrease of lymphocyte and eosinophils values have already been reported in a number of previous investigations, and are prevalently attributable to the well-documented release of catecholamines and cortisol during exercise [8,15,16].

The significant increase of both platelet count (median increase, 17%; IQR, 10–34%) and MPV (median increase, 6%; IQR, 1–9%) recorded immediately after the half-marathon run substantially exceeded the inter-individual biological variation of these parameters (platelet count, 9.1%; MPV, 4.3%) [17], and is also consistent with the well established evidence that aerobic physical activity is effective to enhance circulating activated platelets, as well as platelet-platelet and platelet-leukocyte aggregates [18–22]. More specifically, it has been recently demonstrated that the hyperactive platelets generated during exercise are rapidly cleared by the spleen, which is also a dynamic reservoir of younger and larger platelets (i.e., the human spleen retains one-third of total body platelets, with MPV approximately 20% greater than that of circulating platelets) [23]. The younger platelets are then released into the circulation, thus explaining the significant increase of platelet count and MPV observed after endurance exercise in this and other previous studies [18–22]. Another putative mechanism that may contribute to increase the MPV has been reported by Hilberg et al. [24], who observed that moderate exercise increased both platelet reactivity and platelet-leukocyte conjugate formation, which both contribute to increase the measured value of MPV. Regardless of the underlying mechanism(s), the significant increase of MPV recorded after exercise in this and other studies [18–22] has meaningful clinical implications, suggesting that the enhanced risk of cardiovascular events that is occasionally observed in athletes may be at least in part mediated by platelet hyperreactivity [20]. Indeed, further studies are advisable to define whether an improvement of physical fitness is also accompanied with an increased MPV.

Interestingly, although the pre-run values of hematocrit, hemoglobin, MCH, RDW, MPV, RetCHR, along with the post-run values of MCH, RDW, MPV, monocytes and RetCHR were significantly associated with running time in univariate analysis, only the MPV values before and after the half-marathon remained significantly correlated with running performance in the fully-adjusted model. As predictable, both hemoglobin and hematocrit values were found to be positively correlated with running performance in univariate analysis, but the significance of these associations was lost in the fully adjusted model, especially when VO_2max was entered as covariate. This is plausible, since VO_2max and both hemoglobin and hematocrit clearly interplay in increasing sport performance, and VO_2max is in fact enhanced by approximately 1% for each 3 g/L increase of hemoglobin [25].

As such, this is the first study demonstrating a direct correlation between platelet size and endurance performance to the best of our knowledge. It is noteworthy that the inverse association between pre-run MPV value and half-marathon running time remained significant after adjustment for a number of factors such as age, sex, blood lactate, body mass index, VO_2max, mean training regimen and platelet count, thus confirming the existence of an effective interplay between platelet metabolism and aerobic performance. In univariate analysis, the correlation between running time and pre-run MPV value was the second highest overall, only preceded by that between running time and VO_2max (Table 2). In agreement with a previous study [26], neither the platelet count or the MPV at baseline were significantly associated with VO_2max, thus confirming that the influence of MPV on running performance may be virtually independent from the baseline cardiorespiratory fitness level.

An increased platelet volume is a well established surrogate marker of platelet activation, wherein large platelets are reportedly more active than small platelets [27–29]. The association of this evidence with our data would imply that platelet hyperactivity may be a significant determinant of performance in medium distance running. The use of platelets in sports medicine has risen sharply in recent times. The platelet-rich plasma (PRP), an autologous blood fraction rich in platelets and associated cytokines and growth factors, is mainly used for treatment of sports related

Table 1. Variation of the complete blood cell count after a 21.1 km half-marathon run in 43 amateur runners.

	Pre-run	Post-run	P
Hematocrit	0.45 (0.44–0.47)	0.45 (0.43–0.47)	0.420
Hemoglobin (g/L)	148 (140–155)	148 (138–155)	0.137
RBC (10^{12}/L)	4.8 (4.6–5.0)	4.8 (4.5–5.1)	0.162
MCV (fL)	94 (91–96)	95 (92–97)	**0.004**
MCH (pg)	31 (30–32)	31 (30–32)	0.400
MCHC (g/dL)	32.7 (32.4–33.2)	32.5 (3.19–3.32)	0.068
RDW (%)	13.4 (13.1–13.5)	13.5 (13.1–13.6)	**0.001**
Platelets (10^9/L)	260 (218–299)	321 (287–361)	**<0.001**
MPV (fL)	9.2 (8.6–9.8)	9.5 (8.9–10.1)	**<0.001**
WBC (10^9/L)	5.6 (4.9–6.4)	12.4 (9.8–13.9)	**<0.001**
Neutrophils (10^9/L)	3.1 (2.5–3.6)	9.3 (7.4–11.5)	**<0.001**
Lymphocytes (10^9/L)	2.0 (1.7–2.3)	1.8 (1.5–2.2)	**0.037**
Monocytes (10^9/L)	0.3 (0.2–0.4)	0.5 (0.4–0.6)	**<0.001**
Eosinophils (10^9/L)	0.2 (0.1–0.2)	0.1 (0.0–0.01)	**<0.001**
Basophils (10^9/L)	0.1 (0.1–0.1)	0.1 (0.0–0.1)	0.052
LUC (10^9/L)	0.01 (0.1–0.1)	0.01 (0.1–0.1)	0.063
Reticulocytes (10^9/L)	62 (54–74)	60 (52–73)	0.138
RetCHR (pg)	31 (31–32)	31 (31–32)	0.243

RBC, red blood cell; MCV, mean corpuscular volume; MCH, mean corpuscular hemoglobin (MCH); MCHC, mean corpuscular hemoglobin concentration; (MCHC); RDW, red blood cell distribution width; MPV, mean platelet volume (MPV); WBC, white blood cell; LUC, large unstained cells; RetCHR, reticulocyte hemoglobin concentration.

Table 2. Univariate correlation (r) analysis between running performance and parameters of the complete blood cell count in 43 amateur athletes who completed a 21.1 km half-marathon run.

	Pre-run value		Post-run value	
	r	p	r	p
Hematocrit	−0.329	**0.031**	−0.298	0.052
Hemoglobin	−0.388	**0.010**	−0.291	0.059
RBC	−0.074	0.635	−0.086	0.584
MCV	−0.234	0.131	−0.257	0.097
MCH	−0.306	**0.046**	−0.341	**0.025**
MCHC	−0.240	0.122	−0.199	0.200
RDW	0.316	**0.039**	0.336	**0.027**
Platelets	0.300	0.052	0.256	0.097
MPV	−0.450	**0.002**	−0.476	**0.001**
WBC	−0.208	0.181	0.248	0.109
Neutrophils	−0.142	0.365	0.262	0.090
Lymphocytes	−0.072	0.647	−0.028	0.861
Monocytes	−0.262	0.090	0.361	**0.017**
Eosinophils	−0.143	0.360	−0.258	0.095
Basophils	−0.096	0.538	−0.197	0.207
LUC	−0.039	0.805	0.185	0.234
Ret	0.290	0.059	0.208	0.181
RetCHR	−0.390	**0.001**	−0.379	**0.012**
Blood lactate	–	–	−0.069	0.663
Body mass index	0.092	0.555	-	-
VO2max (mL/min/Kg)	−0.601	**0.001**	-	-

RBC, red blood cell; MCV, mean corpuscular volume; MCH, mean corpuscular hemoglobin (MCH); MCHC, mean corpuscular hemoglobin concentration; (MCHC); RDW, red blood cell distribution width; MPV, mean platelet volume (MPV); WBC, white blood cell; LUC, large unstained cells; RetCHR, reticulocyte hemoglobin concentration; VO2max, maximal aerobic power.

injuries [30–32]. It was recently proven that injection of PRP may also exert some ergogenic effects. In particular, Wasterlain et al. studied the effect of PRP injection on variation of performance-enhancing systemic growth factors in 25 patients [33], and observed that the administration of PRP increased the concentration of insulin-like growth factor-1 (IGF-1), basic fibroblast growth factor (bFGF) and VEGF. Interestingly, Kasuya et al. also showed that a symptom-limited treadmill exercise test was effective to enhance the platelet release of nitric oxide (NO) [34], which would then contribute to raise exercise tolerance and performance [35].

Another mechanism by which platelets may contribute to enhance sport performance is the attenuation of neuropathic pain and/or fatigue during exercise [36]. Kennedy et al. studied platelet activation and function in 17 patients with chronic fatigue

Table 3. Multivariate correlation analysis between running performance and parameters of the complete blood cell count in 43 amateur athletes who completed a 21.1 km half-marathon run.

	Pre-run value	Post-run value
	p	p
Hematocrit	0.338	-
Hemoglobin	0.216	-
MCH	0.512	0.567
RDW	0.272	0.216
MPV	**0.042**	**0.026**
Monocytes	-	0.080
RetCHR	0.967	0.925

Results were also adjusted for age, sex, body mass index, post-run blood lactate, maximal aerobic power (VO_2max) and training regimen.
MCH, mean corpuscular hemoglobin (MCH); RDW, red blood cell distribution width; MPV, mean platelet volume (MPV); RetCHR, reticulocyte hemoglobin concentration.

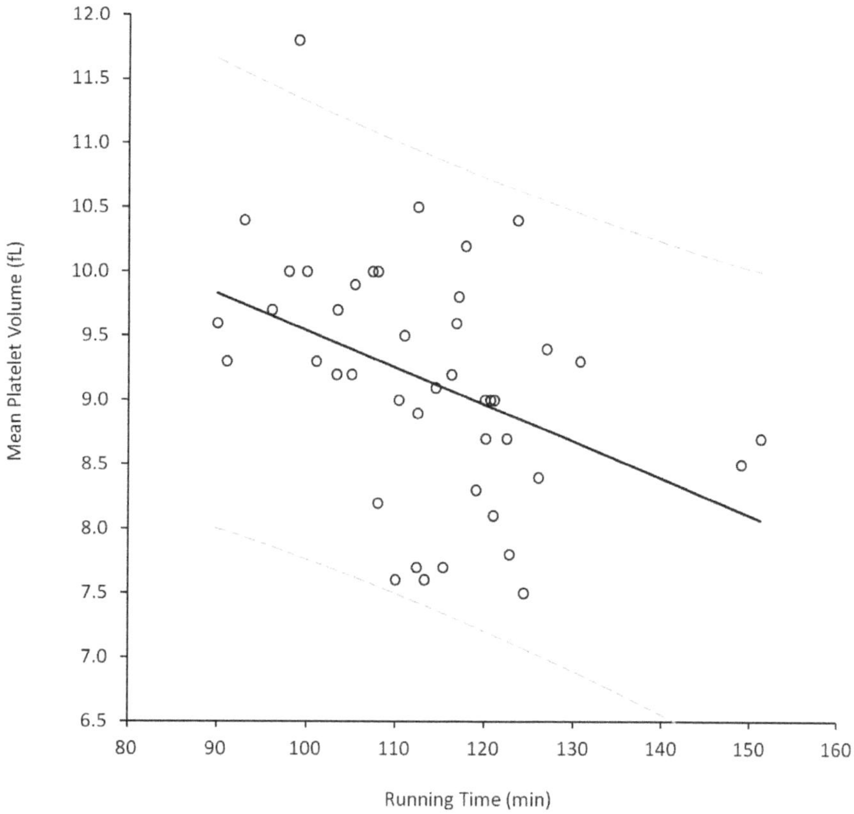

Figure 1. Correlation (and 95% prediction interval, 95% PI) between running performance and baseline value of mean platelet volume (MPV) in 43 amateur athletes completing a 21.1 km half-marathon run.

syndrome and 16 healthy controls [37], reporting that patients displayed lower platelet aggregability and reduced MPV. This would be consistent with the fact that smaller and less active platelets may somehow increase the fatigue threshold, thus conditioning exercise output. A series of studies also demonstrated that platelet gel or autologous platelet tissue graft are effective to lower pain after surgery and are associated with less pain medications and broader range of motion prior to discharge [38–40]. As specifically regards sports, the use of PRP was proven to be effective in reducing pain and promoting function improvement in tennis elbow [41] and other painful tendinopathies [42], as well as for accelerating muscle recovery after acute injury [43].

According to these evidences, it seems hence plausible that hyperactive platelets may exert some pleiotropic effects on endurance sport performance, by both releasing ergogenic mediators as well as by triggering an increase in performance-enhancing substances such as NO into the circulation. Further studies, involving also different running distances, sports and different categories of athletes are needed to confirm these findings and to elucidate the potential underlining mechanisms linking platelet volume and aerobic performance.

Author Contributions

Conceived and designed the experiments: GL CT FS. Performed the experiments: GLS ED SS. Analyzed the data: GL GLS GCG FS. Wrote the paper: GL GCG FS.

References

1. Reuters Press. Americans say they're creatures of simple, solo exercise habits. Available at: http://www.reuters.com/article/2013/09/23/us-fitness-habits-idUSBRE98M0KN20130923. Accessed: 16 August 2014.
2. Knechtle B, Barandun U, Knechtle P, Zingg MA, Rosemann T, et al. (2014) Prediction of half-marathon race time in recreational female and male runners. Springerplus 3:248.
3. Kokkinos P, Myers J (2010) Exercise and physical activity: clinical outcomes and applications. Circulation 122:1637–1648.
4. Brandon LJ (1995) Physiological factors associated with middle distance running performance. Sports Med 19:268–277.
5. Saunders PU, Pyne DB, Telford RD, Hawley JA (2004) Factors affecting running economy in trained distance runners. Sports Med 34:465–485.
6. Williams C, Nute ML (1983) Some physiological demands of a half-marathon race on recreational runners. Br J Sports Med 1983;17:152–161.
7. Knechtle B, Knechtle P, Barandun U, Rosemann T (2011) Anthropometric and training variables related to half-marathon running performance in recreational female runners. Phys Sportsmed 39:158–166.
8. Del Coso J, Fernández D, Abián-Vicen J, Salinero JJ, González-Millán C, et al. (2013) Running pace decrease during a marathon is positively related to blood markers of muscle damage. PLoS One 8:e57602.
9. Kanstrup IL, Ekblom B (1984) Blood volume and hemoglobin concentration as determinants of maximal aerobic power. Med Sci Sports Exerc 16:256–262.
10. Joyner MJ (2003) VO2MAX, blood doping, and erythropoietin. Br J Sports Med 37:190–191.
11. Calbet JA, Lundby C, Koskolou M, Boushel R (2006) Importance of hemoglobin concentration to exercise: acute manipulations. Respir Physiol Neurobiol 151:132–140.
12. Lippi G, Franchini M, Salvagno GL, Guidi GC (2006) Biochemistry, physiology, and complications of blood doping: facts and speculation. Crit Rev Clin Lab Sci 43:349–391.

13. Midgley AW, McNaughton LR, Jones AM (2007) Training to enhance the physiological determinants of long-distance running performance: can valid recommendations be given to runners and coaches based on current scientific knowledge? Sports Med 37:857–880.
14. Joyner MJ, Coyle EF (2008) Endurance exercise performance: the physiology of champions. J Physiol 586:35–44.
15. Lippi G, Schena F, Salvagno GL, Aloe R, Banfi G, et al. (2010) Foot-strike haemolysis after a 60-km ultramarathon. Blood Transfus 10:377–383.
16. Lippi G, Salvagno GL, Danese E, Tarperi C, Guidi GC, et al. (2014) Variation of Red Blood Cell Distribution Width and Mean Platelet Volume after Moderate Endurance Exercise. Adv Hematol 2014:192173. doi:10.1155/2014/192173.
17. Ricós C, Alvarez V, Cava F, García-Lario JV, Hernández A, et al. (1999) Current databases on biological variation: pros, cons and progress. Scand J Clin Lab Invest 59:491–500.
18. Knudsen JB, Brodthagen U, Gormsen J, Jordal R, Nørregaard-Hansen K, et al. (1982) Platelet function and fibrinolytic activity following distance running. Scand J Haematol 29:425–430.
19. Yilmaz MB, Saricam E, Biyikoglu SF, Guray Y, Guray U, et al. (2004) Mean platelet volume and exercise stress test. J Thromb Thrombolysis 17:115–120.
20. Li N, He S, Blombäck M, Hjemdahl P (2007) Platelet activity, coagulation, and fibrinolysis during exercise in healthy males: effects of thrombin inhibition by argatroban and enoxaparin. Arterioscler Thromb Vasc Biol 27:407–413.
21. Whittaker JP, Linden MD, Coffey VG (2013) Effect of aerobic interval training and caffeine on blood platelet function. Med Sci Sports Exerc 45:342–350.
22. Kahan T, Schwieler JH, Wallén H, Nussberger J, Hjemdahl P (2013) Platelet activation during exercise is not attenuated by inhibition of the renin angiotensin system: the role of physical activity. J Hypertens 31:2103–2104.
23. Bakovic D, Pivac N, Eterovic D, Breskovic T, Zubin P, et al. (2013) The effects of low-dose epinephrine infusion on spleen size, central and hepatic circulation and circulating platelets. Clin Physiol Funct Imaging 33:30–37.
24. Hilberg T, Menzel K, Gläser D, Zimmermann S, Gabriel HH (2008) Exercise intensity: platelet function and platelet-leukocyte conjugate formation in untrained subjects. Thromb Res 122:77–84.
25. Otto JM, Montgomery HE, Richards T (2013) Haemoglobin concentration and mass as determinants of exercise performance and of surgical outcome. Extrem Physiol Med 2:33.
26. Cho HC, Kim J, Kim S, Son YH, Lee N, et al. (2012) The concentrations of serum, plasma and platelet BDNF are all increased by treadmill VO_2max performance in healthy college men. Neurosci Lett 519:78–83.
27. Guthikonda S, Alviar CL, Vaduganathan M, Arikan M, Tellez A, et al. (2008) Role of reticulated platelets and platelet size heterogeneity on platelet activity after dual antiplatelet therapy with aspirin and clopidogrel in patients with stable coronary artery disease. J Am Coll Cardiol 52:743–749.
28. Mangalpally KK, Siqueiros-Garcia A, Vaduganathan M, Dong JF, Kleiman NS, et al. (2010) Platelet activation patterns in platelet size sub-populations: differential responses to aspirin in vitro. J Thromb Thrombolysis 30:251–262.
29. Colkesen Y, Muderrisoglu H (2012) The role of mean platelet volume in predicting thrombotic events. Clin Chem Lab Med 50:631–634.
30. Mei-Dan O, Lippi G, Sánchez M, Andia I, Maffulli N (2010) Autologous platelet-rich plasma: a revolution in soft tissue sports injury management? Phys Sportsmed 38:127–135.
31. Mishra A, Harmon K, Woodall J, Vieira A (2012) Sports medicine applications of platelet rich plasma. Curr Pharm Biotechnol 13:1185–1195.
32. World Anti-Doping Agency. The 2014 Prohibited List. International Standard. Available at: http://list.wada-ama.org/. Accessed: 16 August 2014.
33. Wasterlain AS, Braun HJ, Harris AH, Kim HJ, Dragoo JL (2013) The systemic effects of platelet-rich plasma injection. Am J Sports Med 41:186–193.
34. Kasuya N, Kishi Y, Sakita SY, Numano F, Isobe M (2002) Acute vigorous exercise primes enhanced NO release in human platelets. Atherosclerosis 161:225–232.
35. Jones AM (2013) Dietary nitrate supplementation and exercise performance. Sports Med 44 Suppl 1:S35–45.
36. Kuffler DP (2013) Platelet-rich plasma and the elimination of neuropathic pain. Mol Neurobiol 48:315–332.
37. Kennedy G, Norris G, Spence V, McLaren M, Belch JJ (2006) Is chronic fatigue syndrome associated with platelet activation? Blood Coagul Fibrinolysis 17:89–92.
38. Gardner MJ, Demetrakopoulos D, Klepchick PR, Mooar PA (2007) The efficacy of autologous platelet gel in pain control and blood loss in total knee arthroplasty. An analysis of the haemoglobin, narcotic requirement and range of motion. Int Orthop 31:309–313.
39. Everts PA, Devilee RJ, Brown Mahoney C, van Erp A, Oosterbos CJ, et al. (2008) Exogenous application of platelet-leukocyte gel during open subacromial decompression contributes to improved patient outcome. A prospective randomized double-blind study. Eur Surg Res 40:203–210.
40. Fanning J, Murrain L, Flora R, Hutchings T, Johnson JM, et al. (2007) Phase I/II prospective trial of autologous platelet tissue graft in gynecologic surgery. J Minim Invasive Gynecol 14:633–637.
41. Raeissadat SA, Sedighipour L, Rayegani SM, Bahrami MH, Bayat M, et al. (2014) Effect of Platelet-Rich Plasma (PRP) versus Autologous Whole Blood on Pain and Function Improvement in Tennis Elbow: A Randomized Clinical Trial. Pain Res Treat 2014:191525.
42. Andia I, Latorre PM, Gomez MC, Burgos-Alonso N, Abate M, et al. (2014) Platelet-rich plasma in the conservative treatment of painful tendinopathy: a systematic review and meta-analysis of controlled studies. Br Med Bull 110:99–115.
43. Hamid MS, Yusof A, Mohamed Ali MR (2014) Platelet-rich plasma (PRP) for acute muscle injury: a systematic review. PLoS One 9:e90538.

Anti-Atherogenic Effect of Hydrogen Sulfide by Over-Expression of Cystathionine Gamma-Lyase (CSE) Gene

Sau Ha Cheung[1], Wai Kei Kwok[1], Ka Fai To[2], James Yun Wong Lau[1]*

1 Department of Surgery, Faculty of Medicine, the Chinese University of Hong Kong, Hong Kong SAR, People's Republic of China, 2 Department of Anatomical and Cellular Pathology, Faculty of Medicine, the Chinese University of Hong Kong, Hong Kong SAR, People's Republic of China

Abstract

Hydrogen sulfide (H_2S) is an important gaseous signaling molecule that functions in physiological and pathological conditions, such as atherosclerosis. H_2S dilates vessels and therefore has been suggested as an anti-atherogenic molecule. Since cystathionine gamma-lyase (CSE) enzyme is responsible for producing H_2S in the cardiovascular system, we hypothesized that up-regulation of CSE expression *in vivo* with preservation of H_2S bioactivity can slow down plaque formation and, can serve as a therapeutic strategy against atherosclerosis. In this study, C57BL/6 wild type mice (WT), ApoE knockout mice (KO) and transgenic ApoE knockout mice overexpressing CSE (Tg/KO) at four weeks of age were weaned. They were then fed with either normal or atherogenic diet for 12 weeks. At week 16, serial plasma lipid levels, body weight, and blood pressure were measured prior to euthanization of the mice and the size of atherosclerotic plaques at their aortic roots was measured. Tg/KO mice showed an increase in endogenous H_2S production in aortic tissue, reduced atherosclerotic plaque sizes and attenuation in plasma lipid profiles. We also showed an up-regulation in plasma glutathione peroxidase that could indicate reduced oxidative stress. Furthermore, there was an increase in expression of p-p53 and down regulation of inflammatory nuclear factor-kappa B (NF-κB) in aorta. To conclude, alteration of endogenous H_2S by CSE gene activation was associated with reduced atherosclerosis in ApoE-deficient mice. Up-regulation of CSE/H_2S pathway attenuates atherosclerosis and this would be a potential target for therapeutic intervention against its formation.

Editor: John Calvert, Emory University, United States of America

Funding: This work was funded by the Focused Investment Scheme, the Chinese University of Hong Kong (Project number 1903018) and it was received by JYWL. The funders had no role in study design, data collection and analysis, decision to publish, or preparation of the manuscript.

Competing Interests: The authors have declared that no competing interests exist.

* Email: laujyw@surgery.cuhk.edu.hk

Introduction

Atherosclerosis is an inflammatory process that takes place in medium and large sized arteries. It is characterized by plaque formation on the endothelial wall, causing hardening and narrowing of arteries. The process is initiated by accumulation of fatty materials such as cholesterol and triglyceride. Lipid deposition in arteries triggers proliferation of vascular smooth muscle cells (VSMCs) and results in recruitment of circulating inflammatory cells [1]. Macrophages and smooth muscle cells (SMCs) then engulf lipids to form foam cells. With disease progression, VSMCs migrate to intima to form necrotic core which is surrounded by a fibrous cap consisting of VSMCs, collagen and other extracellular matrix (ECM). Plaque rupture occurs by induction of apoptosis of VSMCs and breakdown of collagen and ECM. This causes cerebral or cardiac events [2].

Hydrogen sulfide (H_2S) is a gaso-transmitter along with nitric oxide (NO) and carbon monoxide (CO) [3]. Similar to nitric oxide, H_2S is a potent vasodilator [4] and possesses vasoprotective effects, such as reduction of VSMC proliferations [5]. Cystathionine gamma-lyase (CSE) is one of the key enzymes producing endogenous H_2S and is expressed abundantly in mammalian cardiovascular system [6]. Recently, *in vitro* and *in vivo* studies were carried out to investigate the role of H_2S in the pathogenesis of atherosclerosis. Deficiency of H_2S appears to accelerate atherosclerosis. CSE-knockout mice were shown to have lower aortic H_2S production [7] and were found to develop early fatty streak lesions in the aortic root, elevated plasma levels of cholesterol and low-density lipoprotein cholesterol, hyperhomocysteinemia, increased lesional oxidative stress and adhesion molecule expression, as well as enhanced aortic intimal proliferation after being fed with atherogenic diet [8]. On the contrary, supplementation with H_2S inhibits atherosclerosis. It was found that H_2S inhibited ICAM-1 expression in TNFα-induced HUVECs via the NF-κB pathway in ApoE knockout mice [9] and induced superoxide dismutase (SOD) expression, accompanied by a reduced level of reactive oxygen species (ROS) [10]. H_2S also inhibited macrophage infiltration and reduced lesion size by down-regulation of CX3CR1 and CX3CL1 in macrophages [11,12]. A recent report also showed that ApoE knockout mice with a H_2S-releasing drug administration can decrease vascular inflammation and oxidative stress together with improved endothelial function and reduced atherosclerotic plaque formation [13].

Thus far, the relationship between the metabolism of H_2S and atherosclerosis has been evidenced using CSE knockout mice. CSE gene deletion led to decrease of H_2S production with accelerated atherosclerosis [8] and this can be ameliorated by treatment with NaHS or exogenous H_2S donor [8]. However, this is not clear because the proximal regulation of H_2S at physiological level and toxicological level is ambiguous. Moreover, the *in vivo* level of H_2S is hard to be manipulated since the release of H_2S by exogenous H_2S donor may be time-dependent and/or dose-dependent [14]. CSE inducers or stimulators can be used but little is known.

Therefore, in this study, we hypothesize that endogenous H_2S can alter the development of atherosclerosis by *in vivo* overexpression of CSE. In addition, *in vivo* overexpression of CSE increases endogenous hydrogen sulfide production. Up-regulation of CSE/H_2S system may inhibit atherosclerosis.

Materials and Methods

Animals and Diets

All animal experiments were approved by the Animal Experimentation Ethics Committee (AEEC) of the Chinese University of Hong Kong (Reference Number: 10/083/MIS) and in accordance with the Animals (Control of Experiments) Ordinance (Cap. 340) licensed from the Hong Kong Government Department of Health. ApoE knockout with C57BL/6 background (KO) mice (The Jackson Laboratory, USA) and transgenic (Tg) mice overexpressing cardiac-specific CSE with C57BL/6 background (from Professor Lefer, Emory University School of Medicine) were crossed to generate CSE transgenic ApoE KO mice, i.e. Tg(CSE)$^{+/0}$ApoE$^{-/-}$ mice (Tg/KO). In the present study, Tg/KO littermates were first characterized and confirmed by genotyping before treatment. Mouse tail of littermates was used for the genotyping using Mouse Genotyping Kit (KAPA Biosystems, Woburn, MA, USA). Genotyping for ApoE locus was done according to the provided by the Jackson Laboratory with the use of the forward primer oIMR0180 5′-CCTAGCCGAGGGAGAGCCG-3′, together with the 2 reverse primers oIMR0181 5′-TGTGACTTGGGAGCTCTGCAGC-3′ and oIMR0182 5′-GCCGCCCCGACTGCATCT-3′ where oIMR0180 and oIMR0181 amplify a 155-bp fragment of the WT locus (ApoE$^{+/+}$), and oIMR0180 and oIMR0182 amplify a 245-bp fragment from the targeted allele (ApoE$^{-/-}$). The MHC-CSE transgene was confirmed by PCR reaction using forward primer 5′-TGTTGGATTTCCAGAGCGGCTGTA-3′ and reverse primer 5′-TCTTAGCAAACCTCAGGCACCCTT-3′ to amplify a 420-bp transgene (Tg(CSE)$^{+/0}$).

C57BL/6 mice (WT), ApoE$^{-/-}$ mice (KO) and Tg(CSE)$^{+/0}$ ApoE$^{-/-}$ mice (Tg/KO) were housed in a temperature-controlled room with free access to food and water and maintained on a 12-h light/dark cycle. At 4 weeks of age, mice were weaned and fed either normal diet (Harlan Laboratories, Madison, WI, USA) or atherogenic diet (MP Biomedicals, Aurora, OH, USA) for 3 months. Body weight of each mouse was recorded every week and the weight gain was calculated at the end of the study. Daily food intake to both groups of mice was measured for a week. Blood pressure was also measured at the end of the study using a non-invasive computerized tail cuff system (Kent Scientific Corporation, Litchfield, CT, USA). 6 readings were taken and an average of readings was used. The mice were euthanized at the age of 16 weeks for isolation of tissue for examinations. They were first anaesthetized by injection of ketamine (50 mg/kg im), followed by immediate termination. All efforts were made to minimize suffering.

CSE Quantitation by RT-PCR

Total RNA from aorta and heart tissue were separately homogenized and extracted with Trizol reagent (Invitrogen, Burlington, Ontario, Canada) according to the manufacturer's protocol. The concentration of total RNA was determined by Nanodrop ND-1000 Spectrophotometer (Thermo Fisher Scientific, DE, USA). cDNA synthesis was performed according to the protocol provided with M-MLV reverse transcriptase (Promega Corporation, WI, USA) using 200 units of enzyme, 0.5 μg of random primers (Invitrogen, USA) as primers, and 1 μg of RNA. Real time RT-PCR was carried out using aorta cDNA as template and analyzed in an ABI 7500 Fast Real-Time PCR Systems (Applied Biosystems, Foster City, CA, USA) using fluorescent TaqMan methodology. Real time quantitative RT-PCR was performed using ready-to-use primer and probe sets pre-developed by Applied Biosystems (TaqMan Gene Expression Assays) to quantify mouse CSE and mouse Glyceraldehyde-3-phosphate dehydrogenase (GAPDH). mRNA Ct values for these genes were analyzed on SDS v1.4 Software (Applied Biosystems) and normalized to the house-keeping gene GAPDH. Expression of CSE gene was then validated by running the PCR products on a 2% (w/v) agarose gel.

Protein Expression in Aorta by Western Blotting

Mice aorta was lysed at 4°C in radio-immunoprecipitation assay (RIPA) lysis buffer. The lysate was clarified by centrifugation at 14,000 g for 15 min at 4°C. Protein concentration in the supernatant was determined by BCA protein assay kit (Pierce Biotechnology, IL, USA). Protein samples (50 μg) were separated by 10% SDS-PAGE and then transferred into nitrocellulose membranes (Bio-rad Laboratory, Hercules CA, USA). The membrane was blocked with 3% bovine serum albumin (BSA) in Tris buffered saline (TBS)-Tween buffer and then probed overnight at 4°C with anti-CSE (1:1000; Abnova, Taipei City, Taiwan), anti-phosphorylated p53 (1:1000; Cell Signaling Technology, Danvers, MA, USA), anti-IKK (1:1000, Cell Signaling Technology, Danvers, MA, USA), anti-IκBα (1:1000, Cell Signaling Technology, Danvers, MA, USA), anti-NF-κB p65 (1:1000, Cell Signaling Technology, Danvers, MA, USA) and anti-GAPDH (1:2000; Santa Cruz Biotechnology, CA, USA). It was followed by secondary antibody for 1 h with a 1:2000 dilution of horseradish peroxidase (HRP)-conjugated, goat anti-mouse IgG (Cell Signaling Technology, Danvers, MA, USA) or goat anti-rabbit IgG (Cell Signaling Technology, Danvers, MA, USA). After washing, the membrane was developed with ECL kit (Amersham Pharmacia Biotechnology, Buckinghamshire, UK) and exposed to X-ray films (Amersham Pharmacia Biotechnology, Buckinghamshire, UK). Intensity of bands was quantified using the public domain software, ImageJ software.

Determination of Plasma Lipids and Adiponectin

Mice were fasted for 16 to 20 h prior to sacrifice. Blood samples were drawn by cardiac puncture using 25G needle mounted on a 1 ml syringe and were collected in EDTA tube. Plasma was separated by centrifugation at 2000 g for 10 min and stored at −80°C. Plasma lipid concentrations including total cholesterol and low-density lipoprotein (LDL) cholesterol were measured by quantitative colorimetric techniques according to the manufacturer's procedures (BioAssay Systems, CA, USA). Plasmatic triglyceride level was determined by another commercial assay kit (Wako Pure Chemical Industries Ltd., Osaka, Japan). We measured adiponectin in plasma using an enzyme-linked immunoassay (SPI-BIO Co., Montigny-le-Bretonneux, France).

Hydrogen Sulfide Production in Heart Tissues

Synthesis of hydrogen sulfide (H_2S) in heart tissue homogenates was measured as described by Wallace group [15] with some modifications. Mice heart was quickly isolated and snap-frozen.

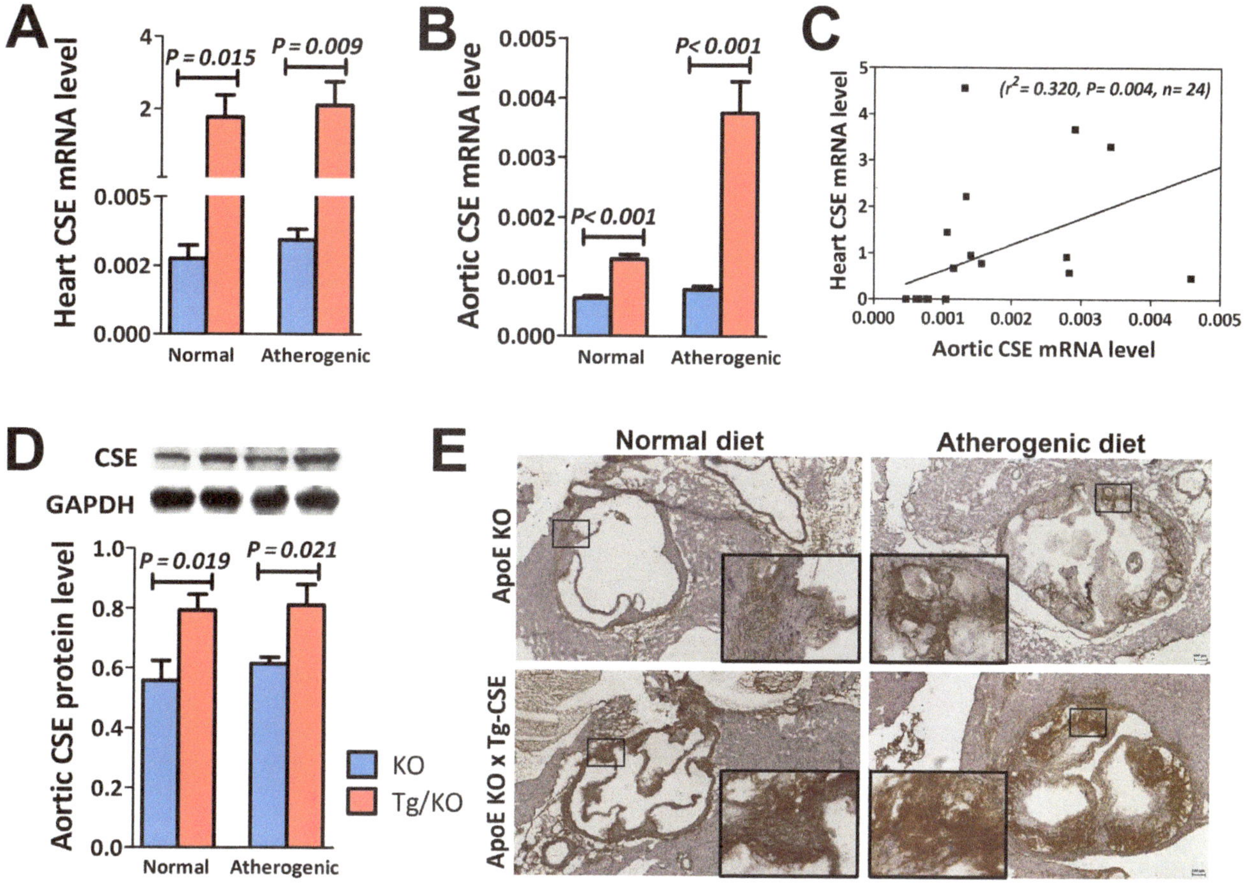

Figure 1. CSE expression in heart and aorta. CSE mRNA levels of (A) heart tissue (n = 6) and (B) aorta (n = 6) in Tg/KO mice were increased when compared to KO mice. (C) The relationship between the heart CSE mRNA level and aortic mRNA level was significantly positive correlated. (D) Besides, protein level (n = 6) was significantly increased in aorta homogenates of Tg/KO mice on either normal or atherogenic diet. (E) Representative immunohistochemical staining also indicated higher CSE expression in aorta root in Tg/KO mice as compared to the KO mice in both diets (Magnification 4×; Insert magnification 20×).

Heart tissue was homogenized in tissue protein extraction reagent (Thermo Pierce, Rockford, IL, USA). The homogenate (0.55 ml) and buffer (0.45 ml) were then cooled on ice for 10 min before l-cysteine (50 µmol/L) and pyridoxal 5′-phosphate (10 mmol/L) were added. The final volume was 1 ml. A smaller 0.5-ml eppendorf containing a piece of filter paper (0.5×2.5 cm) soaked with zinc acetate (1%; 0.5 ml) was put inside the larger vial. The vials were then flushed with nitrogen gas for 20 sec and capped with an airtight serum cap. The vials were then transferred to a 37°C shaking bath for 5 h and stopped by injection of trichloroacetic acid (TCA; 50%; 0.5 ml) into the reaction mixture through the serum cap. The mixture was left to stand for another

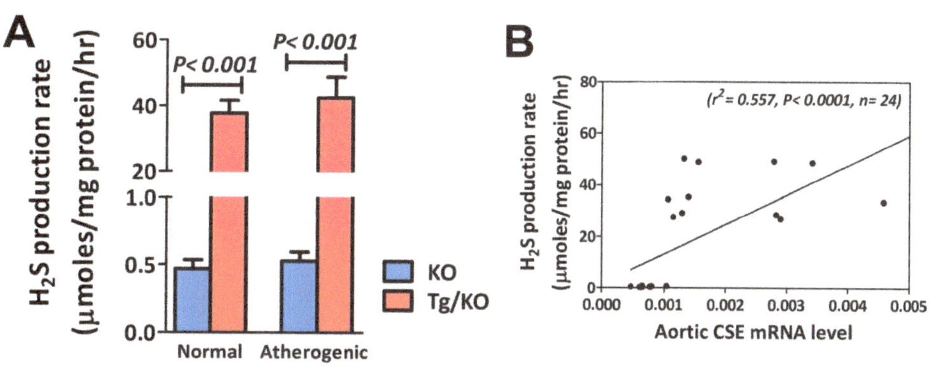

Figure 2. Direct relationship between aortic CSE expression and H_2S production. (A) With overexpression of CSE gene in Tg/KO mice, H_2S production in heart was considerably up-regulated (n = 6). (B) Direct relationship between aorta CSE expression and heart H_2S generation was also revealed, showing significant positive correlation between them.

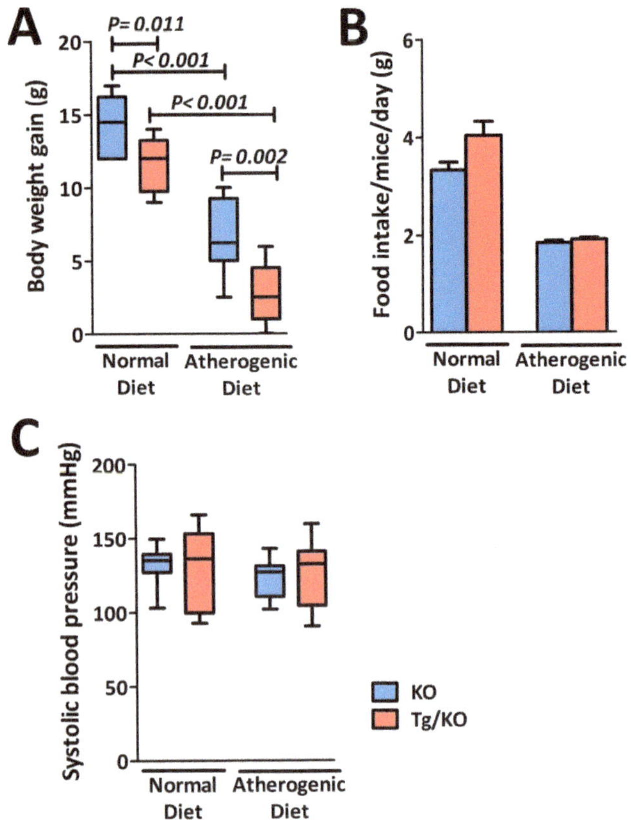

Figure 3. Body weight and systolic blood pressure in CSE transgenic ApoE-KO (Tg/KO) mice. (A) Body weight gain changes during the feeding periods with different diets. Both KO and Tg/KO mice (n = 10) showed increase of body weights with same diet but the weight gain was significantly different. Mice fed with normal diet had higher weight gain than that with atherogenic diet. Moreover, it also showed that Tg/KO mice had fewer weight gains in both normal and atherogenic diets as compared to KO mice. (B) Daily food intake was similar in both KO and Tg/KO (n = 6). (C) Both KO and Tg/KO mice (n = 10) did not have significantly change with the systolic blood pressure, indicating that Tg/KO mice did not cause hypotension after insertion of CSE gene.

60 min to allow for the trapping of evolved H_2S by the Zinc acetate. The serum cap was then removed and N, N-dimethyl-p-phenylenediamine sulfate (20 mmol/L; 50 µl) in 7.2 mol/L HCl and $FeCl_3$ (30 mmol/L; 50 µl) in 1.2 mol/L HCl were added to the inner tube. After 20 min, absorbance at 670 nm was measured with a microplate reader (Bio-Tek Instrument INC., Rockville, MD, USA). The calibration curve of absorbance versus H_2S concentration was obtained by using NaHS solution of varying concentrations (0 to 320 µm). Results were then corrected for the protein content of the tissue sample and expressed as µmoles H_2S generated/mg protein/h.

Quantitation of Atherosclerotic Lesion

To quantify the atherosclerotic lesions in the aortic root, upper part of heart was cut in the ascending aorta and the proximal sample containing the aortic sinus was embedded in Tissue Tek OCT (Optimal Cutting Temperature) compound (Miles Scientific, Naperville, IL, USA) and then stored at −80°C. Serial cryostat sections (6 µm) were prepared on a cryostat (Leica Microsystems, Buffalo, NY, USA). In brief, atherosclerotic lesions in the aortic root were examined at 6 locations and each separated by 90 µm, 9 serial sections were prepared from each location. These sections were stained with oil red O and counterstained with Mayer's hematoxylin. Whole slide images were produced with Leica SCN400 slide scanner (Leica Biosystems, Buffalo Grove, IL, USA), managed with the image server, Digital Image Hub (Leica Biosystems). In each case, average value for 3 serial sections at each of 6 locations of each animal was used for analysis. The lipid composition of the lesion was determined by calculating the percent of the oil red O positive area to the area of aorta root using the public domain software, ImageJ software. The area of aorta root was manually selected and the positive stained area within the aorta root was measured by adjusting the threshold value. The remaining sections were used for immunohistochemical analysis as described below.

Immunohistochemistry of CSE in Aortic Roots

Air-dried cryostat sections (6 µm thickness) of aortic root were fixed with the pre-cooled acetone for 10 min at room temperature and rinsed with PBS three times. Endogenous peroxidase activity was inactivated by treatment in 3% H_2O_2 for 10 min, followed by a wash in PBS. Non-specific staining was blocked by incubation with 2% goat serum in PBS for 30 min and washed in PBS. Slides were then incubated with primary antibody, anti- CSE (Santa Cruz Biotechnology, CA, USA) in a 1:50 dilution at 4°C overnight, followed by secondary antibody in a 1:200 dilution of HRP-conjugated, anti-goat IgG (Cell Signaling Technology, Danvers, MA, USA) for 1 h at room temperature. Immunohistochemical staining was developed by exposure to 3,3′-diaminobenzidine (DAB) and counterstaining was performed with hematoxylin. Whole slide images were produced as described above.

Oxidative Stress Measurement

Commercially available glutathionine peroxidase (GPx) assay kit (Cayman Chemical Company, MI, USA) was used to measure plasma GPx activity according to the manufacturer's instruction. Glutathione and total glutathione were measured using glutathione colorimetric assay (BioVision Incorporated, CA, USA).

Statistical Analysis

All data are presented as the mean ± SEM. Non-parametric t-test was used to compare variables between two groups. For the correlation study, for example CSE expression versus total cholesterol and H_2S production rate versus NF-κB expression, was performed by simple linear regression analysis. For all tests, $P<0.05$ was considered statistically significant. A complete list of the underlying data set was shown in Table S1.

Results

Role of CSE Expression in Hydrogen Sulfide Production Rate in Heart

To investigate the effect of aortic CSE gene activation on endogenous H_2S production in mice heart, CSE expression levels and H_2S production were assessed in CSE transgenic ApoE-KO (Tg/KO) mice and ApoE-KO (KO) mice fed with both normal and atherogenic diets for 12 weeks. As illustrated in Figure 1, CSE gene was detected in heart tissue (Figure 1A) as well as in aorta (Figure 1B). The association of CSE mRNA expression between the heart tissue and aorta was found positive correlated (Figure 1C). This indicates that overexpression of CSE gene can cause an increase of CSE expression in aorta. We then examined CSE protein level in aorta. The protein by western blotting was around 1.3 fold increased (Figure 1D) in Tg/KO mice as

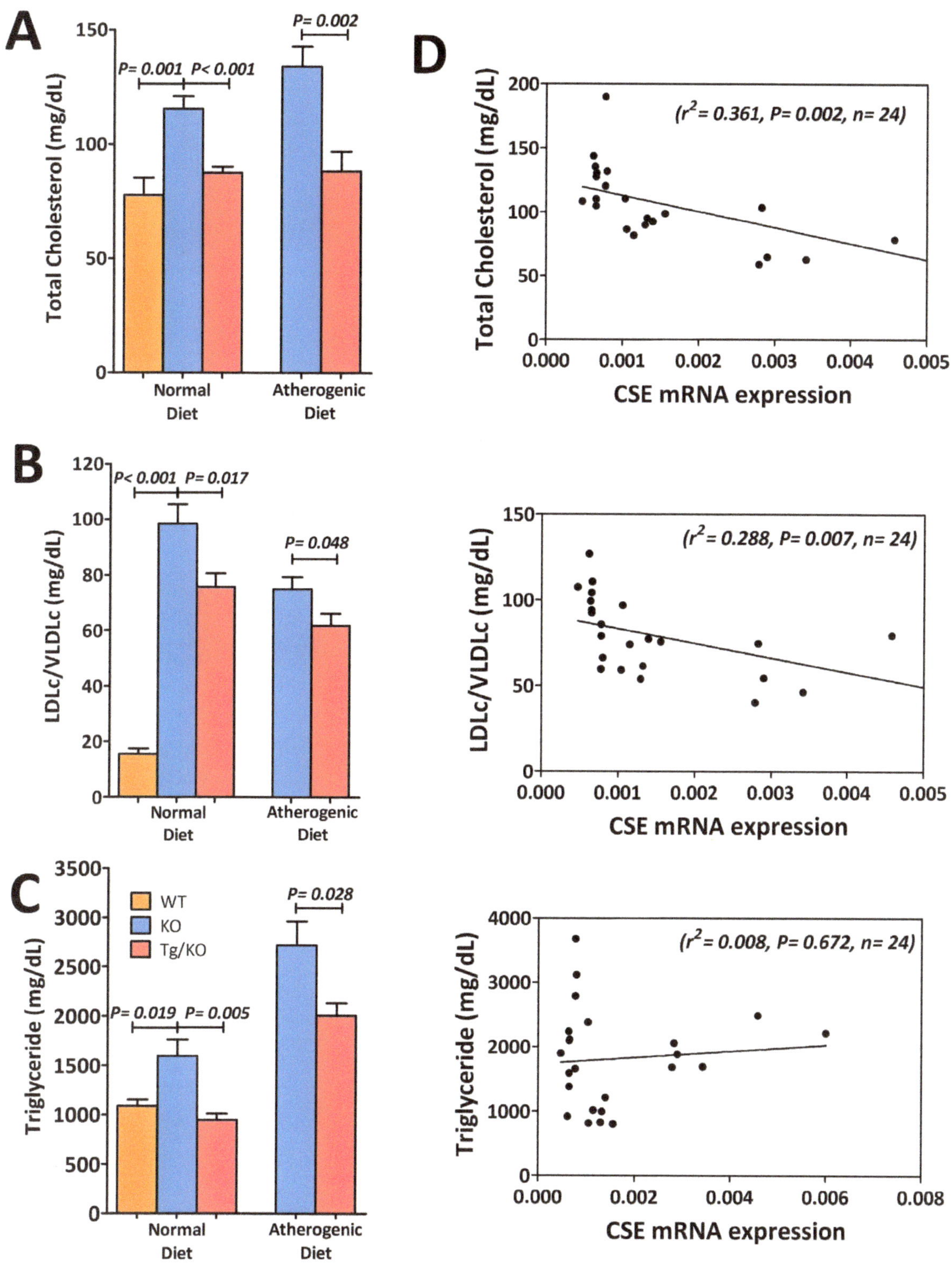

Figure 4. Anti-atherogenic effect of CSE gene activation with higher H_2S production. (A) Plasma total cholesterol (n = 8 to 10), (B) LDL/VLDL cholesterol (n = 8 to 10) and (C) triglyceride level (n = 6) were significantly reduced in Tg/KO mice after feeding with 12 weeks of normal diet or atherogenic diet when comparing to KO mice. (D) Relationship between aortic CSE mRNA expression level and levels of plasma lipids. There was a significant negative relationship between CSE mRNA expression and levels of total cholesterol and LDL/VLDL cholesterol. However, its relationship with triglyceride was not statistically significant.

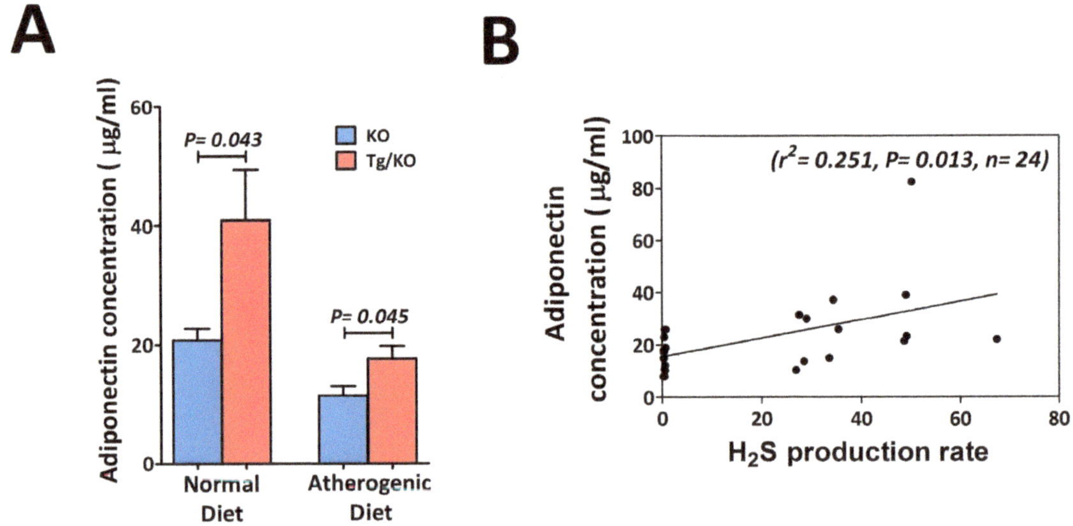

Figure 5. Increased plasma level of adipinectin in CSE transgenic ApoE-KO (Tg/KO) mice. (A) Plasma adiponectin level (n = 6) was higher in Tg/KO mice when compared to the KO mice in both diets. (B) Relationship between plasma level of adiponectin and H_2S production rate was positively correlated.

compared to the corresponding KO mice. Using immunohistochemistry, expression of CSE was detected in the aorta root. CSE was abundantly expressed in aorta of Tg/KO mice in both diets (Figure 1E). To elucidate the role of CSE in H_2S production, H_2S generation from heart was also markedly elevated in Tg/KO mice fed with either normal or atherogenic diets (Figure 2A). The relationship between aorta CSE expression and H_2S production rate from heart also illustrated. There was a significant positive correlation between the aorta CSE expression and the H_2S production in heart (Figure 2B). This indicates that CSE gene is the vital enzyme for the H_2S production in cardiovascular system.

Body weight and blood pressure

During the 12 weeks of diet treatment, both KO and Tg/KO mice increased in their body weight. But their weight gain was significantly reduced once the diets switched from normal to atherogenic at 4 weeks of age (Figure 3A). When comparing Tg/KO mice with KO mice with the same diet, the average weight gain by Tg/KO mice was significant less by about 3 grams (Figure 3A). To demonstrate whether caloric restriction Tg/KO mice could account for cardioprotective effect, food consumption by KO and Tg/KO mice was measured (Table S2). Both KO and Tg/KO mice consumed less in atherogenic diet (Figure 3B). Moreover, the two groups did not differ in the amount of food intake (Figure 3B). Since KO mice shows hypertension in comparison with WT mice groups, it was suspected that overexpression of CSE may lower blood pressure or even cause hypotension in Tg/KO mice. As shown in Figure 3C, CSE gene activation did not significantly change the blood pressure of Tg/KO mice fed with either normal or atherogenic diets. CSE does not appear to affect blood pressure in these mice. Instead, blood pressure seemed to be affected by the level of cholesterol. As shown in Figure 4A, although the total cholesterol of Tg/KO mice was reduced when compared to the KO mice, it was not as low as that of the WT mice.

Anti-atherogenic effects of CSE/H_2S

With the increase of endogenous H_2S, plasma total cholesterol (Figure 4A), LDL/VLDL cholesterol (Figure 4B) and triglyceride (Figure 4C) levels were lowered by 24.1%, 23.1% and 40.7% in respectively in mice fed with normal diet. In mice fed with atherogenic diet, the corresponding decrease were 34.1%, 17.4% and 26.3% respectively. Figure 4D showed that there was a significant negative relationship between aortic CSE expression level and both total cholesterol and LDL/VLDL cholesterol. However, its relationship with triglyceride was not statistically significant. Tg/KO mice were found to have higher plasma adiponectin level as compared to KO mice (Figure 5A). The plasma adiponectin level was positively correlated to the H_2S production (Figure 5B). On the other hand, it was expected that the oxidative stress would be reduced due to the reduced level of LDL/VLDL cholesterol. Therefore, plasma glutathione peroxidase (GPx) activity was determined. In association with attenuation of lipids, markedly elevated plasma GPx activity (Figure 6A), glutathione (GSH) (Figure 6B) and total glutathione/oxidized glutathione (GSH and GSSG) (Figure 6C) were observed in Tg/KO mice fed with both diets, demonstrating that cells are protected from oxidative damages. Overexpression of CSE can help improving plasma lipids and reducing oxidative stress.

CSE overexpression decelerated atherosclerotic development

To gain further insight on the functional role of CSE on the atherosclerosis development, fatty lipids in aorta root were stained with oil red O to show the extent of lesion area in KO mice and Tg/KO mice. As demonstrated in Figure 7A, KO mice fed atherogenic diet for 12 weeks showed significantly more aortic oil red O staining as compared to the KO mice fed with normal diet. Interestingly, Tg/KO mice fed with either normal or atherogenic diet showed diminished of aortic lipid deposition by approximate 50% as comparing with KO mice fed with the same chow (Figure 7B). To show whether overexpression of CSE could reduce lesion area in aorta, correlation between the CSE mRNA expression in aorta and aortic lesion area was performed in respect to different diets. It was shown that activation of CSE gene can significantly attenuate plaque accumulation in aorta in both normal and atherogenic diets (Figure 7C).

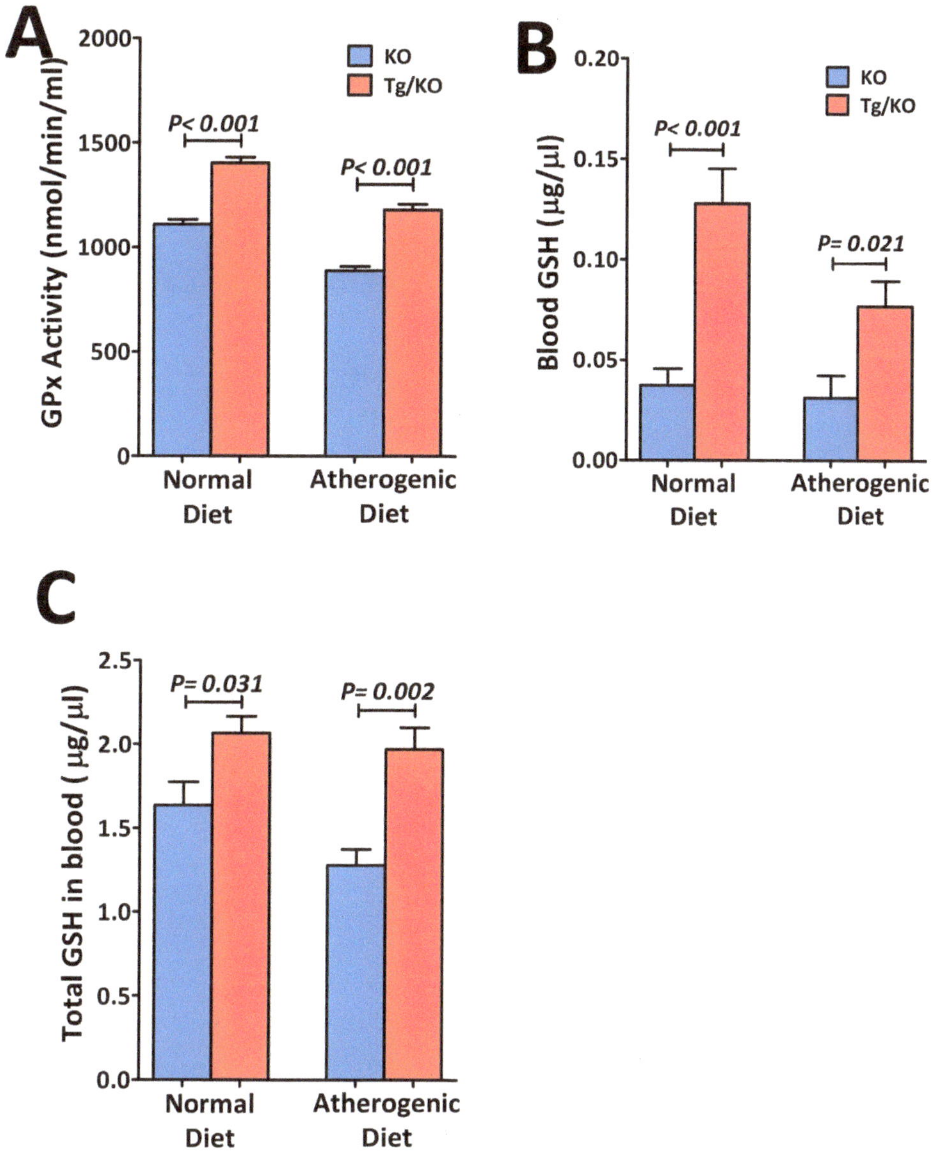

Figure 6. Reduced level of oxidative stress by activation of CSE gene. Improved plasmid lipid levels in Tg/KO mice exhibits reduced level of oxidative stress as indication by higher level of (A) glutathionine peroxidase (GPx) in plasma (n = 6), (B) blood glutathionine (GSH) (n = 6) and (C) total glutathionine (both GSH and GSSG) (n = 6).

Anti-inflammatory response of CSE/H_2S

As an anti-inflammatory molecule of CSE/H_2S, tumor suppressor gene p53 becomes activated to prevent atherosclerosis by inhibition of cell proliferation and promotion of apoptosis in vascular smooth muscle cells. We quantitatively analyzed the expression of aortic p-p53 as shown in Figure 8A. p-p53 was show to be highly expressed in aorta of Tg/KO mice fed with both normal and atherogenic diets. We then examined the involvement of nuclear factor-kappa B (NF-κB) in both KO and Tg/KO mice as markers for vascular inflammation. As shown in immuneblot (Figure 8B), H_2S increased the content of IκBα by activation of IκB kinase (IKK) in Tg/KO mice with both diets. Although expression of IKK (Figure 8C) was not significantly increased in Tg/KO mice, the elevated level of IκBα (Figure 8D) represented a suppression of IκBα degradation and subsequently resulted in significant inhibition of NF-κB (Figure 8E). Between, expression of IκBα and NF-κB were found correlated with the H_2S production (Figure 8F). Activated p-p53 and reduced NF-κB implied anti-inflammatory response induced by CSE/H_2S.

Discussion

CSE/H_2S pathway has been implicated to play an important role in physiologic and pathophysiologic processes of various cardiovascular diseases, including atherosclerosis [10,16]. H_2S has been shown to protect cardiovascular tissue by acting as an anti-inflammatory molecule [17,18]. H_2S deficiency by CSE knockout leads to decrease in endogenous H_2S level and development of advanced atherosclerotic lesion [10]. CSE/H_2S overexpression *in vitro* has been shown to stimulate VSMC apoptosis [19] and inhibit inflammatory response [12]. In this study, we produced CSE transgenic ApoE-KO (Tg/KO) mice to examine the anti-atherogenic effect of H_2S as compared to ApoE-KO (KO) mice, a

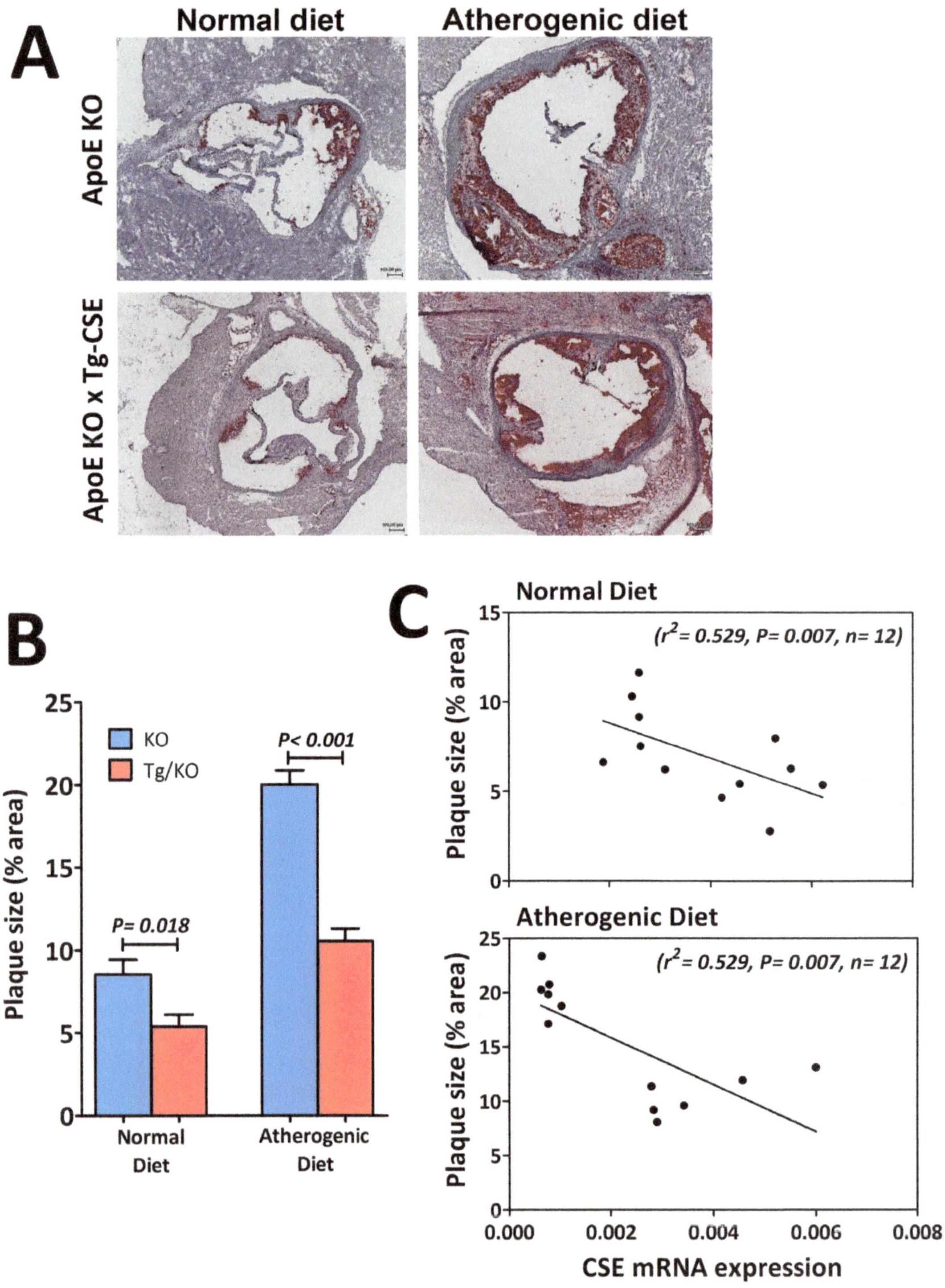

Figure 7. Overexpression of CSE inhibits ApoE deficient mice from atherosclerosis. (A) Atherosclerotic lesion damages in Tg/KO mice improved in both diets when compared to KO mice (Magnification 4×). (B) Quantitative comparisons of the mean percentage of plaque areas in aortic root between KO and Tg/KO mice were calculated using ImageJ software (n = 6). (C) There was a significant negative correlation between aortic CSE mRNA expression and lesion size from aortic root in mice who received both normal diet and atherogenic diet.

mice model for atherosclerosis. Our study shows that *in vivo* CSE/ H_2S overexpression protects ApoE-KO mice from atherosclerosis.

In an earlier study, Yang et al. showed that CSE over-expression of CSE in aortic smooth muscle cells can increase hydrogen sulfide production [19]. We have shown that *in vivo* CSE/H_2S overexpression in ApoE-KO mice can significantly increase CSE mRNA and protein levels in aorta as well as endogenous H_2S production in heart. We also found that the elevated level of H_2S in the heart tissue of Tg/KO mice was associated with the reduced plasma lipids. In healthy subjects, Jain

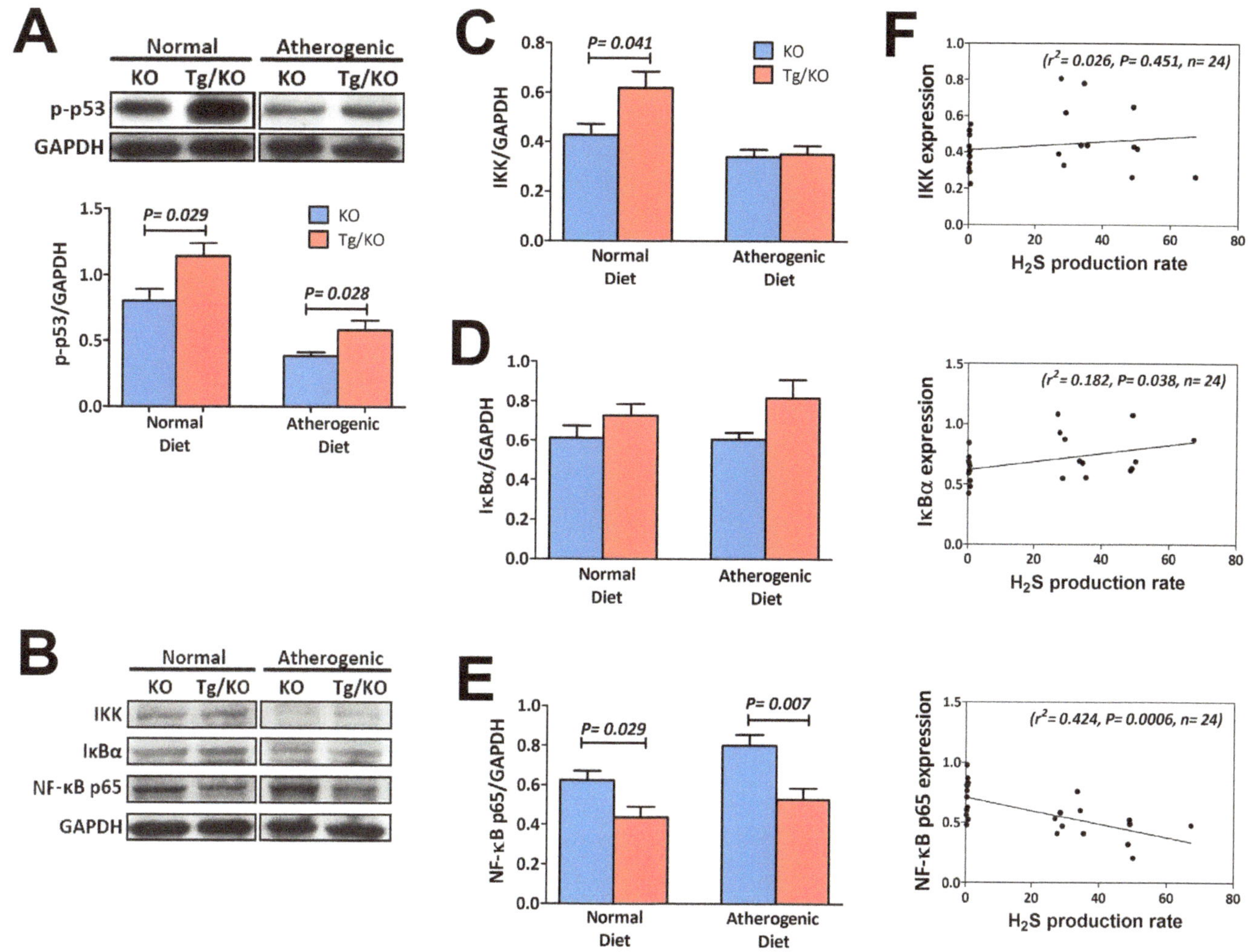

Figure 8. Quantitative analysis of protein expression levels in the aorta of KO and Tg/KO mice. (A) Representative immunoblot showed that p-p53 increased in Tg/KO mice when compared to those in KO mice (n = 6). (B) Immunoblot showed the expression levels of NF-κB pathway including (C) IKK, (D) IκBα and (E) NF-κB p65 (n = 6). Correlation of each protein expression in (B) with H_2S production was shown in (F).

SK et al. measured fasting blood H_2S and cholesterol levels. They found a positive correlation between blood H_2S and HDL-cholesterol [20]. In the same study, blood H_2S positively correlated with adiponectin. In patients with type 2 diabetes mellitus and coronary artery disease, adiponectin level was found to correlate with HDL cholesterol [21]. The effect of H_2S on cholesterol is thought to be mediated through adiponectin. Our results suggest that H_2S regulates plasma lipid metabolism through a high plasma adiponectin level. This may lead to reduced oxidative stress to arterial walls and therefore protects against atherosclerosis. Oxidized LDL is important not only for the formation of fatty streaks but also, along with other physical and/or humoral mediators, for damage to the endothelium. The damaged endothelium allows for continued transport of inflammatory cells and mediators into the vessel wall. These processes generate ROS and increase oxidative stress [22].

With increased level of H_2S in Tg/KO mice, H_2S reacts with ROS and induces increased production of anti-oxidants such as glutathione (GSH) and glutathione peroxidase (GPx) [23]. GSH and GPx are intracellular antioxidants. Increased GPx protects against oxidative stress [24]. In our study, we have shown an elevated level of GPx as well as increased level of GSH and GSSG in Tg/KO mice, indicating reduced oxidative stress by CSE/H_2S. Our findings are consistent with those from another report that H_2S exerts an anti-atherogenic effect in association with elevated plasma GPx [16]. In this study, smaller body weight gain was observed in Tg/KO mice and unfortunately, we could not explain by the dietary experiment. However, interestingly, GSH metabolism has been linked to energy expenditure, insulin sensitivity and body weight regulation [25]. In an earlier placebo-controlled study in healthy subjects, Lands et al. supplemented a whey-based cysteine donor to augment intracellular GSH [26]. They found improved muscular performances in those who received cysteine, which is substrate required for biosynthesis of GSH. In rats, Haraguchi et al. found that whey protein supplements could lead to reduced body and muscle weight gain [27]. In addition, Yang et al. showed a paradoxical relationship between adiponectin and body weight [28]. In another study, adiponectin production in plasma was found to be decreased in obese patients [29]. Adiponectin may therefore inhibit weight gain. Taken together, high plasma adiponectin level and GSH level, which were associated with high H_2S production rate in this study, could at least in part explain the reduced body weight gain in Tg/KO mice when compared to the KO mice.

Tumor suppressor gene p53 plays an important role in protection against atherosclerosis and restenosis [30]. Its expression was found negatively correlated with cell proliferation in human atherosclerosis [31], but directly associated with increased apoptosis [32,33]. With regard to H_2S, many studies have been suggested that H_2S up-regulated p53 expression to activate cell apoptosis and inhibit cell growth [34,35,36]. Baskar and colleagues demonstrated that a H_2S-releasing donor (S-diclofenac) inhibited rat VSMC proliferation associated with induced p53, p53AIP1 and the transcriptional factors of p53 such as p21 and Bax proteins [37]. In gastric cancer cells, a new H_2S-releasing donor (SPRC) has been found to increase the expression of CSE and also induced a pro-apoptotic effect in cancer tissues with elevated expressions of p53 and Bax in tumors and cells [38]. Therefore, it is believed that altered metabolism of CSE/H_2S pathway plays role in cell proliferation of VSMCs and the pro-apoptosis effect of CSE/H_2S on VSMCs may have important implications in the vascular remodeling progress and the development of atherosclerosis [39].

We showed an anti-inflammatory effect of CSE/H_2S overexpression in our Tg/KO mice. Oxidative stress stimulates atherosclerosis by increasing production and translocation of NF-κB [9] which is activated by a multitude of stimuli such as cytokines, oxidized lipids, lipopolysaccharide (LPS). The reduced oxidative stress by CSE/H_2S overexpression may inhibit inflammation via NF-κB signaling pathway. Activation of NF-κB occurs in an IκB kinase complex (IKK)-independent manner and through the tyrosine phosphorylation of IκBα and degradation of IκBα, followed by nuclear translocation of the activated NF-κB dimer to initiate gene transcription [40]. Dysregulation of the NF-κB system is likely to play an important role in inflammatory diseases [41] and also be involved in inflammatory-proliferative process of atherogenesis [42,43]. With increase of oxidative stress in atherosclerosis, ApoE-KO mice showed accumulation of plaque area with increased IκBα degradation and NF-κB expression. Conversely, Tg/KO mice showed inhibited plaque formation and NF-κB expression. There are evidences to show that exogenous H_2S can inhibit NF-κB activation in cells stimulated with TNFα [44] and lipopolysachharides (LPS) [17,18]. Furthermore, overexpression of CSE in macrophage exhibited reduced inflammatory pathway by suppression of IκBα degradation and NF-κB p65 nuclear translocation [13,24]. However, there is no direct evidence showing anti-atherogenic effect of H_2S on suppression of NF-κB except a recent study showed that CSE/H_2S deficiency was associated with increased NF-κB activation [9]. CSE/H_2S overexpression in our study appears to support an anti-inflammatory effect in the protection against atherosclerosis.

In conclusion, we have shown for the first time that H_2S protects against atherosclerosis by CSE gene activation. Endogenous H_2S prevents the progression of atherosclerosis by reducing plasma lipid accumulation, inhibiting oxidative stress and plaque formation and suppressing inflammation in vascular tissues via NF-κB pathway. Therefore, our study provides direct evidence that H_2S is an important mediator in atherosclerosis formation. The CSE/H_2S pathway can be targeted as one of the new therapeutic strategies in prevention of atherosclerosis.

Supporting Information

Table S1 A complete list of data set in this study.

Table S2 Daily food intake per mice.

Author Contributions

Conceived and designed the experiments: WKK JYWL. Performed the experiments: SHC WKK. Analyzed the data: SHC WKK JYWL. Contributed reagents/materials/analysis tools: KFT JYWL. Wrote the paper: SHC JYWL.

References

1. Lusis AJ (2000) Atherosclerosis. Nature 407: 233–241.
2. Libby P (2002) Inflammation in atherosclerosis. Nature 420: 868–874.
3. Sélley E, Kun S, Szijártó IA, Laczy B, Kovács T, et al. (2014) Exenatide induces aortic vasodilation increasing hydrogen sulphide, carbon monoxide and nitric oxide production. Cardiovasc Diabetol 2; 13:69.
4. Köhn C, Schleifenbaum J, Szijártó IA, Markó L, Dubrovska G, et al. (2013) Differential effects of cystathionine-γ-lyase-dependent vasodilatory H2S in periadventitial vasoregulation of rat and mouse aortas. PLoS One 7: e41951.
5. Li H, Mani S, Cao W, Yang G, Lai C, et al. (2012) Interaction of hydrogen sulfide and estrogen on the proliferation of vascular smooth muscle cells. PLoS One 7: e41614.
6. Hu LF, Lu M, Hon Wong PT, Bian JS (2011) Hydrogen sulfide: neurophysiology and neuropathology. Antioxid Redox Signal 15: 405–419.
7. Yang G, Wu L, Jiang B, Yang W, Qi J, et al. (2008) H2S as a physiologic vasorelaxant: hypertension in mice with deletion of cystathionine gamma-lyase. Science 322: 587–590.
8. Mani S, Li H, Untereiner A, Wu L, Yang G, et al. (2013) Decreased endogenous production of hydrogen sulfide accelerates atherosclerosis. Circulation 127: 2523–2534.
9. Wang Y, Zhao X, Jin H, Wei H, Li W, et al. (2009) Role of hydrogen sulfide in the development of atherosclerotic lesions in apolipoprotein E knockout mice. Arterioscler Thromb Vasc Biol 29: 173–179.
10. Wen YD, Wang H, Kho SH, Rinkiko S, Sheng X, et al. (2013) Hydrogen sulfide protects HUVECs against hydrogen peroxide induced mitochondrial dysfunction and oxidative stress. PLoS One 8: e53147.
11. Zhang H, Guo C, Wu D, Zhang A, Gu T, et al. (2012) Hydrogen sulfide inhibits the development of atherosclerosis with suppressing CX3CR1 and CX3CL1 expression. PLoS One 7: e41147.
12. Zhang H, Guo C, Zhang A, Fan Y, Gu T, et al. (2012) Effect of S-aspirin, a novel hydrogen-sulfide-releasing aspirin (ACS14), on atherosclerosis in apoE-deficient mice. Eur J Pharmacol 697: 106–116.
13. Liu Z, Han Y, Li L, Lu H, Meng G, et al. (2013) The Hydrogen sulfide donor, GYY4137, exhibits anti-atherosclerotic activity in high fat fed apolipoprotein $E^{-/-}$ mice. Br J Pharmacol 169: 1795–1809.
14. Wang R (2003) The gasotransmitter role of hydrogen sulfide. Antioxid Redox Signal 5: 493–501.
15. Wallace JL, Dicay M, McKnight W, Martin GR (2007) Hydrogen sulfide enhances ulcer healing in rats. FASEB J 21: 4070–4076.
16. Li W, Tang C, Jin H, Du J (2011) Regulatory effects of sulfur dioxide on the development of atherosclerotic lesions and vascular hydrogen sulfide in atherosclerotic rats. Atherosclerosis 215: 323–330.
17. Li L, Rose P, Moore PK (2011) Hydrogen sulfide and cell signaling. Annu Rev Pharmacol Toxicol 51: 169–187.
18. Pan LL, Liu XH, Gong QH, Zhu YZ (2011) S-Propargyl-cysteine (SPRC) attenuated lipopolysaccharide-induced inflammatory response in H9c2 cells involved in a hydrogen sulfide-dependent mechanism. Amino Acids 41: 205–215.
19. Yang G, Wu L, Wang R (2006) Pro-apoptotic effect of endogenous H2S on human aorta smooth muscle cells. FASEB J 20: 553–555.
20. Jain SK, Micinski D, Lieblong BJ, Stapleton T (2012) Relationship between hydrogen sulfide levels and HDL-cholesterol, adiponectin, and potassium levels in the blood of healthy subjects. Atherosclerosis 225: 242–245.
21. Lautamäki R, Rönnemaa T, Huupponen R, Lehtimäki T, Iozzo P (2007) Low serum adiponectin is associated with high circulating oxidized low-density lipoprotein in patients with type 2 diabetes mellitus and coronary artery disease. Metabolism 56: 881–886.
22. Madamanchi NR, Hakim ZS, Runge MS (2005) Oxidative stress in atherogenesis and arterial thrombosis: the disconnect between cellular studies and clinical outcomes. J Thromb Haemost 3: 254–267.
23. Kimura Y, Goto Y, Kimura H (2010) Hydrogen sulfide increases glutathione production and suppresses oxidative stress in mitochondria. Antioxid Redox Signal 12: 1–13.
24. Pan LL, Liu XH, Gong QH, Yang HB, Zhu YZ (2012) Role of cystathionine γ-lyase/hydrogen sulfide pathway in cardiovascular disease: a novel therapeutic strategy? Antioxid Redox Signal 17: 106–118.
25. Findeisen HM, Gizard F, Zhao Y, Qing H, Jones KL, et al. (2011) Glutathione depletion prevents diet-induced obesity and enhances insulin sensitivity. Obesity (Silver Spring) 19: 2429–2432.

26. Lands LC, Grey VL, Smountas AA (1999) Effect of supplementation with a cysteine donor on muscular performance. J Appl Physiol 87: 1381–1385.
27. Haraguchi FK, Silva ME, Neves LX, dos Santos RC, Pedrosa ML (2011) Whey protein precludes lipid and protein oxidation and improves body weight gain in resistance-exercised rats. Eur J Nutr 50: 331–339.
28. Yang WS, Lee WJ, Funahashi T, Tanaka S, Matsuzawa Y, et al. (2001) Weight reduction increases plasma levels of an adipose-derived anti-inflammatory protein, adiponectin. J Clin Endocrinol Metab 86: 3815–3819.
29. Arita Y, Kihara S, Ouchi N, Takahashi M, Maeda K, et al. (1999) Paradoxical decrease of an adipose-specific protein, adiponectin, in obesity. Biochem Biophys Res Commun 257: 79–83.
30. Mnjoyan ZH, Dutta R, Zhang D, Teng BB, Fujise K (2003) Paradoxical upregulation of tumor suppressor protein p53 in serum-stimulated vascular smooth muscle cells. Circulation 108: 464–471.
31. Ihling C, Menzel G, Wellens E, Monting JS, Schaefer HE, et al. (1997) Topographical association between the cyclin-dependent kinases inhibitor p21, p53 accumulation, and cellular proliferation in human atherosclerotic tissue. Art Thromb Vasc Biol 17: 2218–2224.
32. Li XL, Li BY, Cheng M, Yu F, Yin WB, et al. (2013) PIMT prevents the apoptosis of endothelial cells in response to glycated low density lipoproteins and protective effects of grape seed procyanidin B2. PLoS One 8: e69979.
33. Foster CR, Daniel LL, Daniels CR, Dalal S, Singh M, et al. (2013) Deficiency of ataxia telangiectasia mutated kinase modulates cardiac remodeling following myocardial infarction: involvement in fibrosis and apoptosis. PLoS One 8: e83513.
34. Calenic B, Yaegaki K, Kozhuharova A, Imai T (2010) Oral malodorous compound causes oxidative stress and p53-mediated programmed cell death in keratinocyte stem cells. J Periodontol 81: 1317–1323.
35. Aoyama I, Yaegaki K, Calenic B, Ii H, Ishkitiev N, et al. (2012) The role of p53 in an apoptotic process caused by an oral malodorous compound in periodontal tissues: a review. J Breath Res 6: 017104.
36. Calenic B, Yaegaki K, Ishkitiev N, Kumazawa Y, Imai T, et al. (2013) p53-Pathway activity and apoptosis in hydrogen sulfide-exposed stem cells separated from human gingival epithelium. J Periodontal Res 48: 322–230.
37. Baskar R, Sparatore A, Del Soldato P, Moore PK (2008) Effect of S-diclofenac, a novel hydrogen sulfide releasing derivative inhibit rat vascular smooth muscle cell proliferation. Eur J Pharmacol 594: 1–8.
38. Ma K, Liu Y, Zhu Q, Liu CH, Duan JL, et al. (2011) H2S donor, S-propargyl-cysteine, increases CSE in SGC-7901 and cancer-induced mice: evidence for a novel anti-cancer effect of endogenous H2S? PLoS One 6: e20525.
39. Yang G, Wu L, Bryan S, Khaper N, Mani S, et al. (2010) Cystathionine gamma-lyase deficiency and overproliferation of smooth muscle cells. Cardiovasc Res 86: 487–495.
40. Takada Y, Mukhopadhyay A, Kundu GC, Mahabeleshwar GH, Singh S, et al. (2003) Hydrogen peroxide activates NF-kappa B through tyrosine phosphorylation of I kappa B alpha and serine phosphorylation of p65: evidence for the involvement of I kappa B alpha kinase and Syk protein-tyrosine kinase. J Biol Chem 278: 24233–24241.
41. Li J, Zhong W, Wang W, Hu S, Yuan J, et al. (2014) Ginsenoside metabolite compound K promotes recovery of dextran sulfate sodium-induced colitis and inhibits inflammatory responses by suppressing NF-κB activation. PLoS One 9: e87810.
42. Zhou CH, Liu L, Liu L, Zhang MX, Guo H, et al. (2014) Salusin-β not salusin-α promotes vascular inflammation in ApoE-deficient mice via the I-κBα/NF-κB pathway. PLoS One 9: e91468.
43. Zhuang J, Peng W, Li H, Lu Y, Wang K, et al. (2013) Inhibitory effects of vinpocetine on the progression of atherosclerosis are mediated by Akt/NF-κB dependent mechanisms in apoE-/- mice. PLoS One 8: e82509.
44. Pan LL, Liu XH, Gong QH, Wu D, Zhu YZ (2011) Hydrogen sulfide attenuated tumor necrosis factor-α-induced inflammatory signaling and dysfunction in vascular endothelial cells. PLoS One 6: e19766.

Permissions

All chapters in this book were first published in PLOS ONE, by The Public Library of Science; hereby published with permission under the Creative Commons Attribution License or equivalent. Every chapter published in this book has been scrutinized by our experts. Their significance has been extensively debated. The topics covered herein carry significant findings which will fuel the growth of the discipline. They may even be implemented as practical applications or may be referred to as a beginning point for another development.

The contributors of this book come from diverse backgrounds, making this book a truly international effort. This book will bring forth new frontiers with its revolutionizing research information and detailed analysis of the nascent developments around the world.

We would like to thank all the contributing authors for lending their expertise to make the book truly unique. They have played a crucial role in the development of this book. Without their invaluable contributions this book wouldn't have been possible. They have made vital efforts to compile up to date information on the varied aspects of this subject to make this book a valuable addition to the collection of many professionals and students.

This book was conceptualized with the vision of imparting up-to-date information and advanced data in this field. To ensure the same, a matchless editorial board was set up. Every individual on the board went through rigorous rounds of assessment to prove their worth. After which they invested a large part of their time researching and compiling the most relevant data for our readers.

The editorial board has been involved in producing this book since its inception. They have spent rigorous hours researching and exploring the diverse topics which have resulted in the successful publishing of this book. They have passed on their knowledge of decades through this book. To expedite this challenging task, the publisher supported the team at every step. A small team of assistant editors was also appointed to further simplify the editing procedure and attain best results for the readers.

Apart from the editorial board, the designing team has also invested a significant amount of their time in understanding the subject and creating the most relevant covers. They scrutinized every image to scout for the most suitable representation of the subject and create an appropriate cover for the book.

The publishing team has been an ardent support to the editorial, designing and production team. Their endless efforts to recruit the best for this project, has resulted in the accomplishment of this book. They are a veteran in the field of academics and their pool of knowledge is as vast as their experience in printing. Their expertise and guidance has proved useful at every step. Their uncompromising quality standards have made this book an exceptional effort. Their encouragement from time to time has been an inspiration for everyone.

The publisher and the editorial board hope that this book will prove to be a valuable piece of knowledge for researchers, students, practitioners and scholars across the globe.

List of Contributors

Jieping Yang, Fang Wei, Christopher Schafer and David T. W. Wong
School of Dentistry, University of California Los Angeles, Los Angeles, California, United States of America

Sara Nilsson, Johanna Sjöberg and Matthias Laska
Department of Physics, Chemistry and Biology, Linköping University, Linköping, Sweden

Mats Amundin
Kolmården Wildlife Park, Kolmården, Sweden

Constanze Hartmann and Andrea Buettner
Department of Chemistry and Pharmacy, Friedrich-Alexander-Universität Erlangen-Nürnberg, Erlangen, Germany

Junning Wang, Hong Du, Haitao Yu, Wei Jiang, Ting Zhu, Xuefan Bai and Pingzhong Wang
Department of Infectious Diseases, Tangdu Hospital, Fourth Military Medical University, Xi'an, Shaanxi Province, China

Weijuan Guo
Department of Obstetrics and Gynecology, Chang An Hospital, Xi'an, Shaanxi Province, China

Andreas Wannhoff, Mirja Senner, Karl-Heinz Weiss, Wolfgang Stremmel, Kilian Friedrich, Christian Rupp, Petra Klöters-Plachky, Yvonne Leopold and Daniel N. Gotthardt
Department of Internal Medicine IV, University Hospital Heidelberg, Heidelberg, Germany

Oliver J. Müller and Hugo A. Katus
Department of Internal Medicine III, University Hospital Heidelberg, Heidelberg, Germany

Maik Brune
Department of Internal Medicine I and Clinical Chemistry, University Hospital Heidelberg, Heidelberg, Germany

Peter Schemmer
Department of General and Transplant Surgery, University Hospital Heidelberg, Heidelberg, Germany

Courteney K. Lai, Connie J. Eaves and R. Keith Humphries
Terry Fox Laboratory, BC Cancer Agency Research Centre, Vancouver, BC, Canada
Department of Medicine, Faculty of Medicine, University of British Columbia, Vancouver, BC, Canada

Yeonsook Moon
Department of Laboratory Medicine, Medical School of Inha University, Incheon, Korea

Florian Kuchenbauer
Department of Internal Medicine III, University Hospital of Ulm, Ulm, Germany
Institute of Experimental Cancer Research, Comprehensive Cancer Centre, University Hospital of Ulm, Ulm, Germany

Daniel T. Starzcynowski
Department of ediatrics, Cincinnati Children's Hospital Medical Center, Cincinnati, Ohio, United States of America

Bob Argiropoulos
Department of Medical Genetics, University of Calgary, Calgary, AB, Canada

Eric Yung, Philip Beer, Malina Leung, Grace Lin, Sarah Vollett and Stephen Fung
Terry Fox Laboratory, BC Cancer Agency Research Centre, Vancouver, BC, Canada

Adrian Schwarzer and Amit Sharma
Institute of Experimental Hematology, Hannover Medical School, Hannover, Germany

Gyeongsin Park
Department of Hospital Pathology, Catholic University of Korea, Seoul, Korea

Aly Karsan
Genome Sciences Centre, BC Cancer Agency, Vancouver, BC, Canada
Department of Pathology and Laboratory Medicine, University of British Columbia, Vancouver, BC, Canada

Andrew P. Weng
Terry Fox Laboratory, BC Cancer Agency Research Centre, Vancouver, BC, Canada
Department of Pathology and Laboratory Medicine, University of British Columbia, Vancouver, BC, Canada

Michael Heuser
Department of Hematology, Hemostasis, Oncology, and Stem Cell Transplantation, Hannover Medical School, Hannover, Germany

John W. Newman
USDA, ARS, WHNRC, Obesity and Metabolism Research Unit, Davis, CA, United States of America
Department of Nutrition, University of California Davis, Davis, CA, United States of America

Theresa L. Pedersen
USDA, ARS, WHNRC, Obesity and Metabolism Research Unit, Davis, CA, United States of America

Verdayne R. Brandenburg
Family Medicine, Sanford School of Medicine, University of South Dakota, Sioux Falls, SD, United States of America

William S. Harris
Internal Medicine, Sanford School of Medicine, University of South Dakota, Sioux Falls, SD, United States of America

Courteney K. Lai, R. Keith Humphries and Connie J. Eaves
Terry Fox Laboratory, BC Cancer Agency Research Centre, Vancouver, BC, Canada
Department of Medicine, Faculty of Medicine, University of British Columbia, Vancouver, BC, Canada

Yeonsook Moon
Department of Laboratory Medicine, Medical School of Inha University, Incheon, Korea

Florian Kuchenbauer
Department of Internal Medicine III, University Hospital of Ulm, Ulm, Germany
Institute of Experimental Cancer Research, Comprehensive Cancer Centre, University Hospital of Ulm, Ulm, Germany

Daniel T. Starzcynowski
Department of Pediatrics, Cincinnati Children's Hospital Medical Center, Cincinnati, Ohio, United States of America

Bob Argiropoulos
Department of Medical Genetics, University of Calgary, Calgary, AB, Canada

Eric Yung, Philip Beer, Malina Leung, Grace Lin, Sarah Vollett and Stephen Fung
Terry Fox Laboratory, BC Cancer Agency Research Centre, Vancouver, BC, Canada

Adrian Schwarzer and Amit Sharma
Institute of Experimental Hematology, Hannover Medical School, Hannover, Germany

Gyeongsin Park
Department of Hospital Pathology, Catholic University of Korea, Seoul, Korea

Aly Karsan
Genome Sciences Centre, BC Cancer Agency, Vancouver, BC, Canada
Department of Pathology and Laboratory Medicine, University of British Columbia, Vancouver, BC, Canada

Andrew P. Weng
Terry Fox Laboratory, BC Cancer Agency Research Centre, Vancouver, BC, Canada
Department of Pathology and Laboratory Medicine, University of British Columbia, Vancouver, BC, Canada

Michael Heuser
Department of Hematology, Hemostasis, Oncology, and Stem Cell Transplantation, Hannover Medical School, Hannover, Germany

Gregory C. Shearer
Internal Medicine, Sanford School of Medicine, University of South Dakota, Sioux Falls, SD, United States of America
Basic Biomedical Sciences, Sanford School of Medicine, University of South Dakota, Sioux Falls, SD, United States of America
Cardiovascular Health Research Center, Sanford Research/USD, Sioux Falls, South Dakota, United States of America
Department of Nutritional Sciences, The Pennsylvania State University, University Park, Pennsylvania, United States of America

Eduardo Fuentes, Marcelo Alarcón and Iván Palomo
Department of Clinical Biochemistry and Immunohematology, Faculty of Health Sciences, Interdisciplinary Excellence Research Program on Healthy Aging (PIEI-ES), Universidad de Talca, Talca, Chile

Centro de Estudios en Alimentos Procesados (CEAP), CONICYT-Regional, Gore Maule, Talca, Chile

Jaime Pereira and Diego Mezzano
Department of Hematology-Oncology, School of Medicine, Pontificia Universidad Católica de Chile, Santiago, Chile

Julio Caballero
Center for Bioinformatics and Molecular Simulations, Faculty of Engineering in Bioinformatics, Universidad de Talca, Talca, Chile

Jie Yu, Bing Yu, Jun He, Ping Zheng, Xiangbing Mao and Daiwen Chen
Animal Nutrition Institute, Sichuan Agricultural University, Chengdu, 611130, People's Republic of China
Key Laboratory for Animal Disease-Resistance Nutrition of China Ministry of Education, Sichuan Agricultural University, Chengdu, 611130, People's Republic of China

Guoquan Han
Animal Nutrition Institute, Sichuan Agricultural University, Chengdu, 611130, People's Republic of China
College of Food Science, Sichuan Agricultural University, Ya'an, 625014, People's Republic of China

Ravi Goyal, Dipali Goyal, Nina Chu, Jonathan Van Wickle and Lawrence D. Longo
Center for Perinatal Biology, Department of Basic Sciences, School of Medicine, Loma Linda University, Loma Linda, California, United States of America
Epigenuity LLC, Loma Linda, California, United States of America

Xiao Liu, Zhenze Wang, Ping Zhao, Anqiang Sun, Fan Zhan, Yubo Fan and Xiaoyan Deng
Key Laboratory for Biomechanics and Mechanobiology of the Ministry of Education, School of Biological Science and Medical Engineering, Beihang University, Beijing, China,

Zhanming Fan
Radiologic Department, Beijing Anzhen Hospital, Capital Medical University, Beijing, China

Johanna Maria Eberhard and Silke Kummer
Infectious Diseases Unit, Department of Medicine, University Medical Center Hamburg-Eppendorf, Hamburg, Germany
Heinrich Pette Institute - Leibniz Institute for Experimental Virology, Hamburg, Germany

Philip Hartjen
Infectious Diseases Unit, Department of Medicine, University Medical Center Hamburg-Eppendorf, Hamburg, Germany
Department of Oral and Maxillofacial Surgery, University Medical Center Hamburg-Eppendorf, Hamburg, Germany
Heinrich Pette Institute - Leibniz Institute for Experimental Virology, Hamburg, Germany

Reinhold E. Schmidt
Department of Immunology and Rheumatology, Hannover Medical School, Hanover, Germany
German Center for Infection Research (DZIF), partner site Hamburg and Hannover, Hamburg and Hannover, Germany

Maximilian Bockhorn
Department of General Surgery, University Medical Center Hamburg-Eppendorf, Hamburg, Germany

Clara Lehmann
Department of Internal Medicine I, University Hospital of Cologne, Cologne, Germany

Ashwin Balagopal
School of Medicine, Johns Hopkins University, Baltimore, Maryland, United States of America

Joachim Hauber
Heinrich Pette Institute - Leibniz Institute for Experimental Virology, Hamburg, Germany
German Center for Infection Research (DZIF), partner site Hamburg and Hannover, Hamburg and Hannover, Germany

Jan van Lunzen and Julian Schulze zur Wiesch
Infectious Diseases Unit, Department of Medicine, University Medical Center Hamburg-Eppendorf, Hamburg, Germany
Heinrich Pette Institute - Leibniz Institute for Experimental Virology, Hamburg, Germany
German Center for Infection Research (DZIF), partner site Hamburg and Hannover, Hamburg and Hannover, Germany

Hans Carl Hasselbalch, Lasse Kjær, Morten K. Jensen and Vibe Skov
Department of Hematology, Roskilde Hospital, University of Copenhagen, Roskilde, Denmark

Mads Thomassen and Torben A. Kruse
Department of Clinical Genetics, Odense University Hospital, Odense, Denmark

Caroline Hasselbalch Riley
Department of Hematology L, Herlev Hospital, University of Copenhagen, Herlev, Denmark

Thomas Stauffer Larsen
Department of Hematology X, Odense University Hospital, Odense, Denmark

Ole Weis Bjerrum
Department of Hematology L, Rigshospitalet, University of Copenhagen, Copenhagen, Denmark

Jill Seladi-Schulman, Patricia J. Campbell, Suganthi Suppiah, John Steel and Anice C. Lowen
Department of Microbiology and Immunology, Emory University School of Medicine, Atlanta, Georgia, United States of America

Koji Tanaka, Yuhki Koike, Tadanobu Shimura, Masato Okigami, Shozo Ide, Yuji Toiyama, Yoshinaga Okugawa, Yasuhiro Inoue, Toshimitsu Araki, Keiichi Uchida, Yasuhiko Mohri, and Masato Kusunoki
Departments of Gastrointestinal and Paediatric Surgery, Mie University Graduate School of Medicine, Tsu, Mie, Japan

Akira Mizoguchi
Departments of Neural Regeneration and Cell Communication, Mie University Graduate School of Medicine, Tsu, Mie, Japan

Rodrigo Pessôa, Jaqueline Tomoko Watanabe, Paula Calabria and Alvina Clara Felix
Virology Department, São Paulo Institute of Tropical Medicine, University of São Paulo, São Paulo, Brazil

Paula Loureiro
Pernambuco State Center of Hematology and Hemotherapy, Recife, Pernambuco, Brazil

Ester C. Sabino
Department of Infectious Disease/Institute of Tropical Medicine, University of São Paulo, São Paulo, Brazil

Michael P. Busch
Blood Systems Research Institute, San Francisco, California, United States of America

Sabri S. Sanabani
Clinical Laboratory, Department of Pathology, Hospital das Clínicas, School of Medicine, University of São Paulo, São Paulo, Brazil

Anna Casabianca, Chiara Orlandi, Maddalena Scotti and Mauro Magnani
Department of Biomolecular Sciences, University of Urbino "Carlo Bo", Urbino (PU), Italy

Benedetta Canovari, Marcello Acetoso, Massimo Valentini and Enzo Petrelli
Azienda Ospedaliera Ospedali Riuniti Marche Nord - Presidio Ospedaliero San Salvatore, Pesaro (PU), Italy

Hisayo Jin and Makiko Kashio
Department of Anesthesiology, Chiba University Graduate School of Medicine, Chiba City, Chiba, Japan

Naoya Mimura
Department of Medicine and Clinical Oncology, Chiba University Graduate School of Medicine, Chiba City, Chiba, Japan

Haruhiko Koseki
Laboratory for Developmental Genetics, RIKEN Research Center for Allergy and Immunology, Yokohama, Japan

Tomohiko Aoe
Department of Anesthesiology, Chiba University Graduate School of Medicine, Chiba City, Chiba, Japan
Department of Anesthesiology, Tokyo Women's Medical University, Yachiyo Medical, Center, Yachiyo, Chiba, Japan

Yérali Gandica and Orlando Oliveira
Center for Computational Physics, Department of Physics, University of Coimbra, Coimbra, Portugal

Tobias Schwarz
Center for Computational Physics, Department of Physics, University of Coimbra, Coimbra, Portugal
Heinz-Brandt-Schule, Berlin, Germany

Rui D. M. Travasso
Center for Computational Physics, Department of Physics, University of Coimbra, Coimbra, Portugal
Center of Ophthalmology and Vision Sciences(COCV), Institute for Biomedical Imaging and Life Sciences (IBILI), Faculty of Medicine, University of Coimbra, Coimbra, Portugal

Man Li, Zhen Liang, Xun Sun, Tao Gong and Zhirong Zhang
Key Laboratory of Drug Targeting and Drug Delivery Systems, Ministry of Education, West China School of Pharmacy, Sichuan University, Chengdu, Sichuan, PR China

Giuseppe Lippi
Laboratory of Clinical Chemistry and Hematology, Academic Hospital of Parma, Parma, Italy

Gian Luca Salvagno, Elisa Danese and Gian Cesare Guidi
Laboratory of Clinical Biochemistry, Department of Life and Reproduction Sciences, University of Verona, Verona, Italy

Spyros Skafidas
CeRiSM (Centre for Mountain Sport and Health), Rovereto (TN), Italy

Cantor Tarperi and Federico Schena
Department of Neurological, Neuropsychological, Morphological and Movement Sciences, University of Verona, Verona, Italy

Sau Ha Cheung, Wai Kei Kwok and James Yun Wong Lau
Department of Surgery, Faculty of Medicine, the Chinese University of Hong Kong, Hong Kong SAR, People's Republic of China

Ka Fai To
Department of Anatomical and Cellular Pathology, Faculty of Medicine, the Chinese University of Hong Kong, Hong Kong SAR, People's Republic of China

Index